Football Injuries

Kevin W. Farmer
Editor

James R. Clugston
Associate Editor

Football Injuries

A Clinical Guide to In-Season Management

Springer

Editor
Kevin W. Farmer
Department of Orthopedic Surgery
University of Florida
Gainesville, FL
USA

Team Physician
The University of Florida
Gainesville, FL
USA

Associate Editor
James R. Clugston MD, MS
Departments of Community Health & Family
Medicine and Neurology
Team Physician
University of Florida
Gainesville, FL
USA

ISBN 978-3-030-54874-2 ISBN 978-3-030-54875-9 (eBook)
https://doi.org/10.1007/978-3-030-54875-9

This Springer imprint is published by the registered company Springer Nature Switzerland AG
The registered company address is: Gewerbestrasse 11, 6330 Cham, Switzerland

Foreword

Over the past three decades, sports medicine has evolved as a legitimate subspecialty. To a great extent, the role of the team physician has paralleled that evolution. The single key responsibility of that head team physician has not changed: namely to maintain the short- and long-term good health of the athlete. In fact, improved care of the collegiate student athlete has become an important focal point in many different healthcare specialties.

Of note is the fact that taking care of a student athlete is indeed a unique situation due to the fact that their perceptions and demands are usually influenced by viewing themselves not necessarily as an individual but rather as a member of a team. Occasionally, the goals of that team are not necessarily aligned with what is best medical care for the individual athlete. The team physician must recognize this unique situation and manage it keeping in mind their key responsibility is to the athlete. They may be a "team physician," but when an athlete becomes injured or ill, they are their personal physician.

Due to the exponential scientific growth in sports medicine, the head team physician needs to surround themself with other healthcare providers that recognize the unique role that they play in providing medical care to the athlete. To help accomplish this task, the head team physician must create a "sports medicine healthcare provider team" that, if resources allow, should consist of a certified athletic trainer, physical therapists, nutritionists, medical and surgical subspecialists, strength and conditioning coaches, mental health providers, and other professionals who have a special concern for the student athlete.

Today, the pressure on team physicians to make a quick and accurate diagnosis has never been higher. Musculoskeletal injuries remain the most common problems that most team physicians deal with. The availability of diagnostic aides such as MRIs and other non-invasive technologies help them in this regard. However, medical and psychological issues also can prove challenging to physicians who devote a significant portion of their practice to the care of athletes, thus supporting the establishment of a team of specialist that understand the demands placed on athletes in today's world.

Sometimes, due to the high visibility of these positions, the team physician is frequently "second guessed" by other "experts" who are freely willing to offer their advice without understanding the special circumstances that surround an athlete with a particular injury or illness. It is exactly in this environment that team physicians rely on legitimate outside support for not only making a complete accurate diagnosis but also in implementing a successful treatment program.

In-season management of injuries and illnesses provides a unique set of challenges that may not exist in other forms of medical practices. In situations like this, the luxury of indefinite time as an adjunct to making a diagnosis or managing an injury or illness may not always be a reasonable option. It is for this specific reason a book such as this may prove to be very valuable and timely.

Peter A. Indelicato, MD
Emeritus Professor, The University of Florida
40th President, The American Orthopaedic Society for Sports Medicine

The team physician is an integral part of a team's success. Injuries play such a major role in game planning that having a team physician you can trust is paramount. I have been fortunate to have the pleasure of working with some great team physicians in my career, including Dr. Frank Bassett at Duke, Dr. Peter Indelicato at Florida, and Dr. Jeff Guy at South Carolina. We coaches truly appreciate all you do for our athletes.

Steve Spurrier
Head Ball Coach
Duke University 1987–1989
The University of Florida 1990–2001
The Washington Redskins 2002–2003
The University of South Carolina 2005–2015
The Orlando Apollos 2019

Preface

American football is the most popular contact sport in the United States, and professional football has been the number one watched sport in America for over 30 years. On any given Friday night, millions of high school athletes participate in what has become a big part of the local culture in many parts of our country. Estimates place the number of participants at over 9 million participants annually, with around 1 million football-related injuries annually in high schools alone [1]. In a sampling of a nationwide emergency department (ED) database, representing around 20% of EDs in the country, over a 2-year period from 2010–2011, nearly 400,000 patients presented for injuries related to tackle football. Of those injuries, 26% were for sprains of strains, 21% were for fractures, and 18% were for head injuries. One percent required hospital admission, with a mean length of stay just over 2 days, and there were 11 deaths. Sixteen percent of patients eventually required surgery, mostly for orthopedic injuries [1]. In a 3-year study from 2010–2013 using the same database, over 800,000 injuries were seen due to football injuries, with 80% being in patients less than 17 years of age. Hospital charges extrapolated from that study demonstrate that costs exceed 1.7 billion dollars per year in our country for football-related injuries [2]. Despite the burden placed on the healthcare system, football continues to be extremely popular, and part of the fabric of America.

In the small towns, and big cities, across our great country, as young athletes battle for football supremacy on the gridiron, local physicians cover these games acting as the "team physician." At the highest levels, these physicians are subspecialty trained in sports medicine, often passing certifying exams for a certificate of added qualification. In the high schools around our country, especially in smaller towns, these physicians may have little to no sports medicine experience at all. No matter the level of training, in-season management of injuries presents its own unique set of complexities. Balancing the pressures to return a star athlete to the field for a state title or National Championship run while not setting them up for further injury, or long-term problems, can be very difficult. Add in the concerns about missing time, or playing when not 100%, and college scholarships or the professional football draft, and sport medicine becomes a mine-field many are not prepared to navigate.

The purpose of this textbook is to help physicians working with football athletes make informed decisions about the in-season management of injuries. We will provide the available evidence to help make an informed decision about treatment and a safe, timely return to play. We will also provide recommendations by experts who deal with these issues on a daily basis. As with most injury management and sports medicine, level-one evidence is often sparse. This textbook is in no way the definitive end-all treatment algorithm for all in-season injury management. Team physicians must rely on training and experience to make the most informed decision that is in the best interest of the athlete first, and the team second. This book will hopefully provide a framework that, along with sound medical practice, will help in managing these complex issues that come working with these remarkable athletes.

Gainesville, FL, USA Kevin W. Farmer

References

1. Smart BJ, Haring RS, Asemota AO, Scott JW, Canner JK, Nejim BJ, George BP, Alsulaim H, Kirsch TD, Schneider EB. Tackling causes and costs of ED presentation for American football injuries: a population-level study. Am J Emerg Med. 2016;34(7):1198–204.
2. McGinity MJ, Grandhi R, Michalek JE, Rodriguez JS, Trevino AM, McGinity AC, Seifi A. The impact of tackle football injuries on the American healthcare system with a neurological focus. PLoS One. 2018;13(5):e0195827.

Contents

Contributors

David A. Ajibade, MD Department of Orthopaedic Surgery, University of Missouri, Columbia, MO, USA

Burak Altintas, MD Department of Orthopedics and Sports Medicine, University of Kentucky, Lexington, KY, USA

Scott Anderson, ATC Head Athletic Trainer, The University of Oklahoma, Norman, OK, USA

James Andrews, MD Andrews Institute, Gulf Breeze, FL, USA

Adam Anz, MD Andrews Institute, Gulf Breeze, FL, USA

Breton M. Asken, MD Department of Clinical and Health Psychology, University of Florida, Gainesville, FL, USA

Julian E. Bailes, MD Department of Neurosurgery, NorthShore University HealthSystem, Evanston, IL, USA

Katie Bartush, MD American Sports Medicine Institute, Birmingham, AL, USA

E. Lyle Cain, MD American Sports Medicine Institute, Birmingham, AL, USA

Mark Callanan, MD The Orthopaedic Clinic, Shreveport, LA, USA

Douglas Casa, PhD, ATC Korey Stringer Institute, University of Connecticut, Storrs, CT, USA

Terry Bradly Clay, MD Sports Medicine and Hip Preservation, University of South Alabama, Mobile, AL, USA

James R. Clugston, MD, MS Departments of Community Health & Family Medicine and Neurology, Team Physician, University of Florida, Gainesville, FL, USA

Corey S. Cook, MD Columbia Orthopaedic Group, Columbia, MO, USA

Ron Courson, ATC University of Georgia Athletic Association, Athens, GA, USA

William A. Davis III, MD DuPage Medical Group, Orthopaedic Sports Medicine and Foot and Ankle Injury, North Central College, Naperville, IL, USA

Robert C. Decker, MD Division of Spine Surgery, Department of Orthopedic Surgery, The University of Florida, Gainesville, FL, USA

Dwayne D'Souza, MD Department of Emergency Medicine, Vanderbilt University, Nashville, TN, USA

Katherine M. Edenfield, MD Department of Community Health and Family Medicine, University of Florida, Gainesville, FL, USA

E. Randy Eichner, MD Professor Emeritus of Medicine, University of Oklahoma Health Sciences Center, Oklahoma City, OK, USA

Benton A. Emblom, MD Sports Medicine and Hip Preservation, Andrews Sports Medicine & Orthopaedic Center, Birmingham, AL, USA

Brad Endres, ATC Korey Stringer Institute, University of Connecticut, Storrs, CT, USA

Kevin W. Farmer, MD Department of Orthopedic Surgery, University of Florida, Gainesville, FL, USA

Team Physician, The University of Florida, Gainesville, FL, USA

Erica Filep, MS Korey Stringer Institute, University of Connecticut, Storrs, CT, USA

R. Warne Fitch, MD Department of Emergency Medicine and Department of Orthopaedic Surgery and Rehabilitation, Vanderbilt University, Nashville, TN, USA

Jeremy S. Frank, MD Department of Pediatric Orthopaedic Surgery, Joe DiMaggio Children's Hospital, [U18] Sports Medicine, Hollywood, FL, USA

Michael Goodlett, MD Auburn University, Auburn, AL, USA

Jeffrey Guy, MD University of South Carolina School of Medicine, Prisma Health Department of Orthopedic Surgery, Columbia, SC, USA

Orthopedic Surgery, University of South Carolina, Columbia, SC, USA

Kimberly G. Harmon, MD Departments of Family Medicine and Orthopedics and Sports Medicine, University of Washington, Seattle, WA, USA

Kristopher G. Hooten, MD Department of Neurosurgery, University of Florida, Gainesville, FL, USA

MaryBeth Horodyski, PhD, ATC Department of Orthopedics and Rehabilitation, University of Florida, Gainesville, FL, USA

Robert G. Hosey, MD Department of Orthopedic Surgery and Sports medicine, University of Kentucky College of Medicine, Lexington, KY, USA

Darren L. Johnson, MD Department of Orthopedics and Sports Medicine, University of Kentucky, Lexington, KY, USA

Jennifer Kurowicki, MD Department of Orthopaedic Surgery, St. Joseph's University Medical Center, Seton Hall University, Paterson, NJ, USA

Dennis Timothy Lockney, MD Department of Neurosurgery, University of Florida, Gainesville, FL, USA

Robert C. Matthias, MD Department of Orthopaedic Surgery, Division of Hand, Upper Extremity, and Microvascular Surgery, University of Florida, Gainesville, FL, USA

Timothy Neal, ATC Concordia University, Ann Arbor, MI, USA

Srikanth Nithyanandam, M.B.B.S., MS Exercise Physiology Department of Family and Community Medicine, University of Kentucky College of Medicine, Lexington, KY, USA

Mims G. Ochsner III, MD American Sports Medicine Institute, Birmingham, AL, USA

Fred Reifsteck, MD University of Georgia Athletic Association, Athens, GA, USA

Paul A. Rizk, MD Orthopedic Surgery Resident, The University of Florida, Gainesville, FL, USA

Ryan P. Roach, MD Sports Medicine and Hip Preservation, University of Florida, Gainesville, FL, USA

Thomas P. San Giovanni, MD Miami Orthopedics and Sports Medicine Institute, Department of Orthopedic Surgery, Florida International University College of Medicine, Miami, FL, USA

Samantha E. Scarneo-Miller, PhD West Virginia University, Division of Athletic Training, Health Sciences South, Morgantown, WV, USA

Allen K. Sills, MD Medical Director, The National Football League. Neurosurgery and Orthopedic Surgery, Vanderbilt University Medical Center, Nashville, TN, USA

Brian D. Sindelar, MD Department of Neurosurgery, University of Florida, Gainesville, FL, USA

Michael Seth Smith, MD University of Florida, Department of Orthopedics/Rehabilitation, Division of Sports Medicine, Gainesville, FL, USA

Patrick A. Smith, MD Department of Orthopaedic Surgery, University of Missouri, Columbia, MO, USA

Columbia Orthopaedic Group, Columbia, MO, USA

M. Kyle Smoot, MD Department of Orthopedic Surgery and Sports medicine, University of Kentucky College of Medicine, Lexington, KY, USA

Rebecca Stearns, PhD, ATC Korey Stringer Institute, University of Connecticut, Storrs, CT, USA

Jacob B. Stirton, MD Department of Orthopedics and Sports Medicine, Union General Hospital, Blairsville, GA, USA

Cameron D. Straughn, MD Department of Sports Medicine, James Madison University, Harrisonburg, VA, USA

Alex Wagner, MD Prisma Health/University of South Carolina Sports Medicine Fellowship, Prisma Health Department of Family and Preventative Medicine, Columbia, SC, USA

Norman E. Waldrop III, MD American Sports Medicine Institute, Birmingham, AL, USA

Austin W. Wallace, MD Orthopedic Surgery Resident, The University of Florida, Gainesville, FL, USA

Gautam P. Yagnik, MD Miami Orthopedics and Sports Medicine Institute, Department of Orthopedic Surgery, Florida International University College of Medicine, Miami, FL, USA

Part I

Orthopedic Topics

Shoulder and Elbow Injuries in Football

1

Kevin W. Farmer

Introduction

Shoulder and elbow injuries are commonly seen in football athletes. Approximately 80,000 shoulder injuries occur in high school football players annually, with around 9% of these injuries requiring surgical management [1]. During the 2004 NFL Combine, 49.7% of athletes reported having a shoulder injury during their playing time, with 34% requiring surgical management [2]. Shoulder instability, acromioclavicular (AC) injuries, sternoclavicular (SC) injuries, rotator cuff strains and sprains, and pectoralis injuries are the most common injuries encountered in the shoulder. In regard to the elbow, dislocations, ligamentous sprains, and fractures make up the most commonly encountered diagnoses. Physicians should always keep an eye out for the less commonly seen injuries such as coracoid fractures and physeal fractures, especially around the SC joint in young athletes. Return to play after fractures about the shoulder and elbow should follow sound orthopedic management and healing to avoid re-injury. This chapter focuses on the most commonly encountered in-season football injuries of the shoulder and elbow.

Shoulder

Shoulder Instability/Labral Tears

Shoulder instability is the most common shoulder injury seen on the football field, with anterior instability being more common than posterior instability. The degree of instability ranges from mild instability, or subluxations, to frank dislocations

K. W. Farmer (✉)
Department of Orthopaedic Surgery, University of Florida, Gainesville, FL, USA

Team Physician, The University of Florida, Gainesville, FL, USA
e-mail: farmekw@ortho.ufl.edu

K. W. Farmer (ed.), *Football Injuries*,
https://doi.org/10.1007/978-3-030-54875-9_1

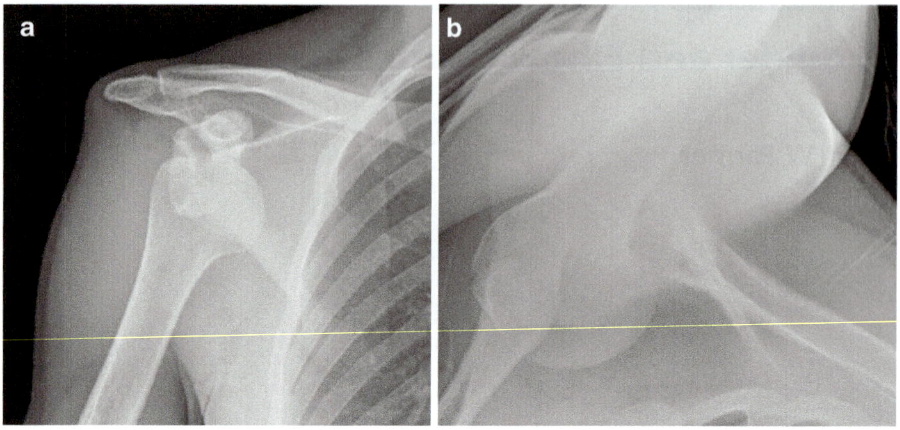

Fig. 1.1 (**a**, **b**) Grashey and axillary images of an anterior shoulder dislocation. Ideally, reduction is performed on the field. Return to play that season is an option based on imaging and degree of instability

requiring a reduction (Fig. 1.1). In collegiate football, the most common time for shoulder instability events occurs during spring practice, with an occurrence of 0.40 events per 1000 athlete exposures (AEs) [3]. During a 10-year time frame with a major Division 1 college team, authors performed 30 Bankart repairs, for around a 3% per year incidence [4]. During the 2004 NFL Combine, 14% of 336 athletes had had a previous Bankart repair during their playing days, indicating just how common this injury is [2].

When managing anterior instability in-season, there are numerous factors that go into the decision-making process, as recurrence rates are exceedingly high in this population, approaching 90%. In a multicenter study of collegiate athletes, 45 athletes were followed after an anterior instability event, and 73% of athletes were able to return that season, at a median of 5 days. Sixty-four percent had recurrent instability that season, and, of those who had recurrent instability, only 67% were able to complete the season. Athletes who had a subluxation were six times more likely to complete the season than those who had a frank dislocation. When looking at time lost and return to play, a Simple Shoulder Test (SST) and a Western Ontario Shoulder Instability Index (WOSI) score were most predictive of return to play, with the SST being inversely predictive of time to return [5]. In looking at off-season surgical repair, collegiate athletes were able to return the following season, with only a 10% recurrence rate. If, after the season, the decision was made to pursue continued nonoperative management, the athlete had a 60% recurrence the following season. This study indicates that the risk of recurrence is still very high, even if the instability is successfully managed for the current season [6]. In looking at management at the professional level, over a 9-year period, 92% of athletes in the NFL were able to return that season following an instability event. Return to play was, on average, the same game for a subluxation and 3 weeks for a dislocation. There was a 55% recurrence rate, which occurred, on average, two and a half weeks after return [7]. In a study of high school athletes, 26 out of 30 (87%) athletes were able to return after shoulder instability, at an average of 10 days. Ten of the 26 athletes (37%) had recurrent events during that season, with an average of 1.4 events during the rest of the season [8].

Posterior instability, although less common than anterior instability, is still a common issue with football players (Fig. 1.2). In an MRI study, football players were 15 times more likely to have a posterior labral tear on MRI than the general population [9]. In an evaluation of athletes with posterior instability at the United States Military Academy, 82% eventually required surgical repair. All athletes who had pain and symptoms with bench press required repair, indicating that this activity may be a good test for those that will fail nonoperative management [10]. Fortunately, outcomes of posterior labral repairs are very good, with 93% returning to football and 96% having excellent American Shoulder and Elbow Surgeon scores and high satisfaction levels [11].

Superior labrum anterior to posterior (SLAP) tears are common injuries in football players (Fig. 1.3). In the NFL, SLAP tears are most common in the offensive lineman, with 28% occurring in this group in one study [12]. Treatment is directed to reducing pain and symptoms. Physical therapy, NSAIDs, and icing are first-line treatments. Modifying the end range of motion can help minimize symptoms, and a Sully brace or harness can often be helpful in that regard. Ultrasound-guided corticosteroid injections can help reduce pain and inflammation and may help in managing an in-season injury. During one NFL season, 60% of players with a SLAP tear were able to be treated nonoperatively initially [12]. If symptoms persist, surgery (arthroscopic repair) after the season has demonstrated good outcomes in football players. If symptoms limit ability to play despite maximizing nonoperative

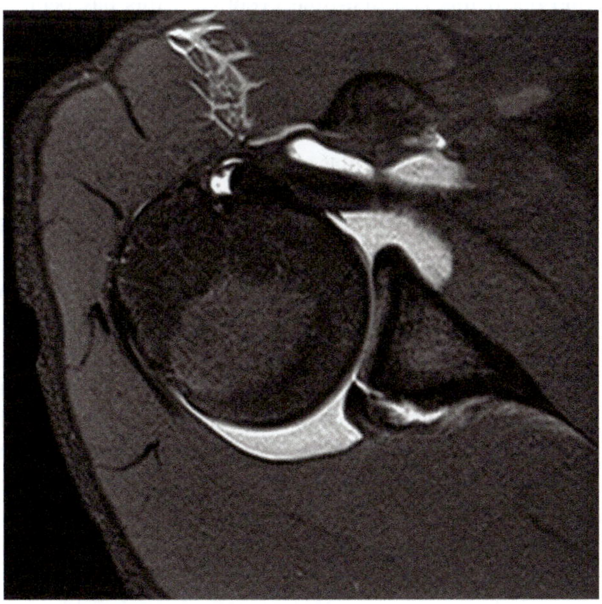

Fig. 1.2 Axillary MR arthrogram image with a large posterior labral tear. Return to play is an option with rehab and bracing. Surgery is typically required after the season

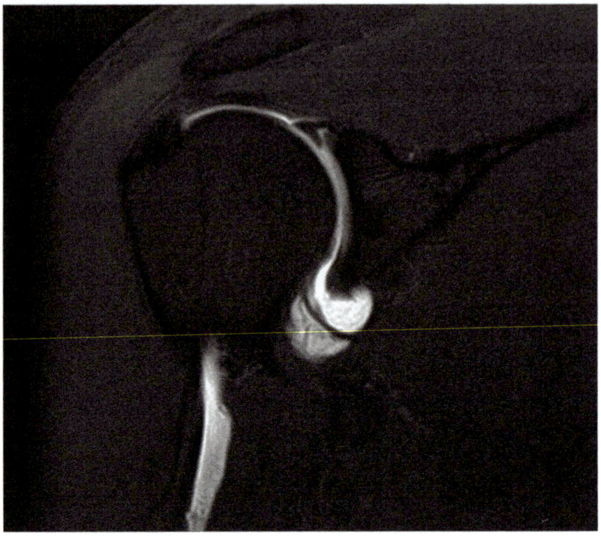

Fig. 1.3 Coronal MR arthrogram image of a superior labral tear (SLAP). The dye can be seen imbibing under the superior labrum. Treatment is based on symptoms

management, in-season repair may be necessary. Wide receivers, quarterbacks, and defensive linemen were the most at-risk positions for needing surgical repair during an NFL season [12]. The time to return to play after a surgical repair is usually around 4–6 months.

Author's Preferred Approach

When dealing with a football player with an in-season shoulder instability event, the evaluation should start with a good history and physical examination. It is important to find out if this is a first-time event or if this has been a recurrent problem. It is also important to investigate the mechanism, as this may direct you toward an anterior or posterior instability. An evaluation of global laxity is important, because patients with increased generalized laxity are at a higher rate of recurrence. A physical examination including range of motion, strength, and tenderness to palpation should be performed. A thorough neurovascular exam should be performed of the upper extremity, and this should be compared to the contralateral side. An evaluation of stability is performed, including an anterior apprehension, a relocation test, and a load and shift, either anterior or posterior, depending on instability. Midrange signs of instability could be a concern for bony involvement, such as a bony Bankart on the glenoid or a large Hill-Sachs lesion on the humerus, and should be investigated further. In the case of a simple subluxation or dislocation, plain radiographs are the first-line imaging modality. Grashey anteroposterior and axillary views are typically all that are needed initially. In an athlete with no signs of fracture or subluxation on radiographs, magnetic resonance imaging (MRI) or, preferably, a magnetic resonance arthrogram (MRA) can be obtained in an elective manner based on schedule availability (Fig. 1.4). For athletes with signs

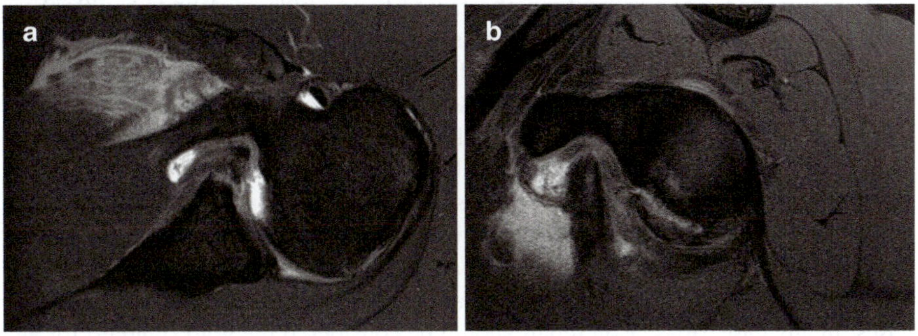

Fig. 1.4 (**a**, **b**) Axillary and sagittal MRI arthrogram images demonstrating an anterior-inferior labral tear and bony Bankart lesion

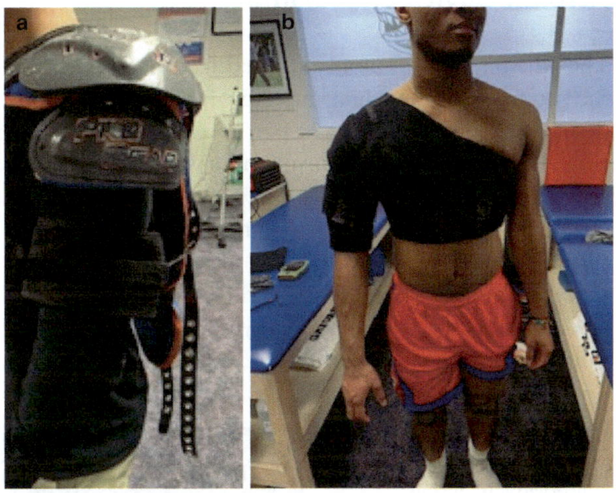

Fig. 1.5 Images of a shoulder harness (**a**) and a Sully brace (**b**) that are used in athletes with shoulder instability

of fracture or evidence of subluxation on radiographs or for concerning physical examination findings, such as midrange instability, further imaging such as MRI or computed tomography (CAT) scan should be obtained prior to returning to play.

Prior to returning to play, a physical therapy regimen should be instituted with the goal of reducing inflammation and achieving a full range of motion and strength. Once this has been achieved, a return to play program is instituted. I prefer a shoulder-stabilizing brace, such as a Sully brace or shoulder harness, and a graduated return to play (Figs. 1.5a. and 5b). That often entails a few "noncontact" practices, followed by a return to play based on progress.

As recurrence is common, it is important to have a plan in place to handle these events. For younger athletes and for teams not in contention for a major title, a "one recurrence rule" is a good rule of thumb. In athletes who do have a recurrence, especially a true dislocation, it is probably best to proceed to surgical repair. For athletes who are competing for a title or who wish to play for college or professional exposure, a conversation should be held with the athlete, their parents, the coaches, and the athletic trainers. All involved parties should be aware that recurrent events may lead to further injury, bone loss, or decreased success of operative repair. At that point, an informed decision can be made about returning. Multiple recurrent events should be discouraged, and surgical treatment should be recommended in those cases. In any case, off-season repair should be considered the gold standard for any athlete returning to contact sports the following season.

Acromioclavicular (AC) Injury

The AC joint is commonly injured from a direct blow to it, often from a tackle on the ground. In an evaluation of professional football players in the NFL, the incidence of AC injuries was 26 per 1000 AEs, with the majority being type 1 injuries (Fig. 1.6). The average return to play was 10 days, with quarterbacks being the most commonly injured, and only 1.7% required surgical intervention [13]. In collegiate football, the incidence was slightly lower, with 3.4 per 1000 AEs, with 96% being type 1 or type 2. Return to sport was 11 days for type 1 or type 2 and 32 days for type 3 or greater [14].

Return to play is typically based on symptoms and tolerability. Anti-inflammatories, physical therapy, icing, and modalities can be helpful in reducing

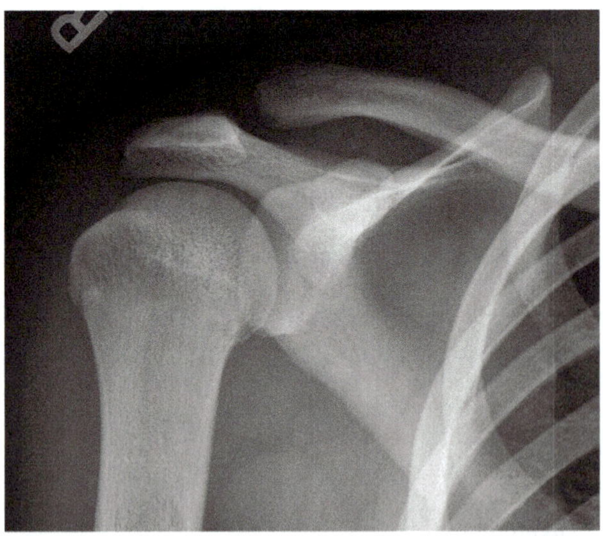

Fig. 1.6 Grade 2 AC separation treated conservatively during the season

symptoms. An intraarticular corticosteroid injection can also be helpful in reducing symptoms but often takes a few days to have an effect. Donut pads and special shoulder pads with AC cutouts can be helpful in reducing symptoms.

Local anesthetic injections, including longer-acting agents such as bupivacaine or ropivacaine, are commonly used at the highest levels, before or during games, to help reduce pain at the joint. Studies have shown little to no long-term detrimental effect on the AC joint by utilizing these injections. In one study of 50 rugby athletes, over ten seasons with an average 60-month follow-up, there were on average 4.6 injections per patient. Seventy-two percent of the athletes perceived the injections as helpful, 3% felt the injections were detrimental, and 0% would not have the injections again [15].

Author's Preferred Approach

For an in-game injury, a physical examination is performed with a special focus for crepitation or step-off of the AC joint, which would necessitate a radiograph of the AC joint to look for fracture or more severe separation. If, based on palpation or x-ray, it is determined to be a mild AC separation, then an intraarticular injection with bupivacaine is utilized. The AC joint is padded, and the athlete is taken through sideline drills to assess symptoms. If symptoms are mild, the athlete can return to play.

Following the game, symptoms are managed with anti-inflammatories, icing, and physical therapy after radiographs of the AC confirm a mild AC separation. A pregame local anesthetic can be considered in certain situations, typically reserved for the highest levels of collegiate and professional football. Donut pads are utilized until symptoms resolve. Although surgery is rarely needed, off-season surgery with a distal clavicle resection can be helpful in cases of type 1 or type 2 with persistent pain. More severe separations, such as type 4 or type 5, will often need acute surgical fixation.

Sternoclavicular Injuries

SC injuries are rare, with only a few cases reported in the literature in football players. Anterior subluxations can be treated symptomatically with rehab, NSAIDs, icing, and padding over the joint. Cortisone shots done under ultrasound can be helpful in minimizing symptoms. A posterior dislocation is an emergency, and prompt evaluation of airway and vascular status is necessary at the time of diagnosis. A CT scan is often necessary to help with diagnosis, and the addition of a CT angiogram can be helpful in assessing for vascular compromise (Fig. 1.7). Emergent reduction, closed versus open, with cardiothoracic backup is the recommended approach. After reduction, a sling for a few weeks and rehabilitation is utilized. Case reports in contact athletes report return to sport in around 4–6 weeks.

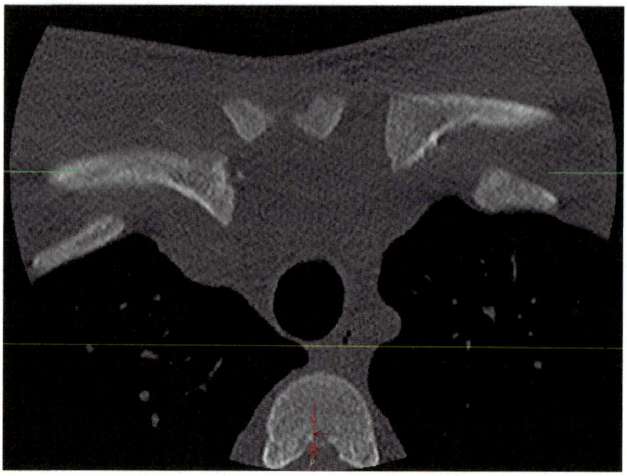

Fig. 1.7 CT scan demonstrating a right posterior SC dislocation

Clavicle Fractures

Clavicle fractures are a common fracture in football players, with football injuries accounting for 10% of clavicle fractures in the National Electronic Injury Surveillance System [16]. Depending on the fracture pattern, location, and displacement, treatment may be either surgical or nonsurgical. In a study of 17 NFL players with clavicle fractures, the average return to play was 3.47 months after injury, with a median missed time of eight games [17]. When looking at nonoperative management of clavicle fractures in NFL players, 96.9% were able to return to sport at a mean of 8 months (244.6 ± 119.6 days). Eight players (27.6%) returned within the same season as their injury [18]. In another study looking at clavicle fractures treated with open reduction and internal fixation, 15 of 17 NFL players (94.1%) were able to return to sport at a mean of two and half months (211.3 ± 144.7) days post surgery. Seven athletes (44%) were able to return in the same season. Operative treatment may slightly improve return to play times, and thus fractures early in the season may be amenable to operative fixation and return to sport toward the end of the season [19] (Fig. 1.8).

Other Soft-Tissue Injuries Around the Shoulder

Rotator cuff injuries are rare in football. In a survey of 86% of NFL team physicians, 51 rotator cuff tears were noted over a 10-year period. Forty-seven of those rotator cuff tears were treated operatively [20]. These injuries are rare in younger athletes, and most cases are rotator cuff contusions. Contusions can be managed with anti-inflammatories, physical therapy, and treatment. An occasional cortisone shot can be helpful, and return to sport is based on symptomatology. Shoulder weakness, pain at night, or failure to improve symptoms should lead to an MRI to evaluate for a tear, which may require surgical repair.

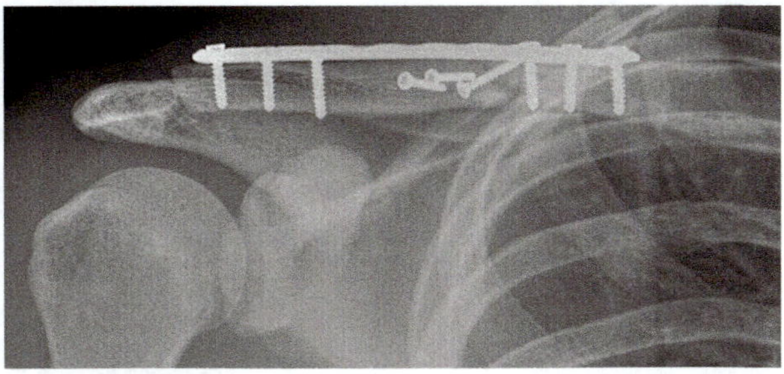

Fig. 1.8 AP clavicle radiograph 3-month status post open reduction and internal fixation of a fracture. The athlete was cleared to return for the last game of the season and play-offs

Pectoralis tears can occur in blocking or, most commonly, during the eccentric phase of bench press. Asymmetry of the pectoralis compared to the contralateral side, bruising, or a palpable defect at the pectoralis insertion may indicate a tear. If there is a suspicion for a pectoralis tear, an MRI should be obtained. An avulsion of the tendon from the humerus should be repaired surgically, as studies have demonstrated improved outcomes with surgical repair compared to nonoperative management. Partial thickness tears or musculotendinous injuries can be managed with physical therapy and modalities. Platelet-rich plasma has been reported in a few case reports. Return to play would be based on healing and symptoms and typically would take about 4–6 weeks.

Elbow

Elbow Dislocation

Around 50% of elbow dislocations in the United States occur during sports, with football being the most common, with an estimated 3000 per year [21] (Fig. 1.9). Between 2000 and 2011, 62 elbow dislocations were documented in professional football, with 65% occurring in defensive linemen. Seventy-six percent were able to return in the same season, at a mean of 25 days. Ninety-four percent were treated nonoperatively, as the vast majority were simple dislocations [22].

Author's Preferred Approach

Ideally, the elbow should be reduced on the field. Elbow radiographs should be obtained to assess reduction and to look for fracture or loose bodies. A lack of a concentric reduction or a displaced coronoid fracture should necessitate further imaging with an MRI or CT scan. If the radiographs are normal, a splint for a few days can be used to reduce the pain and swelling. Within a week, an elbow ROM brace is placed, and extension is gradually progressed to full over a 2–3-week period. Return to play in the brace can be considered once full, painless ROM in the brace is achieved. The brace should be utilized for football activities until 3 months post dislocation.

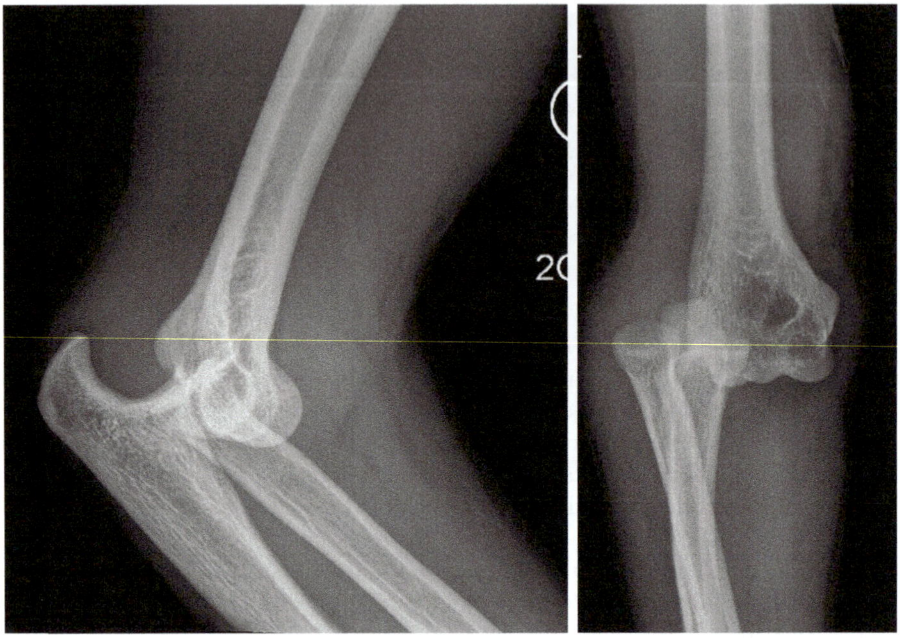

Fig. 1.9 AP and lateral of a posterolateral elbow dislocation. Ideally, these are reduced on the field. Return to play in a brace can be expected once in full range of motion and pain-free if no other pathology is noted

Ulnar Collateral Ligament (UCL) Injuries

UCL injuries have been described in various positions on the football field (Fig. 1.10). Offensive and defensive linemen can typically be treated in a brace, with return to sport as symptoms allow. Surgery is rarely indicated in football players. In a study of ten NFL quarterbacks with UCL tears in their throwing elbow, nine were successfully treated nonoperatively, with an average return to play of 26 days [23]. Treatment with physical therapy is usually the first line. Biologics, such as platelet-rich plasma, have been used with some success in baseball pitchers, but no evidence exists for quarterbacks. It appears that UCL injuries are not as devastating in quarterbacks as they are in pitchers, and nonoperative management should be considered the first-line treatment.

Shoulder and elbow injuries are common in football. Management can be complex and multifactorial. Team physicians must balance the athlete's safety and the pressures of the team. This chapter provides a framework based on the available literature that we have in managing these injuries. Every case is different, with different circumstances. The art of being a team physician entails combining the literature and individual experiences to address each case appropriately.

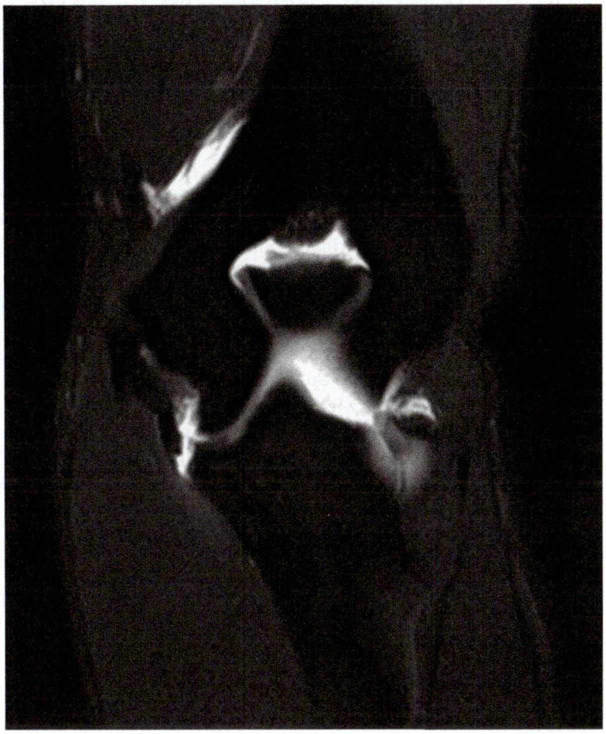

Fig. 1.10 Coronal MR arthrogram of the elbow, demonstrating a distal UCL tear in a defensive lineman. The player was able to return to play in 2 weeks in an elbow brace

References

1. Robinson TW, Corlette J, Collins CL, Comstock RD. Shoulder injuries among US high school athletes, 2005/2006-2011/2012. Pediatrics. 2014;133(2):272–9.
2. Kaplan LD, Flanigan DC, Norwig J, Jost P, Bradley J. Prevalence and variance of shoulder injuries in elite collegiate football players. Am J Sports Med. 2005;33(8):1142–6.
3. Owens BD, Agel J, Mountcastle SB, Cameron KL, Nelson BJ. Incidence of glenohumeral instability in collegiate athletics. Am J Sports Med. 2009;37(9):1750–4.
4. Mehran N, Photopoulos CD, Narvy SJ, Romano R, Gamradt SC, Tibone JE. Epidemiology of operative procedures in an NCAA division I football team over 10 seasons. Orthop J Sports Med. 2016;4(7):1–6.
5. Dickens JF, Owens BD, Cameron KL, Kilcoyne K, Allred CD, Svoboda SJ, Sullivan R, Tokish JM, Peck KY, Rue JP. Return to play and recurrent instability after in-season anterior shoulder instability: a prospective multicenter study. Am J Sports Med. 2014;42(12):2842–50.
6. Dickens JF, Rue JP, Cameron KL, Tokish JM, Peck KY, Allred CD, Svoboda SJ, Sullivan R, Kilcoyne KG, Owens BD. Successful return to sport after arthroscopic shoulder stabilization versus nonoperative management in contact athletes with anterior shoulder instability: a prospective multicenter study. Am J Sports Med. 2017;45(11):2540–6.
7. Okoroha KR, Taylor KA, Marshall NE, Keller RA, Fidai M, Mahan MC, Varma V, Moutzouros V. Return to play after shoulder instability in National Football League athletes. J Shoulder Elb Surg. 2018;27(1):17–22.

8. Buss DD, Lynch GP, Meyer CP, Huber SM, Freehill MQ. Nonoperative management for in-season athletes with anterior shoulder instability. Am J Sports Med. 2004;32(6):1430–3. Epub 2004 Jul 20
9. Escobedo EM1, Richardson ML, Schulz YB, Hunter JC, Green JR 3rd, Messick KJ. Increased risk of posterior glenoid labrum tears in football players. 2007 AJR Am J Roentgenol;188(1):193–197.
10. Lanzi JT Jr, Chandler PJ, Cameron KL, Bader JM, Owens BD. Epidemiology of posterior glenohumeral instability in a young athletic population. Am J Sports Med. 2017;45(14):3315–21.
11. Arner JW, McClincy MP, Bradley JP. Arthroscopic stabilization of posterior shoulder instability is successful in American Football Players. Arthroscopy. 2015;31(8):1466–71.
12. Chambers CC, Lynch TS, Gibbs DB, Ghodasra JH, Sahota S, Franke K, Mack CD, Nuber GW. Superior Labrum anterior-posterior tears in the National Football League. Am J Sports Med. 2017;45(1):167–72.
13. Lynch TS, Saltzman MD, Ghodasra JH, Bilimoria KY, Bowen MK, Nuber GW. Acromioclavicular joint injuries in the National Football League: epidemiology and management. Am J Sports Med. 2013;41(12):2904–8.
14. Dragoo JL, Braun HJ, Bartlinski SE, Harris AH. Acromioclavicular joint injuries in National Collegiate Athletic Association football: data from the 2004–2005 through 2008–2009 National Collegiate Athletic Association Injury Surveillance System. Am J Sports Med. 2012;40(9):2066–71.
15. Orchard JW, Steet E, Massey A, Dan S, Gardiner B, Ibrahim A. Long-term safety of using local anesthetic injections in professional rugby league. Am J Sports Med. 2010;38(11):2259–66.
16. DeFroda SF, Lemme N, Kleiner J, Gil J, Owens BD. Incidence and mechanism of injury of clavicle fractures in the NEISS database: athletic and non athletic injuries. J Clin Orthop Trauma. 2019;10(5):954–8.
17. Vora D1, Baker M, Pandarinath R. Impact of clavicle fractures on return to play and performance ratings in NFL athletes. Clin J Sport Med. 2017;(1):459–64.
18. Jack RA 2nd, Sochacki KR, Navarro SM, McCulloch PC, Lintner DM, Harris JD. Performance and return to sport after nonoperative treatment of clavicle fractures in National Football League Players. Orthopedics 2017;40(5):e836-e843.
19. Jack RA 2nd, Sochacki KR, Navarro SM, McCulloch PC, Lintner DM, Harris JD. Performance and return to sport after clavicle open reduction and internal fixation in National Football League Players Orthop J Sports Med 2017;5(8):2325967117720677. doi: https://doi.org/10.1177/2325967117720677. eCollection 2017 Aug.
20. Foulk DA, Darmelio MP, Rettig AC, Misamore G. Full-thickness rotator-cuff tears in professional football players. Am J Orthop (Belle Mead NJ). 2002;31(11):622–4.
21. Stoneback JW, Owens BD, Sykes J, Athwal GS, Pointer L, Wolf JM. Incidence of elbow dislocations in the United States population. J Bone Joint Surg Am. 2012;94(3):240–5.
22. Chang ES, Bishop ME, Dodson CC, Deluca PF, Ciccotti MG, Cohen SB, Ramsey ML. Management of Elbow Dislocations in the National Football League. Orthop J Sports Med. 2018;6(2):2325967118755451.
23. Dodson CC, Slenker N, Cohen SB, Ciccotti MG, DeLuca P. Ulnar collateral ligament injuries of the elbow in professional football quarterbacks. J Shoulder Elb Surg. 2010;19(8):1276–80.

Forearm, Wrist and Hand Injuries in Football

2

Robert C. Matthias

Football is the most popular spectator sport in the United States and is the top participatory sport for high school boys by a large margin. Given the contact nature of the sport, injury during participation is a risk. Epidemiological studies have demonstrated that 10–30% of football-related injuries involve the upper extremity. Upper extremity injuries range from simple contusions and sprains to complex fractures with potential lifelong sequela. This chapter reviews football injuries of the forearm, wrist, and hand.

Forearm

Forearm injuries are infrequently seen in football with one study demonstrating an occurrence rate of 0.05/1000 athletic exposures, less common than wrist and hand injuries [26]. Minor injuries such as contusions of the forearm are likely common and unreported. The most likely significant forearm injury is a fracture of either the radius, the ulna, or both forearm bones combined.

Radial Shaft

Isolated radial shaft fractures are most commonly displaced and require reduction and surgical fixation to allow for maintenance of reduction and early range of motion. A small percentage of fractures are minimally or non-displaced and may be amenable to treatment with immobilization. These fractures must be closely

R. C. Matthias (✉)
Department of Orthopaedic Surgery, Division of Hand, Upper Extremity, and Microvascular Surgery, University of Florida, Gainesville, FL, USA
e-mail: mattrc@ortho.ufl.edu

K. W. Farmer (ed.), *Football Injuries*,
https://doi.org/10.1007/978-3-030-54875-9_2

followed as the risk of late displacement is high. Prolonged immobilization can result in diminished range of motion, particularly forearm rotation.

Attention must be paid to the wrist joint and distal radioulnar joint (DRUJ) in the setting of a radial shaft fracture as injury to the DRUJ ligaments with resultant instability is possible. A radial shaft fracture with associated DRUJ instability is known as a "Galeazzi fracture" and requires surgical fixation of the fracture with possible ligament repair or reconstruction. DRUJ instability in the setting of a radial shaft fracture has been shown to be more likely if the radial shaft fracture is located within 7.5 cm of the distal radius articular surface [4].

Ulnar Shaft

Isolated ulnar shaft fractures are frequently the result of a direct blow and are commonly referred to as "nightstick" fractures. Unstable ulnar shaft fractures are displaced >50%, have >10-degree angulation, and are located in the proximal third of the ulna. Unstable fractures require surgery while most stable fractures can be treated with immobilization [8].

Careful evaluation of the elbow joint both clinically and radiographically is important in the setting of an isolated ulnar fracture. Dislocation of the radial head is possible and when combined with an ulnar shaft fracture is known as a "Monteggia" fracture. Anatomic reduction of the ulna reduces the radial head dislocation and should be confirmed postreduction with dedicated elbow radiographs [6, 7].

Radius and Ulnar Shaft (Both-Bone Forearm Fracture)

Both-bone forearm fractures can occur from high energy injuries or ground level falls (Fig. 2.1). The most common mechanism is an axial load through the hand. The injury is usually easily identified through exam and standard x-rays. The vast majority of both-bone forearm fractures are displaced and require surgical intervention. No study has evaluated the nonoperative treatment of non-displaced both-bone forearm fractures [5].

Acute Treatment

Suspected forearm fractures should be acutely immobilized and referred for specialized medical care on an urgent basis. A careful neurologic exam should be performed and carefully documented as soon as possible. Serial exams are extremely helpful in diagnosing compartment syndrome. When possible, an objective sensory measurement (i.e., two-point discrimination) should be utilized.

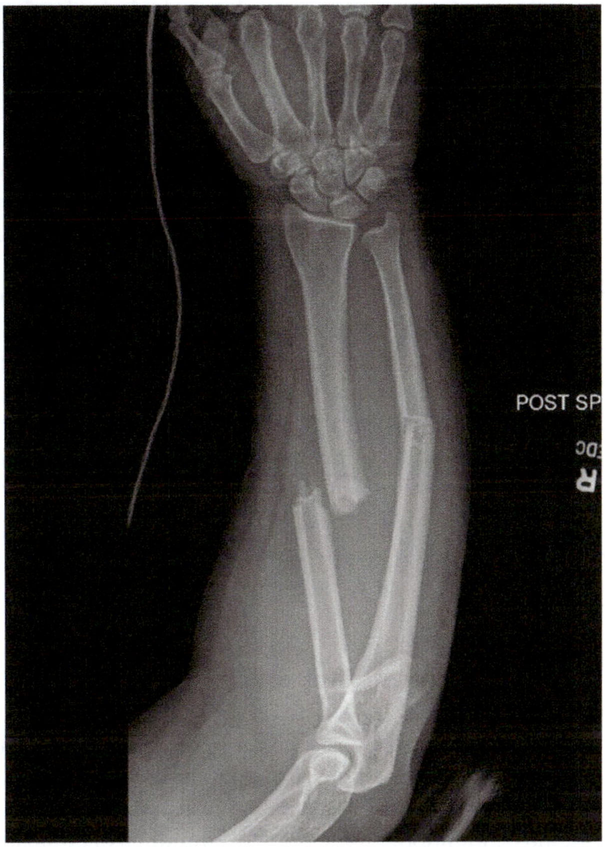

Fig. 2.1 Both-bone forearm fracture

Complications

Both isolated radius and ulna fractures can present as open fractures, but both-bone forearm fractures have a higher incidence of open injuries. Careful examination of the skin overlying these fractures is imperative to identify the injury as open. An open injury requires more urgent treatment, requires irrigation and debridement in addition to fixation of the fracture, and requires additional or alternative perioperative antibiotics when compared to closed injuries. In the field, nearly any open wound near the fracture site should be considered an open injury until it can be more carefully evaluated in a medical facility.

A known and feared complication associated with forearm fractures, particularly both-bone forearm fractures, is compartment syndrome. Acute compartment syndrome occurs when the "interstitial pressure increases with a closed fascial envelope, preventing adequate tissue oxygenation" [9]. Historically the classic signs and symptoms of compartment syndrome include the 5 Ps: pain, paresthesia, pallor, paralysis, and pulselessness. Compartment pressures can be measured in several different ways and different thresholds have been utilized to define compartment syndrome.

In practice, the diagnosis of compartment syndrome is often complex and far from straightforward. The hallmark is pain out of proportion to the exam and severe pain is noted in every patient with compartment syndrome. This pain is often significantly worsened by passive stretch of tendons that pass through the area of increased pressure. In the forearm, passive extension of the fingers stretches the finger flexors within the volar compartment of the forearm eliciting a significant increase in pain. Most who treat compartment syndrome would agree that once pallor, paralysis, and especially pulselessness are present, the diagnosis has been made too late.

When identified in a timely manner, emergent forearm fasciotomies are performed and sequela of compartment syndrome are avoided. When treated too late, compartment syndrome results in dysfunction of some or all contents of the forearm compartments. Muscle death and later necrosis occur relatively early in the process and are irreversible. In its most severe form, forearm compartment syndrome can be devastating with few reasonable salvage options.

Author's Preferred Approach

Acute forearm fractures usually pose little diagnostic dilemma. The forearm should be immobilized in a splint that extends above the elbow. Any laceration of the forearm should be carefully evaluated due to concern for an open fracture. The patient should be monitored for signs and symptoms of compartment syndrome. The patient should be transported to a medical facility for radiographic evaluation.

Isolated radius (Fig. 2.2) and isolated ulna fractures are treated surgically (Fig. 2.3) if displaced and with immobilization only following the criteria outlined above. Monteggia and Galeazzi fractures are treated surgically.

Nearly all both-bone forearm fractures, except in children, are treated with open reduction and internal fixation (Fig. 2.4). Very rarely can a non-displaced both-bone forearm fracture be treated with nonoperatively and then only with close radiographic follow-up.

Return to sport following open reduction and internal fixation is highly variable and based on a number of factors. Surgical wounds should be well healed prior to returning to sport, to avoid an increased risk of wound infection. Cases of high-level athletes returning around 6 weeks after surgical repair have been described. In those cases, custom-fabricated splints, bone stimulators, and medication (parathyroid hormone [*Forteo*], vitamin D, and calcium) were utilized, which would not be a common approach outside of the highest level of football. In most cases, evidence of complete healing is ideal, which often takes anywhere from three to six months.

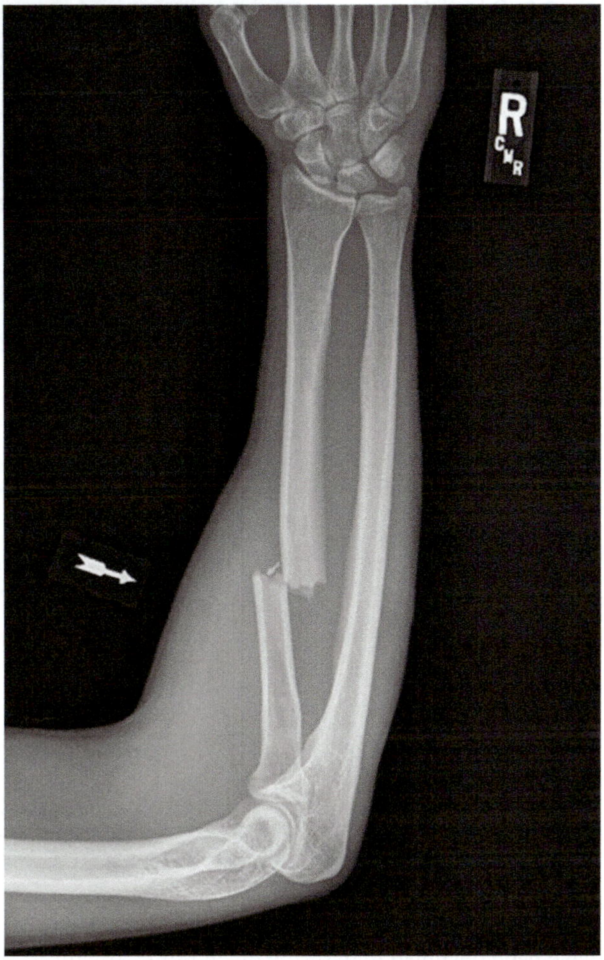

Fig. 2.2 Radial shaft fracture

Wrist

Wrist injuries are more frequently seen in football with approximately 0.11/1000 athletic exposures according to one study [26]. Wrist injuries can involve fractures or soft tissue injuries. Some injuries are mild, treated nonoperatively, and self-limited. Other injuries are higher energy, require surgical intervention, and can lead to lifetime functional deficits.

Distal Radius

Distal radius fractures usually occur from a fall on an outstretched hand (Fig. 2.5). The fracture mechanism varies depending on hand, wrist, and forearm positioning

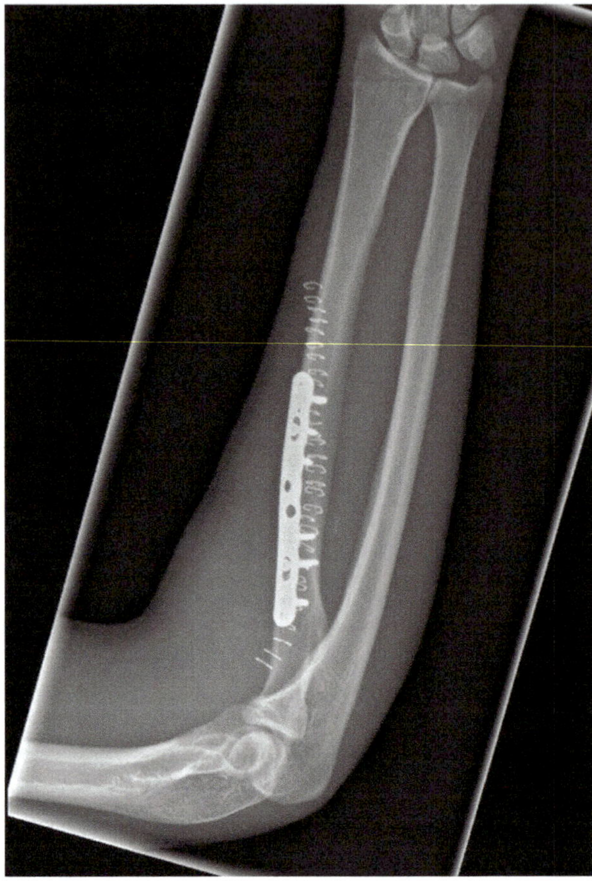

Fig. 2.3 Open reduction, internal fixation of radial shaft fracture

at the time of injury and the amount of force. A multitude of classification systems have been designed to describe distal radius fractures, but these are primarily useful for research purposes. In practice, distal radius fractures are more simply divided by three characteristics: displacement (displaced vs. non-displaced), the number of bony fragments (comminuted vs. non-comminuted), and the location of the fracture in relationship to the joint articular surface (intra- or extra-articular).

Simple fractures are non-displaced or minimally displaced, non-comminuted, and extra-articular. The majority of these fractures are treated nonoperatively with immobilization for 4–6 weeks. Displaced, simple fractures can be reduced (the fracture manipulated and aligned). These fractures must be followed radiographically for signs of delayed displacement. More complex fractures are displaced, comminuted, and intra-articular. These fractures require surgery for reduction and fixation (Fig. 2.6).

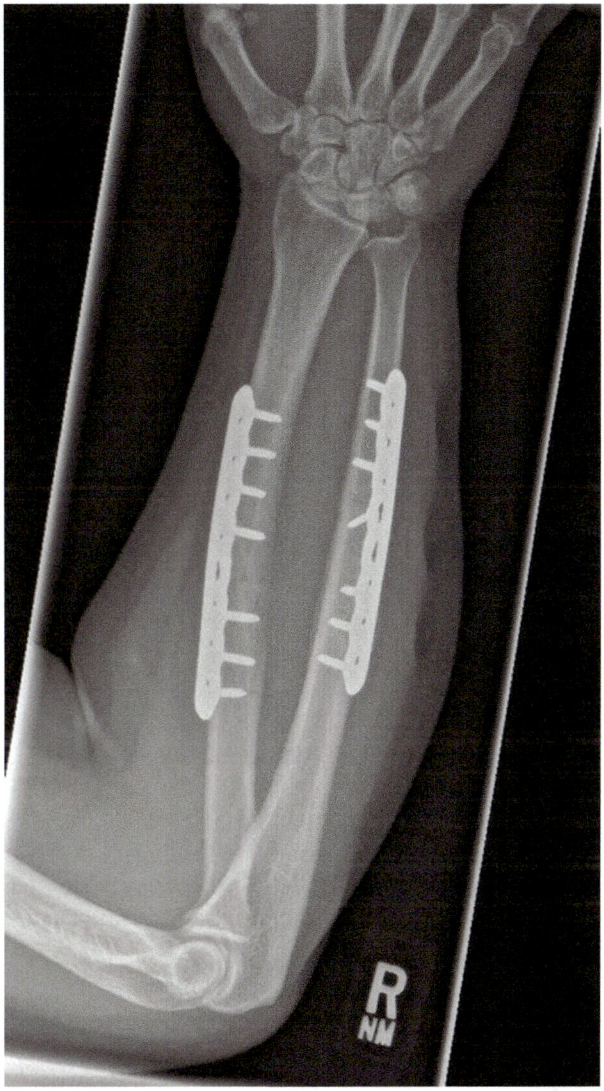

Fig. 2.4 Both-bone forearm fracture following open reduction, internal fixation

Author's Preferred Treatment

Distal radius fractures should be immobilized on the field and patients transferred to a medical facility for radiographic evaluation. Complex, intra-articular fractures may require evaluation with a CT scan. A closed reduction in a medical facility should be attempted on simple, extra-articular fractures as an acceptable reduction can often be accomplished potentially eliminating the need for surgical intervention. Fractures that cannot be acceptably reduced and displaced intra-articular fractures require surgical treatment.

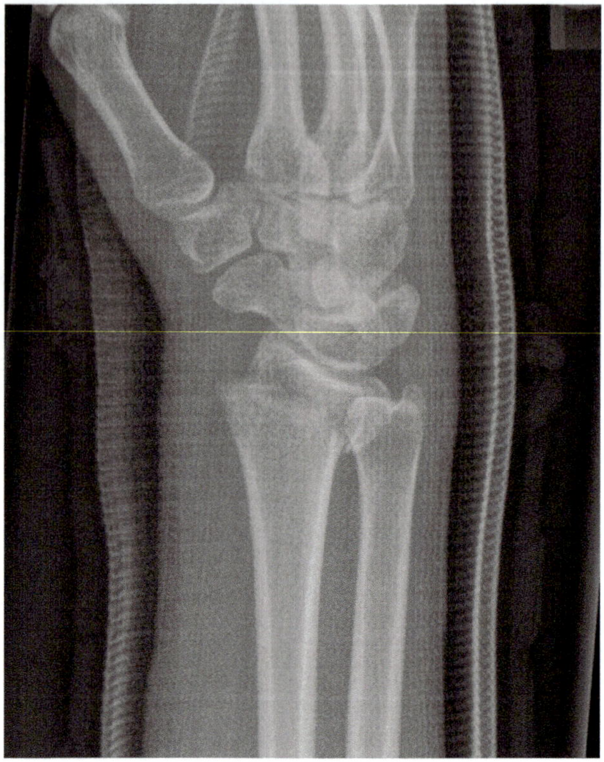

Fig. 2.5 Distal radius fracture

Return to sport is dictated by the degree of articular involvement and stability of fixation. In most cases, complete healing is necessary prior to return. For non-displaced and stable fractures, return to play in a cast a few weeks after the injury is an option, but would also depend on the position and skill level of the athlete.

Scaphoid

Scaphoid fractures are common fractures of the wrist (Figs. 2.7 and 2.8). The scaphoid is the most proximal, radial carpal bone. The fracture is typically caused by a fall on the outstretched hand. The fracture is thought to occur when extension of the carpus allows the scaphoid to impact the distal radius resulting in fracture. Importantly, scaphoid fractures heal less readily and reliably than other bones around the wrist due to their relatively poor blood supply.

Scaphoid blood supply has been studied extensively. In the most common arterial pattern, the blood supply enters through a single dorsal artery which then divides into proximal and distal branches that travel within the scaphoid [33]. A fracture disrupts this blood supply preferentially affecting blood flow to the proximal portion of the scaphoid. Diminished blood flow due to fracture leads to a relatively high nonunion rate. Avascular necrosis of the proximal pole of the scaphoid can also result [29].

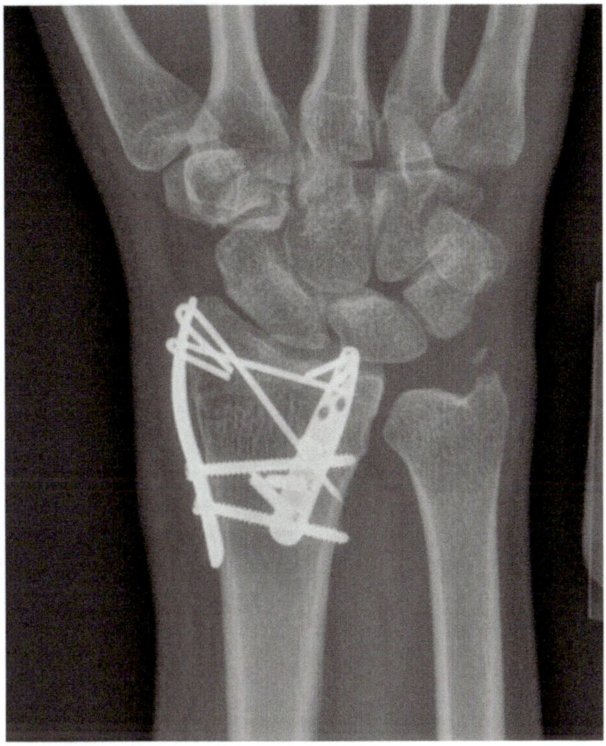

Fig. 2.6 Distal radius following open reduction, internal fixation

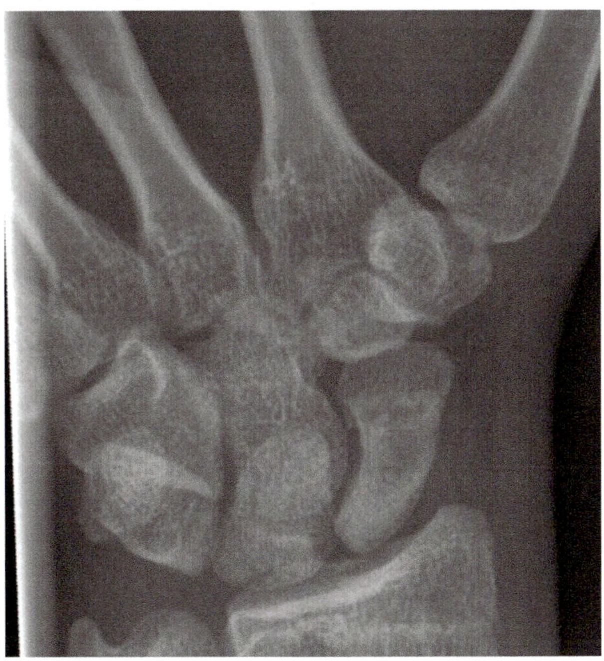

Fig. 2.7 Scaphoid waist fracture

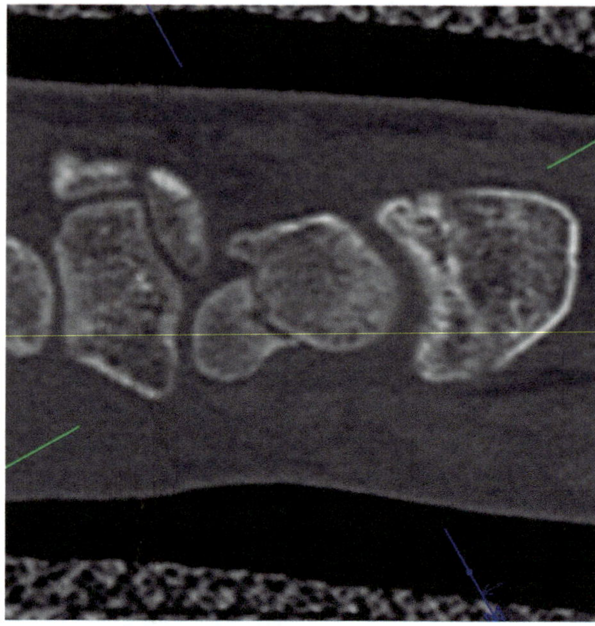

Fig. 2.8 Sagittal CT image of displaced scaphoid fracture

Author's Preferred Treatment

The treatment algorithm for scaphoid fractures is dictated in part by the vascular anatomy. Fractures of the proximal pole have the highest rate of nonunion. Surgical reduction and fixation are recommended for even non-displaced fractures [29]. Scaphoid waist fractures that are non-displaced are treated either with immobilization or open reduction and fixation based on patient preference. Most high-level athletes undergo surgery (Figs. 2.9 and 2.10). Fractures of the distal pole or scaphoid tubercle have the least likelihood of symptomatic nonunion and are treated non-operatively [32, 35].

The evaluation for a patient with a suspected scaphoid fracture includes careful physical exam and radiographic evaluation. Tenderness in the "anatomic snuffbox" is the classic finding, but tenderness over the scapholunate (SL) interval and tenderness over the scaphoid tubercle are also seen. Scaphoid fractures are frequently not visible on initial radiographs. A negative radiograph taken acutely does not rule out the presence of a scaphoid fracture. Any patient with a clinical exam concerning for a scaphoid fracture should be immobilized and subsequently reevaluated clinically and radiographically. Repeat x-rays taken before visible changes of fracture healing could be evident are useless. A delay of at least 3 weeks from injury to repeat imaging is recommended. Alternatively, advanced imaging can be utilized to assess for scaphoid fracture. Both CT and MRI have demonstrated high sensitivity and specificity in identifying acute, occult scaphoid fractures. MRI remains the gold standard [30].

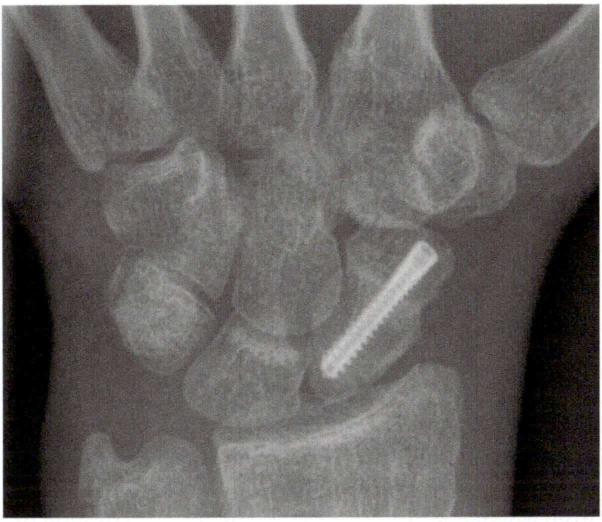

Fig. 2.9 Open reduction, internal fixation scaphoid fracture

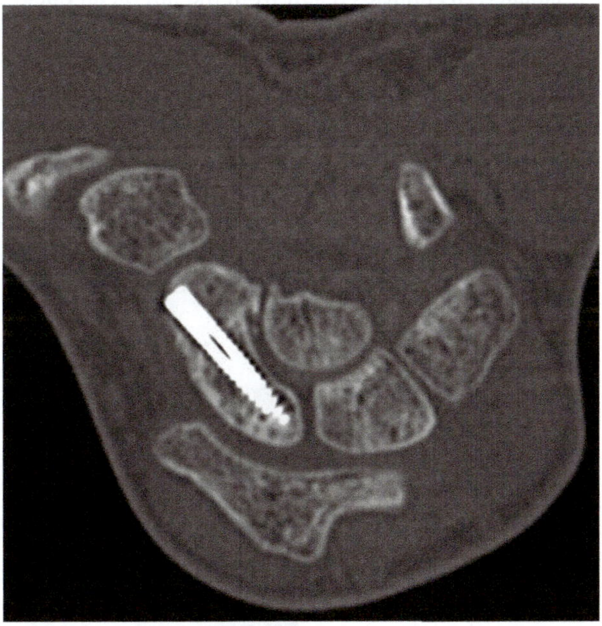

Fig. 2.10 CT following ORIF scaphoid fracture

The importance of an adequate evaluation for scaphoid fracture cannot be overemphasized. When identified and managed appropriately, the union rate for scaphoid fractures is over 90%, and once the fracture is healed patients typically return to preinjury activity levels (Goffin). Missed scaphoid fractures can progress to fracture nonunions. The natural history of scaphoid nonunions has been well described [36] and includes the development of a predictable, progressive, and irreversible pattern of wrist arthritis and commonly lifelong wrist functional limitations.

Following fixation, return to play is allowed once healing of the fracture is noted. In lower-risk cases (non-displaced, stable, etc.), return to play following internal fixation in a thumb-spica cast may be possible a few weeks after surgery [31]. The athlete should be aware that returning to sport prior to complete healing could increase the risk of nonunion and need for further surgery. A thumb-spica cast should be utilized for play for the first 6–12 weeks to minimize stress on the healing fracture.

Wrist Ligament Injuries

The radiocarpal and intercarpal joints are stabilized by robust ligaments that provide stability but allow a wide range of movement. Injuries to these ligaments that are untreated often result in the progressive development of wrist arthritis. The most common pattern of wrist ligament injury was described by Mayfield and progresses from isolated injury to the SL ligament to disruption of multiple intrinsic and extrinsic ligaments resulting in a perilunate dislocation of the carpus.

Isolated SL injuries result from the fall on an outstretched hand. X-rays are usually normal as the development of carpal malalignment can occur late or could show acute SL interval widening (Fig. 2.11). The diagnosis is made by clinical exam often combined with MRI for high-level athletes (Fig. 2.12).

With disruption of the SL ligament, the lunate rotates into hyperextension and the scaphoid rotates into volar flexion (Fig. 2.11). This carpal malalignment is known as dorsal intercalated segment instability (DISI). Identified and treated acutely, the ligament can be repaired or reconstructed returning the wrist to its normal alignment and biomechanics. Untreated, the wrist develops a progressive pattern of arthritis and collapse known as scapholunate advanced collapse (SLAC) [37].

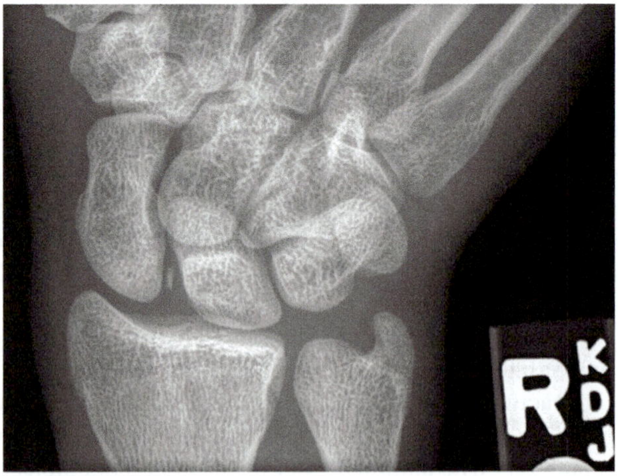

Fig. 2.11 Scapholunate ligament injury with avulsion fracture from the scaphoid

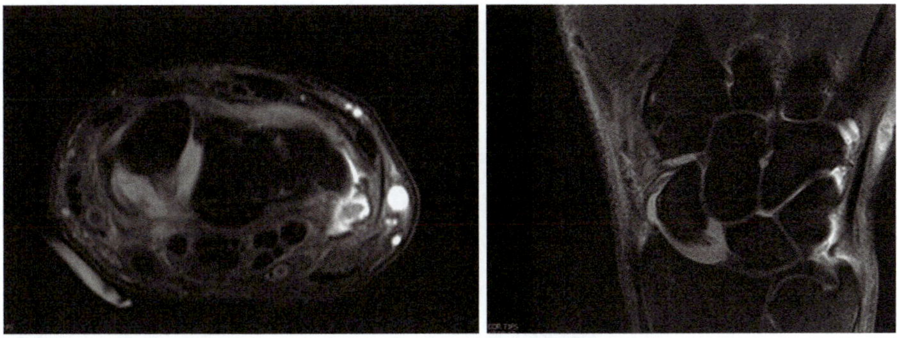

Fig. 2.12 Axial and Coronal images demonstrating scapholunate ligament injury

An injury with greater force can result in disruption of multiple wrist ligaments leading to perilunate dislocation. The lunate remains in position while the carpus dislocates dorsally. In some cases the carpus relocates forcing the lunate to dislocate volarly. Perilunate dislocations are frequently missed on initial radiographs not reviewed by specialists in wrist injuries [38]. Treatment techniques are varied and new surgical procedures are perpetually being developed. In one study of ten NFL players suffering perilunate dislocations, five players were treated with open reduction and pinning while five were treated with closed reduction and pinning. All players experienced diminished wrist ROM and five of ten had either intercarpal widening or degenerative changes on follow-up x-rays. Nine of ten players, however, returned to play within a year and the tenth retired, though his training staff felt his wrist did not limit him from continuing to play [27].

Author's Preferred Treatment

Given the natural history of untreated SL ligament injuries, for acute SL ligament injuries, the author recommends surgical repair and/or reconstruction of the ligament (Fig. 2.13). The timing of surgery is somewhat controversial. In many cases treatment can be delayed until the off-season seemingly without a negative impact on surgical complexity or ultimate outcome. In other cases, however, delayed treatment may result in a fixed deformity of the carpus that is less amenable to surgical reconstruction. An appropriate discussion with the patient regarding the unpredictability of delayed surgery is warranted.

Perilunate dislocations require urgent transport to a capable medical facility where a closed reduction under sedation should be performed. In some cases, closed reduction in the athletic training room has been performed, but can be very difficult in that setting. If a closed reduction is not possible, open reduction and treatment of the injury should be performed within a few days. If the patient is having symptoms of acute carpal tunnel syndrome, a more urgent surgical intervention should be performed.

Return to sport is dependent on the degree of involvement and surgical treatment. In a study of NFL players, return to sport varied from 1.5 weeks to 3 months or the

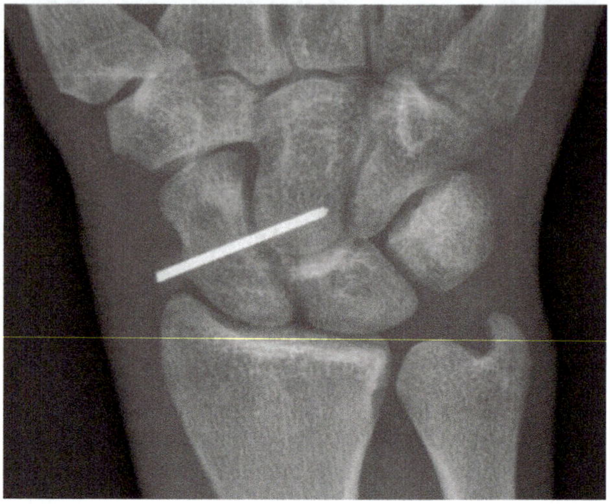

Fig. 2.13 Wrist PA view following scapholunate ligament reconstruction and scaphocapitate pinning

next season. In all cases, immobilization in a cast was utilized for a minimum of 4 weeks. One athlete returned prior to pin removal and sustained a deep wound infection requiring surgical debridement. In all other cases, return to play was delayed until pin removal, and that is the author's recommendation for approaching this injury [27].

Distal Radioulnar Joint (DRUJ)/Triangular Fibrocartilage Complex (TFCC) Injuries

The DRUJ is stabilized by the bony relationship of the sigmoid notch of the radius and the ulnar head and by soft tissue restraints of the volar and dorsal radioulnar ligaments and TFCC. Disruption of the soft tissue stabilizers results in acute dislocation of the DRUJ. Dislocations can be volar or dorsal (most common). Obvious deformity of the ulnar head and diminished pronosupination are seen on exam.

Once reduced, the wrist including the DRUJ is immobilized. An above-elbow splint is used initially to immobilize the DRUJ. By definition the stabilizers of the DRUJ are disrupted during dislocation, but stability can be restored with concentric reduction and immobilization. Chronic instability can be identified with thorough examination, and surgical intervention is warranted.

Author's Preferred Treatment

Closed DRUJ dislocations should be assessed radiographically and then reduced acutely, though the direction of the dislocation of the ulnar head (dorsal or volar) should be noted. If reduction cannot be achieved, open reduction should be performed on an urgent, not emergent, basis. If a successful reduction is achieved, the patient is immobilized in a long arm splint/cast for 6 weeks. If the dislocation was dorsal as is most common, the forearm should be immobilized in supination. If the dislocation was volar, the forearm should be immobilized in pronation. I obtain a CT scan once the patient is immobilized to confirm concentric reduction.

After 6 weeks the cast is removed and the patient is placed in a removable splint which is removed multiple times daily for the patient to work on pronosupination. Usually the patient's forearm rotation is very limited immediately following the casting phase of treatment, but most patients regain motion easily post-casting. I follow the patient clinically until acceptable motion is achieved and an adequate clinical assessment of DRUJ stability can be performed. If the DRUJ is stable, the patient can gradually return to activities as tolerated. If the DRUJ is unstable, an additional MRI is obtained and a plan made for surgical intervention. Due to the length of time of treatment, return to play is often the following season with this injury.

Hand

Fractures

Metacarpal

Metacarpal fractures are the most common hand injury sustained by NFL players (Part 1) and are the most likely hand injury to require surgery with 25% of injuries requiring surgery in one study [2]. Diaphyseal fractures are most common in football players while metacarpal neck, head, and base fractures are seen less commonly [21]. The majority of fractures are treated nonoperatively with immobilization. Open fractures, fractures resulting in unacceptable malalignment or malrotation, and displaced, intra-articular fractures require surgery [16]. Treated with or without surgery, metacarpal fractures can be easily immobilized allowing early return to play. Average return to play for all in-season athletes was 6.3 days with a recommended period of immobilization of 21 days and no reported re-fractures in one study [21]. Geissler et al. reported on ten athletes who underwent ORIF. All returned to play in 1–2 weeks. One patient sustained a refracture 1 year from injury [34].

Bennett's fracture is a fracture of the thumb metacarpal base in which the smaller, ulnar fracture fragment remains in its normal anatomic location due to its attachment to the volar beak ligament of the thumb CMC joint. The remainder of the thumb metacarpal displaces radially due to the pull of the abductor pollicis longus (APL). This fracture frequently displaces requiring reduction and casting or fixation. A similar fracture, a "reverse Bennett's fracture," occurs at the base of the small finger metacarpal. In this case the smaller radial fragment remains reduced while the metacarpal displaces.

Phalanx

Phalangeal fractures are also common injuries among football players and their prevalence is likely underreported as many of these injuries are not severe enough to warrant an x-ray. Unfortunately, phalanx fractures vary widely in severity and sequelae though the clinical presentation may be similar. The pain and clinical findings after a simple, non-displaced fracture that requires no treatment may not be significantly different from an intra-articular fracture of the PIP joint that requires surgery and results in lifelong impairment. Additionally, all the soft tissues critical for finger motion traverse in close proximity to the phalanges, especially the proximal phalanx. Post-injury adhesions and scarring are universal and result in difficulty regaining finger motion. For that reason establishing fracture stability to allow early range of motion is important.

Minimally displaced fractures of the phalangeal shaft are treated nonoperatively with immobilization followed by early motion usually at 2–3 weeks depending on the characteristics of the fracture. Displaced shaft fractures (Fig. 2.14) require either closed or open reduction and fixation (Fig. 2.15). Minimally displaced intra-articular fractures can be treated in the same manner. Some more displaced intra-articular fractures can also be treated nonoperatively. Avulsion fractures of the collateral ligaments and of the tendinous insertions of the central slip and terminal tendon can be treated with immobilization.

Displaced intra-articular fractures involving more than a tendinous insertion require surgery to restore articular congruity. These injuries, particularly involving fracture/dislocations of the PIP joint, can be difficult problems requiring complex operative solutions. In some cases joint reconstruction is accomplished by replacing a portion of the PIP joint with articular autograft from the hamate. Prolonged rehab and recovery and multiple surgical procedures are common in the treatment of these fractures.

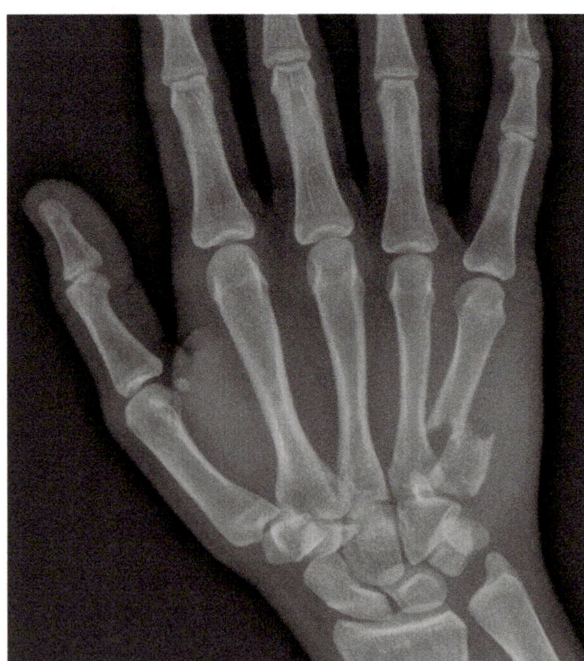

Fig. 2.14 5th metacarpal shaft fracture

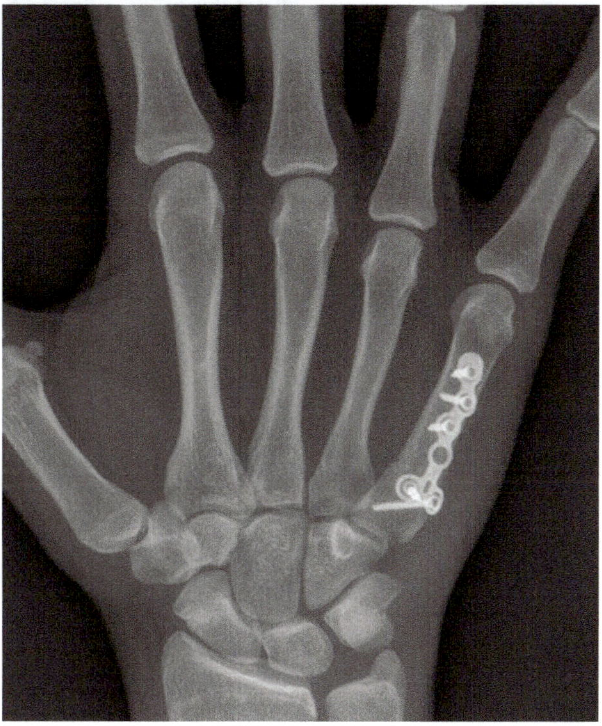

Fig. 2.15 Open reduction, internal fixation of 5th metacarpal fracture

Author's Preferred Treatment

Most hand fractures are minimally or non-displaced and can be treated with a short period of immobilization. Long-term immobilization should be avoided as significant loss of finger range of motion can result. I strictly immobilize most hand fractures for 2–3 weeks from injury and then repeat x-rays. If the fracture has remained stable, I transition the patient to a removable splint to be worn like a cast initially, but for multiple times daily, the split is removed for range of motion exercises. The patient then gradually decreases the amount of time the splint is worn and increases the frequency and aggressiveness of home range of motion exercises over the next 3 weeks, at which time the split is discontinued except during contact drills or play. In non-skill position players, I recommend continued splint immobilization during contact for 3 months post-injury. For skill position players, the risks of earlier, unsplinted return to play are discussed. If the patient wishes to return to play, immobilization options such as buddy taping are used where possible.

For displaced fractures, intra-articular injuries including Bennett's fractures (Fig. 2.16), multiple metacarpal fractures, and open fractures, surgical treatment is necessary (Fig. 2.17). When possible, I preferentially utilize fixation techniques that can be buried under the skin as opposed to percutaneous K-wires, as infection risk and time to return to play are both lessened.

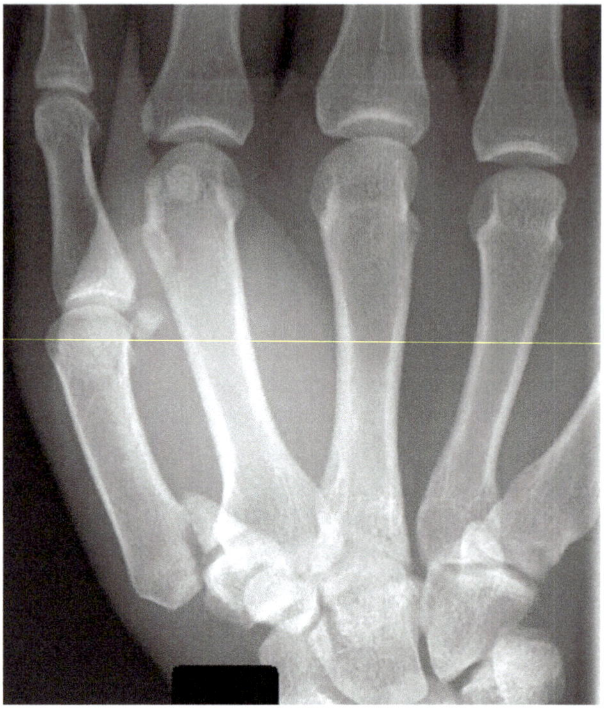

Fig. 2.16 Bennett's fracture

Ligament Injuries

Soft tissue injuries to the fingers occur frequently in football players and are certainly underreported. It is likely that anyone who plays a contact or ball sport will sustain a "jammed" finger at some point. Such injuries involve injury to the soft tissues such as the joint capsule, collateral ligaments, and volar plate that surround the affected joint. Occasionally these injuries result in small bony avulsion fractures either radially or ulnarly (collateral ligament injury) or volarly (volar plate injury) [1]. Swelling and pain with motion ranging from mild to severe are the hallmarks of these injuries. The treatment for these injuries is temporary immobilization for protection of the finger combined with immediate range of motion as pain and swelling allow. Even complete collateral ligament avulsions of the PIP and DIP joints generally are well treated nonoperatively.

Increased soft tissue disruption at a finger joint can result in dislocation. Dislocations of the CMC, MP, PIP, DIP, and IP joint can all occur, but dislocation of the PIP joint is most common [25]. Dorsal displacement of the part of the finger distal to the involved joint occurs most commonly. For most dislocations an acute reduction on the field of sideline is common. A single attempt at reduction is best as the need for multiple reductions likely signals a complex dislocation that requires sedation or surgical intervention to complete. A joint that can be reduced easily but redislocates easily often has additional injury such as a fracture.

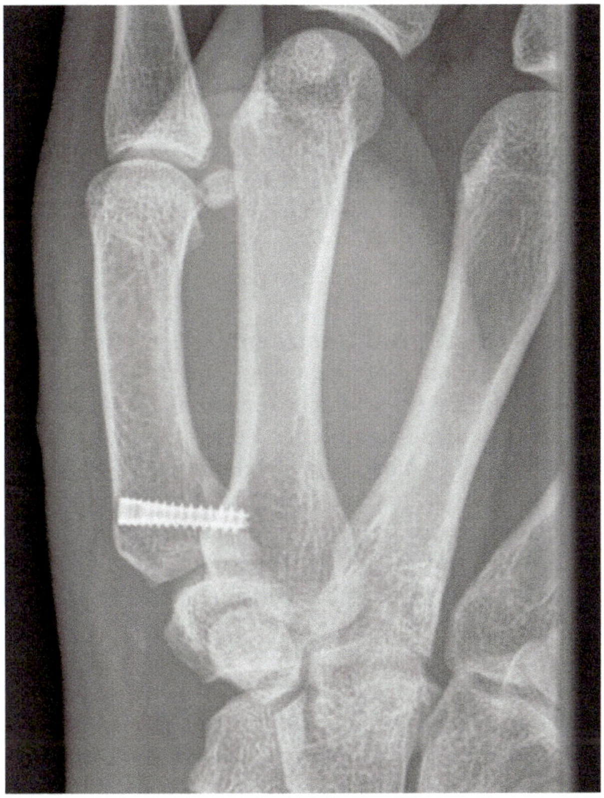

Fig. 2.17 Bennett's fracture following open reduction, internal fixation

A finger joint that is easily reduced should be immobilized with a splint or buddy taping. Immediate return to play as able is not contraindicated but player activity may be reduced by pain [3]. Each dislocation should follow up within a week for x-rays to confirm concentric reduction and assess for additional injuries such as fracture. Finger stiffness can result from these injuries so immobilization with early protected ROM limiting finger terminal extension is warranted.

Ligament injuries of the thumb MP require more attention and intervention than most other soft tissue injures of the hand. The thumb MP joint ulnar collateral ligament (UCL) is injured with forced hyperabduction of the thumb. Resulting injuries can be strains or partial tears in which joint stability is maintained. These injuries are treated with immobilization, usually for approximately 6 weeks. More severe injuries can avulse the ligament from its bony attachment, usually from the proximal phalanx. If the displacement of the ligament is severe enough, the avulsed end is pulled from deep to superficial to the adductor aponeurosis. The interposed adductor aponeurosis prevents the ligament from healing; therefore surgical repair is necessary.

When acutely identified and treated surgically, complete avulsions of the UCL of the MP joint of the thumb can do well. In one study collegiate football players who required surgical repair of the thumb UCL were able to return quickly to play, returned to the same level of play, and had good long-term outcomes. Skill position players had surgery sooner and returned to play later than non-skill position players with no difference in final level of play or clinical outcomes [20]. One study of NFL players found that 25% of players with UCL injuries of the thumb had a combined injury to the radial collateral ligament (RCL) of the thumb as well. High clinical suspicion for this combined injury and the use of MRI when the possibility of a combined injury exists was recommended. All players with isolated UCL or combined UCL/RCL injuries returned to play in the NFL following surgery [15].

Author's Preferred Treatment

The vast majority of soft tissue finger injuries are treated symptomatically with buddy taping and early range of motion. Early motion is important in these injuries as loss of digital motion can be significant and occur rapidly following injury. Deciding which finger injury requires radiographic evaluation can be confusing. Certainly not all "jammed" fingers need an x-ray, but at the same time, missed PIP intra-articular fractures can result in important functional limitation. I recommend reassessment of finger injuries at 1 week. If pain, swelling, and ROM (of which ROM is most important) are all significantly improved from the time of injury, an x-ray is generally not needed. If sufficient improvement is not seen, x-rays are obtained.

Joint dislocations are acutely reduced – sideline reductions are acceptable. Postreduction x-rays must be obtained to rule out a fracture and confirm concentric reduction. Difficult reductions, such as a metacarpal-phalangeal dislocation, may require open reduction (Figs. 2.18, 2.19 and 2.20). Early immobilization is important

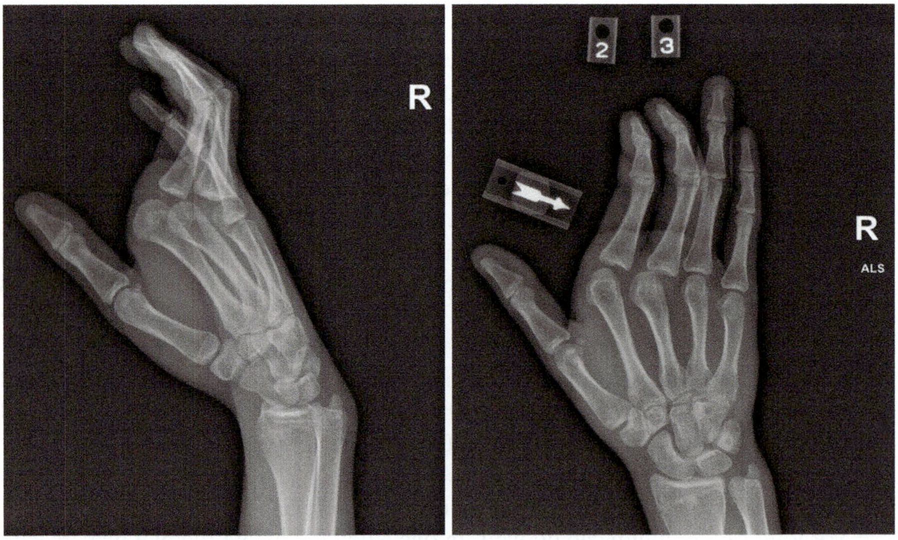

Figs. 2.18 and 2.19 Index and long finger MCP dorsal dislocations

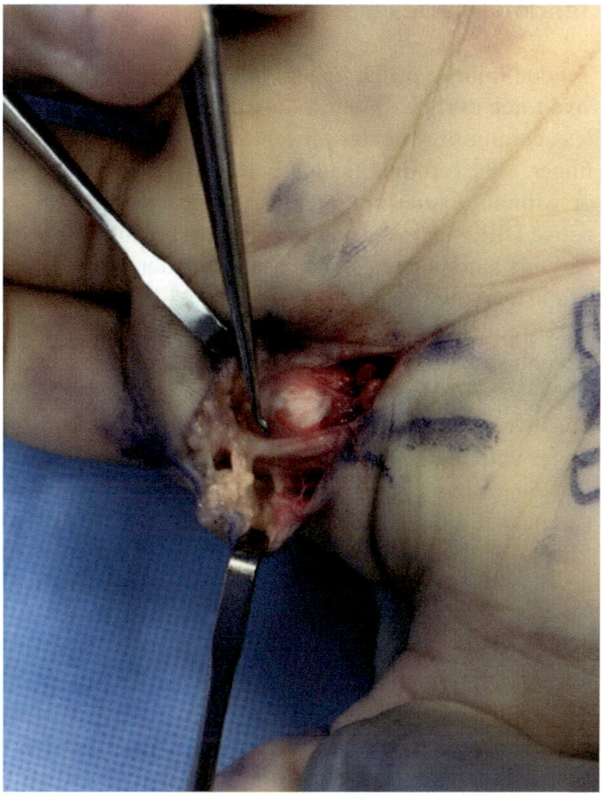

Fig. 2.20 Radial digital nerve of the index finger is subcutaneous and at risk for injury during open reduction of a dorsal MP joint dislocation

and acutely I apply a dorsal block splint for the first 2 weeks followed by a transition to buddy taping only. For dislocations that are clinically stable immediately after reduction and are reduced on x-ray, immediate return to play with buddy taping is allowed with close clinical follow-up.

Stable, partial tears of the thumb collateral ligaments are treated with splint immobilization for 4–6 weeks. The patient is encouraged to remove the splint to work on straight-line thumb flexion and extension during this time as pain improves. At 6 weeks full-time splinting is discontinued, but a splint is worn for contact drills and play for non-skill position players. Skill position players can play unsplinted when pain-free. A soft splint or taping is utilized where possible to provide some level of protection.

Unstable tears of the thumb UCL are treated surgically. If treated acutely, a stable repair is often achieved and return to play with splint immobilization is common for non-skill players. With newer techniques return to play times unsplinted for skill position players is possible, often within a few weeks.

Tendon Injuries

Tendon injuries of the fingers in football players nearly always occur due to excessive force during a blunt traumatic injury. Lacerations to tendons occur but are far less common. An extensor tendon disruption at the DIP joint results in a "mallet finger." The terminal tendon is pulled off of its insertion in the distal phalanx with or without a small fragment of bone. Clinically this tendon results in the loss of active DIP joint extension to neutral. The fingertip will "droop" at the DIP joint at a variable amount but can be passively extended to neutral. Treatment consists of full extension splinting of the DIP joint 24 hours a day for 4–8 weeks. The patient is then weaned from the splint and gentle motion exercises are performed. Results from this treatment have been universally successful [10].

Injury at the insertion site of the central slip of the extensor tendon results in loss of active extension at the PIP joint. The injury occurs in a similar manner to a mallet finger with excessive force resulting in avulsion of the tendon from its insertion in the dorsal base of the middle phalanx. With an acute, complete disruption, the patient will be unable to actively extend at the PIP joint and he will have positive Elson's test. To perform Elson's test, the PIP joint is bent 90 degrees over the end of a table. The PIP joint is held flexed while the patient attempts to extend the finger. A positive test is characterized by a weak PIP extension and rigid DIP joint hyperextension. This injury results in a Boutonniere deformity characterized by PIP flexion and DIP joint hyperextension that can become fixed if the injury is not identified and treated appropriately. Treatment for an acute injury is 4–6 weeks of full-time PIP extension splinting while performing active DIP flexion and extension exercises. Treatment for chronic injuries requires restoration of full passive PIP motion followed by tendon repair or reconstruction. Return to play in splint is an option based on position.

Injuries to the flexor tendons occur less commonly than injuries at the insertions of the extensor tendons. In the general population, tendon injuries are almost always the result of a sharp laceration. In football players, however, a unique injury can occur. A "jersey finger" injury is an avulsion of the flexor digitorum profundus (FDP) tendon from its insertion in the distal phalanx. This was described originally as a football injury usually occurring when a player grabs another player's jersey with the tips of his fingers while that player is running away. The resulting force on the tendon can lead to avulsion of the flexor tendon from its insertion. The ring finger is the injured finger 75% of the time for reasons that are unknown. Several explanations for the propensity for injury to the ring finger have been suggested. One proposed explanation is that during full grip the ring fingertip is 5 mm more prominent than the other fingers in 90% of patients and so is subjected to greater force during pull-away [11]. Another explanation is that the ring finger is uniquely tethered by bipennate lumbrical muscles radially and ulnarly and is therefore more vulnerable to a hyperextension injury [22]. Another is that the ring has less independent motion that the other digits [12]. The FDP insertion of the ring finger is weaker than that of the long finger [13].

The history and clinical exam findings of tenderness over the flexor tendon and absent DIP flexion are usually diagnostic. X-rays should be obtained as in some cases the tendon avulsion is accompanied by fracture of the distal phalanx. The results of surgical treatment are successful but must be undertaken acutely as after approximately 3 weeks, the muscle may have contracted making repair impossible [24]. Multiple studies have demonstrated nearly full DIP flexion and grip strength but some losses of DIP extension after repair [12, 19, 23]. Tendon reconstruction is possible but surgical complexity is greater and the outcome worse than direct repair [18, 23]. Not all patients are functionally limited by absent DIP flexion and elect no intervention, though diminished grip strength will result [14, 17].

Author's Preferred Treatment

Early identification of mallet finger and central slip injuries is imperative and nonoperative treatment for acute injuries is usually successful with many players regaining nearly normal function of the finger. Extension splinting of the DIP and PIP joints for 6–8 weeks is required, but many athletes including skill position players can continue to participate while splinted. When these injuries become chronic, the treatment becomes surgical and the outcomes are usually worse than acutely treated injuries.

Disruption of a flexor tendon such as "Jersey finger" requires surgical treatment to restore to preinjury function. Early classification systems for "Jersey finger" were used to determine surgical urgency with delayed treatment for some injury types deemed acceptable. Additional variants of "Jersey finger" have been more recently identified that make delayed treatment of these injuries unacceptable in my experience. I treat all acute "Jersey finger" injuries with urgent surgical repair and have found some tendons unrepairable at 3 weeks post-injury due to shortening and contracture of the flexor tendon muscle. Post-surgery therapy is critically important including splinting for 6 weeks postoperatively, immediate limited motion, and the avoidance of any gripping activities. Therapy is progressed through a standard protocol and return to full function restricted until 3 months postop at a minimum.

Chronic "Jersey finger" injuries should be approached with caution. Tendon reconstruction is possible, but postoperative adhesions and limited motion are common [39]. For a patient with a chronic "Jersey finger," no pain, and a full MP and PIP motion, the best outcome may result from no additional treatment.

References

1. Carruthers KH, Skie M, Jain M. Jam injuries of the finger: diagnosis and management of injuries to the interphalangeal joints across multiple sports and levels of experience. Sports Health. 2016;8(5):469–78. https://doi.org/10.1177/1941738116658643. Epub 2016 Jul 15.
2. Bartels DW, Hevesi M, Wyles C, Macalena J, Kakar S, Krych AJ. Epidemiology of hand and wrist injuries in ncaa men's football: 2009–2010 to 2013–2014 Orthop J Sports Med. 2019;7(4):1–8.
3. Ellsasser JC, Stein AH. Management of hand injuries in a professional football team. Review of 15 years of experience with one team. Am J Sports Med. 1979;7(3):178–82.
4. Rettig ME, Raskin KB. Galeazzi fracture-dislocation: a new treatment-oriented classification. J Hand Surg Am. 2001;26(2):228–35.
5. Schulte LM, Meals CG, Neviaser RJ. Management of Adult Diaphyseal Both-bone Forearm Fractures. J Am Acad Orthop Surg. 2014;22(7):437–46.
6. Rehim SA, Maynard MA, Sebastin SJ, Chung KC. Monteggia fracture dislocations: a historical review. J Hand Surg Am. 2014;39(7):1384–94.
7. Ring D, Jupiter JB, Waters PM. Monteggia fractures in children and adults. J Am Acad Orthop Surg. 1998;6(4):215–24.
8. Sauder DJ, Athawal GS. Management of isolated ulnar shaft fractures. Hand Clin. 2007;23(2):179–84, vi.
9. Seiler JG, et al. Compartment syndromes of the hand and forearm. J Am Soc Surg Hand. 2003;3(4):184–198.
10. Bachoura A, Ferikes AJ, Lubahn JD. A review of mallet finger and jersey finger injuries in the athlete. Curr Rev Musculoskelet Med. 2017;10(1):1–9.
11. Bynum DK Jr, Gilbert JA. Avulsion of the flexor digitorum profundus: anatomic and biomechanical considerations. J Hand Surg Am. 1988;13(2):222–7.
12. Leddy JP, Packer JW. Avulsion of the profundus tendon insertion in athletes. J Hand Surg Am. 1977;2(1):66–9.
13. Manske PR, Lesker PA. Avulsion of the ring finger flexor digitorum profundus tendon: an experimental study. Hand. 1978;10(1):52–5.
14. Methot J, Chinchalkar SJ, Richards RS. Contribution of the ulnar digits to grip strength. Can J Plast Surg. 2010;18(1):e10–4.
15. Werner BC, Belkin NS, Kennelly S, Weiss L, Barnes RP, Rodeo SA, Warren RF, Hotchkiss RN. Injuries to the collateral ligaments of the metacarpophalangeal joint of the thumb, including simultaneous combined thumb ulnar and radial collateral ligament injuries, in National Football League Athletes. Am J Sports Med. 2017;45(1):195–200.
16. Soong M, Chase S, George Kasparyan N. Metacarpal fractures in the athlete. Curr Rev Musculoskelet Med. 2017;10(1):23–27. https://doi.org/10.1007/s12178-017-9380-0.
17. Talsania JS, Kozin SH. Normal digital contribution to grip strength assessed by a computerized digital dynamometer. J Hand Surg Br. 1998;23(2):162–6.
18. McClinton MA, Curtis RM, Wilgis EF. One hundred tendon grafts for isolated flexor digitorum profundus injuries. J Hand Surg Am. 1982;7(3):224–9.
19. Moiemen NS, Elliot D. Primary flexor tendon repair in zone 1. J Hand Surg Br. 2000;25(1):78–84.
20. Werner BC, Hadeed MM, Lyons ML, Gluck JS, Diduch DR, Chhabra AB. Return to football and long-term clinical outcomes after thumbulnar collateral ligament suture anchor repair in collegiate athletes. J Hand Surg Am. 2014;39(10):1992–8.
21. Etier BE, Scillia AJ, Tessier DD, Aune KT, Emblom BA, Dugas JR, Cain EL. Return to play following metacarpal fractures in footballplayers. Hand (N Y). 2015;10(4):762–6.
22. Lunn PG, Lamb DW. "Rugby finger"—avulsion of profundus of ring finger. J Hand Surg Br. 1984;9(1):69–71.
23. Tuttle HG, Olvey SP, Stern PJ. Tendon avulsion injuries of the distal phalanx. Clin Orthop Relat Res. 2006;445:157–68. Review.

24. Tempelaere C, Brun M, Doursounian L, Feron JM. Traumatic avulsion of the flexor digitorum profundus tendon. Jersey finger, a 29 cases report. Hand Surg Rehabil. 2017;36(5):368–372.
25. Mall NA, Carlisle JC, Matava MJ, Powell JW, Goldfarb CA. Upper extremity injuries in the National Football League: part I: hand and digital injuries. Am J Sports Med. 2008;36(10):1938–44.
26. Carlisle JC, Goldfarb CA, Mall N, Powell JW, Matava MJ. Upper extremity injuries in the National Football League: part II: elbow, forearm, and wrist injuries. Am J Sports Med. 2008;36(10):1945–52.
27. Raab DJ, Fischer DA, Quick DC. Lunate and perilunate dislocations in professional football-players. A five-year retrospective analysis. Am J Sports Med. 1994;22(6):841–5.
28. Rettig AC, Weidenbener EJ, Gloyeske R. Alternative management of midthird scaphoid fractures in the athlete. Am J Sports Med. 1994;22(5):711–4.
29. Krimmer H. Management of acute fractures and nonunions of the proximal pole of the scaphoid. J Hand Surg Br. 2002;27(3):245–8. Review.
30. Garcia RM, Ruch DS. Management of scaphoid fractures in the athlete: open and percutaneous fixation. Sports Med Arthrosc Rev. 2014;22(1):22–8.
31. Goffin JS, Liao Q, Robertson GA. Return to sport following scaphoid fractures: A systematic reviewand meta-analysis. World J Orthop. 2019;10(2):101–14.
32. Winston MJ, Weiland AJ. Scaphoid fractures in the athlete. Curr Rev Musculoskelet Med. 2017;10(1):38–44.
33. Gelberman RH, Menon J. The vascularity of the scaphoid bone. J Hand Surg Am. 1980;5(5):508–13.
34. Geissler WB. Operative fixation of metacarpal and phalangeal fractures in athletes. Hand Clin. 2009;25:409–21.
35. Kawamura K, Chung KC. Treatment of scaphoid fractures and nonunions. J Hand Surg. 2015;33(6):988–97.
36. Vender MI, Watson HK, Wiener BD, Black DM. Degenerative change in symptomatic scaphoid nonunion. J Hand Surg. 1987;12(4):514–19.
37. Watson HK, Ballet FL. The SLAC wrist: scapholunate advanced collapse pattern of degenerative arthritis. J Hand Surg. 1984;9(3):358–65.
38. Herzberg G, Comtet JJ, Linscheid RL, Amadio PC, Cooney WP, Stalder J. Perilunate dislocations and fracture-dislocations: a multicenter study. J Hand Surg. 1993;18(5):768–79.
39. Netscher DT, Badal JJ. Closed flexor tendon ruptures. J Hand Surg. 2014;39(11)2315–23.

Knee Injuries in Football

3

Jacob B. Stirton, Burak Altintas, and Darren L. Johnson

Knee Dislocation

The top priority of the team physician and athletic training staff is always to rule out a medical emergency. Regarding the knee, these emergencies involve vascular injuries which result in a compromise of blood flow to the limb. This is typically associated with knee dislocations or multiligamentous injuries with a large zone of injury. This requires timely recognition with subsequent transport to a hospital for definitive work-up and treatment. The key is to quickly recognize the injury as one that cannot be treated on the sideline and that needs emergent transport to a high-level trauma center where a vascular surgeon is on call.

A typical scenario involves a player being tackled from multiple directions with a planted leg. Observers may even see the knee "bend in the wrong direction" (Fig. 3.1a). It is an injury that will cause most people in the stadium to gasp and instantly know something is very wrong. The player will be writhing in pain – much more so than other knee injuries that we will address later on in this chapter.

Our job is to immediately diagnose, stabilize, and transport our athlete to a higher level of care. A delay in care can result in a loss of limb. The gravity of this statement cannot be overstated.

When approaching the player on the field, an immediate assessment of the knee is required. If the knee is "locked" in a dislocated position, remove the player's shoes and socks and check for a posterior tibial pulse prior to reduction. Once

J. B. Stirton (✉)
Department of Orthopedics and Sports Medicine, Union General Hospital, Blairsville, GA, USA

B. Altintas · D. L. Johnson
Department of Orthopedics and Sports Medicine, University of Kentucky, Lexington, KY, USA
e-mail: dljohns@uky.edu

K. W. Farmer (ed.), *Football Injuries*,
https://doi.org/10.1007/978-3-030-54875-9_3

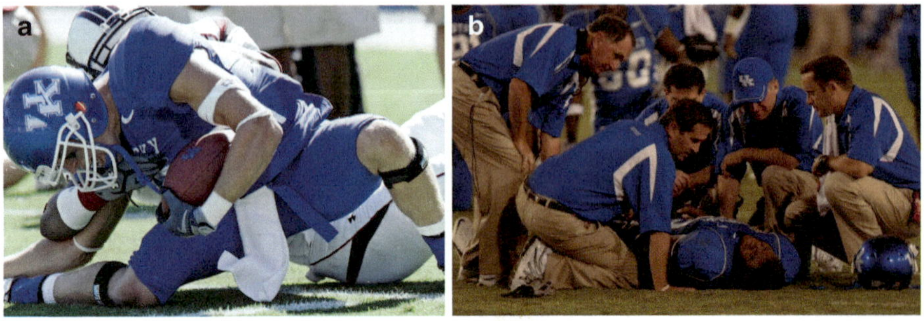

Fig. 3.1 Traumatic knee dislocation (**a**) and on-field evaluation, stabilization, and transport (**b**)

neurovascular status has been assessed, longitudinal traction/countertraction will reduce the joint. This is a multi-person effort, especially with a player who is likely in significant pain. Once reduced, which you will recognize by a more "normal"-appearing knee as well as an ability to now passively range the knee, reassess the pulse. Regardless of the pulses, this is still an emergency that must be transported to the hospital immediately. EMS should be joining you on the field at this point. The assessment of the pulses allows for an accurate description of the timing of events to the treating physicians at the hospital. Limb salvage and vascular repair are time sensitive.

After the knee has been reduced and the neurovascular status has been assessed, there is no need for further examination. Stabilize the knee in extension and immediately transport to the hospital (Fig. 3.1b).

A second scenario (and more common) is the knee dislocation or multiligamentous knee injury that is already reduced when you arrive at the player's side on the field. Most of us can recognize a dislocated knee and know that it is an emergency. The much more dangerous situation is one in which we fail to recognize the dislocation because the knee is already reduced. A failure to recognize the gravity of the situation can cause (and has caused) players to lose their leg due to inadequate treatment. There are three keys to recognizing this injury: have a high index of suspicion based on the violent nature of the injury (knee bent the wrong way or people gasping and looking away), a good examination on the field, and a low threshold for transporting to the hospital immediately.

The first key should be easy. We all know a bad injury when we see it. If you see it, do not second guess yourself, and go onto the field thinking the worst. It is a dislocation until proven otherwise.

Once you are on the field, your assessment is the next key. First document pulses. Any pulse that is absent or diminished when compared to the contralateral side is an emergency. Second, any knee injury that opens to a valgus or varus stress in full extension is unstable and represents either a now reduced knee dislocation or a multiligamentous knee injury. After the neurovascular exam, we would argue that this is the most important on the field examination maneuver of the knee. It will instantly tell you what is the emergency and what can be worked up further on the sideline.

The last key is that if your index of suspicion was high going onto the field and you cannot definitively rule out a knee dislocation and multiligamentous knee injury, then transport the athlete to the hospital. Do not let your pride put their health at risk. Let someone with more expertise, access to advanced imaging, and the ability to definitively treat make the call. No one will fault you for putting your student athlete's health first.

Meniscus Injury

Meniscal injuries, although not as common as MCL or anterior cruciate ligament (ACL) injuries, still account for almost 18% of all knee injuries in the football athlete [1]. Expanding evidence that the meniscus is not only a shock absorber but also an important secondary stabilizer of the knee has led to an even more important role in early diagnosis and treatment of these injuries as it is paramount to the long-term health of the knee joint.

The medial and lateral menisci are c-shaped fibrocartilaginous structures that attach to the tibial plateau anteriorly and posteriorly via their respective roots. They are wedge shaped in cross section and act to increase the congruency between the femoral condyles and tibial plateaus. The difference in shape of the two menisci can be explained by the difference in shape of the bony components of the lateral and medial compartments. The medial meniscus is more c-shaped while the lateral meniscus is more circular. The lateral meniscus is also more mobile than the medial meniscus due to fewer peripheral attachments and the need for greater excursion during knee range of motion. This may also explain the lower incidence of lateral meniscal injuries versus medial meniscus injury [2]. The biomechanical properties of the menisci arise from the arrangement of collagen fibers in a circumferential fashion that disperses the hoop stresses of weight-bearing as well as the radial fibers that resist longitudinal stresses. The lateral compartment of the knee is more dependent on its respective meniscus than the medial compartment due to the difference in shape and size between the lateral and medial meniscus. It is very important to understand that return to play differs in the knee with a simple medial meniscectomy versus lateral meniscectomy. This is because the lateral meniscus transmits more load and covers more surface area of the articular cartilage on the lateral side than the medial meniscus does on the medial side. Both menisci not only provide congruency for load transmission but also add stability to the knee. [3, 4]

The focus of this discussion is on acute meniscus tears in the football player; therefore the typical mechanism of an *acute* injury to the meniscus is a twisting motion of the flexed knee while the foot is planted. The highest-risk athletes therefore are those in cutting sports such as football and soccer with men being almost four times as likely to tear their meniscus as women [5]. And injury to the ACL significantly increases the risk of meniscal pathology (up to 60–70% prevalence in acute ACL ruptures), likely due to their insufficient efforts as secondary stabilizers to the knee after loss of the ACL [6].

On-field examination of the knee should include a brief explanation of injury mechanism, followed by a focused examination to localize tenderness to palpation (usually at the joint line for meniscal pathology) as well as a thorough ligamentous and neurovascular exam. Once ruled stable, the player can be transferred to the sideline or locker room for a more in-depth evaluation.

Once the player is off the field of play, he may be more thoroughly examined by the team physician. Once again, confirm the mechanism of injury with the player. Proceed with a lower-extremity exam focusing on the knee in the usual manner: inspection, palpation, range of motion, assessment of strength, and neurovascular exam, followed by any special tests. In this case, focus on palpation of the joint line as this is the most sensitive and specific physical examination finding for the diagnosis of a meniscus injury [7]. However, it is less so in the setting of a concomitant ACL injury [8]. Special tests for meniscal pathology include the McMurray, Apley grind, and Thessaly tests. The player should also be evaluated for any concomitant ligamentous injury. Over the following 24–48 hours, care should be taken to monitor for any joint effusion that may develop indicating an intraarticular pathology. An isolated meniscus tear in the white-white zone typically does not result in an effusion in the first 48 hours.

If there is high suspicion for meniscal pathology found on physical examination (e.g., effusion, joint line tenderness, positive McMurray test, etc.), advanced imaging is warranted. As with most soft tissue injuries, a non-contrast MRI is the study of choice (Fig. 3.2a), although most typically a complete set of standing plain films of the knee will be ordered first to rule out any osseous pathology or malalignment issues. The menisci should be evaluated on all three planes of the MRI – coronal, sagittal, and axial. The coronal and sagittal views will elucidate the majority of tears, but the axial can be helpful in certain cases of radial or bucket-handle tears if it happens to catch the right cut.

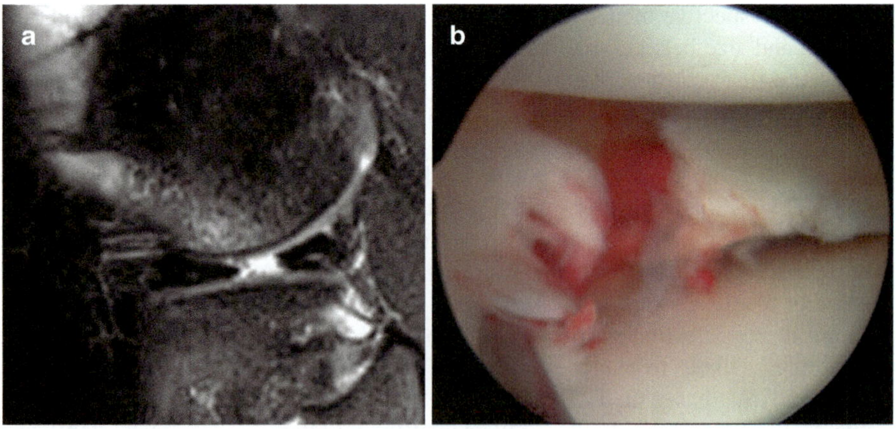

Fig. 3.2 T2-weighted sagittal MRI image of an acute lateral meniscus radial tear (**a**) and corresponding arthroscopic image in preparation of repair (**b**)

The differentiation between exact tear types is beyond the scope of this chapter, but different variations do exist – vertical, horizontal, oblique, radial, etc. For the purpose of nonoperative versus operative treatment, the focus of this chapter will be on stable versus unstable tear types.

Small, stable meniscal tears with no mechanical symptoms (catching, locking) can be treated nonoperatively with rest, activity modification until asymptomatic, NSAIDs, and possibly intraarticular injections of corticosteroids with/without a local anesthetic. The main issue with nonoperative management of meniscal tears, specifically in the high-level athlete, is their risk for re-injury and tear propagation leading to an irreparable tear. This would necessitate the need for partial meniscectomy which has deleterious effects on pressure distribution, load sharing, and stabilization as discussed earlier. Therefore, the authors suggest every effort to preserve meniscal tissue for the overall long-term health of the knee. A non-displaced meniscal tear without effusion or significant mechanical symptoms may be allowed to participate in football until the season is over after a lengthy educational discussion with all involved.

Operative management is necessary in large and unstable tears, patients with mechanical symptoms, and those who have failed to improve with nonoperative treatment. Operative interventions include either repair (Fig. 3.2b) or excision of the torn tissue or a combination of both. While this chapter will not go into an in-depth explanation of operative techniques, it is the authors' opinion that meniscal tissue should be salvaged if at all possible, especially in the young athlete and particularly on the lateral side. The post lateral meniscectomized knee is one of the most common "career-ending" situations seen at the collegiate and NFL level. A truly isolated bucket-handle tear of the medial meniscus is very abnormal, while seeing this injury on the lateral side is quite common. We often repair this lateral bucket-handle tear but the player's season is done. The medial-sided bucket-handle tear is much more controversial with high failure rates of isolated repair. Unless it is the entire medial meniscus, we would recommend meniscectomy on the medial side in the normal knee, while repair of the lateral side is required because of the biomechanical characteristics of each menisci. While very small oblique tears can likely be debrided back to stable tissue, most other tear patterns will necessitate an attempt for repair. Meniscus repair techniques depend on the tear pattern and surgeon preference, but all include repairing a tear with good vascularity and potential for healing in a stable way, whether that be inside-out, outside-in, or all-inside repair technique. It should also be mentioned that evidence has shown that meniscal repairs in the setting of concomitant ACL reconstructions have a higher rate of healing than meniscus repairs performed in isolation. This is possibly secondary to bone marrow stimulation and subsequent influx of bone marrow cells into the joint during the ACL reconstruction [9]. Therefore, the authors advocate microfracture of the intercondylar notch for all meniscus repairs done in isolation in order to potentiate that same healing response.

Rehabilitation for nonoperative treatment of meniscus injuries includes rest, activity modification until asymptomatic, NSAIDs, and possibly intraarticular injections of corticosteroids with/without a local anesthetic. The rehabilitation process for meniscal pathology treated surgically is dependent on the stability of the tear pattern as well as the operative intervention – repair versus debridement. A small stable tear that is simply debrided to a stable border can begin weight-bearing immediately after surgery with therapy to address swelling, ROM, and strengthening. Impact and loaded squatting past 90 degrees of knee flexion is avoided for the first 4 weeks, but initiated soon after. Meniscal tears that are stable but require a repair are treated more conservatively. The authors prefer a 4-week period of weight-bearing as tolerated in a hinged knee brace locked in full extension with immediate postoperative therapy to address swelling, ROM, and strengthening as well. Similarly, loaded knee flexion past 90 degrees and impact are avoided for 8 weeks and then gradually reintroduced. Strengthening and straight-line exercises are continued for the next 2 months at which time cutting drills can be initiated. The most unstable tears (bucket handle, radial) requiring surgical repair are placed on crutches and made toe-touch weight-bearing in a hinged knee brace locked at 30 degrees of knee flexion for the first 4 weeks. They are then transitioned to weight-bearing as tolerated in a hinged knee brace locked in full extension for the following 4 weeks. Therapy to address swelling, ROM, and strengthening are still initiated immediately after surgery with the caveat that ROM not exceed 90 degrees of flexion, even non-weight-bearing, for the first 4 weeks after surgery. They are then progressed similarly to above (only on a 4-week delay). It should be noted that regardless of initial tear stability, all patients are encouraged to come out of their brace while sitting or lying down to work on range of motion immediately after surgery and throughout recovery.

While there is no data supporting strict return to play criteria postoperatively, most surgeons would agree that the patient must have full range of motion and at least 80% strength compared to the contralateral side [10]. Many protocols employ functional testing and single leg hop or crossover hop tests to demonstrate appropriate strength and proprioception. A simple meniscus debridement could return to play within a month (lateral takes longer to return than medial), a stable meniscus repair by 3–4 months, and an unstable meniscus repair by 4–6 months, although each athlete is treated on an individual basis.

MCL and Posteromedial Corner Injuries

Medial collateral ligament (MCL) injuries are the most common ligamentous knee injury in football players as well as the general population (40% of all ligamentous knee injuries). The majority of these are low grade and can be treated nonoperatively, but a thorough examination for concomitant injuries is paramount in protecting our athletes and safely returning them to play.

Valgus forces at the knee are resisted by static stabilizers of the medial knee including the posterior oblique ligament (POL), superficial MCL, and deep MCL. Valgus forces are also resisted by dynamic forces such as the medial head of the gastrocnemius, vastus medialis, pes anserinus, and semimembranosus [11]. The superficial and deep MCLs provide resistance to valgus stress at the knee while the posteromedial corner provides rotational stability to the medial side of the knee. The MCL has a native strength of 4000 N [12].

An MCL injury typically occurs after a contact injury resulting in a valgus force to the knee joint with the foot planted on the ground. This mechanism often leads to a disruption of the deep and superficial MCL. If this is combined with an external rotational force, a disruption of additional restraints such as the ACL and the posteromedial corner is possible. This injury is most commonly seen when a ball carrier is tackled into the lateral aspect of an offensive lineman's knee while he is engaged with a defender [13]. The most commonly associated injuries with a non-isolated MCL tear are injuries to the ACL (95%) followed by the meniscus (5%) [14].

Like most knee injuries, an acute evaluation of an MCL is ideal, prior to any muscle spasms occurring. This initial cursory physical exam and history can take place on the field by the athletic trainer/team physician. A description of the mechanism of injury must be elicited. The examination includes inspection for peripheral hematoma along the medial side of the knee, palpation of the joint line, hamstrings, and the femoral origin and tibial insertion of the MCL, as well as ligamentous stability exams. A thorough evaluation of the neurovascular status of the extremity is necessary to avoid missing a limb-threatening vascular injury. Once it is concluded that the player is stable, he may be removed to the sideline for further in-depth examination.

Once the player is off the field of play, he may be more thoroughly examined by the team physician. Once again, the mechanism of injury needs to be confirmed with the player. Afterward, a lower-extremity examination focusing on the knee in the usual manner should proceed: inspection, palpation, range of motion, assessment of strength, and neurovascular examination, followed by any special tests. In this case, a valgus stress test is performed at full extension and 30 degrees of knee flexion to diagnose MCL injuries: grade 1 (0- to 4-mm medial-sided opening), grade 2 (5- to 9-mm opening), and grade 3 (10- to 15-mm opening). Of note, any medial-sided opening at full extension should alert the examiner to a concomitant ACL or posteromedial corner injury and a possible knee dislocation. Consideration for urgent triage to a medical facility for a definitive work-up is appropriate. Slocum-modified anterior drawer test and an anterior drawer may be considered in external rotation test to evaluate the deep MCL and posteromedial corner, respectively. A thorough examination of the knee should also assess the meniscus with joint line palpation and a McMurray or Thessaly test, the ACL with a Lachman or anterior drawer, the posterior cruciate ligament (PCL) with a posterior drawer, and the patella with the apprehension test. The MCL is most commonly injured on the femoral side of the MCL and is easily diagnosed by simple palpation. Distal MCL tears/avulsions are much less common but tend to be more severe. Any grade 3 opening at 30 or any effusion seen in the first 24 hours requires an urgent MRI.

Isolated grades 1 and 2 MCL injuries can be diagnosed clinically; and generally, an MRI is not necessarily indicated unless the patient has an intra-articular effusion or signs of other ligamentous injuries. If the player has been examined and further imaging is required to confirm the diagnosis, then standing X-rays of the knees can be obtained. The authors typically prefer at least three views – AP, lateral, and sunrise. Plain radiographs are usually not helpful for the diagnosis of an acute MCL injury but can rule out any bony abnormality such as an osseous avulsion or fracture. MRI without contrast is warranted to assess the extent and location of the MCL injury and to rule out any other pathology such as an ACL, posteromedial corner, or meniscus injury.

Acute isolated MCL injuries usually are treated nonoperatively with protective weight-bearing and bracing for 2 to 6 weeks (Fig. 3.3a). In particular, partial tears of the MCL (grade 1 or 2) heal well with conservative treatment [15]. Complete MCL injuries (grade 3 injuries) initially can be treated nonoperatively if they are femoral-based ligament ruptures (Fig. 3.3b) [16].

A complete tibial-sided MCL avulsion with POL extension (knee opens in full extension) is less likely to tighten up with nonoperative management and may require repair or reconstruction. Grade 3 MCL injuries in combination with other ligament injuries of the knee may require acute surgical repair in case of a complete tibial avulsion with POL extension [17]. The rehabilitation and return to play are dictated by the extent of the injuries (e.g., isolated MCL repair could be out 4–6 months while an ACL/MCL reconstruction could be out over 1 year).

Rehabilitation for grade 1 and 2 MCL injuries that are treated nonoperatively consists of a short period of protective weight-bearing and bracing followed by progressive strengthening with quad sets, straight leg raises, and hip adduction exercises. Athletes can work on range of motion and endurance by cycling and adding progressive resistance exercises as tolerated.

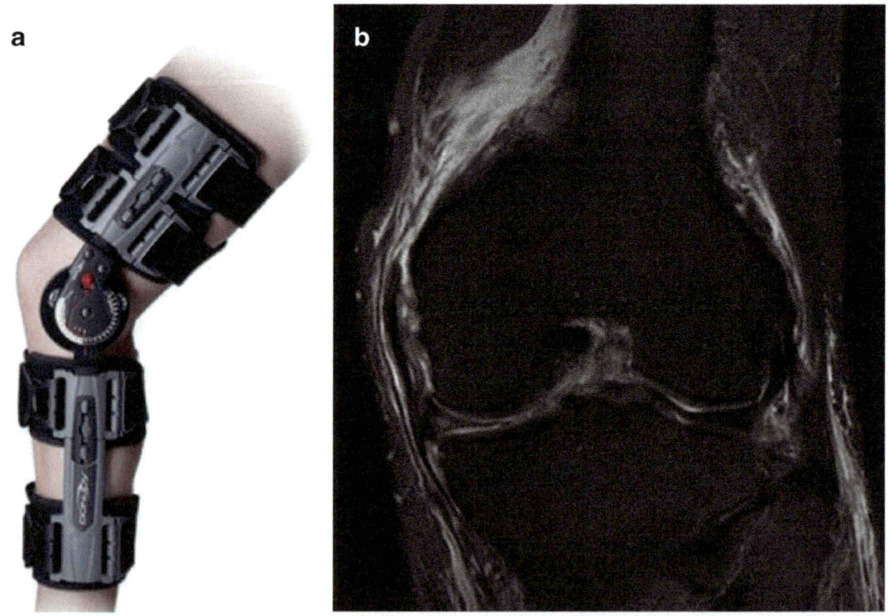

Fig. 3.3 Example of an MCL protecting knee brace from DonJoy (**a**) and T2-weighted coronal MRI image of a femoral-based MCL avulsion injury (**b**)

Grade 1 MCL sprains typically can return to play in 5–7 days, grade 2 in 2–4 weeks, and grade 3 in 4–8 weeks. But these return to play times are completely position dependent. Skill players may require much longer than those who play in the interior of the field. Functional MCL braces can be helpful for offensive linemen and are shown to help prevent MCL injuries in this particular group.

ACL Injury

In the 1970s, Dr. J.C. Kennedy would say that the ACL tear is the most common cause of the ex-athlete [18] meaning and that this was a career-ending injury. While still devastating, this absolutist view is no longer the case. A complete lateral meniscectomy is our most common unsolvable problem in this patient population today. With modern surgical techniques and the current view of rehabilitation, many athletes return to level I sports after ACL injuries.

The ACL's primary function is to resist anterolateral translation of the tibia relative to the femur [19]. It also acts to resist varus displacement of the knee in full extension along with the PCL. The ACL has a native strength of 2200 N [20].

The typical mechanism for an ACL rupture is a noncontact pivoting injury. Although ACL tears are up to 4.5 times as likely in women as in men, they are an extremely common injury in the athlete with over 400,000 reconstructions taking place every year [21]. The most commonly associated injury with a non-isolated ACL rupture is a meniscus tear (up to 75% in acute tears) [6].

As always, an acute evaluation of the knee is ideal as muscle spasm and guarding have often yet to set in. This is the optimal time to assess the stability of the knee and the integrity of the ACL. While on the field, confirm the mechanism of injury with the athlete to determine where to focus your exam. Noncontact pivoting injuries described by an audible "pop" with immediate pain and inability to bear weight are a diagnosis of ACL rupture until proven otherwise. The athlete will typically complain of immediate lateral-sided knee pain (this is because of the pivot mechanism and the large lateral bone bruise that occurs). The player needs to relax as much as possible for a reliable Lachman or anterior drawer test (making sure to compare to the uninjured contralateral side). It is then appropriate to remove the athlete from the field of play and continue a more thorough examination on the sideline or in the locker room. Often the knee effusion (hemarthrosis) is not immediate within 4 hours as opposed to a patellar dislocation where it develops immediately. The ACL-torn knee often "swells up" overnight and the next morning presents to the training room with a large effusion.

Imaging of the knee should consist of three views of plain radiographs to rule out any bony injury and should be followed by an MRI without contrast to confirm the ACL rupture (Fig. 3.4a) and diagnose any other intraarticular pathology such as a meniscus tear or cartilage injury.

ACL ruptures in the athlete are almost certainly treated with surgery. Any high-demand-cutting athlete will be unable to perform to their preinjury level without complete stability of the knee. There is also a high risk of injury to other structures

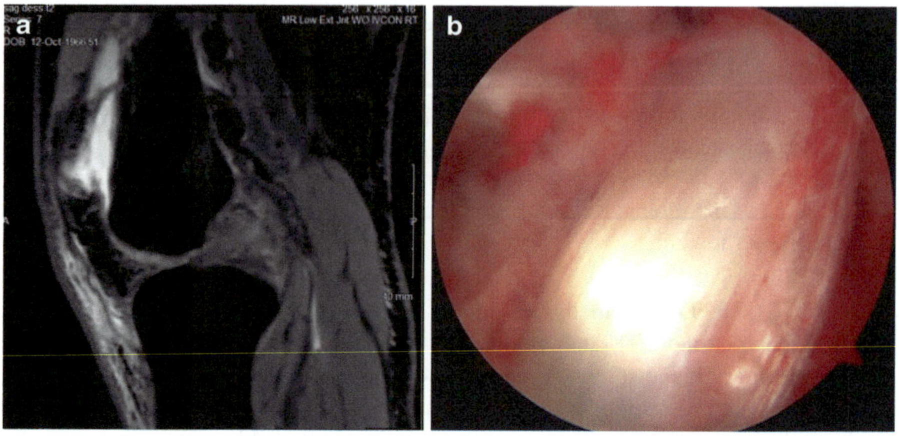

Fig. 3.4 T2-weighted sagittal MRI image of an ACL rupture (**a**) and arthroscopic image of a newly reconstructed ACL using BTB autograft (**b**)

in the ACL-deficient knee such as the medial meniscus which acts as a secondary stabilizer to anterior tibial translation and will endure abnormally high loads of force without an ACL [22]. Nonsurgical management may be considered in a player with a "partial ACL tear" or ACL sprain, which shows a majority of intact fibers on MRI but with some increased edema. If the physical exam confirms a solid endpoint and intact ACL, the athlete can opt fora course of nonoperative treatment which includes a period of rest and progressive rehabilitation. All other unstable ACL ruptures in high-level athletes require surgical treatment for restoration of stability.

The authors' preferred surgical treatment of ACL rupture in the football athlete is reconstruction with bone patella bone (BTB) autograft (Fig. 3.4b). There are varying opinions on the type of graft ranging from hamstring or BTB allografts to hamstring or quadriceps tendon autografts. The longest and most successful track record belongs to the BTB autograft which is why all other grafts are compared to it in high-level studies – e.g., the gold standard – and is this author's preferred technique. Other yet-to-be-proven techniques include ACL repair with new bioscaffolding or "internal bracing" techniques. These lack long-term outcome data and are not advocated by these authors (or senior author). [23, 24]

Rehabilitation from an ACL sprain is treated with activity modification to avoid cutting, pivoting, and impact for a period of 4–6 weeks. During that time focus should remain on range of motion and quad strengthening exercises. Gradual return to activity can resume starting at about 4 weeks from injury.

Postoperative rehabilitation from ACL reconstruction is still a hotly debated topic, but most surgeons agree that early range of motion and quad strengthening are critical components. Disagreement still remains on brace wear and exact return to play criteria and timelines. This author prefers his postoperative patients to begin physical therapy three days after surgery where they will focus on range of motion, patellar mobility, and quad activation. They are placed into a hinged knee brace locked in full extension any time they are ambulating for the first month after surgery. However, the brace comes off when they are sitting or lying down to encourage range of motion. They can wean off their crutches as soon as they are stable and no longer walk with a limp. At 4 weeks postoperatively, the hinged knee brace is unlocked during ambulation and they continue to progress their quad strengthening in physical therapy and at home. At 8 weeks postoperatively, they transition to a low-profile hinged knee sleeve which is worn any time they are in therapy, out of the house in crowded areas, or walking on uneven ground. This knee sleeve is worn for the next several months.

Therapy consists of phases: the immediate postop phase (1–2 weeks), ROM and early strengthening phase (2–4 weeks), the middle strengthening phase (4–12 weeks), the pre-impact and transition to late strengthening phase (3–4 months), and the impact and late strengthening phase (4–9 months).

Return to play is patient specific, but typically is between 9 months to 1 year from surgery. Each athlete will first undergo functional testing and then need to pass all sport-specific drills before being released to return to play. Each patient is counseled regarding the significant risk of graft re-rupture (~15%) as well as rupture of the contralateral ACL (~15%) with return to high-level sport [25].

PCL Injury

The PCL is recognized as an essential stabilizer of the knee. However, the complexity of the ligament has generated controversy about its definitive role and the recommended treatment after injury. A proper understanding of the functional role of the PCL is necessary to minimize residual instability, osteoarthritic progression, and failure of additional concomitant ligament graft reconstructions or meniscal repairs after treatment [26].

The PCL is composed of two bundles, the larger anterolateral bundle (ALB) and the smaller posteromedial bundle (PMB). Classically, the two bundles of the PCL were believed to function independently, with the ALB primarily functioning in flexion and the PMB in extension. However, in light of recent biomechanical investigations, a more synergistic and codominant relationship between the two bundles has been validated [22].

An anterior blow to a flexed knee, which can occur when an athlete falls directly on a hard surface with the knee flexed and foot in plantar flexion, may result in PCL tear [27]. As PCL injuries may be accompanied by concomitant ACL or collateral ligament injuries, leading to a knee dislocation, the on-field examination should focus on joint congruity to start with. If the knee is dislocated, it needs to be reduced on the field prior to transportation as it can be accompanied by a neurovascular injury putting the limb in danger. It is of utmost importance to check the neurovascular status before and after reduction in those cases followed by immobilization of the knee in a brace. The off-field evaluation should assess posterior translation of the knee. Tests used to evaluate the PCL are usually done with the knee flexed 90° since the PCL is the main structure preventing posterior translation of the tibia on the femur in this position [28]. Thus, when the PCL has been torn, posterior translation is increased. If the PCL is injured, a step-off deformity of the proximal tibia will be apparent (positive posterior sag sign). This test can be followed by the quadriceps active test. If the PCL is partially or completely torn, contracting the quadriceps will pull the posteriorly translated proximal tibia forward into a more normal position. Finally, the posterior drawer test (Fig. 3.5a) is done with the examiner sitting on the patient's foot to hold it in a neutral position. The amount of posterior translation is assessed by gently pushing the knee backward with the foot held in neutral rotation with the athlete's quadriceps and hamstrings completely relaxed. Imaging studies include plain radiographs as mentioned above to rule out osseous involvement. Stress radiographs can provide additional diagnostic information to help grade PCL tears [29]. MRI has become the study of choice in acute PCL injuries (Fig. 3.5b). A large prospective study found that MRI was 99% accurate in diagnosing the presence of PCL injury, confirmed by arthroscopy [30]. MRI is useful as it can also assess menisci, articular surfaces, and other ligaments of the knee.

Typically, acute, truly isolated PCL injuries (grades I and II) are treated nonsurgically. Most of these patients are able to return to sports within 4–6 weeks of nonoperative treatment [31]. The goal of a comprehensive rehabilitation program should be to strengthen the musculature about the knee while minimizing forces across the patellofemoral and tibiofemoral compartments. Exact rehabilitation protocols have been very nonspecific and varied. It has been shown that tibiofemoral compression forces are reduced with closed kinetic chain exercises, and open kinetic chain quadriceps exercises exert an anterior pull on the tibia [32].

Operative management (fairly uncommon) is usually indicated in isolated grade 3 PCL tears that remain symptomatic despite an adequate course of conservative therapy and for PCL injuries in the setting of concomitant-associated injuries. These include PLC injury or in the presence of a repairable meniscal body/root tear or MCL insufficiency [27]. There are two prevalent techniques that exist for PCL reconstruction based on the tibial insertion site: the transtibial and the tibial inlay techniques [27]. While there are multiple graft options, a recent systematic review did not show a significant difference in postoperative functional outcomes between patients treated with autograft and those treated with allograft [33]. There is no

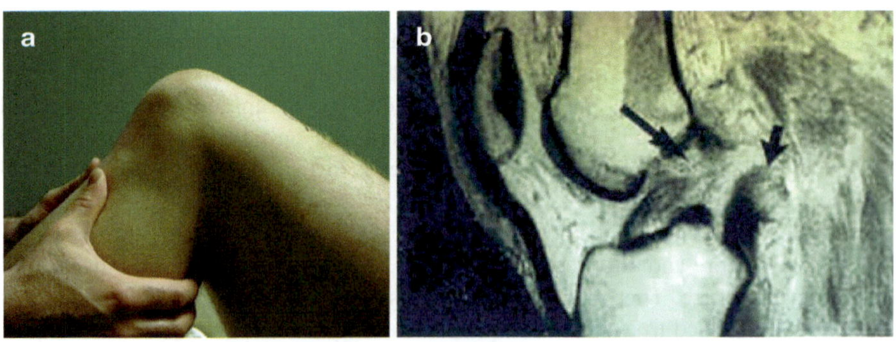

Fig. 3.5 Posterior drawer test signifying a PCL rupture (**a**) T1-weighted sagittal MRI image of a proximal PCL avulsion (**b**)

consensus in the postoperative rehabilitation in the current literature. The senior author of this article prefers toe-touch weight-bearing for four weeks with the brace locked in 30 degrees of flexion for the first four weeks after the surgery but enforces ROM as tolerated with the athlete in supine or sitting position. Afterward the athlete can be transitioned into weight-bearing as tolerated with the brace locked in extension for another four weeks. Starting in the ninth postoperative week, the athlete may continue weight-bearing with the brace unlocked for another month. The expected return to play after PCL reconstruction is similar to ACL reconstruction depending on the athlete's symptoms, ROM, stability, and strength. There are no clear guidelines regarding return to play after PCL reconstruction [34].

LCL and Posterolateral Corner Injuries

A varus load or blow inside of the knee may result in lateral collateral ligament (LCL) tears [35]. The majority of posterolateral knee injuries are caused by a blow to the anteromedial aspect of the knee, a contact or noncontact hyperextension injury, or a varus noncontact injury [36]. Approximately 60% of PCL injuries are associated with tears of the PLC structures, including the LCL, coronary ligament, popliteo-fibular ligament, popliteus tendon, and arcuate ligament [31]. An overseen LCL or PLC injury may lead to varus-thrust gait pattern which may be debilitating.

The LCL is the primary static stabilizer to varus opening of the knee [32]. The popliteus muscle and tendon complex on the posterolateral aspect of the knee has many components that provide a static and dynamic stabilizing effect to the posterolateral rotation of the knee. The midthird lateral capsular ligament is a thickening of the lateral capsule of the knee. The superficial layer consists of the iliotibial band and the biceps femoris.

The on-field examination of the injured athlete should again as stated above focus on ruling out a knee dislocation. If this is the case, the knee should be reduced immediately, and the athlete should be sent to the closest emergency room for further management. The delay in the ER presentation may result in serious long-term vascular complications which may even lead to loss of limb. Thus, these injuries should be taken very seriously. Most PLC injuries present with concomitant ACL or PCL injuries and isolated cases are rare. The off-field examination of the athlete should focus on determining the extent of the injury and understanding concomitant injuries. Especially the peroneal nerve can be injured. The correct diagnosis and documentation of this involvement are crucial for further management of the athlete as a severe peroneal nerve involvement with foot drop will necessitate an ankle-foot orthosis (AFO) to prevent long-term flexion contracture of the foot.

The severity of collateral ligament injury is generally indicated by the amount of joint-line opening with varus stress: less than 5-mm opening is indicative of grade 1 (minor sprain) injury while 6–10-mm opening is suggestive of a grade 2 (partial tear) injury. If the knee opens more than 1 cm without solid endpoint, a grade 3 (complete tear) is expected. However, the amount of joint-line opening in a varus stress test varies among patients, so it is essential to compare the injured knee with the uninjured knee. The dial test assesses posterolateral rotation of the tibia on the femur and injuries to the posterolateral knee. While the test is often described as being done with the patient prone, it can be performed in a supine position as well. This is especially more convenient for off-field examination. As the athlete's feet are externally rotated, the amount of rotation of the two limbs is compared by observing the tibial tubercles. An increased passive external rotation in 30 degrees of knee flexion is indicative of a PLC injury while a positive dial test in 90 degrees of knee flexion shows a combined PLC and PCL injury.

The imaging consists of radiographs of the injured knee. Special attention should be paid to Segond fracture which is a cortical avulsion at the tibial insertion of the lateral capsule in its mid-portion and is indicative of severe ligamentous damage. Moreover, the arcuate sign may be present on standard AP radiograph indicating avulsion fracture of the fibular head (Fig. 3.6a) [31]. Ultimately, an MRI of the knee should be obtained to assess the extent of the damage.

The recommended treatment for patients with grade 1 to 2 isolated PLC/LCL injuries (partial injuries) initially is nonoperative. This involves RICE, weight-bearing as tolerated, temporary bracing, and closed chain quadriceps exercises. The athlete may ambulate off crutches when he/she can walk without a limp. The estimated return to play is approximately 1 week for grade 1 injuries while it may take 1–4 weeks for grade 2 injuries.

Grade 3 injuries usually require surgical treatment. Of note, it is extremely unusual to have an isolated grade 3 injury of the PLC and is much more common to be combined with an ACL tear, PCL tear, or both. Based on the time from injury to surgery as well as injury severity, the surgical treatment may range from direct

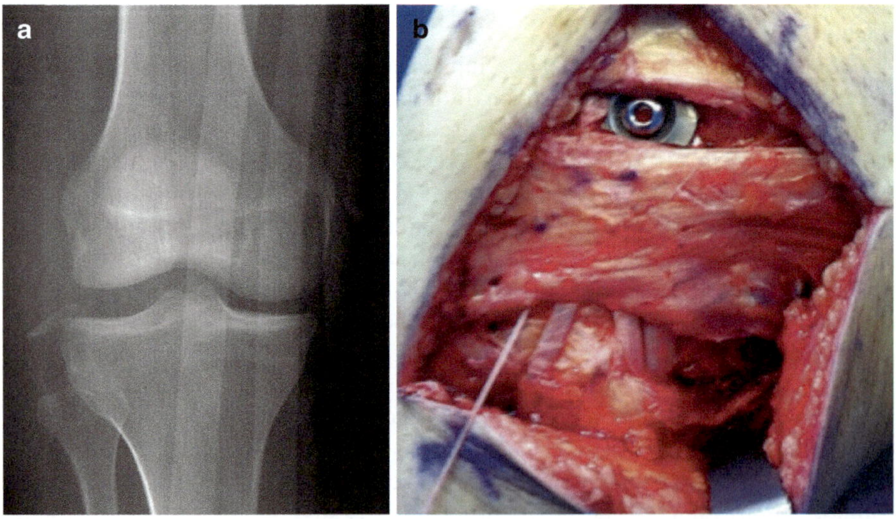

Fig. 3.6 AP plain film illustrating the fibular avulsion fracture, or "arcuate sign," as well as lateral joint space widening (**a**) and clinical image of a newly reconstructed PLC using a modified Larson technique using a hamstring allograft (**b**)

repair to reconstruction using auto- or allografts. The senior author prefers the modified Larson technique using a hamstring graft (Fig. 3.6b). The postoperative rehabilitation is the same as in PCL injuries. Regarding the return to play, there are no high-level evidence-based guidelines. The postoperative timeline is dependent on the athlete's subjective and objective assessment as mentioned above for the PCL injuries.

Patellar Dislocation Injury

Fifty to 60% of initial first-time lateral patellar dislocations will occur secondary to a sports-related injury and will involve a compromised medial patellofemoral ligament (MPFL) and medial retinaculum at least 80% of the time. [37, 38] The MPFL is a thin fascial band approximately 53 (ranging 45–64) mm long that links from the region of the medial epicondyle of the femur to the proximal part of the medial border of the patella. It is the primary passive restraint that resists lateral translation of the patella [39].

Lateral patellar dislocations may occur after lateral blow to the knee (Fig. 3.7a). The on-the-field management relies on the correct recognition and diagnosis followed by reducing it using a medial reduction maneuver while moving the knee into full extension; this will always reduce the patella if it is still dislocated in flexion "on the field." The off-field evaluation includes a more thorough examination with palpation along the MPFL and retinacular structures followed by performing the patellar apprehension test. With the athlete seated or supine and the knee flexed to 45°, the patella is pushed laterally. Apparent increased laxity and apprehension indicate the possibility of patellar subluxation or dislocation. Although rare, other injuries such as quadriceps tendon tears should be evaluated as well. A single leg raise test is usually sufficient for this. A large effusion hemarthrosis will develop in the first 12 hours which is typically much quicker than an ACL tear.

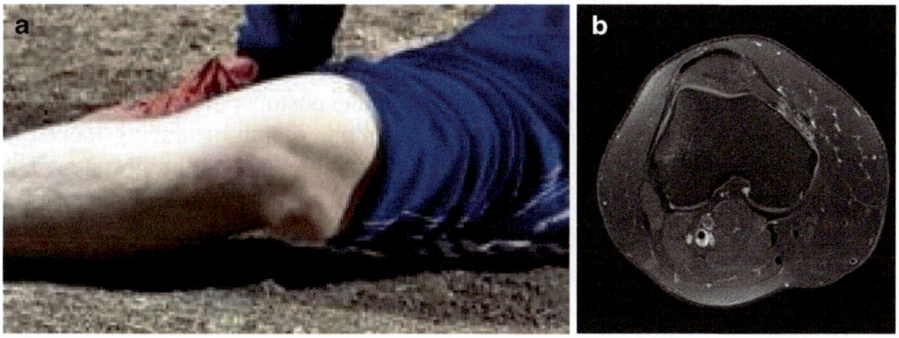

Fig. 3.7 Acute lateral patellar dislocation (**a**) and T2-weighted axial MRI image demonstrating an MPFL rupture (**b**)

The imaging should include radiographs to rule out fractures or osteochondral lesions. Moreover, an MRI of the knee needs to be obtained to assess the MPFL integrity as well as any chondral lesions with or without loose bodies or concomitant ligamentous damage (Fig. 3.7b). While recurrent lateral patellar dislocation is known to lead to degenerative process, a single first-time or infrequently recurring traumatic lateral patellar dislocation also seems to be associated with gradual cartilage deterioration [40]. Measurement of the Caton-Deschamps index and the tibial tubercle trochlear groove distance as well as the assessment of the trochlear groove is important to understand the anatomy and guide treatment. The bone bruise of the medial patella along with the lateral trochlea may be signs of patellar instability.

First-time patellar dislocations are commonly treated nonoperatively. Once this decision is made, aspiration of the hemarthrosis and injection of corticosteroid are performed to eliminate the knee effusion as quickly as possible and to allow for early range of motion and rehabilitation. Rehabilitation of the major muscle group of the thigh simply cannot move forward with a knee effusion. The biology of the knee, or an effusion, dictates how fast we can move in therapy and eventually return to play. However, a recent study suggests that the surgical MPFL reconstruction achieved better clinical outcomes than nonsurgical treatment for the acute primary patellar dislocation in the skeletally mature patients with the presence of abnormal patellofemoral anatomy. Thus, surgery may be considered as the better choice for these specific patients. [41, 42] Trochlear dysplasia, elevated TT–TG distance, patella alta, complete MPFL tear at its isolated femoral side, and complete combined MPFL tear in the first-time dislocation are independently associated with a higher incidence rate of the second-time dislocation [37]. Thus these factors should be weighted in the decision making. The nonoperative treatment includes mobilization with a brace locked in extension with weight-bearing as tolerated for one month with moving the knee as tolerated up to 90 degrees of flexion. If the patella remains stable after one month, the brace may be transitioned into a hinged patellar knee sleeve without any ROM restrictions. The sleeve can be discontinued by symptom relief and clinical patellar stability after 2 months.

Operative treatment includes the repair versus reconstruction of the MPFL. A recent systematic review showed that a double-bundle MPFL reconstruction seems to provide more favorable outcomes than a single-bundle MPFL reconstruction [43]. The senior author prefers reconstruction using a hamstring autograft for the treatment of recurrent dislocators. The postoperative rehabilitation is similar to the ACL reconstruction and involves one month of bracing locked in extension with weight-bearing as tolerated followed by gradual progression. The best available studies to date would suggest high return to play rates (84%–100%) and a highly variable timeframe for return (3–12 months) after patellar stabilization surgery [34].

References

1. Loughran GJ, et al. Incidence of knee injuries on artificial turf versus natural grass in National Collegiate Athletic Association American Football: 2004-2005 through 2013-2014 seasons. Am J Sports Med. 2019;47(6):1294–301.
2. Thompson WO, Thaete FL, Fu FH, et al. Tibial meniscal dynamics using three-dimensional reconstruction of magnetic resonance images. Am J Sports Med. 1991;19:210–6.
3. Greis PE, Bardana DD, Holmstrom MC, et al. Meniscal injury: I. Basic science and evaluation. J Am Acad Orthop Surg. 2002;10:168–76.
4. McDermott ID, Amis AA. The consequences of meniscectomy. J Bone Joint Surg Br. 2006;88:1549–56.
5. Baker BE, Peckham AC, Pupparo F, et al. Review of meniscal injury and associated sports. Am J Sports Med. 1985;13:1–4.
6. Spindler KP, Schils JP, Bergfeld JA, et al. Prospective study of osseous, articular, and meniscal lesions in recent anterior cruciate ligament tears by magnetic resonance imaging and arthroscopy. Am J Sports Med. 1993;21:551–7.
7. Fowler PJ, Lubliner JA. The predictive value of five clinical signs in the evaluation of meniscal pathology. Arthroscopy. 1989;5:184–6.
8. Shelbourne KD, Martini DJ, McCarroll JR, et al. Correlation of joint line tenderness and meniscal lesions in patients with acute anterior cruciate ligament tears. Am J Sports Med. 1995;23:166–9.
9. Krych AJ, et al. Surgical repair of meniscal tears with concomitant anterior cruciate ligament reconstruction in patients 18 years and younger. Am J Sports Med. 2010;38(5):976–82.
10. Kozlowski EJ, Barcia AM, Tokish JM. Meniscus repair: the role of accelerated rehabilitation in return to sport. Sports Med Arthrosc Rev. 2012;20:121–6.
11. LaPrade RF, Engebretson AH, Ly TY, et al. The anatomy of the medial part of the knee. J Bone Joint Surg Am. 2007;89(9):2000–10.
12. Smeets K, et al. Mechanical analysis of extra-articular knee ligaments. Part one: native knee ligaments. Knee. 2017;24(5):949–56.
13. Peterson L, et al. Incidence of football injuries and complaints in different age groups and skill-level groups. Am J Sports Med. 2000;28(5 Suppl):S51–7.
14. Fetto JF, Marshall JL. Medial collateral ligament injuries of the knee: a rationale for treatment. Clin Orthop. 1978;132:206–18.
15. Andrews K, Lu A, Mckean L, Ebraheim N. Review: medial collateral ligament injuries. J Orthop. 2017;14(4):550–4.
16. Giannotti BF, Rudy T, Graziano J. The non-surgical management of isolated medial collateral ligament injuries of the knee. Sports Med Arthrosc Rev. 2006;14:74–7.
17. Wilson TC, Satterfield WH, Johnson DL. Medial collateral ligament "tibial" injuries: indication for acute repair. Orthopedics. 2004;27:389–93.
18. Fowler PJ, Snyder-Mackler L. Commentary. J Orthop Sports Phys Ther. 2001;31(11):661.
19. Brandsson S, Karlsson J, Sward L, et al. Kinematics and laxity of the knee joint after anterior cruciate ligament reconstruction: pre- and postoperative radiostereometric studies. Am J Sports Med. 2002;30:361–7.
20. Dienst M, Burks RT, Greis PE. Anatomy and biomechanics of the anterior cruciate ligament. Orthop Clin North Am. 2002;33:605–20.
21. Gans I, et al. Epidemiology of recurrent anterior cruciate ligament injuries in National Collegiate Athletic Association Sports: the injury surveillance program, 2004–2014. Orthop J Sports Med. 2018;6(6).

22. Hirschman HP, Daniel DM, Miyasaka K. The fate of unoperated knee ligament injuries. Knee ligaments: structure, function, injury, and repair. New York: Raven Press; 1990.
23. Andersson C, Odensten M, Gillquist J. Knee function after surgical or nonsurgical treatment of acute rupture of the anterior cruciate ligament: a randomized study with a long-term follow-up period. Clin Orthop Relat Res. 1991:255–63.
24. Grontvedt T, Engebretsen L, Benum P, Fasting O, Molster A, Strand T. A prospective, randomized study of three operations for acute rupture of the anterior cruciate ligament. Five-year follow-up of one hundred and thirty-one patients. J Bone Joint Surg Am. 1996;78:159–68.
25. Wiggins AJ, et al. Risk of secondary injury in younger athletes after anterior cruciate ligament reconstruction a systematic review and meta-analysis. Am J Sports Med. 2016;44(7):1861–76.
26. Laprade CM, et al. Emerging updates on the posterior cruciate ligament. Am J Sports Med. 2015;43(12):3077–92.
27. Laprade RF, Wentorf F. Acute knee injuries; on-the-field and Sideline evaluation. Phys Sportsmed. 1999;27(10):55–61.
28. Grood ES, Stowers SF, Noyes FR. Limits of movement in the human knee: effect of sectioning the posterior cruciate ligament and posterolateral structures. J Bone Joint Surg Am. 1988;70(1):88–97.
29. Fanelli GC, Beck JD, Edson CJ. Current concepts review: the posterior cruciate ligament. J Knee Surg. 2010;23(2):61–72.
30. Gross ML, Grover JS, Bassett LW, Seeger LL, Finerman GA. Magnetic resonance imaging of the posterior cruciate ligament. Clinical use to improve diagnostic accuracy. Am J Sports Med. 1992;20:732–7.
31. Johnson P, Mitchell SM, Görtz S. Graft considerations in posterior cruciate ligament reconstruction. Curr Rev Musculoskelet Med. 2018;11(3):521–7.
32. Lutz GE, Palmitier RA, An KN, Chao EYS. Comparison of tibiofemoral joint forces during open-kinetic-chain and closed-kinetic-chain exercises. J Bone Joint Surg Am. 1993;75:732–9.
33. Ansari AS, et al. Influence of graft source on postoperative activity and joint laxity in posterior cruciate ligament reconstruction: a systematic review. Arthroscopy. 2019;35(1):262–74.
34. Bedi A, Musahl V, Cowan JB. Management of posterior cruciate ligament injuries: an evidence-based review. J Am Acad Orthop Surg. 2016;24(5):277–89.
35. Nannaparaju M, et al. Posterolateral corner injuries: epidemiology, anatomy, biomechanics and diagnosis. Injury. 2018;49(6):1024–31.
36. LaPrade RF, Wentorf F. Diagnosis and treatment of posterolateral knee injuries. Clin Orthop Relat Res. 2002;402:110–21.
37. Laidlaw MS, Diduch DR. Current concepts in the management of patellar instability. Indian J Orthop. 2017;51(5):493–504.
38. Sherman SL, et al. Return to play after patellar stabilization. Curr Rev Musculoskelet Med. 2018;11(2):280–4.
39. Amis AA, et al. Anatomy and biomechanics of the medial patellofemoral ligament. Knee. 2003;10(3):215–20.
40. Salonen EE, et al. Traumatic patellar dislocation and cartilage injury a follow-up study of long-term cartilage deterioration. Am J Sports Med. 2017;45(6):1376–82.
41. Zheng X, et al. Surgical medial patellofemoral ligament reconstruction versus non-surgical treatment of acute primary patellar dislocation: a prospective controlled trial. Int Orthop. 2019;43(6):1495–501.
42. Longo UG, et al. Treatment of primary acute patellar dislocation: systematic review and quantitative synthesis of the literature. Clin J Sport Med. 2017;27(6):511–23.
43. Lee DY, et al. Which technique is better for treating patellar dislocation? A systematic review and meta-analysis. Arthroscopy. 2018;34(11):3082–93.

Ankle Injuries in Football

4

Norman E. Waldrop III, E. Lyle Cain, Katie Bartush, and Mims G. Ochsner III

Lateral Ankle Sprains

The seemingly benign "ankle sprain" has become commonplace is sports, especially in football. Players of all ages sustain these injuries and most parents, coaches, and players have some knowledge of "rolling" an ankle and sustaining a "sprain." Certainly, some of the general public's knowledge stems from the fact that ankle sprains are so common. At the high school level, ankle sprains are the most common injury during practice and competition and more likely to occur during practice than in games [1]. This may be due in part to the fact that there are more exposures during practices each season than in games. In 2006, the most common foot and ankle injuries among former collegiate football players participating in the Combine were lateral ankle sprains. Several epidemiological studies have been performed to characterize the incidence of ankle injuries in National Football League (NFL) players [2]. The foot and ankle are involved in roughly 17% of NFL injuries and occur most frequently in linemen [2]. Among foot and ankle injuries, lateral ankle sprains are increasingly common.

Lateral ankle sprains are important not only because of the frequency with which they occur but also because of their potential to cause long-term ankle instability. In fact, approximately 20–40% of lateral ankle sprains will lead to persistent symptoms, including pain and instability, if left untreated [3]. This chapter will focus on ways to minimize time lost from competition and how to prevent chronic instability.

The osseous anatomy of the ankle consists of the tibia medially, fibula laterally, and talus distally. It is a sickle-shaped joint with cartilage on both sides. While the tibial surface is commonly convex, it can be concave in approximately 16% of individuals. It is wider anteriorly than posteriorly.

N. E. Waldrop III (✉) · E. L. Cain · K. Bartush · M. G. Ochsner III
American Sports Medicine Institute, Birmingham, AL, USA
e-mail: norman.waldrop@andrewssm.com

K. W. Farmer (ed.), *Football Injuries*,
https://doi.org/10.1007/978-3-030-54875-9_4

The lateral ankle complex is made up of the anterior talofibular ligament (ATFL), calcaneofibular ligament (CFL), and posterior talofibular ligament (PTFL) [4]. The ATFL arises from the distal fibula and inserts onto the lateral aspect of the talar body (Fig. 4.1). The CFL connects the lateral fibula to the calcaneal tubercle. The PTFL runs from the posterior aspect of the lateral fibula to the posterior process of the talus.

The effect each ligament has on ankle mechanics depends on the position of the talus relative to the tibia. With the talus in neutral or dorsiflexion, the wider anterior border sits between the malleoli and imparts stability to the mortise. As the talus is plantarflexed, the mortise is no longer filled with bony anatomy and stability depends on ligamentous structures. The ATFL is taut with the ankle in plantarflexion, while the CFL is taut with subtalar inversion and the ankle in a neutral or dorsiflexed position. Perhaps the most well-known study on lateral ankle sprains was performed by Brostrom in 1965, who found that the ATFL was the most commonly injured lateral ankle ligament and, in fact, lateral ankle sprains occur most commonly when the ankle is in this plantarflexed and inverted position [5]. Oftentimes an injured player describes a "pop" or twisted ankle. While a player's injury mechanism can be a clue to diagnosis, many times the injury is not observed and/or the athlete cannot recall exactly what happened.

In these cases, practitioners must rely more heavily on their physical exam. When examining a patient with a suspected lateral ankle sprain, approach the exam systematically. The first portion of the exam begins with an analysis of the athlete's gait. This can be performed as they come off the field, and complete inability to bear weight may signify a more severe injury. Once sidelined, have the player sit and remove his cleats. After inspection and a brief assessment of neurovascular status,

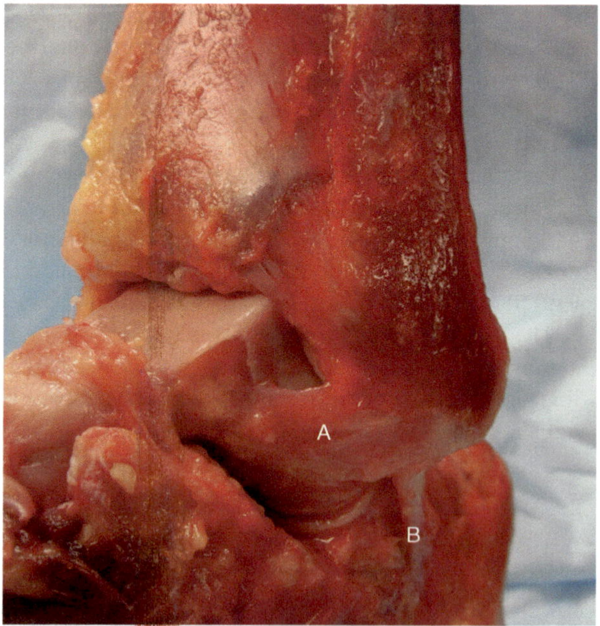

Fig. 4.1 ATFL (**a**) and CFL (**b**) are the main structures of the lateral ligament complex. These ligaments provide the lateral ankle ligamentous stability. The ATFL and its broad insertion are well visualized. The CFL provides stability to both the tibiotalar and subtalar joints

assess the alignment of the hindfoot. A cavus foot can be a risk factor for ankle sprains. Test active and passive plantarflexion and dorsiflexion as well as subtalar inversion and eversion. Palpate the malleoli and ligamentous structures. Be sure to begin away from the area of tenderness to gain an athlete's trust and obtain a more precise exam.

After this is complete, move to dynamic tests of ankle stability. The anterior drawer test is a test of the ATFL and is performed with an anterior force placed on a dorsiflexed talus (Fig. 4.2a). While this can be compared to the contralateral foot for a baseline level of laxity, it is more helpful in anesthetized patients. Depending on the rules of participation, you can inject the tibiotalar joint with a local anesthetic to temporarily anesthetize the patient on the sidelines. This will allow you to perform these tests without causing pain and differentiate pain from instability.

The talar tilt test evaluates the function of the CFL. The examiner places one hand above the malleoli with the ankle slightly plantarflexed and holds the calcaneus in the other hand in order to use it to invert the foot (Fig. 4.2b).

These dynamic tests are difficult to objectively measure. Several grading systems have been used to characterize lateral ankle sprains. However, much of this relies on experience, with comparison to the athlete's contralateral side, and is largely subjective [6–8]. The most widely used classification system has three grades. The first is mild and involves little tenderness, no instability, and no loss of function. A grade 2, or moderate injury, consists of moderate swelling, tenderness, and instability, with a decrease in function. Grade 3 injuries are the most severe (Table 4.1). Grade 3 injury implies a complete ATFL rupture and has edema and ecchymosis that may be

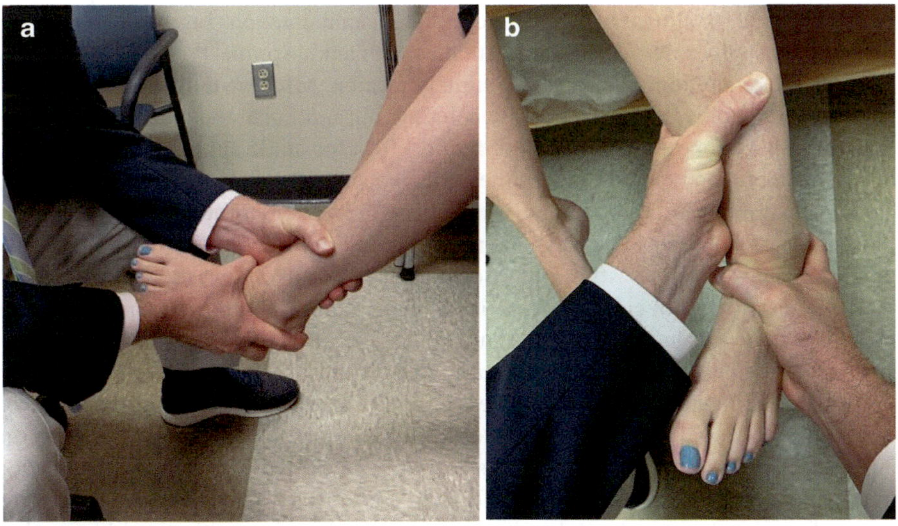

Fig. 4.2 (**a**) Anterior drawer test, using an anterior force on the calcaneus with the leg stabilized. (**b**) Varus Tilt test, a varus force is applied to the calcaneus and talus while stabilizing the subtalar joint

Table 4.1 Classification systems of lateral ankle sprains

Classification system of lateral ankle sprains
Anatomic system
Grade I: ATF sprain
Grade II: ATF and CF sprain
Grade III: ATF, CF, and PTF sprains
AMA standard nomenclature system
Grade 1: ligament stretched/attenuated
Grade 2: ligament partially torn
Grade 3: ligament completely torn

AMA American Medical Association, *ATF* anterior talofibular, CF calcaneofibular, *PTF* posterior talofibular

visible on the skin, very limited motion, frank instability, and is unable to participate [8].

Remember that there can be numerous associated injuries with low ankle sprains. Be wary of syndesmosis injuries (discussed subsequently), deltoid ligament sprains, subtalar subluxations or dislocations, lateral process of the talus fractures, peroneal tendon subluxations, underlying subtalar coalitions, avulsion fractures, or osteochondral lesions. Adequate radiographs can help identify most of these.

Obtain AP, lateral, and oblique or mortise images of the ankle. It is prudent to obtain full-length images of the tibia and antero-posterior, lateral, and oblique images of the foot. If at all possible, have the player standing when these are taken because this will demonstrate limb alignment and foot position more accurately. These weight-bearing views can also show instability such as talar tilt if a player has had many ankle sprains and chronic instability. Contralateral comparison views may be useful. Stress x-rays themselves or those where the examiner is using their hand to perform the external rotation, anterior drawer, or talar tilt tests listed above are less helpful with decisions about treatment but serve as excellent documentation (Fig. 4.3).

MRI is usually reserved for those athletes with ankle sprains that do not progress through the rehabilitation process in a timely fashion. MRI can delineate reasons for an athlete's inability to return to play including intraarticular and soft-tissue pathology as well as bone edema. When ordering MRIs for ankle sprains, most orthopedists consider many factors such as the performance of the athlete, time since injury, resources of the institution, and position during the season. Remember that many of the causes of slow return to play can be evaluated intra-operatively by arthroscopy, and MRI may not always provide useful information. Perhaps more importantly, MRI findings may not correlate with instability findings on physical exam becuase MRI is a static test, not a dynamic exam.

After diagnosis, focus begins on returning the athlete safely to the field as quickly as possible. In some cases, the athlete can return to play during the same game or practice. Additional stability is imparted with a lace-up ankle brace or taping by an athletic trainer. After competition, he/she should be treated with "RICE therapy" or rest, ice, compression, and elevation [9]. Rest can consist of non-weight-bearing for a few days in a splint or boot, brace, or limiting high-impact activities like running and cutting. Remember that during recovery, supportive athletic shoes with laces are better than sandals and slip-on shoes. Anti-inflammatory medications are

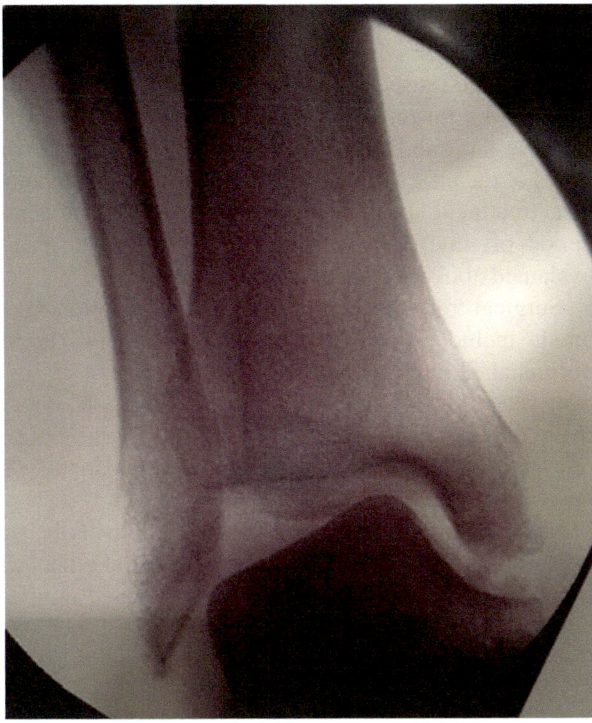

Fig. 4.3 Stress fluoroscopy of right ankle demonstrating significant instability with talar tilt test. Incongruency of the lateral tibiotalar joint is noted

excellent for pain control during this time. When the athlete is able to bear weight without pain, begin active range of motion exercises and progress through a proprioception training. Many of these exercises include single-leg standing activities on uneven surfaces or balance boards. Single-leg hops can be a quick tool to assess their progress. In our experience, once the player can do 15 consecutive single-leg hops, they can usually return to play. Finally, the player can resume noncontact football-specific drills. Progression should be based on the player's progression, not strictly based on time.

Surgical treatment is usually reserved for chronic instability. Clinically, these players have more instability and less pain than acute ankle sprains. It is not advisable to operate during the season unless absolutely necessary, as this would most likely preclude the player from participating for the remainder of the season. There are several operative repair techniques, many are of only historical interest, as they have fallen out of favor. Most surgeons today prefer an anatomic repair; however, there are still surgeons employing non-anatomic repairs, such as Evans technique, which uses a portion of the peroneus brevis tendon to stabilize the lateral ankle and prevent inversion.

Today, the author's preferred technique is to anatomically repair both the ATFL and CFL (Brostrom-Gould procedure) while often employing a newer augment technique utilizing an internal brace (Arthrex, Naples, FL). This augmentation is valuable in high-level collegiate and NFL players, whose ankles see tremendous stress. It is also indicated for players who have had prior failed ankle instability surgery or those who have baseline hypermobility [10]. Salvage options include anatomic reconstruction of the ATFL and CFL with allograft tissue. However, these are reserved for refractory cases of chronic instability. During surgery, arthroscopy can assess instability, remove hematoma and debris from the joint, characterize the status of the articular cartilage, and allow for intervention if needed. Following surgical treatment, the player is placed in a splint and is non-weight-bearing for a short period of time (2–4 weeks). Subsequently, the rehabilitation is similar to that explained above for nonoperative treatment.

Surgical treatment is not without complication. Early complications most commonly include issues with wound healing and superficial peroneal nerve injury. Technical failures intraoperatively can present as immediate recurrent instability from inadequate fixation or failures in fixation. Poor range of motion postoperatively may represent over-constraint of the joint. Late complications include recurrent chronic lateral ankle instability. Be aware that athletes sometimes describe instability as pain.

While most lateral ankle sprains are relatively benign injuries that allow players to return to play quickly, remember to rule out other causes of pain in these athletes. In addition, begin considering these associated injuries when a player is unable to return to the field in a reasonable timeframe. These may signal associated injuries that require surgical treatment to preserve their long-term function.

Syndesmosis Injuries

Syndesmosis sprains of the ankle in the athlete often result in a significant amount of lost playing time. This injury has garnered significant attention in the sports medicine realm over the past decade as the frequency of these injuries has increased and the treatment algorithms have changed. Colloquially referred to as *high ankle sprains*, syndesmotic injuries can result in a greater level of impairment than isolated injuries to the lateral ligamentous complex. The reported incidence of syndesmosis sprains ranges from 1% to 16% of ankle injuries [11–15]. These injuries are often missed or undiagnosed, and occur less frequently than isolated lateral ankle sprains [16].

The ankle syndesmosis contains a bony congruence between the distal tibia and fibula with ligament reinforcement. This ligamentous complex provides the majority of stability to the syndesmosis and consists of three distinct entities: the anterior inferior tibiofibular ligament (AITFL), the posterior inferior tibiofibular ligament (PITFL), and the interosseous tibiofibular ligament or membrane (ITFL) [17].

The AITFL has a broad fanlike origin on the anterolateral tubercle of the tibia that travels obliquely, tapering off as it travels toward its insertion on the longitudinal tubercle of the lateral malleolus. This gives the AITFL a triangular or trapezoidal appearance [18]. The AITFL often consists of several bands, and some consider the most inferior band a separate entity entirely: the accessory AITFL. These fibers can be seen during ankle arthroscopy [19].

The PITFL consists of the deeper transverse tibiofibular ligament and a superficial PITFL. The superficial PITFL originates on the posterior aspect of the tibia at the posterolateral tubercle and travels obliquely down the posterior fibula. The deep portion originates distally on the posterior tibia and has a more transverse course, inserting anterior to its superficial counterpart. Some consider this portion its own entity, the transverse ligament (Fig. 4.4). The PITFL is the strongest ligament of the syndesmotic complex and therefore is usually the last to tear. Given its inherent strength, injuries to PITFL commonly result in an avulsion, rather than midsubstance tear [17, 20]. The ITFL originates approximately 1–1.5 cm proximal to the tibiotalar joint and runs the majority of the course of the tibia and fibula [17].

The syndesmosis is best thought of as a dynamic structure that moves in three dimensions. Several cadaveric studies have illustrated the importance of the syndesmosis complex to ankle stability. When the AITFL is sectioned, there is an additional 4–12 mm of sagittal translation between the tibia and fibula [12, 21, 22]. Xenos et al. described a 2.3 mm increase in translation with isolated AITFL transection. When both the distal most 8 cm of the ITFL and 8 cm of PITFL were transected, a total of 7.3 mm of translation between the tibia and fibula occurred [23]. Rotational instability also occurs with disruption of the syndesmosis. With isolated AITFL resection, there is an average increase of 2.7 deg. of rotation. With complete disruption of the complex, this number increased to 10.2 deg. of rotation [24, 25].

Several classification systems exist when describing syndesmosis injuries. In the acute setting, the practitioner must differentiate between stable and unstable syndesmoses. Furthermore, an ankle may possess latent versus frank instability. The ankle

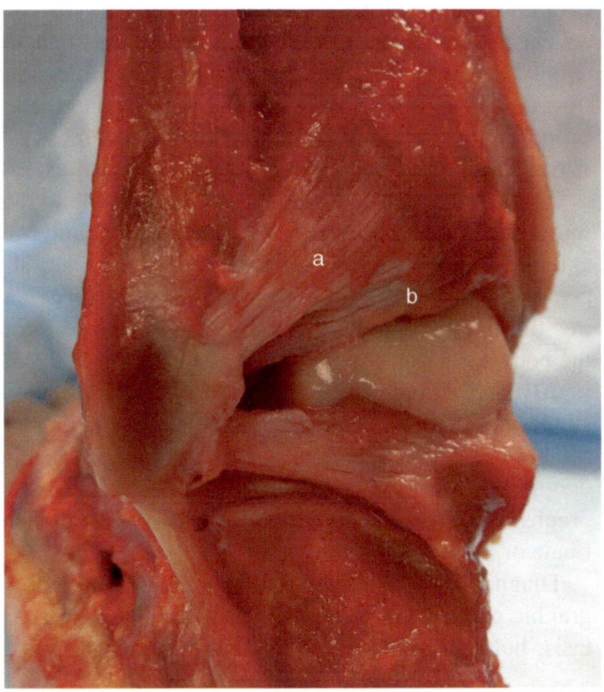

Fig. 4.4 Posterior tibiofibular ligament (**a**) is a large, strong ligament connecting the posterior tibia and fibula. The most inferior band of this ligament, often a separate band itself, is often called the transverse ligament (**b**). These bands both contribute to the significant overall strength of the posterior ligamentous complex

with latent instability will have normal-appearing radiographs but will reveal instability with stress views or dynamic image evaluation. Frank diastasis occurs when widening is present on routine ankle imaging [26]. The graded ankle sprain classification is also commonly used. A grade I injury describes a stable ankle with mild distal tibiofibular joint tenderness. A grade II injury results in a partial tear to the syndesmosis complex with a positive squeeze test and external rotation test. A grade III injury is a complete disruption of the syndesmosis plus or minus deltoid injury [27].

An isolated acute ligamentous syndesmotic injury oftentimes goes undiagnosed; therefore the practitioner must maintain a high level of suspicion, employ a detailed physical exam, and obtain appropriate imaging. High ankle sprain injuries range from a mild injury to the syndesmotic complex to a complete diastasis of the distal tib-fib joint. Diastasis is defined as "any loosening in the attachment of the fibula to the tibia at the inferior tibiofibular joint, and is not confined to a wide separation of the bones" [28].

These injuries most commonly occur secondary to an external rotation force but can also result from a hyper-abduction force if the deltoid ligament is compromised. Hyper-dorsiflexion injuries can lead to diastasis as the anterior talus drives into the mortise [29, 30].

Upon examination, an individual with a syndesmotic injury will typically complain of anterolateral ankle tenderness, oftentimes with minimal tenderness over the ATFL or CFL. Tenderness over the deltoid ligament may indicate an abduction component to the injury mechanism. Palpation of the entire length of the fibula must occur to identify a proximal fibula fracture, and the severe swelling and ecchymosis common to a lateral ankle sprain are often less severe.

The *squeeze test* is a common clinical exam maneuver indicative of a high ankle sprain. A positive result occurs when the examiner squeezes between the fibula and tibia at the level of the mid-calf, eliciting pain at the level of the ankle. Miller et al. proposed that the height of anterolateral tenderness relative to the tibiofibular joint correlates with the severity of a syndesmotic injury [31].

The *external rotation test* is the most reliable to diagnostic test for syndesmotic injuries. With the knee flexed 90 degrees, one hand stabilizes the distal leg while an external rotation force is applied to the foot. Pain at the syndesmosis indicates a positive result. If able to bear weight, this test is dynamically reproducible by having the patient stand on the affected extremity alone while externally rotating the body.

AP, lateral, and oblique views of the ankle should be obtained in the suspected syndesmotic injury. Up to 50% of patients may have a bony avulsion off the anterior tibia or posterior malleolus, making radiographic evaluation an essential part of the diagnostic workup [11, 28, 32]. If tender at the proximal tibia, AP and lateral radiographs of the knee should be obtained to rule out a spiral fracture of the proximal fibula or *Maisonneuve* fracture.

Diagnosis of tibiofibular diastasis can be made by measuring several radiographic parameters. Widening of the medial clear space >4 mm may indicate diastasis, but there is often significant variability with this measurement, putting to question its reliability [28]. Several studies have advocated the use of tibiofibular overlap, with 5 mm on the AP and 1 mm on the mortise view representing normal findings [33]. The tibiofibular clear space is another parameter used, with a normal value ranging from 3 mm to 6 mm on an AP radiograph [34–37]. There is no single radiographic parameter that best identifies diastasis on routine radiographic imaging. Therefore, stress radiographs are an important part of the high ankle sprain workup (Fig. 4.5). An external rotation and abduction force are applied to the ankle to potentially reveal diastasis. When stress radiographs are inconclusive, advanced imaging in the form of a weight-bearing CT or MRI should be performed.

MRI is an excellent test for the diagnosis of syndesmotic injuries. Kazunori et al. showed that an MRI containing syndesmotic ligament discontinuity, a curved or wavy appearance of the ligament, or ligamentous non-visualization resulted in 100% sensitivity, 93% specificity, and 97% accuracy (Fig. 4.6) [38]. Although MRI is quite accurate with regard to syndesmotic injury identification, it is a static test. Thus, one might argue that weight-bearing CT has the advantage over MRI in that it can identify dynamic instability. CT scans, however, are often used to evaluate the syndesmosis in the chronic setting, not in the acute injury phase.

Arthroscopic evaluation of the distal tibiofibular joint has become the gold standard for diagnosing a syndesmosis injury. Calder et al. proposed that syndesmotic instability is present when a 2.9 mm shaver can fit within the distal tibiofibular joint [39]. The arthroscopic "drive-through sign" is another method to identify instability arthroscopically. If a 2.9 mm shaver can easily fit through the medial gutter during arthroscopy, one must have a high suspicion for syndesmotic and deltoid injury [40].

Syndesmotic sprains without diastasis are nonoperative and may be treated with proprioceptive rehabilitation, functional brace wear, and short-term activity modification. West Point cadets that suffered a stable sprain returned to full activity at an average of 43 days [14]. In the elite athlete, platelet-rich plasma or "PRP" is a

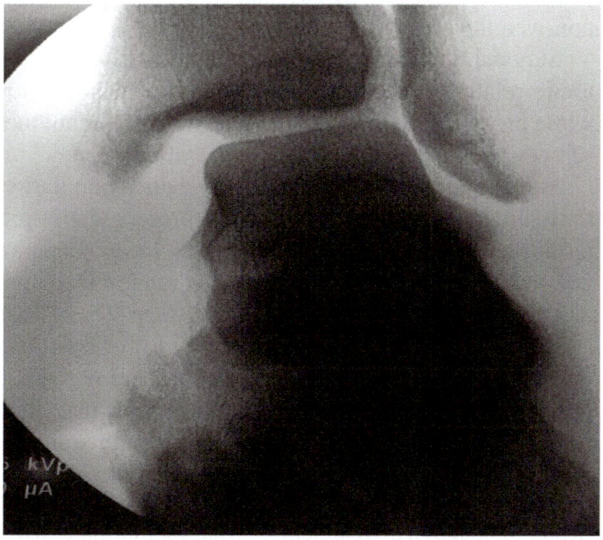

Fig. 4.5 Stress fluoroscopic image of syndesmosis injury indicating widened medial tibial clear space and loss of normal tibiofibular overlap

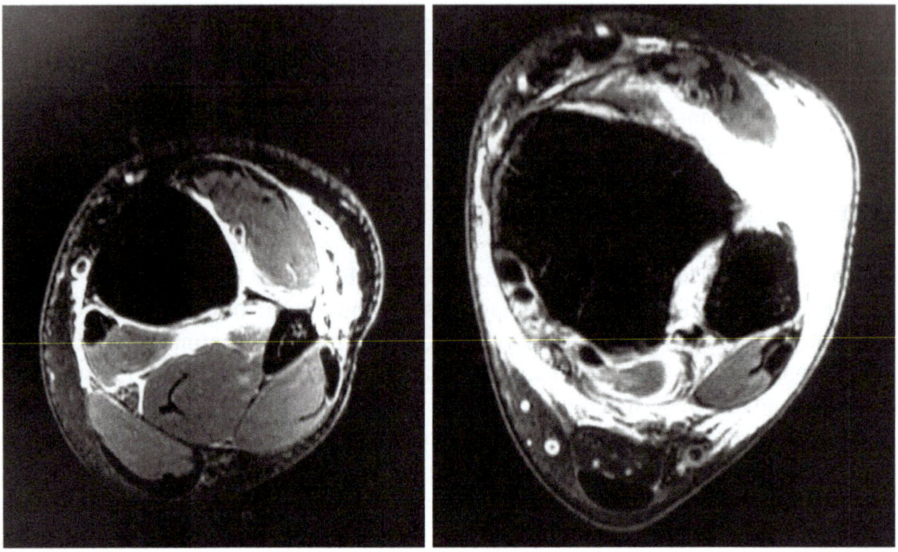

Fig. 4.6 Axial T2-weighted MR images indicating a significant syndesmosis injury with incongruence of the fibula and tearing of the interosseous membrane on the proximal axial cut and both the AITFL and the PITFL near the ankle

common adjunct to conservative management. Laver et al. performed an RCT comparing PRP to controls in elite athletes with AITFL injuries. Those receiving PRP had a significantly shorter ($p = 0.0006$) return to play time ($n = 41$ days) than the control group ($n = 60$ days) [41].

In patients with latent or dynamic instability, conservative treatment is an option if advanced imaging confirms anatomic reduction in the incisura fibularis. These patients typically require cast and boot immobilization for 8 weeks, with 4 weeks of non-weight-bearing.

Surgical fixation of high ankle sprains focuses on restoration of the normal anatomic relationship of the tibiofibular ligament to allow for early and full motion while increasing stability. Typically, fixation techniques are broken down into rigid screw versus dynamic suture button stabilization.

Suture button fixation has recently gained popularity because there is a lower risk for malreduction of the syndesmosis, preserved physiologic micromotion at the distal tibiofibular joint, and a significantly lower reoperation rate without failure [14, 26, 42–44]. Colcuc et al. performed a randomized controlled trial comparing rigid and dynamic fixation with 1-year follow-up. Those treated with dynamic suture button fixation experienced a significantly lower complication rate and a faster return to sport (14 vs. 19 weeks, $p = 0.0006$). There was no difference with regard to pain or clinical outcomes [45]. A meta-analysis of three RCTs and seven cohort studies performed by Gan et al. revealed no difference in clinical outcome, syndesmosis malreduction rate, and complication rate. There was a significantly lower need for hardware removal in the suture button fixation group. Ultimately, insufficient definitive evidence exists to consider either technique superior [46].

In our experience, surgical intervention is reserved for the athlete who cannot bear weight and has a positive squeeze test and significant pain with external rotation exam. Those with tenderness greater than 5 cm proximal to the ankle joint may have a more severe injury, likely warranting surgical intervention. In athletes with this subset of symptoms, we routinely order an MRI to evaluate the integrity of the syndesmotic complex. The MRI is obtained primarily to evaluate for the integrity of the AITFL and PITFL. If more than one ligament is compromised, it is considered a potentially unstable joint. In the face of positive MRI findings, a stress exam should be performed to correlate the static MRI test and confer the presence of dynamic instability. If multiple ligaments are involved, intraoperative fluoroscopic evaluation is performed and often confirms any latent instability. Arthroscopic evaluation is then performed. Any hematoma within the ankle joint is evacuated, and the distal tibiofibular joint is debrided to allow for anatomic reduction of the syndesmosis. Any additional cartilage injury is addressed at this time.

After arthroscopic evaluation, a small incision is made over the fibula, and a two-hole plate is used in conjunction with two suture button fixation devices. The plate assists with force dissipation of the construct. The tight ropes are placed in a divergent manner to maximize the pullout strength of our fixation (Fig. 4.7).

Immediately postoperatively the patient is placed in a boot with cold compression and IV NSAIDs. During the first 72 hours postop, treatment focuses on a range

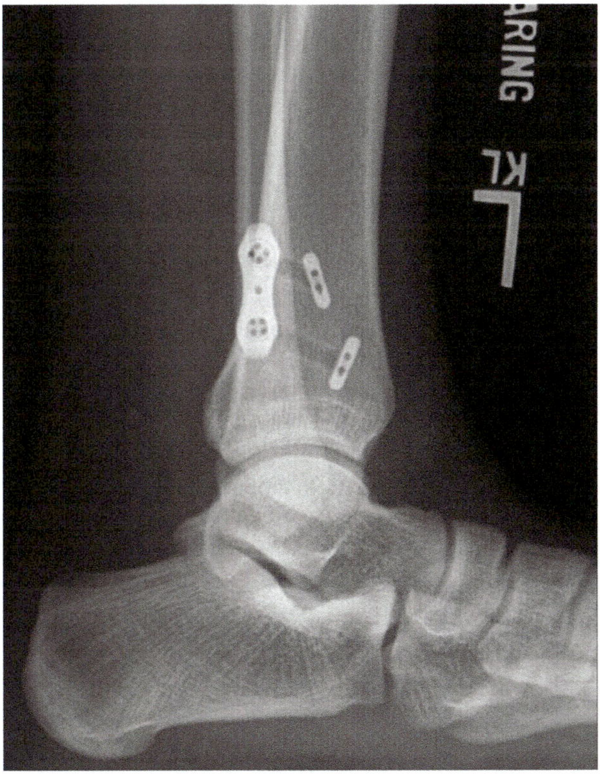

Fig. 4.7 AP and lateral radiographic views of an offensive lineman treated with dual suture button stabilization for a high-grade syndesmotic injury

of motion exercises, swelling control, and non-weight-bearing of the involved extremity. Weight-bearing begins POD 4 in a CAM walker. At POD 7–9, the patient is transitioned to Alter-G treadmill or pool work. Subjects then progress to land exercises when able, usually between POD 10 and POD 15. Return to play is allowed when the athlete can pass return to sport testing.

In summary, syndesmotic injuries must be diagnosed early to avoid a prolonged treatment course. Anatomic reduction and stability must be confirmed to manage these injuries appropriately. If instability exists, surgical intervention focuses on anatomic restoration of the distal tibiotalar joint and allows for faster return to play in the elite athlete. Postoperative management focuses on early range of motion with a brief period of non-weight-bearing, followed by gradual resumption of weight-bearing activity and eventual return to sport when strength and agility are restored.

Ankle Fractures

While less common than ankle sprains, ankle fractures are frequent injuries that lead to significant time loss for athletes. When this type of injury occurs, ankle fractures sideline most athletes immediately. The injuries that cause these fractures are usually associated with higher energy than those that cause avulsion fractures and sprains. Because players are exposed to higher amounts of energy when they sustain ankle fractures, these injuries are more traumatic and can cause significant morbidity. Some authors report that return to play at a competitive level can be staggeringly low. In one study, 88% of recreational athletes had returned to sports, while only 11.6% of competitive athletes had returned to sports 1 year after an ankle fracture [47]. This chapter focuses on ways to improve in-season and long-term outcomes. The ankle mortise consists of the tibia medially, fibula laterally, and talus distally. It is a sickle-shaped joint with cartilage on both sides. Approximately 10–15% of body weight is transmitted through the fibula during the normal gait cycle. Athletes commonly subject their ankles to higher stresses during the run of play. The tibia ends distally as the medial malleolus while the fibula extends further distally and comprises the lateral malleolus. This relationship is important in assessing the length of the fibula while identifying fractures during diagnosis and evaluating the quality of a reduction during treatment. The ligaments that attach to these malleoli provide the ankle with their primary soft tissue stability. Specifically, the deltoid ligament arises on the medial malleolus and inserts on the talus, navicular, and calcaneus. It is an important stabilizer of the mortise and knowledge of its anatomy and function is important during treatment decisions for ankle fractures.

Ankle fractures typically occur in football players when the foot is rotated about the ankle. An inversion mechanism is the most common mechanism leading to fracture, although many different mechanisms can lead to fracture. Oftentimes, in the fast-paced nature of a football game, the athlete is unable to adequately describe the mechanism leading to the injury. They usually occur in a skilled-position player or lineman whose foot is planted on the field when he contacts the ground or an opponent. Players will endorse pain isolated to the ankle. Commonly, they will be unable to bear weight immediately after the injury, though it is not uncommon for the athlete to be able to bear weight, even with a fracture. The medical staff evaluating the player on the field or sideline after injury often get the most complete physical exam before the ankle becomes swollen.

Identification of an ankle fracture on the field may be obvious if the ankle is subluxated or dislocated. Gently reducing the ankle will help the athlete feel more comfortable and help the medical staff completely assess the players' neurovascular status. There is no value in obtaining x-rays prior to reduction. Trained personnel should reduce a dislocation as quickly as possible. Be sure to look for abrasions, tenting, and pallor. These skin changes can signal an open fracture and players with such injuries should be taken to an orthopedic surgeon for treatment immediately. Unfortunately, open fractures that are reduced on initial presentation may be more difficult to recognize.

To begin the exam, check for active ankle flexion, extension, inversion, and eversion. While most players will have some weakness due to pain, complete inability to perform these motions may signal a more serious injury. Next, check for sensation in all dermatomes of the foot. Most players will have some paresthesias from the injury that resolve quickly.

Finally, reserve palpation until the end of the exam as this helps build a player's trust in the medical staff. Palpate the medial and lateral malleoli, tibiotalar joint line, deltoid ligament, and fibular head. Pain at the fibular head, just distal to the proximal tibiofibular joint, can signal that the syndesmosis may be injured. Aside from obvious dislocations, point tenderness and inability to bear weight should signal practitioners to obtain radiographs.

Basic images consist of antero-posterior, lateral, and mortise radiographs of the ankle. Most fractures will be readily apparent on these views. If suspicion for a fracture is high and it is not evident on unilateral x-rays alone, bilateral weight-bearing views of the contralateral extremity can serve as a comparison. It is prudent to image the entire tibia and foot to rule out concomitant injuries. Image ankle injuries without any splinting material, braces, or boots as these can obscure osseous anatomy. Obtaining as much information as possible during an exam and with imaging can help facilitate treatment decisions.

If an ankle fracture is not readily apparent, scrutinize radiographs for small avulsion fractures. For example, fractures of the lateral process of the talus can mimic lateral ankle sprains and are often misdiagnosed. Avulsion fractures from the posterior tibia can signal a syndesmosis injury. Using dynamic imaging and/or stress x-rays is also a useful tool to assess stability and is discussed in greater detail below. After all necessary images have been performed, place the athlete in a well-padded splint or immobilizing boot. Remember that ankle fractures may swell quickly and pressure on tenuous skin can change a relatively benign fracture pattern with intact skin into a more serious open fracture.

There are several classification systems examiners use to characterize ankle fractures. Younger teenage players are subject to "transitional fractures" because their physes are still closing. Transitional fractures are also known as triplane and tillaux fractures. A triplane fracture involves disruption through the physes of the tibia in the sagittal, axial, and coronal planes. As these athletes age and their physes continue closing, injuries more often result in tillaux fractures. These tillaux fractures are avulsions of the anterolateral tibia distal to the physis, and they are most easily seen on antero-posterior x-rays. After players' physes close, they are subject to different fracture patterns. Consequently, there are also many adult fracture pattern classifications.

These adult-type ankle fractures in football players have been studied primarily in the NFL. By far the most common ankle fracture in the NFL is isolated distal fibula fractures. The predominant descriptive tool for these injuries is the Weber classification, and it describes a distal fibula fracture line based on its relationship to the syndesmosis. Weber A fractures are distal to the syndesmosis, Weber B fractures are at the level of the syndesmosis, and Weber C are all those above the syndesmosis.

Fibula fractures also occur in combination with other fracture patterns about the ankle (Table 4.2). A second classification system, called the Lauge-Hansen system, is based on injury mechanisms that cause fractures. Although its reliability has not been established, this system is useful to those on the field who witness the injury. It serves as a convention among providers to help communicate injury severity and

Table 4.2 Ankle fracture classification systems

Classification systems of ankle fractures			
Fibula fracture location	Danis-Weber classification	Lauge-Hansen classification	Stage description
Infrasyndesmotic	Type A	Supination adduction (SA)	Transverse fracture of the distal fibula Vertical fracture of the medial malleolus
Transsyndesmotic	Type B	Supination external rotation (SER)	Injury to the AITFL Oblique/spiral fracture of the distal fibula Injury to the PITFL or avulsion fracture of the posterior malleolus Medial malleolus fracture or sprain of the deltoid ligament
Suprasyndesmotic	Type C	Pronation external rotation (PER)	Medial malleolus fracture or sprain of the deltoid ligament AITFL injury Oblique fracture of the fibula proximal to the tibial plafond Injury to the PITFL or avulsion fracture of the posterior malleolus
		Pronation Adduction (PA)	Medial malleolus fracture or sprain of the deltoid ligament Injury to the AITFL Transverse/comminuted fracture of the fibula proximal to the tibial plafond

guide treatment plans. There are four main categories within the Lauge-Hansen classification: supination-adduction, supination-external rotation, pronation-abduction, and pronation-external rotation. The first word of these mechanisms describes the position of the foot, while the second word denotes the force that is applied to the extremity. Regardless of the classification systems used to characterize these injuries, they are useful because they help medical staff communicate clearly about an athlete's injury.

There are many classification systems; however, the most important characteristic of ankle fractures is stability. While some fracture patterns are inherently stable and may not require surgery, others are unstable and most likely will require surgery. Instability in the ankle mortise is defined as asymmetry in the articulation of the talus, tibia, and fibula. Most commonly this occurs from disruption of the syndesmosis. Identifying unstable ankle fracture patterns can be difficult. When used alone, plain x-rays have limited use in diagnosing associated syndesmosis injuries, especially when they occur with low fibula fractures. Dynamic or stress x-rays can aid in these scenarios. As previous described, the syndesmosis can be interrupted in association with a wide variety of ankle fractures. External rotation stress views help assess the syndesmosis and deltoid complex. However, there is much variation in the normal anatomic appearance of syndesmosis. Any views that are suspicious for a widened mortise or isolated medial malleolus fracture should have full-length tibia x-rays performed to assess the proximal fibula for a Maisonneuve injury. Advanced imaging is useful for some fractures, and an orthopedic surgeon can decide if they are needed. CT scans are useful to assess the size and fracture plane for posterior malleoli fractures, and MRI assesses the syndesmosis, other ligamentous injuries, and the state of the articular cartilage.

After a complete physical exam and imaging, treatment decisions are made. Some ankle fractures are treated conservatively without exposing an athlete to the risks of surgery while still allowing him to return to play quickly and safely. For example, an oblique fibula fracture with negative stress x-rays indicating stability can be treated without surgery and progress as symptoms allow. Most authors believe stable, nondisplaced Weber A and B lateral malleolus fractures can be treated conservatively [48].

Unfortunately, nearly half of ankle fractures are associated with disruptions of the syndesmosis and studies show they are being treated surgically with increasing frequency. From 2000 to 2014, nearly half of all distal fibula fractures were treated with surgery [49]. On the lateral side of the ankle, Tornetta et al. have used a more individualized algorithm for surgical decision making [48]. However, the authors believe fibula fractures associated with any instability of the mortise on the stress x-rays should be treated with open reduction and internal fixation. This includes all ligamentous supination external rotation type 4 injuries.

As described above, the deep deltoid ligament attaches to the colliculi of the medial malleoli and provides stability to the mortise. Therefore, supracollicular fractures are unstable and should be treated with surgery. Operative indications for medial malleolus fractures also extend to those with an articular component or vertical fracture pattern, which are most commonly associated with supination adduction injuries. The supination adduction fracture pattern should receive extra consideration as it is associated with plafond impaction which should be addressed with adequate visualization during surgery and may require bone grafting.

Avulsion fractures on the medial side of the ankle usually occur at the anterior colliculus. While commonly treated nonoperatively in recreational athletes, these superficial deltoid complex avulsions which occur during high-energy ankle fractures in athletes are a distinct injury pattern and should be recognized as such. Deltoid avulsion may benefit from primary open repair. The majority of NFL players treated surgically for deltoid avulsion injuries are able to return to play after surgery with no reported complications or persistent medial ankle pain or instability [35].

Some posterior avulsions can be treated conservatively. However, fractures of the posterior malleolus that are displaced, greater than one-third of the articular surface, and those with syndesmosis disruption require surgical intervention [50].

While many treatment algorithms are agreed upon in the literature, there is still debate about particular fracture patterns. For example, the management of nondisplaced, radiologically unstable fractures (i.e., nondisplaced bimalleolar fractures and nondisplaced Weber C fractures) is a topic of discussion [50]. Some advocate primary surgical fixation to facilitate early return to sport and others advocate attempted conservative management. Robertson et al. found that conservative management of nondisplaced bimalleolar fracture resulted in quicker return to play with fewer persistent symptoms. As such, current recommendations advise attempted conservative management of these fracture types, with close follow-up and surgical intervention if displacement occurs [50].

Once a decision has been made to proceed with surgery, there are several reduction and fixation options for osseous injuries. Reduction can be achieved with either open or percutaneous techniques. Open reduction internal fixation with lag screws and tubular plates is most commonly employed. The typical construct utilizes a lateral fibular plate to avoid peroneal irritation, though there are advocates of posterior fibular anti-glide fixation. Medial malleolus fixation typically utilizes a partially threaded cannulated screw.

Intramedullary fixation is gaining popularity in athletes because it can reduce an athlete's risk of symptomatic hardware [50]. It is best suited for unstable fibula fractures [51] but does not control length without adequate fracture opposition.

Repair of soft tissue injuries during initial operative intervention remains debatable in elite athletes, particularly in regard to management of the deltoid. Some clinicians only advise repair in settings when soft tissue blocks fracture reduction [52]. Athletes who received repair compared to those without repair did not show improvements in long-term follow-up. Short-term results are critical in the athletic population; therefore we advocate for deltoid ligament repair regardless of its effect on fracture reduction. For the syndesmosis, we prefer endobutton fixation through a well-contoured plate; a construct that has been studied in the NFL did not result in any residual pain or stiffness. Screw fixation for the syndesmosis has been the standard; however, emerging literature over recent years has supported the use of suture button constructs for syndesmosis stabilization [53].

Treating ankle fractures surgically can facilitate early return to football. However, it can also be associated with an increased rate of persistent symptoms, most frequently pain. Many causes of chronic pain after ankle injuries occur due to the injury itself and are recognized as pain generators after an athlete has not returned in a reasonable timeframe. For example, chondral injuries to the talar dome commonly cause chronic pain. Ankle arthroscopy, at the time of primary surgical intervention, can help treat chondral lesions and improve healing and long-term outcomes.

The role of arthroscopy is increasing in conjunction with ankle fractures. There are multiple factors associated with the use of arthroscopy as an adjunct to ankle fracture fixation. Some surgeons have advocated that you can better predict instability with arthroscopy. It allows better assessment of instability in multiple planes as well as reduction once the fixation is complete. Studies show that intra-articular lavage is beneficial to the patient. It significantly reduces the inflammatory cytokines in the joint, which may provide short-term pain relief as well as lower the risk of long-term posttraumatic arthritis. Visualization of the entire joint allows full assessment of associated injuries (Fig. 4.8). Arthroscopy allows the surgeon to fully assess the cartilage surfaces and address any acute cartilage damage. At the very least, it allows the surgeon to fully counsel the patient on the extent of their injury, which can help guide their postoperative course.

Proponents of ankle arthroscopy cite the ability to inspect the joint, educate the athlete, address intra-articular chondral lesions, or debride hematomas and debris as good reasons to routinely perform arthroscopy during the treatment of ankle fractures, although others argue that it does not change the acute management. Even if arthroscopy does not change the acute management of such injuries, we believe it is a valuable tool for documenting the severity of articular damage and as a prognostic tool. If a player returns to the office and has not progressed appropriately during rehabilitation, the status of the joint space during arthroscopy becomes valuable

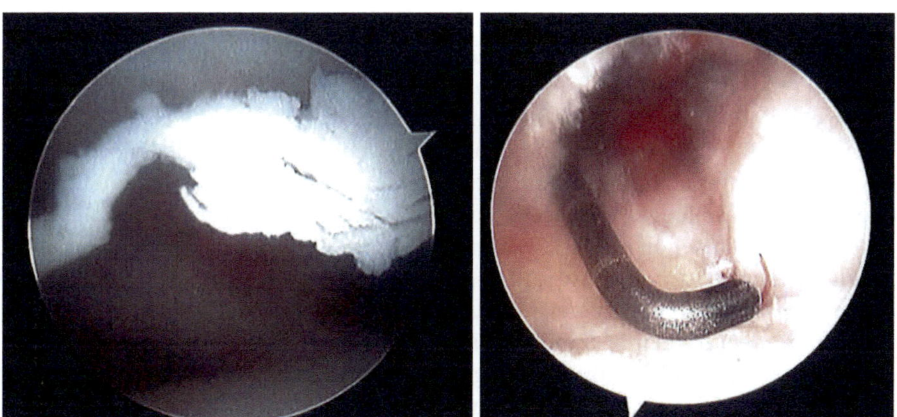

Fig. 4.8 Arthroscopic photos in a Weber C ankle fracture with cartilage debris and resultant 1 cm traumatic OCL on the lateral talar shoulder

information. Therefore, arthroscopy is a valuable tool in "identifying and treating intra-articular damage that would otherwise remain unrecognized and may provide prognostic information regarding the functional outcome of these injuries." [54]

The goal of all treatment decisions both surgical and nonsurgical is to safely and quickly return to football without compromising the longevity of an injured ankle. Naturally, more severe injuries usually require prolonged recovery times. Isolated fibula fractures result in fewer days missed than any other ankle fracture pattern. The mean time missed is approximately 90 days [49]. Predictors of return to sporting activities at 1 year include younger age, male gender, no or mild systemic disease, and a less severe ankle fracture [47]. The evaluation and management of ankle fractures discussed above can be very objective; in contrast, return to play criteria have been notoriously individual and subjective. There are, however, some general guidelines practitioners can use to collaborate with ATCs and PTs when deciding how quickly a player can return. For ankle fractures treated nonoperatively, we begin noncontact football including jogging, weightlifting, footwork, or "shadow" drills around 6–8 weeks post-injury. Return to contact football drills can usually begin around 12–16 weeks post-injury. Special consideration should be given to those treated surgically and who undergo syndesmotic fixation. In these cases, weight-bearing should not begin until 8 weeks after surgery and sport-specific drills adjusted accordingly.

While infrequent, complications do occur and can delay a full return to play. The medical team should be aware of several common complications. The skin of the ankle is thin, especially over the medial malleolus, and concerns about the healing of surgical incisions should be addressed in a timely fashion. In the early postoperative period, non-unions can be a source of pain. This is particularly true of medial malleolus non-unions. Non-union can continue to cause pain months after surgery, but it is more likely that they are found in the first 8 weeks. Complications from syndesmosis fixation are more likely to occur after 8 weeks. The most common of these is syndesmosis screw irritation or decreased range of motion [55]. Oftentimes players with these symptoms will ask that their hardware be removed. We recommend that only intact screws which have not broken be removed after 4–6 months after all other causes of persistent symptoms have been ruled out. A diagnostic and therapeutic injection at the site of the screw head can aid in this decision. CT scans are useful in the chronic setting to evaluate for malreduction of the fibula. Remember, the fibula can be malreduced in the transverse plane (most commonly shortened from its original length). Lastly, as mentioned above in regard to routine ankle arthroscopy, osteochondral lesions can be a source of prolonged pain. While ankle fractures are a common source of missed playing time for football players, most will return to play. It is important to recognize, examine, image, and treat each players with respect to their specific fracture. Some will return to play almost immediately, while others will make a more gradual return. In rare cases, players with the most severe fractures may only return to their baseline at 2–3 years after surgery [56].

Ankle injuries occur commonly in the football player. Systematic evaluation of the lateral ligamentous complex and syndesmosis should occur in each patient.

Radiographic evaluation should be performed to rule out fracture and to assess for possible dynamic instability. Surgery should address instability and obtain anatomic restoration of the ankle joint. Ankle arthroscopy is a useful adjunct to ligamentous repair or fracture fixation that identifies cartilage injury often missed with diagnostic imaging. Return to play should be tailored to each individual injury but should focus on early range of motion and graduated return to play.

References

1. Nelson AJ, Collins CL, Yard EE, Fields SK, Comstock RD. Ankle injuries among United States high school sports athletes, 2005-2006. J Athl Train. 2007;42(3):381–7.
2. Mulcahey MK, Bernhardson AS, Murphy CP, Chang A, Zajac T, Sanchez G, et al. The epidemiology of ankle injuries identified at the national football league combine, 2009-2015. Orthop J Sports Med. 2018;6(7):2325967118786227.
3. Matheny LM, Johnson NS, Liechti DJ, Clanton TO. Activity level and function after lateral ankle ligament repair versus reconstruction. Am J Sports Med. 2016;44(5):1301–8.
4. Miller M, DeLee TS. Drez & Miller's orthopaedic sports medicine. 5th ed. Philadelphia, PA: Elsevier; 2020.
5. Brostrom L. Sprained ankles. 3. Clinical observations in recent ligament ruptures. Acta Chir Scand. 1965;130(6):560–9.
6. Balduini FC, Tetzlaff J. Historical perspectives on injuries of the ligaments of the ankle. Clin Sports Med. 1982;1:3–12.
7. Balduini FC, Vegso JJ, Torg JS, Torg E. Management and rehabilitation of ligamentous injuries to the ankle. Sports Med. 1987;4:364–80.
8. Lynch SA. Assessment of the injured ankle in the athlete. J Athl Train. 2002;37(4):406–12.
9. Kerkhoffs GM, van den Bekerom M, Elders LA, van Beek PA, Hullegie WA, Bloemers GM, et al. Diagnosis, treatment and prevention of ankle sprains: an evidence-based clinical guideline. Br J Sports Med. 2012;46(12):854–60.
10. Clanton, T et al. Internal brace ligament augmentation repair, faculty forum virtual roundtable. Arthrex. 2017. LB1-00022-EN_C.
11. Boytim MJ, Fischer DA, Neumann L. Syndesmotic ankle sprains. Am J Sports Med. 1991;19:294–8.
12. Cedell C. Supination–outward rotation injuries of the ankle: a clinical and roentgenological study with special reference to the operative treatment. Acta Orthop Scand Suppl. 1967;110:1–148.
13. Gerber JP, Williams GN, Scoville CR, et al. Persistent disability with ankle sprains: a prospective examination of an athletic population. Foot Ankle Int. 1998;19(10):653–60.
14. Hopkinson WJ, St Pierre P, Ryan JB, et al. Syndesmosis sprainsof the ankle. Foot Ankle. 1990;10:325–30.
15. Hunt KJ, George E, Harris AH, et al. Epidemiology of syndesmosis injuries in intercollegiate football: incidence and risk factors from the National Collegiate Athletic Association Injury Surveillance System data from 2004-2005 to 2008-2009. Clin J Sport Med. 2013;23(4):278–82.
16. Maehlum S, Daljord OA. Acute sports injuries in Oslo: a one year study. Br J Sports Med. 1984;18:181–5.
17. Kelikian AS, editor. Sarrafian's anatomy of the foot and ankle: descriptive, topographic, functional. 3rd ed. Philadelphia: Lippincott Williams & Wilkins; 2011.
18. Molinari A, Stolley M, Amendola A. High ankle sprains (syndesmotic) in athletes: diagnostic challenges and review of the literature. Iowa Orthop J. 2009;29:130.
19. Bassett FH III, Gates HS III, Billys JB, et al. Talar impingement by the anteroinferior tibiofibular ligament: a cause of chronic pain in the ankle after inversion sprain. J Bone Joint Surg Am. 1990;72:55–9.

20. Beumer A, van Hemert WLW, Swierstra BA, et al. A biomechanical evaluation of the tibiofibular and tibiotalar ligaments of the ankle. Foot Ankle Int. 2003;24(5):426–9.
21. Ashhurst APC, Bromer RS. Classification and mechanism of fractures of the leg bones involving the ankle. Arch Surg. 1922;4:51–129.
22. Broström L. Sprained ankles. III. Clinical observations in recent ligament ruptures. Acta Chir Scand. 1965;130:560–9.
23. Xenos JS, Hopkinson WJ, Mulligan ME, et al. The tibiofibular syndesmosis: evaluation of the ligamentous structures, methods of fixation, and radiographic assessment. J Bone Joint Surg Am. 1995;77:847–56.
24. Close JR. Some applications of the functional anatomy of the ankle joint. J Bone Joint Surg Am. 1956;38:761–81.
25. Rasmussen O. Stability of the ankle joint: analysis of the function and traumatology of the ankle ligaments. Acta Orthop Scand Suppl. 1985;211:1–75.
26. van Dijk CN, et al. Classification and diagnosis of acute isolated syndesmotic injuries: ESSKA-AFAS consensus and guidelines. Knee Surg Sports Traumatol Arthrosc. 2016;24(4):1200–16. https://doi.org/10.1007/s00167-015-3942-8.
27. Jelinek JA, Porter DA. Management of unstable ankle fractures and syndesmosis injuries in athletes. Foot Ankle Clin. 2009;14(2):277–98.
28. Bonnin JG. Injuries to the ligaments of the ankle. J Bone Joint Surg Br. 1965;47(4):609–11.
29. Edwards GS Jr, DeLee JC. Ankle diastasis without fracture. Foot Ankle. 1984;4:305–12.
30. Hsu AR, Gross CE, Lee S. Intraoperative O-arm computed tomography evaluation of syndesmotic reduction. Foot Ankle Int. 2013;34:753–9.
31. Miller BS, Downie BK, Johnson PD, Schmidt PW, Nordwall SJ, Kijek TG, Jacobson JA, Carpenter JE. Time to return to play after high ankle sprains in collegiate football players: a prediction model. Sports Health. 2012;4(6):504–9.
32. Fritschy D. An unusual ankle injury in top skiers. Am J Sports Med. 1989;17:282–6.
33. Pettrone FA, Gail M, Pee D, et al. Quantitative criteria for prediction of the results after displaced fracture of the ankle. J Bone Joint Surg Am. 1983;65:667–77.
34. Harper MC, Keller TS. A radiographic evaluation of the tibiofibular syndesmosis. Foot Ankle. 1989;10:156–60.
35. Hsu AR, Lareau CR, Anderson RB. Repair of acute superficial deltoid complex avulsion during ankle fracture fixation in national football league players. Foot Ankle Int. 2015;36(11):1272–8.
36. Outland T. Sprains and separations of inferior tibiofibular joint without important fracture. Am J Surg. 1943;59:320–9.
37. Sclafani SJA. Ligamentous injury of the lower tibiofibular syn desmosis: radiographic evidence. Radiology. 1985;156:21–7.
38. Kazunori O, Masato T, Kohei N, et al. Injury of the tibiofibular syndesmosis: value of MR imaging for diagnosis. Radiology. 2003;227(1):155–61.
39. Calder JD, et al. Stable versus unstable grade II high ankle sprains: a prospective study predicting the need for surgical stabilization and time to return to sports. Arthroscopy. 2016;32(4):634–42.
40. Schairer WW, et al. Arthroscopically assisted open reduction-internal fixation of ankle fractures: significance of the arthroscopic ankle drive-through sign. Arthrosc Tech. 2016;5(2):e407–12.
41. Laver L, et al. Plasma rich in growth factors (PRGF) as a treatment for high ankle sprain in elite athletes: a randomized control trial. Knee Surg Sports Traumatol Arthrosc. 2015;23(11):3383–92. https://doi.org/10.1007/s00167-014-3119-x.
42. Gould JS. Operative foot surgery. Philadelphia, PA: WB Saunders; 1994.
43. Qamar F, Kadakia A, Venkateswaran B. An anatomical way of treating ankle syndesmotic injuries. J Foot Ankle Surg. 2011;50(6):762–5. https://doi.org/10.1053/j.jfas.2011.07.001.
44. Rigby RB, Cottom JM. Does the Arthrex TightRope(R) provide maintenance of the distal tibiofibular syndesmosis? A 2-year follow-up of 64 TightRopes(R) in 37 patients. J Foot Ankle Surg. 2013;52(5):563–7.
45. Colcuc C, Blank M, Stein T, et al. Lower complication rate and faster return to sports in patients with acute syndesmotic rupture treated with a new knotless suture button device. Knee Surg Sports Traumatol Arthrosc. 2018;26(10):3156–64.

46. Gan K, et al. Dynamic fixation versus static fixation for distal tibiofibular syndesmosis injuries: a meta-analysis. Med Sci Monit. 2019;25:1314–22.
47. Colvin AC, et al. Return to sports following operatively treated ankle fractures. Foot Ankle Int. 2009;30(4):292–6.
48. Tornetta P 3rd, Axelrad TW, Sibai TA, Creevy WR. Treatment of the stress positive ligamentous SE4 ankle fracture: incidence of syndesmotic injury and clinical decision making. J Orthop Trauma. 2012;26(11):659–61. https://doi.org/10.1097/BOT.0b013e31825cf39c.
49. Werner BC, et al. Distal fibula fractures in national football league athletes. Orthop J Sports Med. 2017;5(9):2325967117726515.
50. Robertson GA, Wood AM. Fractures in sport: Optimising their management and outcome. World J Orthop. 2015;6(11):850–63.
51. Bugler KE, et al. The treatment of unstable fractures of the ankle using the Acumed fibular nail: development of a technique. J Bone Joint Surg Br. 2012;94(8):1107–12.
52. Stromsoe K, et al. The repair of a ruptured deltoid ligament is not necessary in ankle fractures. J Bone Joint Surg Br. 1995;77(6):920–1.
53. Donley BG, et al. Pronation-external rotation ankle fractures in 3 professional football players. Am J Orthop (Belle Mead NJ). 2005;34(11):547–50.
54. Loren GJ, Ferkel RD. Arthroscopic assessment of occult intra-articular injury in acute ankle fractures. Arthroscopy. 2002;18(4):412–21.
55. Schepers T. To retain or remove the syndesmotic screw: a review of literature. Arch Orthop Trauma Surg. 2011;131(7):879–83.
56. Mai H. The NFL orthopaedic surgery outcomes database (NO-SOD): the effect of common orthopaedic procedures on football careers. Am J Sports Med. 2016;44(9):2255–62.

Foot Injuries in Football

5

William A. Davis III, Gautam P. Yagnik,
and Thomas P. San Giovanni

Introduction

Injuries of the foot in athletes have a wide range of mechanisms, acuteness, severity, and long-term disability. In this chapter, we will discuss several of the most common injuries occurring in athletes. Many injuries of the foot can be managed during the season with nonoperative measures. We will review pertinent anatomy, presentation, work-up, and management for these injuries. While the details of any surgical procedures are beyond the scope of this chapter, indications for nonsurgical and surgical treatment will be reviewed.

Turf Toe

Turf toe describes a spectrum of injuries involving the structures associated with the first metatarsophalangeal (MTP) joint. Injured structures can include the plantar plate and capsule, the plantar musculature, the sesamoid complex, and the articular surface of the metatarsal head to variable degrees. The injury was initially described by Bowers and Martin in 1976 occurring in American football players [1]. Following the introduction of artificial playing surfaces (AstroTurf), the injury became more common, with a 1990 study noting a 45% prevalence among active professional

W. A. Davis III (✉)
DuPage Medical Group, Orthopaedic Sports Medicine and Foot and Ankle Surgery, North Central College, Naperville, IL, USA

G. P. Yagnik · T. P. San Giovanni
Miami Orthopedics and Sports Medicine Institute, Department of Orthopedic Surgery, Florida International University College of Medicine, Miami, FL, USA

K. W. Farmer (ed.), *Football Injuries*,
https://doi.org/10.1007/978-3-030-54875-9_5

football players and the vast majority of those occurring on artificial turf [2]. More recent data suggests that the incidence of the injury is decreasing, presumably due to improvements in artificial turf designs [3].

Anatomy

On the plantar aspect of the first MTP joint, two hallucal sesamoids are embedded within the flexor hallucis brevis (FHB) tendon. These lie directly below and articulate with the plantar aspect of the first metatarsal head. Connecting the sesamoids to the plantar base of the first proximal phalanx is a dense fibrous band of soft tissue known as the plantar plate. The plantar plate plays an essential role to the stability of the first MTP joint resisting the ground reactive forces seen by the hallux which otherwise would lead to repetitive dorsal translation or subluxation. Surrounding musculature includes the abductor and adductor hallucis tendons, which insert on the medial and lateral aspects of the first proximal phalanx base. Varus and valgus stability to the first MTP joint is conferred by medial and lateral capsule along with the integrity of the medial and lateral metatarsosesamoid ligaments and sesamoidophalangeal ligaments. The flexor hallucis longus (FHL) tendon lies just plantar to the plantar plate and passes deep to and in between the medial and lateral sesamoid. The sesamoids are connected to each other by the intersesamoid ligament. Any combination of injury to the above structures has been seen with turf toe injuries, particularly those of higher grades.

Presentation

The injury most commonly presents following a hyperextension injury in which the first MTP joint experiences an axial load with the foot in equinus. This is commonly seen during an active push off or when the forefoot is fixed with the heel elevated and another player lands on the back of the heel. With this mechanism, anything from a mild sprain of the plantar plate complex to a complete dorsal dislocation of the MTP joint can occur [3]. An additional valgus force may result in greater injury to the medial sesamoid component, medial ligaments, and medial capsule, which can lead to a traumatic hallux valgus deformity over time [4, 5].

Following the described mechanism, players may present with swelling, plantar ecchymosis, and pain with the push-off phase of gait. On examination, the player will exhibit point tenderness over the plantar plate, dorsal capsule, and collateral ligaments. Varus and valgus testing of the MTP joint should be performed to test the collateral ligaments, and a dorsoplantar drawer test should be performed to assess the integrity of the plantar plate aiding in the determination of a grossly unstable injury [6]. The contralateral foot should always be used for comparison noting any asymmetric findings of alignment, motion, stability, and function.

Sideline Management

If any instability is detected on physical exam, the player should be held out from participation for the rest of that practice or game. Initial clinical evaluation on the sideline or locker room should assess whether an obvious fracture is present (crepitus) and whether the first MTP joint is located, subluxed, or dislocated. If dislocation of the joint is obvious, a closed reduction can be attempted yet may require a local block at the hallux or regional at the ankle. If plain radiographs are available at the sports facility, then these should be obtained. Otherwise, a closed reduction of a dislocation may need to be performed prior to x-rays if gross deformity is noted to avoid delays in joint realignment. If a closed reduction is performed, the opportune time to assess stability is at that moment with a dorsal-plantar drawer sign, as this information may prove valuable to the player's injury management. A spectrum exists from grossly unstable with drawer (easily dislocated dorsally) to stable (resistance to dislocation provided by the joint anatomy and resting tension of the surround soft tissue structures).

Initial treatment should include rest, ice, elevation, and immobilization. A walking boot, cast shoe, or short leg cast with the hallux MTP joint in slight plantarflexion is recommended to allow for soft tissue rest [5]. Various modifications of DME and injury-specific taping techniques can be employed. A cut out under the hallux can be created within the foam insole of a boot or cast shoe to maintain the desired position of the hallux. Additionally, layered taping over the dorsal aspect of the first proximal phalanx can provide a strong block to dorsal translation. Control of any varus or valgus or rotational malalignment may be incorporated into taping technique to address specific components to the injury.

Work-up

Appropriate imaging should be obtained to evaluate the extent of the injury and thus formulate a treatment plan and return to play goals. Radiographs include weight-bearing anteroposterior (AP), lateral (LAT), and oblique (OBQ) radiographs of the foot and an axial sesamoid view if possible. Additionally, an AP radiograph of the contralateral foot should be obtained for the comparison of sesamoid position or other signs of significant asymmetry. Ideally the weight-bearing AP views should be performed with pressure on a single limb rather than shared as with a bilateral AP view. If pain does not allow for this, a bilateral AP would suffice for demonstration of any obvious asymmetry. Radiographs may reveal sesamoid fractures, bony flecks indicating capsular avulsion, sesamoid diastasis, or sesamoid retraction. Proximal migration of one or both sesamoids is suggestive of a plantar plate rupture [7].

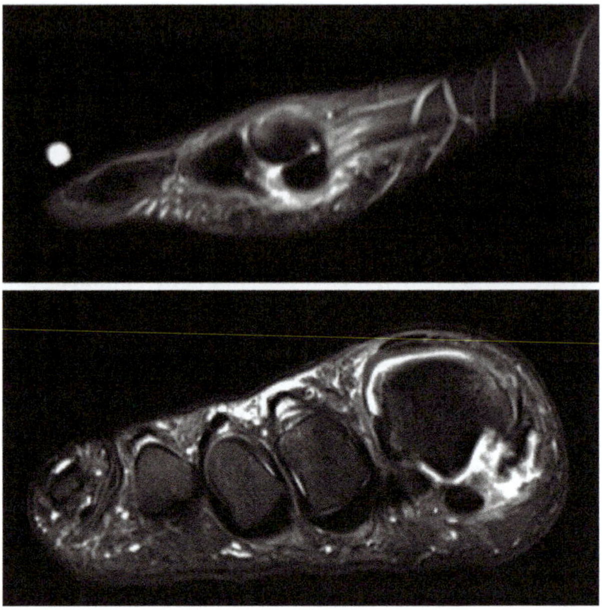

Fig. 5.1 Turf toe. T2-weighted MRI sagittal and axial images demonstrating rupture of the plantar plate from the distal aspect of the medial sesamoid (top) and disruption of the intersesamoid ligament (bottom)

Advanced imaging should be obtained in the event of a suggested plantar plate rupture on plain radiographs. MRI can delineate the pattern of injury and provide information on surrounding soft tissue disruption [1] (Fig. 5.1). MRI may also demonstrate bone marrow edema, osteochondral lesion, or intraarticular loose body that may be impossible or difficult to visualize on plain radiographs. Depending on the circumstances and imaging findings, this additional information may provide useful information for injury management, particularly if surgical intervention is contemplated.

Classification and Treatment

Injury classification, initially described by Clanton and later modified by Anderson, is as follows [5, 6]:

Grade I – capsular sprain without disruption, normal range of motion, no ecchymosis, ability to bear weight, normal radiographs, and intact soft tissue on MRI with surrounding edema.

Grade II – partial plantar plate and capsule tearing, presence of swelling and ecchymosis, painful range of motion, difficulty weight-bearing, possibly normal radiographs, and high signal intensity on MRI that does not extend all the way through the plantar plate.

Grade III – complete tear through plantar plate and capsule, significant swelling and loss of motion, abnormal radiographs, and full thickness tear on MRI.

Initial treatment is as described above for sideline management. For grade I injuries, players will benefit from slight plantarflexion taping and the use of a stiff soled shoes or Morton extension orthotic. With a medial sided injury, a toe spacer may be used to decrease the chance of developing posttraumatic hallux valgus. After the resolution of soft tissue swelling, generally in 3–5 days, athletes may return to low-impact activities as tolerated [8]. Taping or strapping to limit the degree of hallux dorsiflexion may be continued as the player initially returns to play.

For grade II injuries, initial treatment is the same as for grade I. The player will likely lose on average 2 weeks of playing time with this injury. Again, following the resolution of acute pain and swelling, low-impact activities may be initiated as tolerated, and toe protection is recommended. Once the athlete is tolerating low-impact activities, gradual advancement of running, jumping, and push-off activities may proceed [1].

With grade III injuries, initial treatment remains the same; however, 8 weeks of immobilization may be required before returning to sports activities. In severe cases, complete resolution of symptoms may not occur for 6 months [5].

Conclusion

Surgical treatment for turf toe injuries is rarely indicated and is beyond the scope of this chapter. It is typically reserved for severe grade III injuries, especially with concomitant injuries around the first MTP joint (Fig. 5.2). Prospective studies comparing treatment options are lacking, and most evidence is based on retrospective case series. Regardless of treatment strategy, turf toe may be a significant injury to

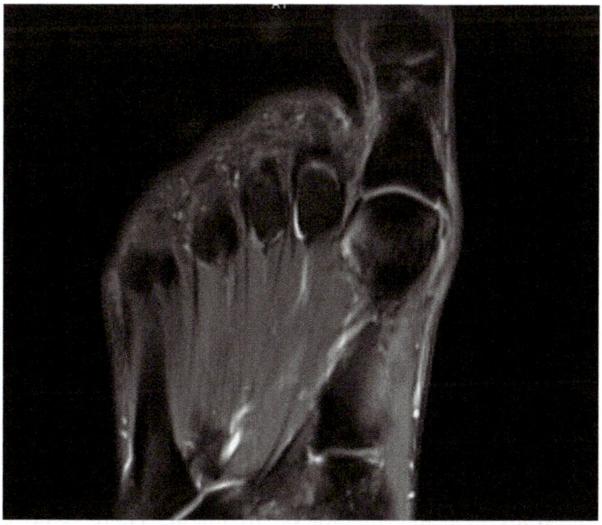

Fig. 5.2 Grade III turf toe. T2 MRI image demonstrating disruption of the medial collateral ligaments and capsule. Additionally, this high-grade injury results in the associated bone contusion seen in the metatarsal head, as well as surrounding soft tissue edema

an athlete that can disrupt a season and cause significant pain and disability. Recognition and treatment is important for these injuries can lead to varying degrees of persistent pain, stiffness, posttraumatic arthritis, or deformity in the form of hallux rigidus and/or traumatic hallux valgus (traumatic bunion). Furthermore, athletic performance and career longevity can be negatively impacted. It is common for the injured hallux MTP joint to display some degree of limited motion in the long term. Radiographic signs of hallux rigidus, whether symptomatic or asymptomatic, are also a common finding years following significant turf toe injury. Prompt diagnosis and appropriate treatment can allow most athletes to return to pre-injury level of performance.

Lisfranc Injuries

The Lisfranc joint complex of the midfoot has a unique combination of osseous anatomy and stout ligamentous support that allows for effective force transfer from the hindfoot to the forefoot during ambulation. It is, therefore, of critical importance in push-off activities in sports.

Lisfranc injuries are uncommon, and they present as a broad spectrum of injuries, ranging from low-energy sprains to high-energy fracture dislocations. Their uncommon occurrence and potential for subtle presentation contribute to 20–40% of Lisfranc injuries being missed initially [9]. A high level of scrutiny is indicated in any midfoot sprain. Recognition of this high rate of missed injury has, therefore, led to improved early detection. If left untreated, players may develop posttraumatic arthritis and arch collapse [10]. Even with recognition and treatment, years following the injury, posttraumatic arthritis can ensue.

Anatomy

The Lisfranc joint complex is composed of the tarsometatarsal (TMT), intercuneiform, and proximal intermetatarsal joints. The first, second, and third metatarsals articulate with the medial, middle, and lateral cuneiform bones. This is commonly referred to as the 1st, 2nd, and 3rd TMT joints. The fourth and fifth metatarsals articulate with the cuboid as the 4th and 5th TMT joints. The osseous anatomy of the trapezoidal cuneiforms creates a "Roman arch" structure in the coronal plane, with the middle cuneiform serving as the keystone for the second metatarsal base. Additionally, the second metatarsal–middle cuneiform articulation is recessed proximally, conferring further osseous structural stability [10].

Ligamentous support also contributes to the stability of the Lisfranc joint. Dorsal, interosseous, and plantar ligaments attach the recessed second metatarsal base to the medial cuneiform. The interosseous ligament is the strongest and is often referred to as the Lisfranc ligament. The second through the fifth metatarsals are stabilized by the transverse intermetatarsal ligament. There is no intermetatarsal ligament that exists between the first and second metatarsals; therefore, this is a vulnerable region

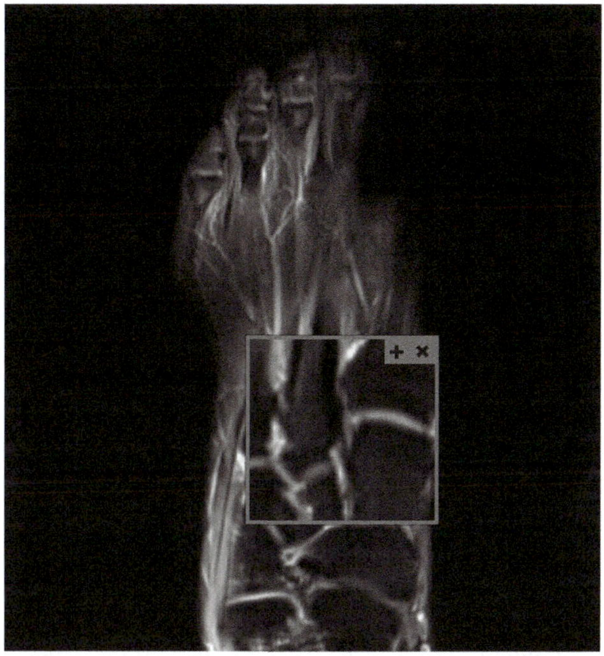

Fig. 5.3 Lisfranc ligament. The interosseous ligament runs obliquely from the plantar lateral base of the medial cuneiform to the plantar medial base of the second metatarsal

within the complex. The Lisfranc ligament runs obliquely from the plantar lateral base of the medial cuneiform to the plantar medial base of the second metatarsal (Fig. 5.3). This ligament is a dense, strong ligament that confers stability through this zone. Further dynamic stability is conferred by the insertions of the tibialis anterior and the peroneus longus tendons [10].

Aside from the classically described Lisfranc injury involving a shift between the second metatarsal base and medial cuneiform, the interval between the 1st and 2nd metatarsal bases and 1st–2nd intercuneiform joint are of particular importance anatomically. This region represents a Lisfranc variant injury pattern noted with athletes.

Presentation

Injuries to the Lisfranc joint can occur through multiple mechanisms. Crush injuries can cause significant osseous and soft tissue damage. In sports, Lisfranc injuries can occur through two common mechanisms. One mechanism occurs when the hindfoot is anchored and a forceful rotation occurs about the midfoot, such as an equestrian who falls with the foot strapped. More commonly, a player with a plantarflexed forefoot and MTP joints in maximal dorsiflexion has an axial load applied to the hindfoot, such as when another player falls on the heel [11].

Subtle Lisfranc injuries may be difficult to diagnose, particularly on the sideline. Players will typically have difficulty bearing weight following a Lisfranc injury.

There may be swelling over the dorsomedial midfoot [10]. The presence of plantar ecchymosis is strongly associated with a Lisfranc injury [12]. The midfoot should be palpated for tenderness with particular attention to the metatarsal bases, TMT joints, naviculocuneiform joint, and navicular tuberosity. Pain elicited with a passive pronation-abduction stress maneuver through the junction of the forefoot-midfoot is suggestive of injury. Dorsoplantar drawer testing of the individual 1st, 2nd and 3rd TMT joints may reveal TMT instability or elicit pain upon testing.

Sideline Management

If a Lisfranc injury is suspected due to swelling, tenderness, and difficulty bearing weight, the player should be made non-weight-bearing. Swelling can be significant; therefore, ice should be applied and the extremity elevated. Immobilization should be in a splint or CAM boot.

Work-up

Imaging of a suspected Lisfranc imaging begins with weight-bearing AP, lateral, and oblique views of the foot. On the AP view, the medial borders of the second metatarsal and the middle cuneiform should align. On the oblique view, the medial borders of the fourth metatarsal and cuboid should align. On the lateral view, there should be no dorsal or plantar subluxation of the metatarsals at the TMT joint. If there is a question of subtle irregularity, comparisons with the contralateral foot should be made. Greater than 2 mm of translation is suggestive of injury [10] (Fig. 5.4). Additionally, a "fleck sign," which is an avulsion of the base of the second metatarsal, is indicative of a Lisfranc ligament injury [13] (Fig. 5.5).

If plain radiographs are normal in a player with a suspected midfoot injury, stress radiographs and advanced imaging can be useful. Stress radiographs are performed with an abduction-pronation stress maneuver but can be painful to the patient [14]. To perform this, an ankle block would likely be required to perform adequately or under IV sedation/general anesthesia. In our experience, however, this is rarely performed. CT scan may show bony abnormalities such as avulsion fractures or comminution. With the advent of weight-bearing CT scan technology, a weight-bearing CT scan with comparison may prove helpful (Fig. 5.6). The scan should reveal greater detail of subtle abnormalities and has the potential to become an effective tool in those with a dynamic instability or equivocal weight-bearing x-ray findings. MRI can be useful for demonstrating ligamentous disruption and has been correlated with intraoperative instability [15]. MRI may also give findings consistent with injury pattern such as disruption or partial tear of the Lisfranc ligament, signal intensity through the zones of the intercuneiform region, and bone contusions of the metatarsal bases and or cuboid (Fig. 5.7). The cuboid can be injured at times secondary to compression from the abduction force.

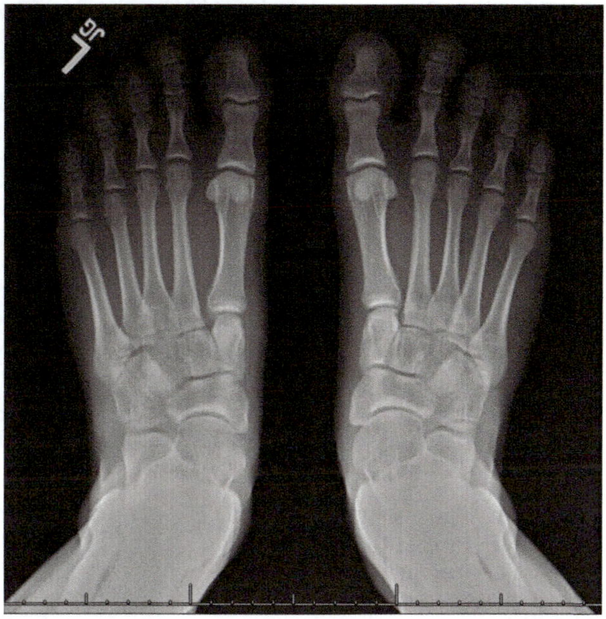

Fig. 5.4 Lisfranc injury. Bilateral weight-bearing AP radiographs demonstrating irregularity of the second metatarsal–middle cuneiform border and widening of the interval between the second metatarsal base and medial cuneiform of the left foot

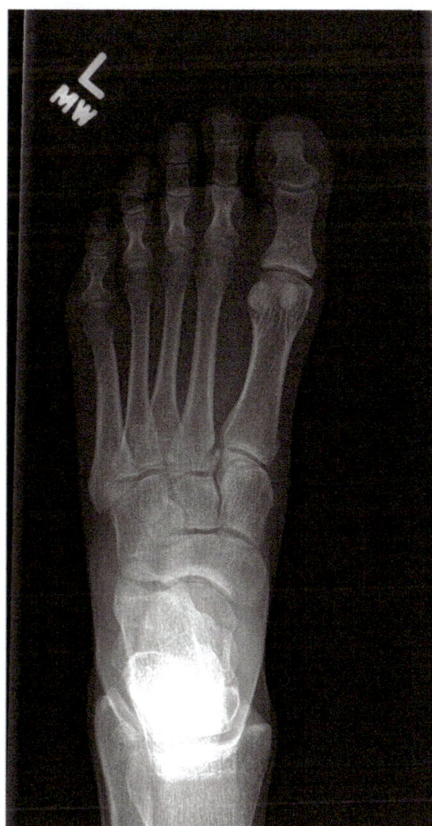

Fig. 5.5 "Fleck sign." AP radiograph demonstrating an avulsion of the base of the second metatarsal, indicating a Lisfranc injury

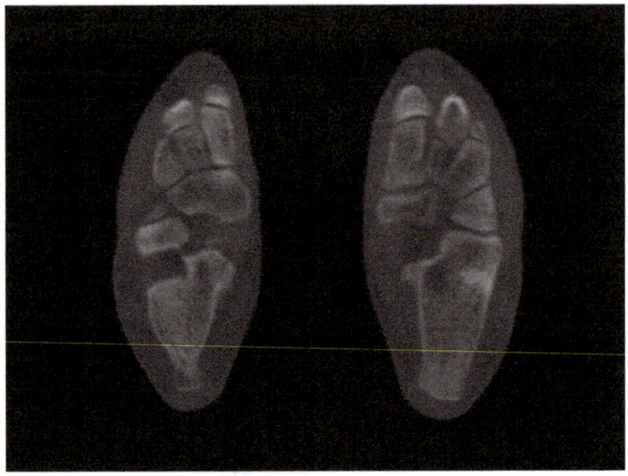

Fig. 5.6 Bilateral weight-bearing CT scan demonstrating diastasis between the medial cuneiform and second metatarsal base

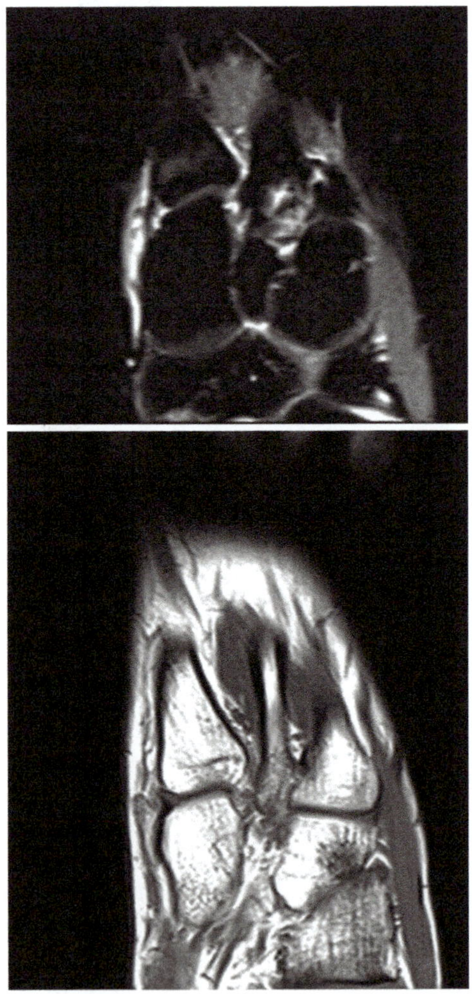

Fig. 5.7 T2 (top)- and T1 (bottom)-weighted MRI scan of a Lisfranc injury demonstrating a tear of the Lisfranc ligament as well as associated soft tissue edema and bone contusion at the base of the second metatarsal

Treatment

Several classification schemes have been proposed, and while they are useful for descriptive purposes, none predict outcomes or guide treatment. A mild Lisfranc injury can be treated successfully nonoperatively if subtle instability is ruled out. With appropriate plain radiographs and advanced imaging, if clinical findings are still suggestive of injury, an examination under anesthesia may be performed [10].

For stable injuries, nonoperative treatment consists of 4–6 weeks of non-weight-bearing immobilization. A short leg cast or CAM boot with arch support is recommended. After this period of immobilization, the player may benefit from a course of physical therapy to improve gait and balance. Return to play can occur after resolution of pain and swelling and may take 4–6 months or longer [10].

For unstable injuries, surgical management is indicated. Definitive management is delayed until the soft tissue envelope can accommodate surgical incisions. The details of operative treatment are beyond the scope of this chapter but generally involve closed versus open reduction depending upon the injury pattern, with rigid anatomic fixation of the medial and middle columns of the foot and possible flexible temporary fixation for the lateral column if necessary. An ongoing debate in the literature revolves around whether these injuries are best treated with ORIF or with primary arthrodesis. Future research is needed to delineate indications for each treatment option, particularly as it pertains to the athlete and ability to return to the same functional level [10].

Hardware removal is at times planned for 4–6 months following surgery or may be left in if asymptomatic. Controversy exists regarding hardware removal in the setting of an aligned yet unfused Lisfranc joints for athletes. Some advocate leaving hardware, while others remove it routinely. Some surgeons base the decision on individual circumstances. There has been no true consensus yet with respect to hardware removal with the exception that it should not be removed within 4 months to allow for adequate healing of this region due to the forces that are generated through it.

Posttraumatic arthritis can occur with nonoperative treatment and operative treatment years later, whether anatomical alignment is restored or not. This has a much lower occurrence with anatomical alignment; however, the initial impact forces to the articular cartilage at the time of the injury must be taken into account and the individual's biological cartilage response to that injury would be outside the control of the treating physician. Explaining these factors to the athlete may prove helpful so they have an understanding of some of the potential long-term implications following the trauma they sustained.

Conclusions

Lisfranc injuries, while uncommon, have the potential to be missed due to subtle presentations. A high index of suspicion is needed when a player suffers a midfoot injury with a corresponding mechanism. Missed diagnosis can lead to posttraumatic arthritis, persistent pain, and arch collapse. Determination of stability is necessary to guide operative versus nonoperative treatment and requires careful evaluation of advanced imaging and provocative testing if there is any question in the case of subtle injuries.

Jones Fractures

Fifth metatarsal base fractures are common injuries in athletes. Approximately 70% of metatarsal fractures are fifth metatarsal fractures, and 80% of these occur in the proximal end [16, 17]. Basketball, American football, and soccer are among the three highest-risk sports for fifth metatarsal base fractures [18]. Fractures may be acute fractures, stress fractures, or refracture through an incomplete union.

There are distinct anatomic zones of the proximal fifth metatarsal that are necessary to consider when classifying a given fracture. The anatomy has implications for treatment and outcomes due to the vascular supply and the biomechanical forces that passed through that region. The Jones fracture, described by Sir Robert Jones in 1902 [19] and popularized by modern media attention of elite athlete injuries, is one type of proximal fifth metatarsal fracture. Proximal fifth metatarsal tuberosity avulsion fractures ("pseudo-Jones" fractures) and diaphyseal stress fractures (proximal shaft fractures) are the other two types that will be discussed.

Anatomy

The fifth metatarsal is typically divided anatomically into the tuberosity, the metaphyseal-diaphyseal junction, and the proximal shaft. Lawrence and Botte described them as Zones I, II, and III, respectively [20].

The tuberosity is extraarticular and serves as the insertion of the lateral plantar fascia and peroneus brevis tendon just distal to that. These Zone I fractures are generally considered to be avulsion fractures by the lateral band of the plantar fascia (more common) or peroneus brevis tendon (less common) upon a sudden contractile force (Fig. 5.8).

The metaphyseal-diaphyseal area, or Zone II, includes the fourth-fifth metatarsal articulation and is considered a vascular watershed area between proximal and distal osseous blood supplies. This area of relative hypovascularity predisposes fractures in this area, Jones fractures, to delayed union or nonunion [21] (Fig. 5.9).

The proximal diaphysis, or Zone III, is the area just distal to the fourth-fifth metatarsal articulation and is a common site of stress fractures in athletes [22] (Fig. 5.10). Players with pes cavus or hindfoot varus may be at increased risk of these fractures due to increased lateral column weight-bearing [23, 24], often referred to as "lateral column overload."

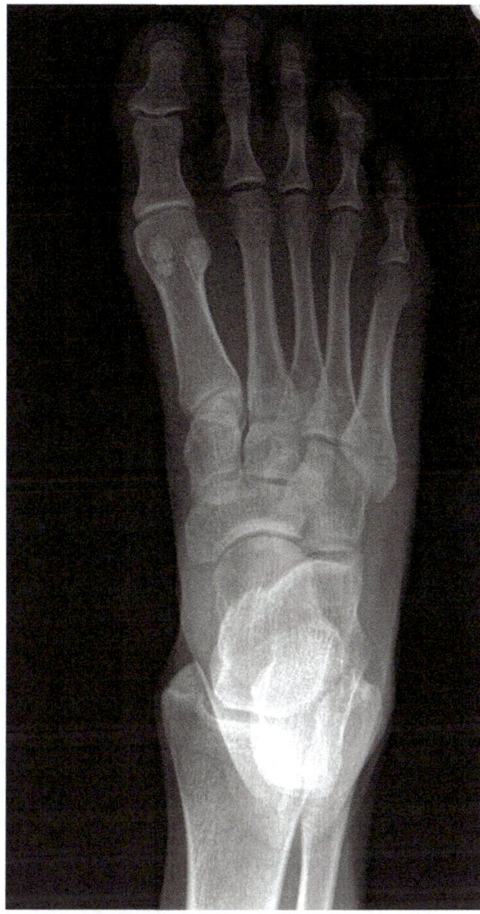

Fig. 5.8 Zone I (tuberosity) fracture of the base of the fifth metatarsal. This extraarticular fracture is an avulsion fracture by the lateral band of the plantar fascia or possibly the peroneus brevis tendon

Presentation

Fractures of the fifth metatarsal base may be either acute injuries or stress fractures. Players who sustain an acute fracture will usually present with pain, swelling, and difficulty bearing weight following a sudden inversion injury or pure adduction force upon a loaded foot. There will typically be tenderness over the fracture site. The foot may exhibit erythema and bruising as well. Players who experience stress fractures will typically experience prodromal symptoms, such as activity-related pain over the lateral aspect of the foot followed by a sudden increase in symptoms once the cortical bone finally fails [18].

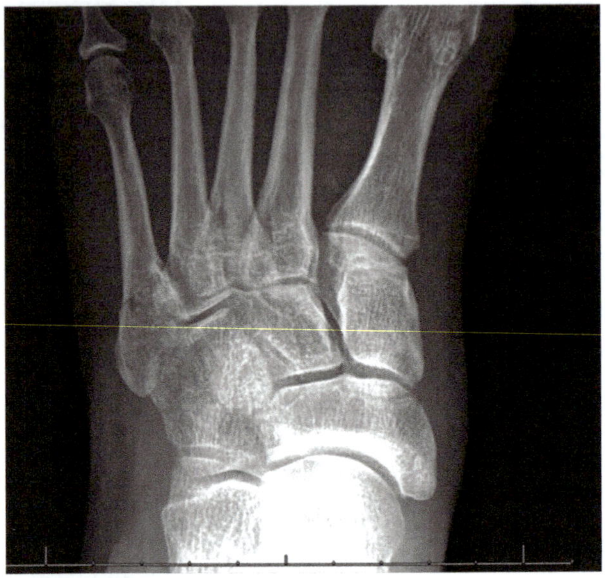

Fig. 5.9 Jones fracture (Zone II) of the fifth metatarsal. AP radiograph of the foot demonstrates an acute Jones fracture with the fracture line extending into the articulation of the fourth and fifth metatarsal bases

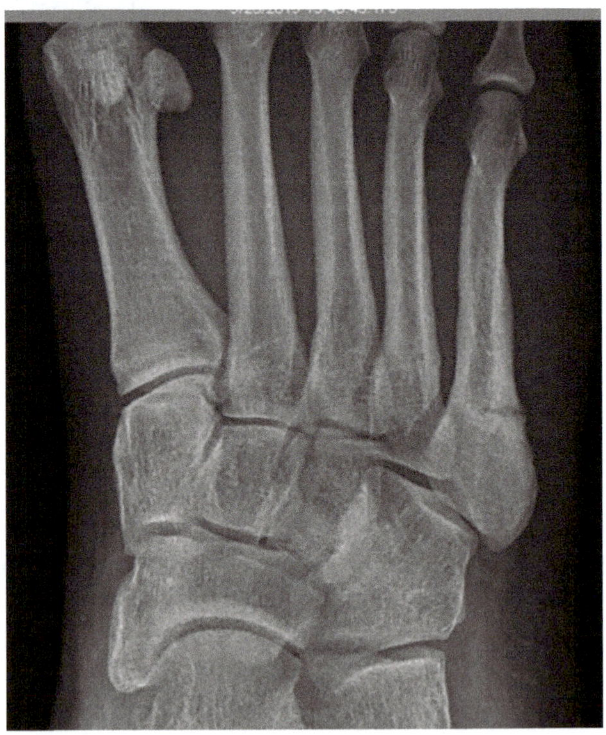

Fig. 5.10 Zone III fifth metatarsal fracture, immediately distal to the fourth-fifth metatarsal articulation. This radiograph demonstrates a fracture in a 20-year-old collegiate football player sustained during a game. Subtle thickening and beaking at the lateral cortex indicates a stress reaction in this chronic injury, which finally failed acutely during competition

Refracture may occasionally occur through a previous site of incompletely healed fracture or reveal that a nonunion had occurred through a relative biomechanically weak zone. If this does occur, both biologic and biomechanical sources should be reassessed. It would be prudent to investigate potential contributory factors that are intrinsic to the bone (e.g., vitamin D deficiency or endocrine factors) and extrinsic to the bone (i.e., varus hindfoot alignment contributing to lateral column overload).

Sideline Management

Following an acute injury, the ice, elevation, and pain control should be initiated. Immobilization in a CAM boot or splint will allow for soft tissue rest.

Work-up

It is important to assess their overall foot and ankle alignment. This is easy to perform but often not done in the case of an acute fracture. Simply by having the player stand and viewing them front, side, and back may allow the treating physician to have a better understanding of predisposing factors, such as a varus hindfoot or cavovarus foot shape, which may aid in the treatment of this condition and prevention of future issues with the contralateral foot.

Radiographic imaging should include weight-bearing AP, lateral, and oblique views of the weight-bearing foot. Contralateral comparison views are not typically needed but may be helpful in a skeletally immature foot. Additionally imaging, such as MRI or bone scan, may be helpful in the diagnosis of an early stress fracture. Bone scans have become less common over the years with the improvements that have occurred within the field magnetic resonance imaging. Additionally the MRI scan does not involve radiation to the patient. Computed tomography (CT) scan does expose the patient to radiation but can aid in the diagnosis of nonunion [25].

Treatment

Zone I injuries have been shown to heal predictably well with nonoperative treatment. The original report by Dameron in 1975 demonstrated healing in 99 of 100 patients with nonoperative treatment [26]. Multiple studies have shown similar results, even with slight comminution. Even fractures extending into the cuboid-metatarsal joint and those with >2 mm displacement have been shown to heal predictably and with equivalent functional outcomes as nondisplaced, extraarticular Zone I fractures [27]. Nonoperative treatment should consist of a hard-soled shoe and early weight-bearing, as delayed weight-bearing has been shown to be a predictor of poorer functional outcome [28].

There are certain Zone I fractures for which operative treatment should be considered. Those with significant displacement, comminution, or intraarticular involvement >30% of the cuboid-metatarsal joint are recommended by some authors to be treated operatively [18].

Zone II fractures, true Jones fractures, treated with ORIF have been shown to have higher union rates, earlier demonstration of radiographic healing, and therefore earlier return to baseline athletic activity. The typical form of ORIF has been intramedullary screw fixation. A systematic review from 2013 [29] of 26 studies on treatment and return to sport following Jones fractures found a union rate of 76% for nonoperative treatment and 96% for screw fixation. Operative treatment allowed a return to sport between 4 and 18 weeks as compared to 9–22 weeks with nonoperative treatment. When considering allowing full return to sport, the physician should observe adequate bony bridging on plain radiographs and confirm on thin cut CT scan if there is questionable healing.

Use of a bone growth stimulator with immobilization has had mixed results as a treatment option for acute fracture, and no recommendations exist specifically for athletes. As such, the bone stimulator may be considered as an adjunctive therapy in combination with intramedullary screw fixation, though no specific literature has been presented to advocate its combined use.

If nonoperative treatment is chosen for Zone II fracture, a slightly more frequent interval follow-up would be recommended. Four-week non-weight-bearing AP, lateral, and oblique foot radiographs could be obtained. Although fracture healing would not be anticipated at that time, certain radiographic signs, such as widening of the fracture line representing bone resorption, can be prognostic indicators of fracture healing and suggest potential development of delayed or nonunion. If this should occur, a CT scan can determine if callus formation is noted or absent and may help the treating physician in decision-making of either continued nonoperative management versus changing strategy to operative management. Assessment of patient compliance, reassessment of biological factors, and treatment plan alteration may be required.

Stress fractures of Zone III are at increased risk of nonunion in athletes, especially those with cavovarus deformities. Similar to Zone II fractures, these players should undergo intramedullary screw fixation, as there is a 33% risk of refracture of Zone III injuries with nonoperative treatment when the fracture is stress related [22]. This high refracture rate may once again represent intrinsic or extrinsic predisposing factors. Therefore, the authors' recommendation would be for the treating physician to have a higher degree of suspicion when evaluating a player with a Zone III fracture; treat the acute fracture but also seek to determine why it occurred in this particular player.

Conclusions

The majority of tuberosity fractures (Zone I) have been shown to heal reliably with nonoperative treatment consisting of a hard shoe and early weight-bearing. Proximal shaft fractures (Zone III) and refractures through a previous Jones (Zone II) warrant higher level of investigation for biologic and biomechanical contributing factors. In the setting of acute Jones fractures (Zone II) and proximal shaft fractures (Zone III), operative treatment remains the preferred treatment in athletes. Operative treatment with an intramedullary screw yields higher union rates and an earlier return to sport than nonoperative treatment. While successfully treated fractures may not be career threatening, missed time due to injury during the season can be significant.

Navicular Stress Fractures

Stress fracture of the navicular bone is not a common injury in the general population, but there is an increased prevalence in athletes. Those at particular risk include athletes engaging in explosive running or cutting sports [30]. One study found that as high as 73% of stress fractures in track athletes involved the navicular [31], whereas the injury is uncommon in endurance runners.

Anatomy

The navicular bone of the midfoot is a component of the Chopart joints (also referred to as transverse tarsal joints). These joints consist of the more mobile talonavicular joint and the relatively stiffer calcaneocuboid joint. The posterior tibial tendon has an insertion on the plantar aspect of the navicular and produces inversion of the hindfoot when activated. Hindfoot inversion allows locking of the transverse tarsal joint, creating a rigid lever arm during the push-off phase of gait.

The vascular anatomy of the navicular likely contributes to the development of stress fractures. A recent cadaveric study demonstrated dorsal and plantar blood supplies, with only 56% having a diffuse intraosseous blood supply and 11.8% having an avascular zone [32].

Presentation

Athletes may have variable presentations of navicular stress fractures. Initially, the fractures are often only painful during sports, but eventually this can progress to

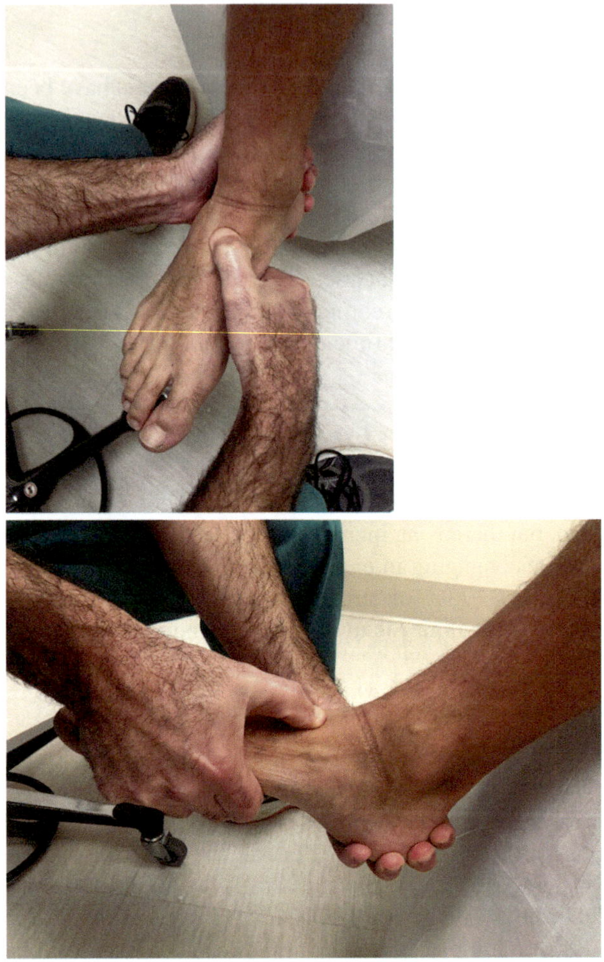

Fig. 5.11 "N-Spot." Clinical examination of the foot demonstrating palpation of the dorsal navicular prominence. Players with a navicular stress fracture will often exhibit a maximal point of tenderness at this specific location

pain with daily activities or even pain at night. Tenderness over the dorsal navicular prominence is a common finding [33] and has been referred to as the "N spot" (Fig. 5.11). Palpation of this region with maximal point of tenderness should raise suspicion for navicular stress fractures particularly in athletes with unexplained ongoing midfoot pain with activity. This is quite different from tenderness along the medial navicular tuberosity, which may represent either insertional posterior tibial tendon tendinitis or stress reaction through the synchondrosis bridge of an accessory navicular. Patients may have pain with a single-leg hop or a heel raise. Because of the insidious onset and vague symptoms, delay in diagnosis can range from 4 to 7 months from the onset of symptoms [30].

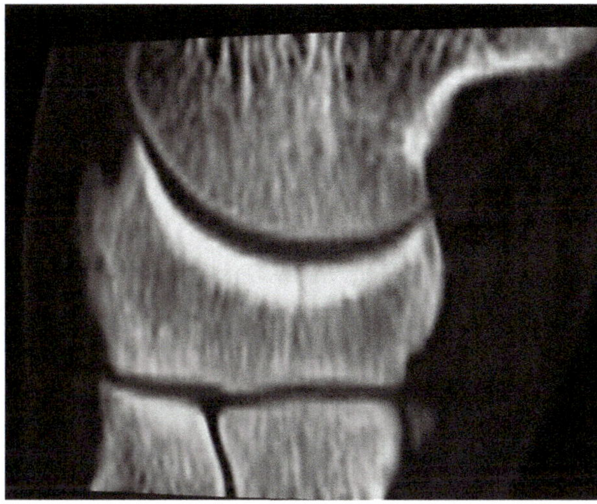

Fig. 5.12 Navicular stress fracture. CT image demonstrating sagittal fracture line in the midportion of the navicular

Work-up

Appropriate imaging begins with plain radiographs; however, these are often normal. Almost all navicular stress fractures are nondisplaced. A true fracture line does not become apparent until late in the condition and, therefore, would not be demonstrated on early plain radiographs. One study found that only 18% of stress fractures diagnosed on CT scan were visible on plain radiographs [34]. CT scan is an excellent diagnostic tool for these fractures (Fig. 5.12). It is lower in cost than MRI, has excellent sensitivity, and provides detail of the fracture and surrounding bony involvement. MRI can be useful for identifying navicular stress reactions before the development of a fracture.

Treatment

There is a paucity of high-quality evidence in the literature to guide the treatment of navicular stress fractures. Historically, nonoperative treatment has been favored except in cases where a complete fracture line is noted on radiographs or CT scan. Identification of sclerotic edges at stress fracture zone or any displaced fractures would mandate surgical repair. One meta-analysis found that non-weight-bearing immobilization in a cast for 6 weeks yielded a 96% success rate with return to sport of 4.9 months in patients with nondisplaced navicular stress fractures [35]. However, similar to Jones fractures, in the setting of a high-level athlete, operative treatment may be considered to minimize the time of immobility and improved the predictability of healing in a shorter timeframe. Stability and compression across the fracture site appear to improve the speed of fracture healing.

Early weight-bearing and early surgical intervention have both been investigated as a means to speed up the return to sport. Early weight-bearing has been shown to have worse results and longer return to sport than delayed weight-bearing immobilization [34–36]. Early surgical intervention has been shown to have similar return to sport times as 6-week cast immobilization [35]. One study, however, demonstrated a faster return to sport with early ORIF compared to nonoperative treatment for complete fractures [37]. Factors contributing to a faster recuperation with ORIF include less time immobilized in a cast, less muscle atrophy, and earlier range of motion. The recuperation following these injuries has a significant component that can be attributed to restoring the strength and proprioception lost from prolonged pain and periods of immobilization that these patients experience prior to being diagnosed.

Conclusions

Although navicular stress fractures are uncommon in the general population, physicians should maintain a high index of suspicion when dealing with nontraumatic midfoot pain in athletes, particularly track athletes or those doing explosive running and jumping. A delay in diagnosis is common, and combined with a significant return to sport time for all treatment strategies, players may be out of full participation for many months. While larger, high-quality studies are needed determine optimal treatments for navicular stress fractures, most of these fractures can be safely and effectively treated nonoperatively. In the high-level athlete, a lower threshold for operative treatment may exist due to the timeframe and desire for earlier return to sport.

Plantar Fasciitis

Plantar fasciitis is a common condition characterized by infra-calcaneal heel pain. In 80% of individuals with plantar heel pain, the underlying cause is plantar fasciitis . The lifetime prevalence of plantar fasciitis has been estimated at around 10% in the United States [38]. Athletes, particularly runners, are at higher risk than the general population. Plantar fasciitis has been considered an overuse injury in which tissue degeneration occurs from repetitive microtrauma and irregular blood flow. The terms fasciitis, fasciosis, and fasciopathy are all used clinically and in the literature with distinctions relating to chronicity [39]. For the purposes of this chapter, the general condition will be referred to as plantar fasciitis.

Anatomy

The plantar fascia or aponeurosis is composed of densely packed collaged fibers. It arises from the medial calcaneal tuberosity and attaches distally to the plantar forefoot and medial and lateral intermuscular septa. The anatomy allows for the plantar fascia to resist tensile forces during stance and gait, thus maintaining the arch of the foot. During push-off, the plantar fascia is important for the function of the windlass mechanism, where MTPJ dorsiflexion results in shortening of the plantar fascia and increasing tension to resist arch collapse [40].

Although the word fasciitis implies an inflammatory process, plantar fasciitis is histologically more of a degenerative process as a result of repetitive microtrauma to the origin of the plantar fascia [41]. Myxoid degeneration, fascial microtears, collagen necrosis, and angiofibroblastic hyperplasia are characteristic [42].

Presentation

Athletes with plantar fasciitis will usually complain of gradual onset inferior heel pain. It is typically most painful for the first few steps in the morning, improves throughout the day, and then may worsen again in the evening. The pain quality is often described as a sharp knifelike pain that gradually improves after walking for period of time. Bilateral involvement has been reported in up to 30% of cases [43]. Tenderness will be localized to the medial tuberosity of the calcaneus at the origin of the plantar fascia; however, patients may be tender further distally and laterally as well. Passive dorsiflexion of the toes tightens the windlass mechanism and will usually exacerbate pain [41]. If partial rupture occurs, it is typically at the medial tuberosity origin. There will be a sudden onset of intense pain with difficulty bearing weight on the plantar surface of the heel. Ecchymosis may be seen along the plantar aspect of the hindfoot and extending to the midfoot due to the hematoma tracking along the fascial planes. The maximal point of tenderness would be at the calcaneal origin or slightly proximal to its insertion, rather than the plantar midfoot.

Work-up

Important in the work-up is considering the other possibilities on the differential diagnosis, as several other entities may cause inferior heel pain.

Tarsal tunnel syndrome is characterized by pain along the medial, plantar aspect of the foot. These patients, however, typically report burning and tingling symptoms, have a positive Tinel sign, and do not have exacerbation of pain with passive toe dorsiflexion [41]. The history will also be different for a tarsal tunnel compressive nerve syndrome for the pain gradually increases while walking and upright or any prolonged standing. Gravity will increase the venous pressure, which will reduce the available space within the tarsal tunnel and cause a gradual increasing pressure-type pain rather than the sharp knifelike pain that warms up over a short period of time of walking. Distinction on history alone is important.

Baxter neuritis is a compression of the first branch of the lateral plantar nerve (nerve to the abductor digiti quinti) and typically presents with plantar medial heel pain similar to plantar fasciitis. Some authors believe that the conditions are often occurring simultaneously. Failure of treatment of plantar fasciitis may necessitate EMG and or MRI evaluation to evaluate Baxter nerve compression and muscular fatty infiltration.

Calcaneal stress fractures can cause significant heel pain but will likely present with swelling and hindfoot warmth. A calcaneal squeeze test with medial and lateral pressure will be painful in a patient with a calcaneal stress fracture, differentiating it from plantar fasciitis [41]. At times the radiologist may read the bone edema at the inferior calcaneal bone spur as a stress fracture or stress reaction, yet this represents more of inflammation of the bony origin of the plantar fascia rather than a stress fracture. Stress fracture of the calcaneus is a different entity, which occurs through the body of the calcaneus. It is a rather rare condition to occur in the athlete. Bone contusions and fat pad contusions can occur in the plantar heel region and have a different presentation to that of plantar fasciitis.

Imaging has a limited role in the diagnosis of plantar fasciitis and is therefore reserved for failures of normal treatment and atypical presentations. X-rays will often be normal, but approximately 50% will demonstrate an infra-calcaneal heel spur [44]. While patients often believe the spur causes plantar fascial pain, it has been demonstrated in cadaveric dissections to occur in the flexor digitorum brevis origin rather than the plantar fascia.

After 4–6 months of nonoperative treatment of plantar fasciitis, advanced imagining should be considered to rule out other pathologies. Ultrasound has been shown to be effective in diagnosing plantar fasciitis and will demonstrate hypoechoic fascia [45]. MRI is arguably most effective and will demonstrate fascial thickening and increased signal intensity in the plantar fascia [46] (Fig. 5.13). MRI can also demonstrate an acute tear and should be obtained if sudden intense symptoms develop, particularly when ecchymosis is noted.

Treatment

For the in-season athlete, treatment of plantar fasciitis is initially nonoperative. Multiple treatments have been studied with variable results, and most clinicians will employ several treatment modalities. It is important to counsel the player from the beginning that plantar fasciitis does typically improve (85–90% of cases) with nonoperative treatments [47, 48], but that complete recovery can take 6–12 months.

Orthoses, physical therapy for Achilles tendon and plantar fascial stretching, injections, night splints, and cast or boot immobilization have all been studied and show varying successes in the literature.

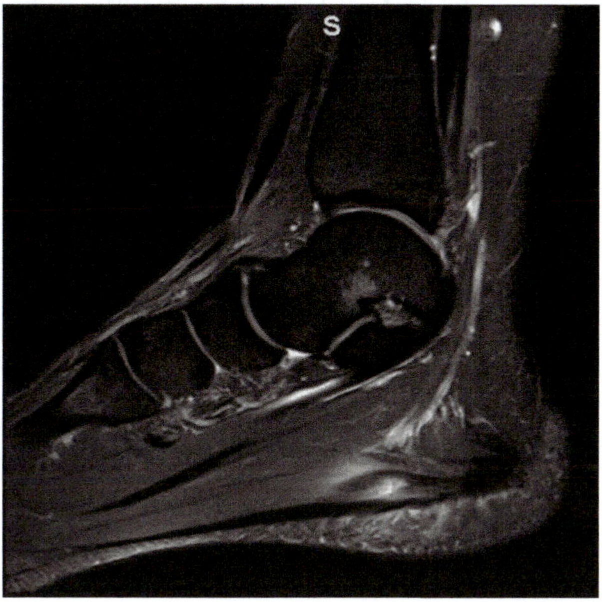

Fig. 5.13 Plantar fasciitis. T2-weighted MRI demonstrating thickening of the plantar fascia with surrounding edema

A reasonable treatment strategy for the in-season athlete would be to begin with over-the-counter cushioned heel inserts, nonsteroidal anti-inflammatories, and a home exercise program of heel cord and plantar fascia-specific stretching. Athletes should do the stretches several times a day but particularly in the morning before getting out of bed and any time after prolonged sitting or lying down. If the athlete would like, a night splint that keeps the ankle and foot dorsiflexed can be tried as well.

If there is no improvement in symptoms after several weeks of these initial management strategies, custom orthoses can be ordered and formal physical therapy can be initiated. Additionally, a corticosteroid injection can be attempted. It is important to note, however, that evidence of effectiveness is limited, and there are risks of plantar fascial rupture and heel pad atrophy [49]. After an injection, the player should be briefly immobilized in a CAM boot to protect from rupture. The player may require several weeks off and immobilization in the boot for protected weight-bearing until symptoms decrease. The exact timing of return to activity depends upon symptom reduction with a gradual return as tolerated.

If symptoms are not improving after several months of nonoperative management, an MRI should be considered to confirm the diagnosis of plantar fasciitis and evaluate for other pathology. If the pain and functional impairment are significant, surgical release can be considered. Surgery involves a partial release of the plantar fascia with or without a decompression of the Baxter nerve. Prior to embarking on a decompression of the distal tarsal tunnel, the authors recommend that objective evidence of nerve compression be proven, for the dissection to decompress this nerve can also lead to additional scarring. Therefore, EMG and nerve conduction studies confirming a nerve compression syndrome should be obtained prior to contemplating a tarsal tunnel release. Release of the plantar fascia alone can be performed endoscopically yet is reserved for chronic cases were significant pain persists despite exhausting nonoperative treatment modalities.

Conclusions

Plantar fasciitis is common in athletes and especially runners. As it is more of a fasciopathy than a true fasciitis, basic treatments aimed at decreasing inflammation are not always effective, and the duration of symptoms can be many months. A combined approach of stretching programs, shoe inserts, physical therapy, and night splints can typically be effective and surgical procedures avoided. However, the athlete should be counseled as to the often-prolonged course, and the clinician should be careful to consider other pathologies.

References

1. Bowers KD, Martin RB. Turf-toe: a shoe-surface related football injury. Med Sci Sports. 1976;8:81–3.
2. Rodeo SA, O'Brien S, Warren RF, Barnes R, Wickiewicz TL, Dillingham MF. Turf-toe: an analysis of metatarsophalangeal joint sprains in professional football players. Am J Sports Med. 1990;18:280–5.
3. Clough TM, Majeed H. Turf toe injury - current concepts and an updated review of literature. Foot Ankle Clin. 2018;23:693–701.
4. George E, Harris AHS, Dragoo JL, Hunt KJ. Incidence and risk factors for turf toe injuries in intercollegiate football: data from the national collegiate athletic association injury surveillance system. Foot Ankle Int. 2014;35:108–15.
5. Clanton TO, Ford JJ. Turf toe injury. Clin Sports Med. 1994;13:731–41.
6. McCormick JJ, Anderson RB. Turf toe: anatomy, diagnosis, and treatment. Sports Health. 2010;2:487–94.
7. Prieskorn D, Graves SC, Smith RA. Morphometric analysis of the plantar plate apparatus of the first metatarsophalangeal joint. Foot Ankle. 1993;14:204–7.
8. McCormick JJ, Anderson RB. The great toe: failed turf toe, chronic turf toe, and complicated sesamoid injuries. Foot Ankle Clin. 2009;14:135–50.
9. Aronow MS. Treatment of the missed Lisfranc injury. Foot Ankle Clin. 2006;11:127–42. ix
10. Weatherford BM, Anderson JG, Bohay DR. Management of tarsometatarsal joint injuries. J Am Acad Orthop Surg. 2017;25:469–79.
11. Eleftheriou KI, Rosenfeld PF. Lisfranc injury in the athlete: evidence supporting management from sprain to fracture dislocation. Foot Ankle Clin. 2013;18:219–36.
12. Ross G, Cronin R, Hauzenblas J, Juliano P. Plantar ecchymosis sign: a clinical aid to diagnosis of occult Lisfranc tarsometatarsal injuries. J Orthop Trauma. 1996;10:119–22.
13. Myerson MS, Fisher RT, Burgess AR, Kenzora JE. Fracture dislocations of the tarsometatarsal joints: end results correlated with pathology and treatment. Foot Ankle. 1986;6:225–42.
14. Coss HS, Manos RE, Buoncristiani A, Mills WJ. Abduction stress and AP weightbearing radiography of purely ligamentous injury in the tarsometatarsal joint. Foot Ankle Int. 1998;19:537–41.

15. Raikin SM, Elias I, Dheer S, Besser MP, Morrison WB, Zoga AC. Prediction of midfoot instability in the subtle Lisfranc injury. Comparison of magnetic resonance imaging with intraoperative findings. J Bone Joint Surg Am. 2009;91:892–9.
16. Petrisor BA, Ekrol I, Court-Brown C. The epidemiology of metatarsal fractures. Foot Ankle Int. 2006;27:172–4.
17. Hasselman CT, Vogt MT, Stone KL, Cauley JA, Conti SF. Foot and ankle fractures in elderly white women. Incidence and risk factors. J Bone Joint Surg Am. 2003;85:820–4.
18. Hong CC, Pearce CJ, Ballal MS, Calder JDF. Management of sports injuries of the foot and ankle: an update. Bone Joint J. 2016;98-B:1299–311.
19. Jones R. I. Fracture of the base of the fifth metatarsal bone by indirect violence. Ann Surg. 1902;35:697–700.2.
20. Lawrence SJ, Botte MJ. Jones' fractures and related fractures of the proximal fifth metatarsal. Foot Ankle. 1993;14:358–65.
21. Smith JW, Arnoczky SP, Hersh A. The intraosseous blood supply of the fifth metatarsal: implications for proximal fracture healing. Foot Ankle. 1992;13:143–52.
22. Miller MD, Thompson SR, editors. Miller's review of orthopaedics. 7th ed. Philadelphia, PA: Elsevier; 2016.
23. Williams DS, McClay IS, Hamill J. Arch structure and injury patterns in runners. Clin Biomech (Bristol, Avon). 2001;16:341–7.
24. Kaufman KR, Brodine SK, Shaffer RA, Johnson CW, Cullison TR. The effect of foot structure and range of motion on musculoskeletal overuse injuries. Am J Sports Med. 1999;27:585–93.
25. Porter DA. Fifth metatarsal jones fractures in the athlete. Foot Ankle Int. 2018;39:250–8.
26. Dameron TB. Fractures and anatomical variations of the proximal portion of the fifth metatarsal. J Bone Joint Surg Am. 1975;57:788–92.
27. Egol K, Walsh M, Rosenblatt K, Capla E, Koval KJ. Avulsion fractures of the fifth metatarsal base: a prospective outcome study. Foot Ankle Int. 2007;28:581–3.
28. Vorlat P, Achtergael W, Haentjens P. Predictors of outcome of non-displaced fractures of the base of the fifth metatarsal. Int Orthop. 2007;31:5–10.
29. Roche AJ, Calder JDF. Treatment and return to sport following a Jones fracture of the fifth metatarsal: a systematic review. Knee Surg Sports Traumatol Arthrosc. 2013;21:1307–15.
30. Ramadorai MUE, Beuchel MW, Sangeorzan BJ. Fractures and dislocations of the tarsal navicular. J Am Acad Orthop Surg. 2016;24:379–89.
31. Brukner P, Bradshaw C, Khan KM, White S, Crossley K. Stress fractures: a review of 180 cases. Clin J Sport Med. 1996;6:85–9.
32. McKeon KE, McCormick JJ, Johnson JE, Klein SE. Intraosseous and extraosseous arterial anatomy of the adult navicular. Foot Ankle Int. 2012;33:857–61.
33. Burne SG, Mahoney CM, Forster BB, Koehle MS, Taunton JE, Khan KM. Tarsal navicular stress injury: long-term outcome and clinicoradiological correlation using both computed tomography and magnetic resonance imaging. Am J Sports Med. 2005;33:1875–81.
34. Khan KM, Fuller PJ, Brukner PD, Kearney C, Burry HC. Outcome of conservative and surgical management of navicular stress fracture in athletes. Eighty-six cases proven with computerized tomography. Am J Sports Med. 1992;20:657–66.
35. Torg JS, Moyer J, Gaughan JP, Boden BP. Management of tarsal navicular stress fractures: conservative versus surgical treatment: a meta-analysis. Am J Sports Med. 2010;38:1048–53.
36. Potter NJ, Brukner PD, Makdissi M, Crossley K, Kiss ZS, Bradshaw C. Navicular stress fractures: outcomes of surgical and conservative management. Br J Sports Med. 2006;40:692–5; discussion 695
37. Saxena A, Fullem B. Navicular stress fractures: a prospective study on athletes. Foot Ankle Int. 2006;27:917–21.
38. Crawford F, Thomson C. Interventions for treating plantar heel pain. Cochrane Database Syst Rev. 2003:CD000416.

39. Schneider HP, Baca JM, Carpenter BB, Dayton PD, Fleischer AE, Sachs BD. American college of foot and ankle surgeons clinical consensus statement: diagnosis and treatment of adult acquired infracalcaneal heel pain. J Foot Ankle Surg. 2018;57:370–81.
40. Sarrafian SK. Functional characteristics of the foot and plantar aponeurosis under tibiotalar loading. Foot Ankle. 1987;8:4–18.
41. Neufeld SK, Cerrato R. Plantar fasciitis: evaluation and treatment. J Am Acad Orthop Surg. 2008;16:338–46.
42. Lemont H, Ammirati KM, Usen N. Plantar fasciitis: a degenerative process (fasciosis) without inflammation. J Am Podiatr Med Assoc. 2003;93:234–7.
43. Buchbinder R. Clinical practice. Plantar fasciitis. N Engl J Med. 2004;350:2159–66.
44. Davies MS, Weiss GA, Saxby TS. Plantar fasciitis: how successful is surgical intervention? Foot Ankle Int. 1999;20:803–7.
45. Akfirat M, Sen C, Günes T. Ultrasonographic appearance of the plantar fasciitis. Clin Imaging. 2003;27:353–7.
46. Berkowitz JF, Kier R, Rudicel S. Plantar fasciitis: MR imaging. Radiology. 1991;179:665–7.
47. null G. Plantar fasciitis: diagnosis and conservative management. J Am Acad Orthop Surg. 1997;5:109–17.
48. Martin RL, Irrgang JJ, Conti SF. Outcome study of subjects with insertional plantar fasciitis. Foot Ankle Int. 1998;19:803–11.
49. Acevedo JI, Beskin JL. Complications of plantar fascia rupture associated with corticosteroid injection. Foot Ankle Int. 1998;19:91–7.

Muscle Strains in Football

6

Jeffrey Guy and Alex Wagner

Introduction

Epidemiology

American football is an extremely popular sport involving sudden bursts of maximal exertion, high-impact collisions, frequent direction changes, and intense training workloads. American football remains popular with more than 100,000 collegiate athletes and 1 million high school athletes [1]. At the collegiate level, the national estimate of athlete exposures exceeds 5 million [2]. American football remains one of the highest-risk sports for injuries. A surveillance of injuries from 2009–2010 through 2013–2014 estimated an average annual number of injuries of 47,199, accounting for an estimated injury rate per 1000 athlete exposures of 9.2 (9.0–9.4) (cdc mmw article). Injury surveillance shows that muscle strains are the third most common injury in competition, accounting for 12.1% of injuries, the second most common injury in scrimmages accounting for 15.7% of injuries, and the most common injury in regular practices accounting for 26% of injuries [3]. It is interesting to note that compared to all football injuries, which have high rates in competition, muscle strain injuries are more common in practice [3].

Second to strains, muscle contusions are the most frequent muscle injury. Current injury surveillance systems do not delineate muscle from soft tissue contusions, but it is well known that contusions account for a large proportion of injuries. NCAA data shows that contusions account for 16.3% of injuries in competition, 12.5% of

J. Guy (✉)
University of South Carolina School of Medicine, Prisma Health Department of Orthopedic Surgery, Columbia, SC, USA

Orthopedic Surgery, University of South Carolina, Columbia, SC, USA

A. Wagner
Prisma Health/University of South Carolina Sports Medicine Fellowship, Prisma Health Department of Family and Preventative Medicine, Columbia, SC, USA

K. W. Farmer (ed.), *Football Injuries*,
https://doi.org/10.1007/978-3-030-54875-9_6

injuries in scrimmage, and 10.1% of injuries in regular practice [3]. Epidemiological studies of high school football players demonstrate consistent data with contusions being the second most common injury, accounting for 12.7–15.9% of injuries [4].

Data regarding muscle injury in the NFL is similar to the reported high school and collegiate level. In a single NFL team, 46% of practice injuries were muscle strains [5]. Injuries to hamstring and quadriceps muscle account for 13% of all injuries among NFL players [5]. Surveillance of one NFL team over 10 years revealed a hamstring injury rate of 1.79 per 1000 athlete exposures for practices and 4.07 per 1000 athlete exposures for games [6].

Cumulatively, muscle strain and injuries account for 53–65% of all injuries sustained at high level of football participation [1]. The injury severity of muscle strains and contusions vary based on location. Lower-extremity injuries are the most common, accounting for approximately 28% of all injuries [1]. The burden of injury is varied based on the location. In a study of one NFL team's training camp injuries, hamstring strains led to the most days lost at 8.3, second only to knee sprains. Additionally, both hip flexor strains (6.6 days) and quadricep strains (5.4 days) accounted for greater than 5 days missed [1]. Additional muscle injuries leading to lost days include lumbar strain (4.9 days), groin strain (4.8 days), Achilles strain (3.8 days), and contusions (3.2 days) [1].

Based on the frequency and burden of muscle injuries, timely and accurate diagnosis is important in order to promptly institute.

Etiology and Risk Factors

The underlying etiology of muscle injuries is multifactorial. As indicated by the incidence, certain muscles are more prone to injuries. Muscles at the highest risk of injury share common underlying characteristics. Muscles in which the origin crosses two joints are at increased risk of muscle injury [7]. The increased susceptibility to injury is due to the muscle's activity on limiting range of motion of the joint they cross. Additionally, muscles that are used for rapid acceleration and quick movements have a higher percentage of type II fibers and are at increased risk of injury [7]. Since football mainly consists of these types of movements and plays, the incidence of muscle injuries is not surprising.

There are additional modifiable risk factors for muscle injuries that are important to identify. Inadequate preparation due to deconditioning, inadequate warm-up, fatigue, and dehydration are all important modifiable risk factors [8]. Specific lower-extremity muscle strains have been found to share similar risk factors. Previous injuries to hamstrings, quadriceps, and calf muscles, both recent (<8 weeks ago) and remote, are significant risk factors for repeat injury in the same, previously injured muscle [9]. Additionally, past calf injury has been implicated in muscle injuries to both the quadriceps muscles and hamstring muscles [9].

Biomechanics of Injury

Muscle injury typically occurs via two main mechanisms, either direct injury or indirect injury. Direct injury, including direct trauma to the muscle, causes compression against underlying bone which can lead to a spectrum of muscle injuries [MRI]. A three-stage clinical grading system has been defined categorizing contusions as mild, moderate, and severe [10]. Mild contusion consists of loss of range of motion of one-third normal motion, moderate contusion has a loss of range of motion by one-third to two-thirds normal motion, and severe contusion accounts for a greater than two-thirds loss of normal motion [10].

Indirect injury occurs through forcible stretching of muscle fibers. This stretching disrupts the normal architecture of muscle fibers. This most commonly occurs at the musculotendinous junction, which, in skeletally mature patients, is the weakest and most vulnerable site for muscle strain [11]. Muscle strain more commonly occurs during the eccentric phase of contraction when the muscle is lengthening as it contracts. The eccentric contraction generates greater forces than concentric contraction disrupting the normal connective tissue architecture and leading to injury [11].

No universal grading system for muscle strains has been developed. A three-stage grading system was originally described for the classification of quadriceps injury and has been adapted to classify injuries to other muscles. This original grading system describes a grade I injury as a tear of a few muscle fibers with the fascia remaining intact. Grade II injuries describe a tear of a moderate number of fibers without disrupting the fascia. Grade III injuries are a tear of many fibers with partial tearing of the fascia [12]. This initial grading system has been refined, with the most commonly used system incorporating loss of function. This grading system describes a grade I injury as a small tear with <5% loss of function, a grade II injury as a larger tear with 5–50% loss of function, and a grade III injury as >50% loss of function [10].

Clinical Evaluation

Obtaining a relevant clinical history is important in diagnosing acute muscle injuries. A typical history of muscle strain will involve an acute painful episode during an episode of intense exertion [11]. The history for a muscle contusion will typically include a history of a direct blow to the muscle. Not all acute injuries will cause cessation of activity. Ability to continue to participate is typically dependent on severity [11]. History should also focus on the listed risk factors above to help provide a complete clinical picture.

Physical examination of acute muscle injuries should include general inspection, range of motion, and strength. General inspection may reveal superficial ecchymosis and swelling. This is not always present as muscle contusions tend to occur at the muscle-bone interface [MRI]. In the setting of complete muscle tears, a palpable defect may be present. Less severe injuries may have less drastic physical exam findings. Range of motion and strength compared to the unaffected side are important physical exam findings to note. Depending on the severity of injury, range of motion may only be minimally affected. It is important to monitor for pain with active range of motion, especially in the eccentric phase. The affected side will demonstrate weakness compared to the unaffected side, more attributable to decreased central drive due to pain compared to actual muscle damage [11].

Imaging

Plain radiographs and computed tomography have only limited capability in evaluation of acute muscle injuries due to their general poor visualization of soft tissue. Subtle findings such as soft tissue swelling on plain radiographs may be present but has limited diagnostic utility. CT imaging may potentially show acute hemorrhage into injured muscles, but imaging of acute muscle injuries is better pursued through alternative modalities. Ultrasound and magnetic resonance imaging (MRI) are the typically preferred imaging modality due to their ability to detect and localize acute injuries.

Ultrasound

Prior to the development of MRI, ultrasound was the best available tool for evaluation of muscle injury [13]. Due to the clear disadvantage of user dependence, MRI has become more popular in the imaging of musculoskeletal disorders, including sports-related muscle injury [14]. However, due to increased availability and portability of ultrasound, as well as increased education on ultrasound, sonography has become increasingly popular in the evaluation of acute muscle injuries. Advantages of ultrasound compared to MRI include superior spatial resolution, cost, convenience, portability, dynamic evaluation of the injury, and the ability to perform simultaneous intervention [10, 14].

Identification of muscle contusions on ultrasound demonstrates an ill-defined area of hyperechogenicity [10]. Comparison with contralateral muscles of similar location can be useful in identifying the general hyperechoic nature of a contused muscle. In the acute phase of the injury, the area of injury within the muscle may be isoechoic with adjacent unaffected muscle [15]. In the setting of significant direct trauma, muscle hematoma is likely. On ultrasound, this is identified as a hypoechoic fluid collection surrounded by irregular muscle fibers. In the first 24–48 hours, the muscle tissue surrounding the fluid collection may have increased reflectivity, but after 48–72 hours, the hematoma organizes demonstrating a clear echogenic margin [10]. Because of this, the ideal timing of initial ultrasound examination is between 2 and 48 hours [13].

In the evaluation of indirect muscle injuries, ultrasound has been proven to be equivalent to MRI in the sensitivity of detection of acute muscle injury [16]. A three-stage grading system for identification of muscle strain injury has been well established [13]. Grade I injury can be normal on ultrasound or can demonstrate focal or general areas of increased echogenicity involving <5% of the muscle substance [13]. Grade II injury involves a disruption of >5% but <100% of muscle fibers on a cross-sectional view and typically is accompanied by an intramuscular fluid collection [13]. In a grade III injury, or a complete rupture, there is complete discontinuity of the muscle at the musculotendinous junction with the presence of intermuscular and perifascial fluid as well as hyperechogenicity of surrounding muscle [10].

In addition to acute evaluation of suspected muscle injuries, ultrasound can be used to dynamically guide therapeutic interventions. Ultrasound-guided hematoma evacuation allows for increased accuracy and needle placement to minimize procedural pain. Ultrasound-guided needle placement is useful to ensure appropriate site delivery of biologics which have shown a recent increased role in treatment of muscle injuries.

Additionally, recent data has suggested sonography as a tool to guide clinical progression and reduce recurrent rate of thigh muscle strains. A muscle injury return to play protocol has been proposed to use ultrasound, not only in the initial diagnostic setting but also once an athlete has rehabbed to 80% of speed/power to evaluate the presence of residual hematoma, lack of functional contraction, or presence of hyperemia. High-risk ultrasound findings at 80% speed/power including residual hematoma or lack of functional contraction would prevent an athlete from progressing, mitigating risk for reinjury. Presence of persistent hyperemia is only considered an intermediate risk factor allowing an athlete to progress slowly under careful supervision. The development of this protocol was admittedly based on experiential data and the authors acknowledge the need for a prospective study to validate this approach [14].

Magnetic Resonance Imaging

Used in increasing frequency for muscular injuries, MRI provides excellent lesion detection and localization of injury [10]. MRI has been shown to have high-contrast resolution, high sensitivity, and the ability to image in multiple planes. MRI is the imaging modality of choice to confirm and evaluate the extent and severity of injury [16]. MRI imaging protocols vary from institution to institution. Necessary imaging sequences should include a fat-suppressed fluid-sensitive sequence, such as a short tau inversion recovery (STIR), fat-saturated proton density-weighted imaging, or T2-weighted imaging [10, 17]. These images are more sensitive for the identification of muscle edema or hemorrhage [10].

In the identification of muscle contusions and hematomas, there is a characteristic feather-like high signal with the muscle on fat-suppressed fluid-sensitive sequences. There is diffusely high signal present on fluid-sensitive sequences of

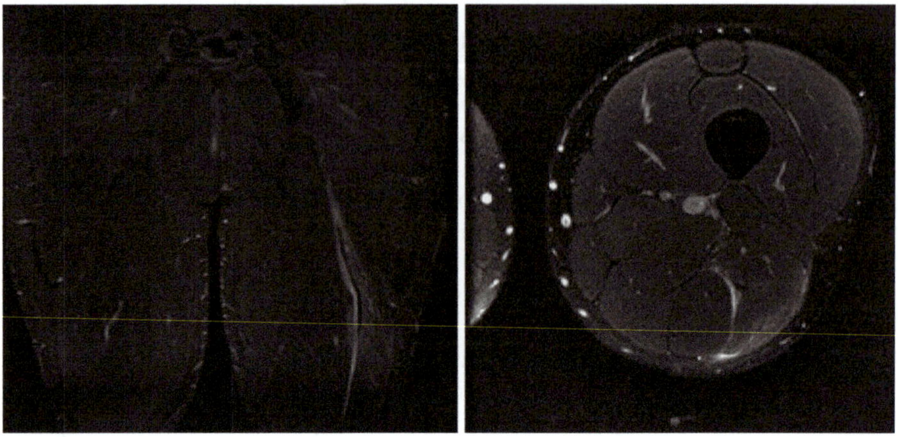

Fig. 6.1 Coronal and axial views of a grade I semitendinosus muscle tear. Note the perifascial fluid without disruption of normal muscular architecture

images obtained after 48 hours after acute injury. Grading of muscle strain injury on MRI follows the general principles outlined above in clinical grading and imaging with ultrasound. Grade I strains, as shown in Fig. 6.1, demonstrate increased signal on fluid-sensitive sequences due to edema in the muscle as well as potential perifascial fluid. The hallmark of grade I strains include the lack of significant disruption of muscle architect, <5% on cross-sectional area. Grade II strains demonstrate a distortion of normal muscle architecture with associated muscular hematoma. Grade III strains demonstrate complete disruption of the musculotendinous junction with accumulation of hematoma between the two [10].

Recent reviews have looked to assess the prognostic ability of MRI in determining reinjury risk as well as identifying predictors for return to play and performance [17, 18]. Based on current evidence, there is no strong evidence for any MRI findings at the time of injury or at the time of return to play as a predictor for hamstring reinjury risk [18]. There is, however, moderate evidence that intratendinous injuries on MRI at the time of injury are associated with higher reinjury risk [18].

In the evaluation of predicting return to play of calf muscle injuries, more extensive involvement of connective tissue is associated with prolonged time to return to play [19]. Current evidence indicates that injuries involving large muscle volume, length, or surface as well as those with central tendon involvement result in a longer return to play [17]. A study specifically on football players who do not have MR evidence of injury but only clinical findings (those with grade 0 to grade I injuries) shows a shorter period of return to play. Unfortunately, there is limited evidence on MRI factors on predicting return to play in grade II–III muscle injuries [17].

Treatment

As noted above, acute muscle injuries can lead to prolonged loss of football participation. Minor injuries can be healed in 1 week but more severe injuries can require 4–8 weeks of healing [11]. Because of this potential for prolonged healing, the identification and utilization of proper treatment modalities are important to try and maximize an athlete's in-season participation. Additionally, it is important to utilize proper therapy in order to ensure adequate healing to prevent repeat injury. One study showed that recurrent or repeat injuries are more severe than the initial injury and cause the most time lost from sports participation [20].

Acute management with relative immobilization, rest, ice, compression, and elevation have been utilized as the initial treatment modalities based mostly on experiential data without significant clinical studies. Despite logical and physiological basis for their use, there is no significant scientific evidence for these initial treatment modalities.

RICE – Rest, Ice, Compression, and Elevation

The concept of rest after an acute muscle injury promotes pain control. A brief period of relative immobilization should be utilized to allow scar tissue to begin forming connections between the injured muscle fibers. Prolonged immobilization, however, leads to decreased muscle volume, structure, and function with reorganization of sarcomeres [7]. Clinical studies have shown a 20% decrease in muscle strength after only 1 week of immobilization [7]. Additionally, a high incidence of myositis ossificans has been demonstrated with prolonged immobilization [21]. Conversely, mobilization of the injured muscle too early does not allow adequate scar formation to provide the scaffolding for muscle healing and increases the risk of repeat injury [22].

Ideally, relative immobilization and rest for less than 1 week should be employed and gradual return to submaximal activity and motion should be initiated, limited on the basis of pain. Injuries to the lower extremity should be supported with crutches for limited to non-weight-bearing during the time of rest. After this brief period of immobilization, supervised, cautious active mobility should be started. It has been shown that early tensile loading stimulates collagen fiber growth and realignment and early mobilization promotes decreased muscle adhesion formation and more rapid recovery of proprioception [7].

In addition to early immobilization and relative rest, cryotherapy, or the application of ice, plays an important role in the management of muscle injuries. There has been controversy on the true physiologic effect of cryotherapy. Studies have shown that the application of ice to below 15 °C leads to increased permeability causing increased swelling [7]. Additional studies have shown that cryotherapy leads to vasoconstriction with decreased transient perfusion but without long-term changes on muscular microcirculation [23]. In addition, several studies have looked at the role of cryotherapy on inflammation without development of a consensus. Some studies have shown that ice decreases inflammation while other studies have demonstrated an increase in inflammation with ice [7]. Despite this controversy on the effect of cryotherapy on swelling and inflammation, application of ice has been consistently shown to provide an analgesic effect. This analgesic effect can be helpful for early mobilization of the injured extremity to allow for participation in early rehab. Due to its simplicity and relative low risk of treatment, as well as its analgesic benefit, cryotherapy in the initial phase of treatment is still recommended and a mainstay of muscle injury treatment.

Compression and elevation are mainstays of treatment of many, if not all, musculoskeletal injuries. In the setting of acute muscle injuries, it is thought that the application of compression leads to decreased hematoma formation and promotes hematoma reabsorption. This has not been systematically studied but does have logical and physiologic basis for use. Studies have proven decreased muscular blood flow with compression but no sound evidence relating this to accelerated healing [24]. Compression with cryotherapy compared to cryotherapy alone has shown benefit in improved pain control in patients post-ACL reconstruction, but no studies have been performed in the evaluation of muscle injuries. The low risk of harm, the simplicity of the intervention, and the understanding of the benefits of compression make compression an important treatment intervention in the management of acute muscle injury.

Physical Therapy

As previously discussed, a limited period of immobilization with relative early motion is optimal for muscle injury recovery. Early rehabilitation has been shown to be crucial for a faster clinical recovery to sports [25]. One study in recreational athletes with lower-extremity muscle strains demonstrated a decreased return to sport interval by 3 weeks in a group starting rehabilitation at 2 days post injury compared to 9 days post injury [25]. The overall goals of physical therapy are to promote healing, restore full range of motion and strength, and prepare for return to sports specific training. Typically, rehab has focused on four main stages static stretching, isometric loading, dynamic loading with increased resistance, and functional exercises combined with heavy strength training [25].

Therapy protocols can typically be divided into five phases: phase I or the acute phase, phase II or the subacute phase, phase III or the remodeling phase, phase IV or the functional phase, and phase V which is return to competition. The duration in each stage is variable. The acute phase focuses on RICE therapy as discussed above and is utilized for approximately 1–7 days until signs of inflammation begin to resolve. The subacute phase can begin when swelling and pain begin to resolve or improve. This phase focuses on the return of full range of motion and, once without pain, can progress to regular concentric strength exercises. Submaximal isometric contraction is utilized in this phase and begins at 3 days to >3 weeks of injury. The remodeling phase is when hamstring stretching can begin and occurs at 1–6 weeks after injury during severity. During this phase, range of motion needs to be pain-free and the focus is on strengthening and flexibility. Frequent daily stretching at this phase has been shown to regain full range of motion and have a decreased total rehabilitation program. In this third phase of therapy, eccentric exercises can be performed. The functional phase of rehab occurs at 2 weeks to 6 months after injury with the goal to return to sport. Further increases in hamstring flexibility and strength are developed to reach normal values. In this stage, a progression from pain-free jogging to sprinting is utilized. Phase V, return to competition, typically occurs at 3 weeks to 6 months and focuses on maintaining strength and flexibility to prevent reinjury [26].

In addition to these injury location specific exercises, data has shown the importance of programs focused on trunk stabilization and progressive agility training [27]. Programs focused on trunk stabilization and progressive agility training have been shown to be more effective in promoting return to sports and preventing reinjury in hamstring injuries [27]. Thus, rehab that incorporates trunk stabilization and progressive agility training should be an important part of treatment.

Pharmacologic Treatment

Inflammation is an important factor in the setting of acute muscle injuries. It is thought that inflammation produces signals that trigger the healing cascade. However, it is well known that inflammation can be a contributing factor to pain. Management with anti-inflammatories is a reasonable treatment option. There have been few randomized control trials looking at the use of both nonsteroidal anti-inflammatories (NSAIDs) and glucocorticoids in the treatment of muscle injuries [22].

NSAIDs are commonly used in acute muscle injuries. A systematic review of the literature in human studies shows that acute use of NSAIDs can improve the recovery from acute muscle injury by reducing strength loss, soreness, and blood CK level [28]. Additionally, in experimental models, short-term use of NSAIDs has been demonstrated to decrease the inflammatory cell reaction without adverse effects on the healing process, tensile strength, ability of the injured muscle to contract, or myofiber regeneration [22]. Experimental data in animal models suggest that NSAID administration may have adverse effects in the healing of acute muscle injuries; however, there is no evidence to suggest such effects in human studies [28]. Based on this data, it is therefore reasonable to utilize NSAIDs both in the acute management of acute muscle injuries to decrease acute inflammation and throughout the rehabilitation process in an as needed fashion.

Corticosteroid use in acute injury seems to have negative effects in the healing process of acute muscle injuries. A study of systemic corticosteroids has shown initial benefit in muscle injury with decreased initial inflammation and increased force generating capacity but, in later effects, included delayed clearing of necrotic tissue and normal healing response as well as delayed muscle regeneration [21]. Intramuscular corticosteroid injection has also not been well studied. A retrospective study without objective results did demonstrate that in NFL athletes with hamstring strains, corticosteroids did not produce any adverse effects [29]. This study only highlights the potential safety of intra-injury injections but is unable to draw any conclusions regarding efficacy. At this time, the body of evidence supporting corticosteroid use for acute muscle injuries is insufficient.

Platelet-Rich Plasma Therapy

An evolving therapeutic modality, platelet-rich plasma (PRP) therapy, has an exciting potential for treatment of acute muscle injuries to expedite the healing process. Animal model studies have theorized that the abundance of growth factors and cytokines in PRP induces cell proliferation and migration, increases angiogenesis, and enhances muscle tissue regeneration [30–32]. A systematic review by Kunze et al. evaluated 21 studies looking at the basic science effects of PRP in vitro and in vivo models [33]. The review of these basic science studies shows that PRP treatment leads to an increased myocyte proliferation, growth factor expression, leukocyte recruitment, and angiogenesis in muscle model which demonstrates that PRP has the potential to serve as an effective treatment modality to expedite healing of the muscular pathology [33].

Clinical studies, however, have shown conflicting results. A systematic review by Grassi et al. evaluated eight randomized control trials using PRP for muscle injuries. Significant study outcomes for PRP treatment included return to sport, reinjuries, pain, strength, and complications. Of the reviewed studies reporting each outcome, there was no significant difference in reinjury, reported complications, and strength. Conflicting results for pain were reported with three studies reporting better pain outcomes with PRP compared to control and two studies demonstrating no difference. Most interestingly, across six reviewed studies, a random-effect meta-analysis revealed a significant mean difference −7.17 days in favor of PRP. This effect was noted to be not statistically significant when comparing the data from the only two double-blinded studies [34].

While promising basic science evidence exists for the use of PRP for muscle injuries, clinical application lacks robust evidence. The difficulty with extrapolating PRP research into clinical practice is multifactorial. First, the term PRP has a wide definition across the literature in regard to formulation including preparation and contents. Oftentimes, studies either fail to report the preparation and composition of their PRP or they are not an easily reproducible formulation making translation to clinical utility difficult. Additionally, current clinical research is underpowered. While RTP was able to demonstrate a significantly improved time to return, the overall quality of this evidence according to the grade guidelines was reported as low due the limited number of studies and their biases [34].

As PRP continues to be studied, there may be an increase in evidence for its clinical utility. Despite observed anecdotal success, the evidence recommending treatment of muscle injuries with PRP is considered low quality.

Surgical Management

While muscle injuries continue to plague the sport of football, early identification and severity of injury remain critical to the safe return of play of the athlete. Early evaluation in terms of mechanism of injury, physical exam, and imaging including possible ultrasound, CAT scans, and/or an MRI may be necessary to qualify an injury and determine timing for a safe return to play. The interpretation of results is key to not only determine a safe return to play but also minimize the risk of reinjury. Given the difficulty in qualifying muscle injuries as well as the inherent pressure from athletes and the coaching staff to return to play, we will continue to see muscle injuries near the top of our injury lists.

While the majority of muscle injuries can be managed adequately with conservative treatments there are occasions where surgical interventions may have to be considered. There is no consensus as to when a surgical approach should be implemented; however, most common seem to be centered around an intra/intermuscular hematoma and/or the development of subsequent compartment syndrome. Reports of primary repair of muscle fibers are rare and technically challenging. Myositis ossificans is a late complication of muscle injury may also result in surgical necessity.

Muscle injuries resulting in hematoma formation can occur with either a direct trauma or contusion or indirectly following a tear of muscle fibers most commonly during an eccentric load to the muscle fibers. The resulting localized bleeding can form a hematoma as demonstrated in Fig. 6.2 below. They also generate increased pressure in the area. Early evaluation at the time of injury is typically characterized by a sensation of a "pop" by the athletes as well as an immediate termination of

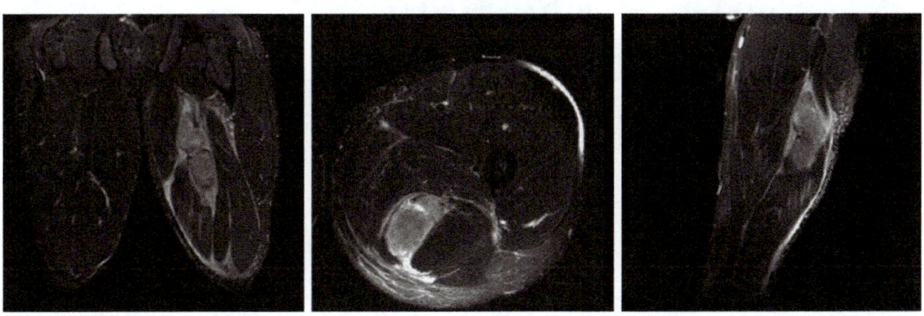

Fig. 6.2 MRI findings consistent with a high grade II vs. grade III adductor tear with large hematoma collection

activity and disability requiring assisted mobilization. Physical exam may result in a palpable defect and then inability to sustain a contraction of the involved muscle group. High grade II (partial tear) or grade III (complete tear) are at risk for bleeding and hematoma formation [35, 36]. Repeat injury to a muscle that was previously considered a lower grade injury is also at great risk. Hematoma formation should be considered in an extremity with increasing girth of the extremity over the first 24 hours as well as increasing pain. Further imaging may be necessary if this level of disability exists.

The prognosis of muscular hematoma is generally good; however, poor prognosis indicators include the increasing size and fluctuating muscle swelling after 24 hours, persistent swelling after 48–72 hours, increasing pain intensity, extension of tenderness from the site of injury, and/or persistent restricted motion of the limb involved [37].

In the event of worsening symptoms, surgical hematoma decompression should be considered. Operative drainage of the hematoma can typically be done with a small incision, therefore minimizing the chance for further or recurrent bleeding (Fig. 6.3). CT or MRI of the extremity can be helpful in determining the best surgical approach. While there is no specific rule to the timing of surgical intervention, allowing the bleeding to stabilize prior to surgical intervention would be optimal. In the event the athlete developed increasing pain, diminished pulses, and/or paresthesia, a development compartment syndrome should be considered. Surgical intervention in this setting should be considered immediate and may also require a compartment release fasciotomy.

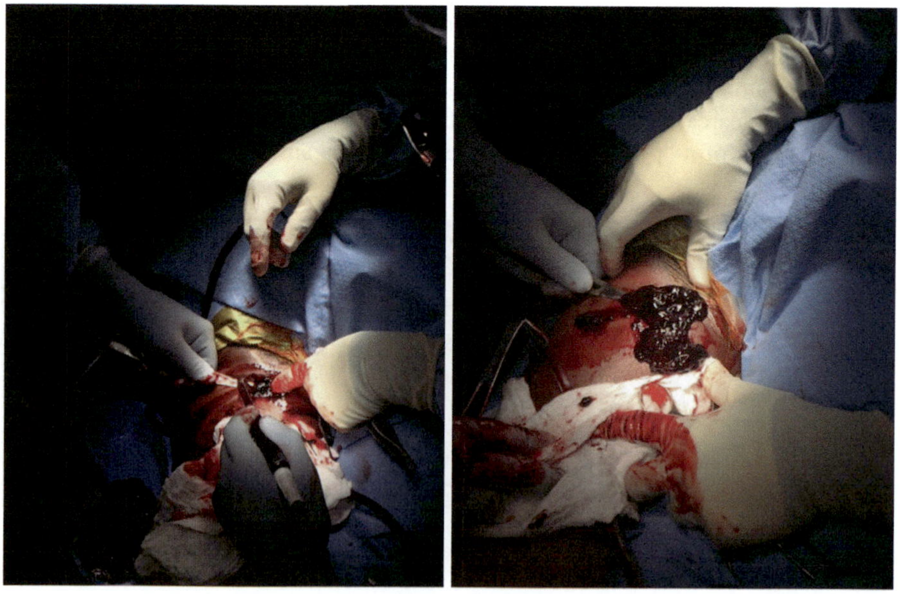

Fig. 6.3 Surgical exploration and decompression of large hematoma from hamstring tendon

Myositis ossificans can be a serious and painful complication after muscle injury. The offending injury can occur from a single blow to the extremity or repeated lower-level injuries to the same area. The periosteal calcifications within the muscle can be diagnosed on serial X-rays usually seen 4–6 weeks after the injury. Athletes typically experience moderate tenderness, swelling, loss of motion, and palpable hardening of the tissues in the area [38]. While typically myositis ossificans is managed conservatively, some athletes develop permanent limitations of motion, persistent pain, and loss of function. These athletes may require surgical intervention to remove the bone. Surgery is not typically attempted prior to 4–6 months after the offending injury to allow for complete maturation of the excess bone in order to minimize recurrence [39].

References

1. Feeley BT, Kennelly S, Barnes RP, Muller MS, Kelly BT, Rodeo SA, et al. Epidemiology of national football league training camp injuries from 1998 to 2007. Am J Sports Med. 2008;36(8):1597–603.
2. Kerr ZY, Marshall SW, Dompier TP, Corlette J, Klossner DA, Gilchrist J. College sports-related injuries - United States, 2009-2010 through 2013-14 academic years. MMWR Morb Mortal Wkly Rep. 2015;64(48):1330–6.
3. Kerr ZY, Simon JE, Grooms DR, Roos KG, Cohen RP, Dompier TP. Epidemiology of football injuries in the national collegiate athletic association, 2004-2005 to 2008-2009. Orthop J Sports Med. 2016;4(9):232596711666450.
4. Rechel JA, Yard EE, Comstock RD. An epidemiologic comparison of high school sports injuries sustained in practice and competition. J Athl Train. 2008;43(2):197–204.
5. Lawrence DW, Hutchison MG, Comper P. Descriptive epidemiology of musculoskeletal injuries and concussions in the national football league, 2012-2014. Orthop J Sports Med. 2015;3(5):232596711558365.
6. Elliott MCCW, Zarins B, Powell JW, Kenyon CD. Hamstring muscle strains in professional football players: a 10-year review. Am J Sports Med. 2011;39(4):843–50.
7. Noonan TJ, Garrett WE. Muscle strain injury: diagnosis and treatment. J Am Acad Orthop Surg. 1999;7(4):262–9.
8. Arner JW, McClincy MP, Bradley JP. Hamstring injuries in athletes: evidence-based treatment. J Am Acad Orthop Surg. 2019;27(23):868–77.
9. Orchard JW. Intrinsic and extrinsic risk factors for muscle strains in Australian football. Am J Sports Med. 2001;29(3):300–3.
10. Lee JC, Mitchell AWM, Healy JC. Imaging of muscle injury in the elite athlete. BJR. 2012;85(1016):1173–85.
11. Garrett WE. Muscle strain injuries: clinical and basic aspects. Med Sci Sports Exerc. 1990;22(3):436–43.
12. Ryan AJ. Quadriceps strain, rupture, and charlie horse. Med Sci Sports. 1969;1(2):106–11.
13. Peetrons P. Ultrasound of muscles. Eur Radiol. 2002 Jan;12(1):35–43.
14. Hall MM. Return to play after thigh muscle injury: utility of serial ultrasound in guiding clinical progression. Curr Sports Med Rep. 2018;17(9):296–301.
15. Aspelin P, Ekberg O, Thorsson O, Wilhelmsson M, Westlin N. Ultrasound examination of soft tissue injury of the lower limb in athletes. Am J Sports Med. 1992;20(5):601–3.
16. Connell DA, Schneider-Kolsky ME, Hoving JL, Malara F, Buchbinder R, Koulouris G, et al. Longitudinal study comparing sonographic and MRI assessments of acute and healing hamstring injuries. Am J Roentgenol. 2004;183(4):975–84.

17. Kumaravel M, Bawa P, Murai N. Magnetic resonance imaging of muscle injury in elite American football players: predictors for return to play and performance. Eur J Radiol. 2018;108:155–64.
18. van Heumen M, Tol JL, de Vos R-J, Moen MH, Weir A, Orchard J, et al. The prognostic value of MRI in determining reinjury risk following acute hamstring injury: a systematic review. Br J Sports Med. 2017;51(18):1355–63.
19. Prakash A, Entwisle T, Schneider M, Brukner P, Connell D. Connective tissue injury in calf muscle tears and return to play: MRI correlation. Br J Sports Med. 2018;52(14):929–33.
20. Brooks JHM, Fuller CW, Kemp SPT, Reddin DB. Incidence, risk, and prevention of hamstring muscle injuries in professional rugby union. Am J Sports Med. 2006;34(8):1297–306.
21. Beiner JM, Jokl P. Muscle contusion injuries: current treatment options. J Am Acad Orthop Surg. 2001;9(4):227–37.
22. Järvinen TAH, Järvinen TLN, Kääriäinen M, Äärimaa V, Vaittinen S, Kalimo H, et al. Muscle injuries: optimising recovery. Best Pract Res Clin Rheumatol. 2007;21(2):317–31.
23. Smith TL, Curl WW, George C, Rosencrance E. Effects of contusion and cryotherapy on microvascular perfusion in rat dorsal skeletal muscle. Pathophysiology. 1994;1(4):229–33.
24. Thorsson O, Lilja B, Nilsson P, Westlin N. Immediate external compression in the management of an acute muscle injury. Scand J Med Sci Sports. 2007;7(3):182–90.
25. Bayer ML, Magnusson SP, Kjaer M. Early versus delayed rehabilitation after acute muscle injury. N Engl J Med. 2017;377(13):1300–1.
26. Petersen J. Evidence based prevention of hamstring injuries in sport. Br J Sports Med. 2005;39(6):319–23.
27. Sherry MA, Best TM. A comparison of 2 rehabilitation programs in the treatment of acute hamstring strains. J Orthop Sports Phys Ther. 2004;34(3):10.
28. Morelli KM, Brown LB, Warren GL. Effect of NSAIDs on recovery from acute skeletal muscle injury: a systematic review and meta-analysis. Am J Sports Med. 2018;46(1):224–33.
29. Levine WN, Bergfeld JA, Tessendorf W, Moorman CT. Intramuscular corticosteroid injection for hamstring injuries: a 13-year experience in the national football league. Am J Sports Med. 2000;28(3):297–300.
30. Hammond JW, Hinton RY, Curl LA, Muriel JM, Lovering RM. Use of autologous platelet-rich plasma to treat muscle strain injuries. Am J Sports Med. 2009;37:1135–42.
31. Mazzocca AD, McCarthy MB, Chowaniec DM, Dugdale EM, Hansen D, Cote MP, Bradley JP, Romeo AA, Arciero RA, Beitzel K. The positive effects of different platelet-rich plasma methods on human muscle, bone, and tendon cells. Am J Sports Med. 2012;40:1742–9.
32. Quarteiro ML, Tognini JR, de Oliveira EL, Silveira I. The effect of platelet-rich plasma on the repair of muscle injuries in rats. Rev Bras Ortop. 2015;50:586–95.
33. Nunze KN, Hannon CP, Fialkoff JD, Frank RM, Cole BJ. Platelet-rich plasma for muscle injuries: a systematic review of the basic science literature. World J Orthop. 2019;10(7):278–91.
34. Grassi A, Napoli G, Romandini I, Samuelsson K, Zaffagnini S, Candrian C, Filardo G. Is Platelet-Rich Plasma (PRP) effective in the treatment of acute muscle injuries? A systematic review and meta-analysis. Sports Med. 2018;48:971–89.
35. Almakinders LC. Results of surgical repair versus splinting of experimentally transected muscle. J Orthop Trauma. 1991;5:173–6.
36. Kujala UM, Orava S, Jarvinen M. Hamstring injuries: current trends in treatment and prevention. Sports Med. 1997;23:397–404.
37. Klein JH. Muscular hematomas: diagnosis and management. J Manipulativ Physio Ther. 1990;13:96–100.
38. Larson CM, Almakinders KSG, Garrett WE. Evaluating and managing muscle contusions and myositis ossificans. Phys Sports Med. 2002;30:41–50.
39. Miller AE, Davis BA, Beckley OA. Bilateral an recurrent myositis ossificans in an athlete: a case report and review of treatment options. Arch Phys Med Rehabil. 2006;87:286–90.

Lumbar Spine Injuries in Football

7

Paul A. Rizk, Austin W. Wallace, and Robert C. Decker

Introduction

Football is a high-impact game and injuries to the spine are common and, on rare occasions, can be catastrophic. Meron, over a 10-year period, found an injury rate of 10.10 per 100,000 athlete exposures in high school football. As a comparison, the risk was 3.04 per 100,000 for all sports [1]. Chung found the risks were increased in college football, particularly in Division I [2].

Brophy, in a review of the National Football League (NFL) Combine data over 14 years, found an increasing numbers of injuries detected over time. Low back pain occurred at an incidence of 8.3 per 100 players and spondylolisthesis at 1.01 per 100 players [3]. Mall reported that injuries to the axial skeleton accounted for 7% of all injuries in the NFL [4]. Spine injuries can result in missed playing time and shortened careers at any level. Within this chapter, we present the most common injuries to the lumbar spine and their basic management to help guide team medical professionals.

Spine injuries, when they occur, require proper evaluation and management. For catastrophic injuries, safe expedited transport to a hospital equipped to manage spine trauma is important. It is important to have a protocol and the proper medical equipment available as well a person responsible for evaluating the injured player and another for activating emergency services if needed. This individual or staff should be well versed on managing facemasks, helmets, shoulder pads, immobilization techniques, and transfer techniques [5–8]. The protocols for spine boarding and

P. A. Rizk · A. W. Wallace
Orthopedic Surgery Resident, The University of Florida, Gainesville, FL, USA

R. C. Decker (✉)
Division of Spine Surgery, Department of Orthopedic Surgery, The University of Florida, Gainesville, FL, USA
e-mail: deckerc@ortho.ufl.edu

K. W. Farmer (ed.), *Football Injuries*,
https://doi.org/10.1007/978-3-030-54875-9_7

transport are the same as described in detail in Chap. 9 and should be followed for a suspected unstable lumbar spine fracture as well.

Training and planning should consist of reviewing various spine injuries so medical staff are competent to provide safe care and not to further injure the athlete. First steps in evaluation should include a thorough history including nature of injury as well as a physical exam in order to understand the injury mechanism and any neurological defects that may be present.

Lumbar Spine Fractures

Minor fractures of the lumbar spine are often due to repetitive activity or low energy impact. They include injuries to the transverse process, spinous process, articular process, or pars interarticularis. Most of these injuries can be treated nonoperatively [9].

Compression fractures occur from an axial load on a straightened spine. In this position, the force is transmitted through the vertebral bodies without the posterior structures offloading axial force as they normally do in lordosis. In compression fractures, the anterior column of the vertebrae fails leading to fracture. Neurological sequelae are not associated with compression fractures and management is usually with immobilization in a brace followed by therapy as a bridge to return to play once the fracture has healed and the patient is asymptomatic [10, 11].

When the anterior and middle columns of the spine fail, a burst fracture occurs. A burst fracture has a higher risk of neurologic and spinal cord injury due to potential displacement of the middle column into the vertebral canal. Based on the fracture, neurologic exam, and symptoms, management can range from nonoperative management with immobilization to surgical management with decompression and fusion [11]. Fractures can also occur with translation or rotation of the spine that often causes injury to the disco-ligamentous structures that creates increased instability of the spine often requiring surgical management.

Return to play is complicated as no high-quality evidence is available and is predominantly based on expert opinion. After fracture, return is based on bony healing on CT or mature fusion after surgery, painless range of motion, absence of neurologic deficits, and full strength of the extremities and lumbar muscles. Potential contraindications to returning to play include residual neurologic deficit, malalignment of the spine, narrowing of the spinal canal, loss of range of motion, and multilevel surgery.

Disk Herniation

Disk herniations occur commonly in the lumbar spine (Fig. 7.1). Common symptoms are back pain with radiating pain down an extremity and sometimes neurologic deficits including numbness and weakness. Whenever suspected, a thorough

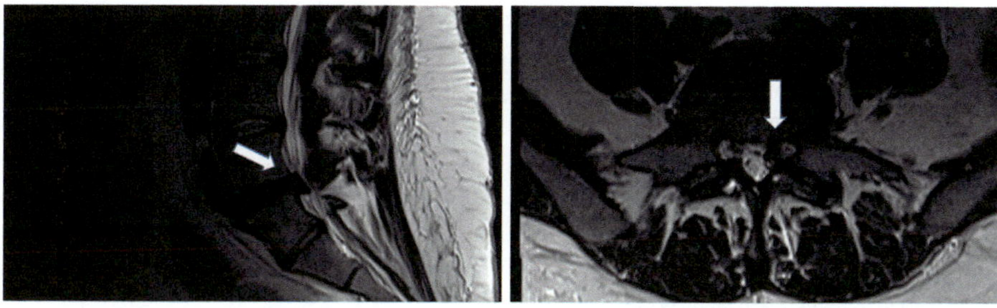

Fig. 7.1 Sagittal and MRI of the lumbar spine with arrows pointing to a posterolateral disk herniation

history and neurologic exam should be performed. MRI is the most appropriate non-invasive test to confirm the presence of a disk herniation. Gray, in a retrospective review of NFL players, found disk herniations represented 13% of all spine injuries. Most of the disk herniations occurred in the lumbar spine, and most frequently at L5–S1 followed by L4–L5. Lumbar disk injuries occurred most commonly in offensive lineman while blocking, though they can occur without contact [12].

Overall, disk herniations led to the second highest mean number of days lost of all spine injuries with spinal cord injuries accounting for the most missed days. Gray found that players suffering disk herniations missed a mean of 11 games due to injury [12]. Unfortunately, the database does not record injury grading, severity, or treatment provided. Additionally, it does not provide athletes' past history of disk pathology to help determine if the disk herniation is a new or older injury as disk herniations can be asymptomatic and predate injury [13, 14].

Treatment for disk herniation is often conservative to start including short-term rest, activity modification, medications, physical therapy, chiropractor treatment, and epidural steroid injections (ESIs). Medications commonly utilized include non-steroidal anti-inflammatory drugs (NSAIDs), oral steroids, and gabapentin [15].

ESIs have been considered a part of a lower back pain and radicular treatment in the young athlete since the 1950s (Fig. 7.2). Advanced imaging and higher demand of high-level athletes have changed the utilization of ESI over time. In 1980, Jackson evaluated 32 athletes who had low back pain associated with radiculopathy treated with ESI. Duration of symptoms prior to injection varied significantly ranging from 2 weeks to 18 months. ESI was successful in 44% of athletes. Other studies in the 1950s reporting on the general population reported a 67–70% success [16–18].

More recently and promising, Krych reviewed 17 NFL players who had 27 lumbar disk herniation episodes and underwent ESI. All diagnoses were confirmed by MRI and injections were performed within 14 days of onset of symptoms. Krych reported 89% return to play with only 2.8 practices and 0.6 games lost on average. The manner of injection did not affect the return to play. Risk for failure was associated with a sequestered disk fragment and weakness on physical exam. This study demonstrates how acute ESIs, a relatively low-risk procedure, can be efficacious in return to play for athletes [19]. Individual treatment plans should be customized

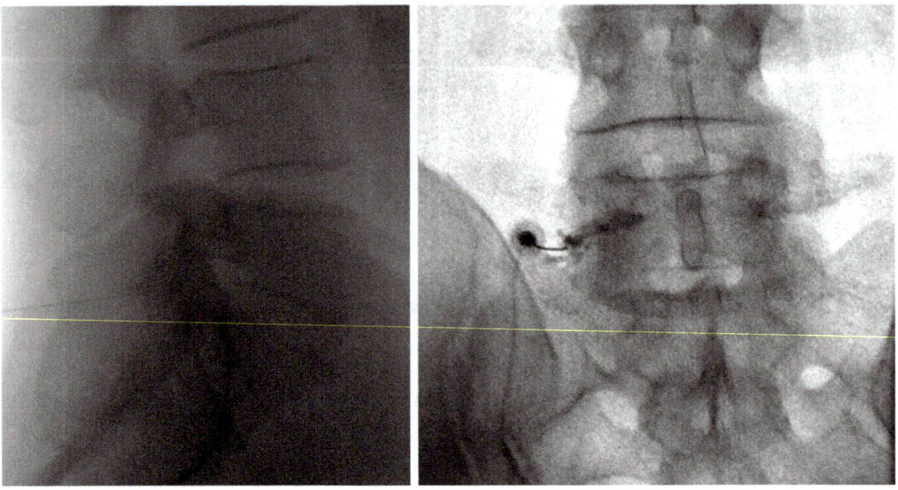

Fig. 7.2 Lateral and AP of the lumbar spine demonstrating a L5–S1 transforaminal epidural injection with contrast on the AP running along the L5 nerve root

based on the patient's symptoms and circumstances. If the patient is not sufficiently improved after a trial of conservative treatment including an ESI, then surgical removal of the disk may be an option [20].

Linemen have been shown to have increased risks of lumbar disk herniation compared to other position groups. Moorman reported on a higher incidence of lumbar endplate concavity in lineman compared to age-matched controls, theorized to be secondary to repetitive axial loading with extension during blocking. Athletes with endplate concavity had less general lumbar complaints than their age-matched controls. However, there was no difference in playing professional football, years played, games played, or games started with or without hyperconcavity of the lumbar spine endplates [21]. Additionally, Paxton noted that lineman endplate changes did not provide an advantage or disadvantage [22].

Hsu found that 82% of athletes were able to return to play after lumbar herniations. Offensive and defensive linemen were the most commonly affected positions. Eighty percent of professional football players treated surgically were able to return to play, while only 59% of those treated conservatively without surgery were able to return. These results were based on information made publicly available so they may represent an incomplete picture, as injury severity, nor treatment algorithms, were available [23]. Schroeder in his review of NFL Combine data looked at players diagnosed with lumbar disk herniations. For those treated nonoperatively or surgically, there was no difference in years played, games played, games started, or performance score compared to matched controls without a disk herniation. The affected level did not have an effect on career longevity, performance, or need for future lumbar surgery. No difference was seen based on the lumbar level herniated, which had been a concern as different levels innervate different muscles [24].

Current studies suggest a return to sport is possible following lumbar disk herniation with both conservative and surgical treatments. Most recommendations of return to play are based on expert opinion and should be tailored to the individual based on their symptoms, functional needs, and situation [25].

Low Back Pain

Half of adults will experience back pain within a given year. Likewise, back pain is common in football. Injuries can occur from trauma, overuse, or deviating from optimal kinematics. Hasselbrock estimated, from NCAA Injury Surveillance Program, an injury rate of 24.62 per 1000 athletic exposure for football. That was the highest rate of all college sports and more than double the next sport – female gymnastics. Most football lumbar injuries were strains followed by unspecified pain. Most athletes miss less than 24 hours of participation due to their injury [26]. However, low back pain can linger and effect play.

All instances of low back pain should have a detailed history and performance of an orthopedic and neurologic exam. History should include onset, chronicity, and location of the pain. Conservative management often includes NSAIDs, cold, heat, activity modification, and rest. Bracing can be used for short periods for pain relief or longer term for fractures. Physical therapy should be initiated once severe acute symptoms have subsided [9, 27]. Abdelraouf demonstrated a link between lower trunk musculature endurance and increased risk of low back pain when compared to healthy athletes. They recommended rehabilitation strategies that emphasized endurance of the trunk extensors and flexors [28]. Flexibility of hamstring and gluteal muscles should be addressed as well. When therapy is initiated, proper mechanics should be supervised closely.

Lumbar facet syndrome (LFS) can be suspected as a significant contributing factor to low back pain in athletes who perform repetitive extension and twisting motions [29]. Repetitive facet joint loading is suspected to result in facet joint capsule hypertrophy and inflammation resulting in activation of the numerous nociceptors and mechanoreceptors leading to localized and radicular pain [30]. Much like those suffering from lumbar disk herniation, patients will complain of localized low back pain exacerbated by twisting motions or hyperextension with pain that may radiate into the buttocks or posterior thighs. In cases of LFS, MRI can demonstrate a wide spectrum of findings from normal anatomy to subchondral edema at the joint space to severe degenerative facet joint changes and cysts.

Much debate exists regarding the correlation between radiographic degenerative changes and clinical symptoms [31]. As such, if conservative management with cessation of aggravating activity, NSAIDs, and physical therapy fails, then diagnostic fluoroscopically guided injection of the facet capsule or medial branch nerve could be pursued [32]. Significant symptomatic relief, typically defined as 80% reduction of pain and the ability to perform previously painful activities, corroborates the diagnosis of LFS [33]. These patients can then be referred for facet joint denervation [31]. When performed in the appropriate patient and for the appropriate condition, facet joint neurolysis provides significant pain relief, reduces the need for analgesics, and minimizes disability. The relief from neurolysis typically plateaus between 3 and 6 months after the procedure and then diminishes thereafter due to nerve regeneration. The procedure can then be safely repeated and pain relief reliably again obtained [34].

While the literature is replete with studies examining the effects of lumbar facet neurolysis on low back pain in the general population, relatively little has been published specifically investigating the success in athletes. In 2003, Vad performed a prospective study examining the results of radiofrequency denervation in professional baseball pitchers. Twelve pitchers who had failed conservative management, including physical therapy and oral anti-inflammatories, underwent diagnostic medial branch blocks and subsequent neurolysis of the bilateral L4–L5 and L5–S1 zygapophyseal joints. This was followed by a graduated physical therapy regimen with progressive return to competitive pitching. The study reports that 83% returned to a pre-procedural pitching level and all experienced statistically significant lumbar pain relief [35]. While only a single study and a limited number of participants, the results are promising and suggest that athletes suffering from lumbar facet joint syndrome can be safely and successfully treated with facet joint neurolysis.

Spondylolysis can be a cause of low back pain. Spondylolysis is a bone defect of the pars interarticularis, a part of the vertebrae between the facet joints (Fig. 7.3). Fredrickson noted that in the asymptomatic general population, spondylolysis is present in 4.4% of children and 6% of adults [36].

The defect is believed to be created by repetitive trauma from shear loading of the posterior elements, particularly from lumbar hyperextension. Genetic predisposition is also believed to play a role as well. It most commonly occurs at L5 and can be associated with spondylolisthesis. Fatigue stress can lead to fracture and spondylolisthesis. Spondylolisthesis is a translation of one vertebral body on the adjacent

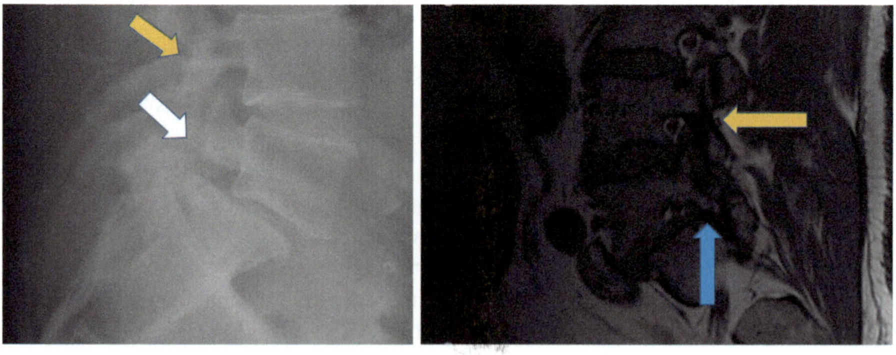

Fig. 7.3 Lateral XR and sagittal MRI of the lumbar spine in a patient with spondylolysis (pars defect) and spondylolisthesis. The white arrow is pointing to the spondylolysis at L5 on the lateral XR. You can see the break in the posterior elements at the pars interarticularis. The blue arrow illustrates the same disruption of the posterior elements on MRI. The orange arrows illustrate the normal anatomy at L4 on both the XR and MRI

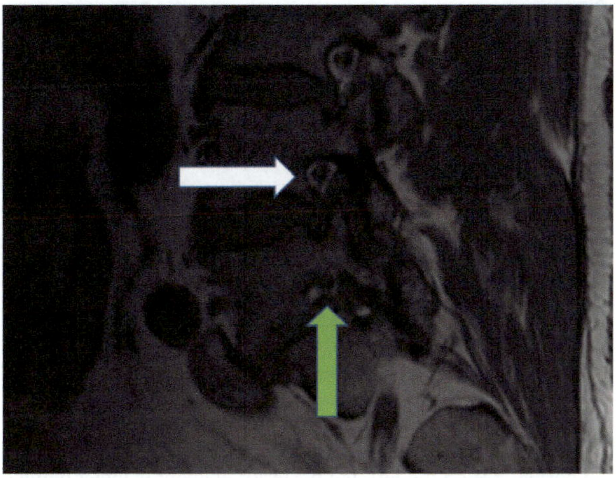

Fig. 7.4 Sagittal MRI image showing the exiting nerve roots at each level. The green arrow illustrates the compressed exiting L5 nerve root due to the spondylolisthesis. The white arrow demonstrates the normal exiting L4 nerve root surrounded by white fat indicating no nerve compression

vertebral body [37]. Low back pain is the main symptom, which can occur in the midline or over the facet joints laterally. Pain can also radiate to the buttock and posterior thigh. Symptoms can be exacerbated with rotation and hyperextension. Neurological symptoms may be present in cases where spondylolisthesis is present often correlating with the nerve root that exits at the involved level, usually L5 (Fig. 7.4).

Establishing a diagnosis can improve the chances of healing. Iwamoto stated that the primary goal for athletes with acute spondylolysis is healing and higher healing rates are seen if detected early [38]. Yamazaki found that high defect stage (stage related to how progressed the spondylolysis was with the lowest only showing a stress reaction on MRI and the highest defect demonstrating pseudoarthrosis on CT), stage of contralateral pars defect stage, and poor flexibility were negative prognostic factors for bone healing [39].

Lumbar radiographs can be performed to evaluate for spondylolysis. Iwamoto found that 69% of high school and college football players with low back pain had at least one abnormality on their radiographs [40].

Radiographic presence of spondylolysis was the single most important predictor of low back pain. High school players with spondylolysis had low back pain at a rate of 79.8% while only 37.1% of those without spondylolysis had back pain [40]. While athletes with spondylolysis may have pain, the presence of spondylolysis does not mean that it is going to be painful in the future. McCarroll found that spondylolysis was asymptomatic in 80% of NCAA football players [41].

Grodahl in review of published studies could not recommend patient history for diagnosing spondylolysis or spondylolisthesis. Palpation of step deformity may be useful for spondylolisthesis but one-legged hyperextension test was not supported for the diagnosis of spondylolysis [42]. Therefore, if suspected, imaging is the best way to confirm. The best initial radiographic study is a two-view plain film due to efficacy, low cost, and low radiation exposure (Fig. 7.5). MRI is helpful for early imaging looking for edema within and around the pars area, particularly in the

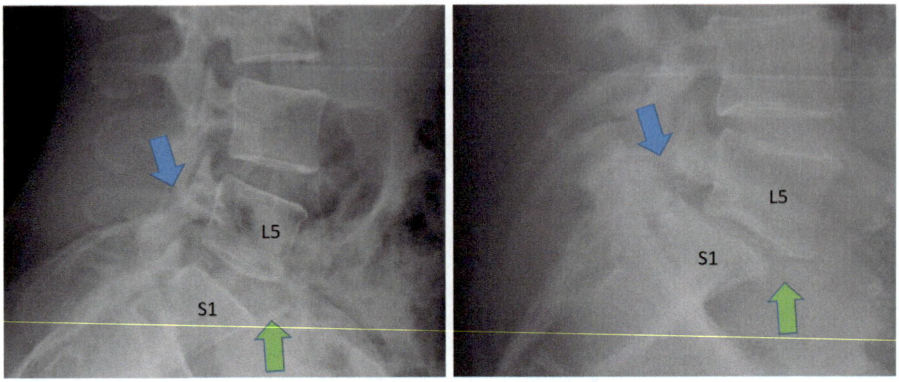

Fig. 7.5 Lateral XR of the lumbar spine showing the normal anatomy on the left and the spondylolysis and spondylolisthesis on the right. The blue arrows point to the posterior elements of L5. In the normal XR on the left, the posterior element is intact while on the right the posterior element is disrupted by the spondylolysis. The green arrows point to the anterior L5–S1 disk. The normal anatomy is demonstrated on the left while the right demonstrates a spondylolisthesis (slip) at L5–S1. With a spondylolisthesis, the anterior portions of the vertebral bodies are not aligned

ipsilateral pedicle, while CT scan is helpful in identifying spondylolysis, though with greater radiation exposure [43, 44]. Chronic pars defects will not show uptake on bone scan or MRI and CT scan can show bone definition and healing.

Most athletes can be managed with conservative measures leading to good-to-excellent long-term outcomes. With spondylolysis, the first question that needs to be answered is if the lesion is acute or chronic. That can be determined by age, history, exam, and imaging. If acute, treatment is aimed at healing the injury and preventing nonunion. Rest with competition restriction is the initial mainstay of treatment with length of rest being dependent on age, acuity of injury, and symptoms.

In skeletally mature patients, recreational athletes, or chronic conditions with an acute flare, bracing can be used for pain control and as an adjuvant to activity modification during the inflammatory state and is discontinued once the patient's pain is improved to start physical therapy. In a mature or chronic patient, the goal should be symptom management without an expectation of defect union. Bracing may be contraindicated in a high-level athlete due to functional and strength loses while in the brace.

This period of rest can be longer than 3 months depending on clinical circumstances. Once symptoms improve, rehabilitation is added to the treatment with particular attention towards hamstring flexibility [39]. Older, advanced athletes may return faster depending on athletic requirements. Rehabilitation is started with low-impact aerobic conditioning and muscular stabilization. Once this is tolerated, the athlete is advanced to sport-specific training with attention focused on improving playing technique in a closely supervised fashion. Studies have shown healing between 3 and 6 months in skeletally immature patients, and this can be assessed by CT scan [38, 45]. If there is a question regarding back pain in adolescents, early referral to an orthopedic provider is warranted as Nielsen found earlier presentation to orthopedic providers decreased the time to diagnosis that can help with initiating appropriate treatment [46].

Both nonsurgical and surgical treatments of symptomatic spondylolysis can be effective in relieving pain and returning the athlete to play. An extended trial of nonoperative management is undertaken prior to operative consideration which is commonly a fusion or a direct repair of the pars defect [47]. Overley found that adolescent athletes return to play 92.2% of the time when treated nonoperatively. When surgery is required, the return to play afterwards decreases to 90.3%. Return to play can occur when symptoms have abated and fusion is mature [48]. For the advanced athlete, return can occur in the absence of neurologic symptoms and if they have demonstrated return to preinjury functional level even with continued symptoms. In general, treatment of spondylolysis and spondylolisthesis should be individualized based on the age, symptoms, sport, and level of competition [49].

Return to Play and Outcomes

Schroeder reviewed combined data on lumbar spine diagnoses as a predictor of outcome in professional football. Of the 2965 athletes reviewed, 14% were identified as having a preexisting lumbar condition with the most common being spondylosis, herniated disk, spondylolysis, and strain (followed by stenosis, fracture, SI joint pain, scoliosis, and kyphosis). Players without a lumbar diagnosis were more likely to be drafted. Players with a preexisting diagnosis, that were drafted, played for a shorter period of time, played less games, and started less games. However, there was no performance difference noted. Players with spondylosis, lumbar herniated disk, or spondylolysis were less likely to be drafted than controls, though there was no difference in career performance. Players with spondylolysis were associated with a shorter playing career, in both years played and games played. In further analysis between athletes who had been treated with nonoperative care versus micro discectomy for lumbar disk herniation, there was no difference in years played, games played, games started, or performance. Athletes treated with surgery, when compared to matched controls, did not demonstrate differences in years played, games played, games started, or performance [24].

Conclusion

The game of football places a tremendous amount of stress on the spine and injuries are common. Most injuries are minor and, with some basic treatment, an athlete can return to play quickly. However, catastrophic injuries do occur. Therefore, it is imperative to have a medical team that is aware of possible injuries, the treatment of injuries, a plan of care, and knowledge as to when to activate emergency services.

References

1. Meron A, McMullen C, Laker SR, Currie D, Cornstock RD. Epidemiology of cervical spine injuries in high school athletes over a ten-year period. PM R. 2018;10:355–72.
2. Chung AS, Makovicka JL, Hassebrock JD, Patel KA, Tummala SV, Deckey DG, et al. Epidemiology of cervical injuries in NCAA football players. Spine. 2019;44(12):848–54.
3. Brophy RH, Barnes R, Rodeo SA, Warren RF. Prevalence of musculoskeletal disorders at the NFL combine – trends 1987 to 2000. Med Sci Sports Exerc. 2007;37(1):22–7.
4. Mall NA, Buchowski J, Zebala L, Brophy RH, Wright RW, Matava M. Spine and axial skeleton injuries in the National Football League. Am J Sports Med. 2012;40:1755–61.
5. Swartz EE, Boden BP, Courson RW, Decoster LC, Horodyski MB, Norkus SA, et al. National athletic trainers' association position statement: acute management of the cervical spine–injured athlete. J Athl Train. 2009;44(3):306–31.
6. National Athletic Trainers Association [Internet]. Carrollton: appropriate prehospital management of the spine-injured athlete updated from 1998 document. Available from: https://www.nata.org/sites/default/files/Executive-Summary-Spine-Injury-updated.pdf.
7. Waninger KM. Management of the helmeted athlete with suspected cervical spine injury. Am J Sports Med. 2004;32(5):1331–50.
8. Prasarn ML, Horodyski MB, DiPaola MJ, Dipaola CP, Del Rossi G, Conrad BP. Controlled laboratory comparison study of motion with football equipment in a destabilized cervical spine. Orthop J Sports Med. 2015;3(9):1–5.
9. Ball JR, Harris CB, Lee J, Vives MJ. Lumbar spine injuries in sports: review of the literature and current treatment recommendations. Sports Med Open. 2019;5(1):26–36.
10. Allen BL Jr, Ferguson RL, Lehmann TR, O'Brien RP. A mechanistic classification of closed, indirect fractures and dislocations of the lower cervical spine. Spine. 1982;7(1):1–27.
11. Vaccaro AR, Koerner JD, Radcliff KE, Oner C, Reinhold M, Schnake KJ, et al. AOSpine subaxial cervical spine injury classification system. Eur Spine J. 2016;25:2173–84.
12. Gray BL, Buchowski JM, Bumpass DB, Lehman RA, Mall NA, Matava MJ. Disc herniations in the National Football League. Spine. 2013;38(22):1934–8.
13. Boden SD, Davis DO, Dina TS, Patronas NJ, Wiesel SW. Abnormal magnetic-resonance scans of the lumbar spine in asymptomatic subjects. A prospective investigation. J Bone Joint Surg Am. 1990;72:403–8.
14. Boden SD, McCowin PR, Davis DO, Dina TS, Mark AS, Wiesel SW. Abnormal magnetic-resonance scans of the cervical spine in asymptomatic subjects. A prospective investigation. J Bone Joint Surg Am. 1990;72:1178–84.
15. Mortazavi J. Low back pain in athletes. Asian J Sports Med. 2015;6(2):e24718.
16. Cappio M. Sacral epidural administration of hydrocortisone in therapy of lumbar sciatica: study of 80 cases. Reumatismo. 1957;1:60–70.
17. Jackson DW, Rettig A, Wiltse LL. Epidural cortisone injections in the young athletic adult. Am J Sports Med. 1980;4:239–43.
18. Gardner WJ, Goebert HW Jr, Sehgal AD. Intraspinal corticosteroids in the treatment of sciatica. Trans Am Neurol Assoc. 1961;86:214–5.
19. Krych AJ, Richman D, Drakos M, Weiss L, Barnes R, Cammisa F, et al. Epidural steroid injection for lumbar disc herniation in NFL athletes. Med Sci Sports Exerc. 2012;44:193–8.
20. Kreiner DA, Hwang SW, Easa JE, Resnick DK, Baisden JL, Bess S, et al. An evidence-based clinical guideline for the diagnosis and treatment of lumbar disc herniation with radiculopathy. Spine J. 2014;14:180–91.
21. Moorman CT 3rd, Johnson DC, Pavlov H, Barnes R, Warren RF, Speer KP, et al. Hyperconcavity of the lumbar vertebral endplates in the elite football lineman. Am J Sports Med. 2004;32(6):1434–9.
22. Paxton ES, Moorman CT, Chehab EL, Barnes RP, Warren RF, Brophy RH. Effect of hyperconcavity of the lumbar vertebral endplates on the playing careers of professional American football linemen. Am J Sports Med. 2010;38(11):2255–8.

23. Hsu WK. Performance-based outcomes following lumbar discectomy in professional athletes in the National Football League. Spine. 2010;35:1247–51.
24. Schroeder GD, Lynch TS, Gibbs DS, Chow I, Labelle M, Patel AA, et al. Pre-existing lumbar spine diagnosis as a predictor of outcomes in National Football League athletes. Am J Sports Med. 2015;43(4):972–8.
25. Reiman MP, Sylvain J, Loudon JK, Goode A. Return to sport after open and microdiscectomy surgery versus conservative treatment for lumbar disc herniation: a systemic review with meta-analysis. Br J Sports Med. 2016;50:221–30.
26. Hasselbrock JD, Patel KA, Makovicka JL, Chung AS, Tummala SV, Pena AJ, et al. Lumbar spine injuries in national collegiate athletic association athletes. Ortho J Sports Med. 2019;7(1):1–10.
27. Dizdarevic I, Bishop M, Sgromolo N, Hammoud S, Atanda A Jr. Approach to the pediatric athlete with back pain: more than just the pars. Phys Sports Med. 2015;43(4):421–31.
28. Abdelraouf OR, Abdel-aziem AA. The relationship between core endurance and back dysfunction in collegiate male athletes with and without nonspecific low back pain. Int J Sports Phys Ther. 2016;11(3):337–44.
29. Watkins RG, Dillin WH. Lumbar spine injury in the athlete. Clin Sports Med. 1990;9:419–48.
30. Cavanaugh JM, Ozaktay AC, Yamashita HT, King AI. Lumbar facet pain: biomechanics, neuroanatomy and neurophysiology. J Biomech. 1996;29:1117–29.
31. Perolat R, Kastler A, Nicot B, Pellat JM, Tahon F, Attye A, et al. Facet joint syndrome: from diagnosis to interventional management. Insights Imaging. 2018;9:773–89.
32. Filippiadis DK, Kelekis A. A review of percutaneous techniques for low back pain and neuralgia: current trends in epidural infiltrations, intervertebral disk and facet joint therapies. Br J Radiol. 2015;89:1–10.
33. Manchikanti L, Manchikanti KN, Manchukonda R, Cash KA, Damron KS, Pampati V, et al. Evaluation of lumbar facet joint nerve blocks in the management of chronic low back pain: preliminary report of a randomized, double-blind controlled trial: clinical trial NCT00355914. Pain Physician. 2007;10:425–40.
34. Bogduk N, Dreyfuss P, Govind J. A narrative review of lumbar medial branch neurotomy for the treatment of back pain. Pain Med. 2009;10:1035–45.
35. Vad VB, Cano WG, Basrai D, Lutz GE, Bhat AL. Role of radiofrequency denervation in lumbar zygapophyseal joint synovitis in baseball pitchers: a clinical experience. Pain Physician. 2003;6:307–12.
36. Fredrickson BE, Baker D, McHolick WJ, Yuan HA, Lubicky JP. The natural history of spondylolisthesis and spondylolisthesis. J Bone Jt Surg Am. 1984;66(5):699–707.
37. Jackson DW, Wiltse LL, Dingeman RD, Hayes M. Stress reactions involving the pars interarticularis in young athletes. Am J Sports Med. 1981;9(5):304–12.
38. Fujii K, Katoh S, Sairyo K, Kata T, Yasui N. Union of defects in the pars interarticularis of the lumbar spine in children and adolescents. The radiological outcome after conservative treatment. J Bone Jt Surg Br. 2004;86(2):225–31.
39. Yamazaki K, Kota S, Oikawa D, Suzuki Y. High defect stage, contralateral defects, and poor flexibility are negative predictive factors of bone union in pediatric and adolescent athletes with spondylolysis. J Med Investig. 2018;65:126–30.
40. Iwamoto J, Abe H, Tsukimura Y, Wakano K. Relationship between radiographic abnormalities of the lumbar spine and incidence of low back pain in high school and college football players: a prospective study. Am J Sports Med. 2004;32(3):781–6.
41. McCarroll JR, Miller JM, Ritter MA. Lumbar spondylolysis and spondylolisthesis in college football players. A prospective study. Am J Sports Med. 1986;14(5):404–6.
42. Grodahl LH, Fawcett L, Nazareth M, Smith R, Spencer S, Heneghan N, et al. Diagnostic utility of patient history and physical examination data to detect spondylolysis and spondylolisthesis in athletes with low back pain: a systematic review. Man Ther. 2016;24:7–17.
43. Tofte JN, CarlLee TL, Holte AJ, Sitton SE, Weinstein SL. Imaging pediatric spondylolysis: a systematic review. Spine. 2017;42:777–82.

44. Sairyo K, Katoh S, Takata Y, Terai T, Yasui N, Goel VK, et al. MRI signal changes of the pedicle as an indicator for early diagnosis of spondylolysis in children and adolescents: a clinical and biomechanical study. Spine. 2006;31(2):206–11.
45. Miller SF, Congeni J, Swanson K. Long term functional and anatomical follow-up of early detected spondylolysis in young athletes. Am J Sports Med. 2004;32:928–33.
46. Nielsen E, Andras LM, Skaggs DL. Diagnosis of spondylolysis and spondylolisthesis is delayed six months after seeing nonorthopedic providers. Spine Deform. 2018;6(3):263–6.
47. Crawford CH, Ledonio CG, Bess RS, Buchowski JM, Burton DC, Hu SS, et al. Current evidence regarding the etiology, prevalence, natural history, and prognosis of pediatric lumbar spondylolysis: a report from the scoliosis research society evidence based medicine committee. Spine Deform. 2015;3(1):12–9.
48. Overley SC, McAnany SJ, Andelman S, Kim J, Merrill RK, Cho SK, et al. Return to play in adolescent athletes with symptomatic spondylolysis without listhesis: a meta-analysis. Global Spine J. 2018;8(2):190–7.
49. Tallarico RA, Madom IA, Palumbo MA. Spondylolysis and spondylolisthesis in the athlete. Sports Med Arthrosc Rev. 2008;16:32–8.

Cervical Spine Conditions in Football

8

Brian D. Sindelar, Dennis Timothy Lockney, MaryBeth Horodyski, Kristopher G. Hooten, and Allen K. Sills

Epidemiology

It is estimated that 17,000 spinal cord injuries (SCIs) occur annually, with over a quarter of a million people living in the United States with the associated sequela. Of those 17,000, roughly 40% are due to motor vehicle accidents, 30% due to falls, 14% due to violence, and only 10% due to sports-related accidents [1]. Though those attributable to sports-related activities pale in comparison to the grand total, sports-related SCIs typically occur in our youth and are therefore a significant event in a healthy individual early in his or her life. This affliction becomes a substantial physical and financial burden not only on the patient and family, but also on the healthcare system with estimations of roughly 1.5–3 million dollars over a lifetime to care for a person suffering with an SCI [2].

Within the United States, football is the second most common cause of sports-related SCI yearly, surpassed only by diving [3]. But due to the sheer volume of youth, high school, collegiate, and professional football players in comparison to other sports, football has the highest incidence of SCI per athlete exposures [4, 5]. Among multiple reviews, a catastrophic injury has been estimated to occur in

B. D. Sindelar (✉) · D. T. Lockney · K. G. Hooten
Department of Neurosurgery, University of Florida, Gainesville, FL, USA
e-mail: DennisTimothy.Lockney@neurosurgery.ufl.edu

M. Horodyski
Department of Orthopedics and Rehabilitation, University of Florida, Gainesville, FL, USA
e-mail: horodmb@ortho.ufl.edu

A. K. Sills
Neurosurgery and Orthopedic Surgery, Vanderbilt University Medical Center, Nashville, TN, USA

Chief Medical Officer, The National Football League, Nashville, TN, USA

K. W. Farmer (ed.), *Football Injuries*,
https://doi.org/10.1007/978-3-030-54875-9_8

roughly 0.52–10 per 100,000 athlete exposures within high school participants, 1.55–4.72 per 100,000 athlete exposures within collegiate players, and 14 per 100,000 athlete exposures among professionals [5–7].

Aside from significant neurological injury following an SCI, football players are also prone to the many more "benign" spinal injuries including nonoperative fractures, ligamentous strains, myofascial injuries, and disc herniations. A 10-year reivew of the National Football League by Mall et al., demonstrated 44% of spinal injuries occur within the cervical spine, 31% within the lumbar spine, and 4% within the thoracic spine [9]. A retrospective review by Delaney et al. reported that there were a total of 169 cervical fractures of the 11,000 total neck injuries (contusions, sprains/strains, dislocations) that presented to an emergency department within the United States from hockey, football, and soccer from 1990 to 1999 [8]. This chapter focuses on cervical spine injuries because though they make up just around half of all spine injuries, they are associated with 96% of all catastrophic spinal injuries [3, 9].

A historical appreciation of the evolving prevalence over the past half century helps shed light on specific high-risk behaviors within football and the response by the associated governing bodies to make football a safer sport. Through the early nineteenth century, cranial protection for the collegiate football player advanced from thick hair, to leather football helmets, and then finally to the more modern helmets seen today. Modern helmet designs were developed in the 1970s in response to the significant cranial and intracranial injuries that were occurring in the sport of football [10]. Though the institution of modern helmets significantly reduced skull fractures and intracranial hemorrhages, there was a reciprocal increase in total cervical spine injuries by 204% and, specifically, an increase in quadriplegia by 116% [11, 12]. This may be due to a sense of invincibility by the helmeted players altering their tackling style from wrapping up the opposing player, to the defensive player using their body as a weapon and leading with the crown of their head to make the tackle.

Known as "spearing," this form of tackling was initially defined in the 1960s as "intentionally and maliciously striking the opponent with one's helmet after the opponent had been downed" [12]. With greater awareness of the direct relation of spearing to the cause of cervical spine injuries, the National Collegiate Athletic Association (NCAA) and the National Federation of State High School Associations moved to eliminate this by removing the terms "intentional" and "deliberate" from the description of spearing in 1976, to then renouncing a needed intent to "punish" an opposing player in '05-'06, to ultimately banning any form of striking another player with the top of one's helmet in '08. Stating, "when in question, it is a foul" [7, 12–14]. This removed all subjectivity between what should and should not be considered an illegal form of tackling. This important rule implementation and subsequent adjustment in the definition led to a 270% reduction in SCIs from the mid-1970s to 2000 [6, 11, 14–16] (Fig. 8.1). In more

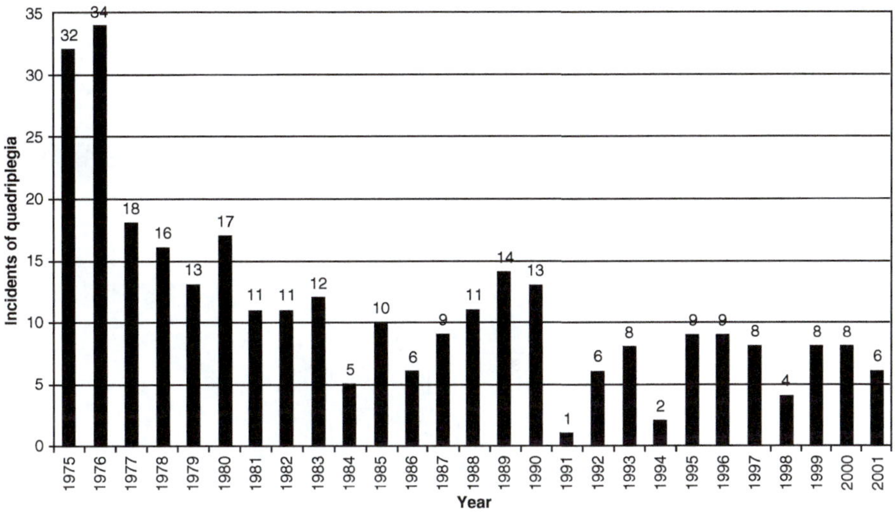

Fig. 8.1 Incidence of quadriplegia in high school and college athletes. Data from the National Football Head and Neck Injury Registry (1976–1991) and the National Center for Catastrophic Sports injury Research (1992–present). (With permission from Heck et al. [12])

detail, in 1976, the risk of spinal cord injury in high school was 7.72 per 100,000 athlete exposures and 30.66 per 100,000 athlete exposures in collegiate athletes. By 1987, this dropped significantly to 2.31 per 100,000 athlete exposures among high school athletes and 10.66 per 100,000 athlete exposures in collegiate football players [13].

Roughly 70–80% of all spinal injuries in football are due to tackling, specifically spear tackling with a player's head down (Fig. 8.2) [6, 7, 9, 12, 16]. Therefore, the attempt to completely eliminate spear tackling dramatically reduced the incidence of both SCI and quadriplegia in the sport of football. As anticipated, other risk factors associated with development of SCI are in those who perform more tackling and are exposed to higher velocities during collisions with opposing players. Therefore, it is understandable why SCI is more likely in defensive backs, linebackers, and special team players, but less likely in preseason and practice versus in-season games, and more likely in collegiate players rather than high school athletes [5–7, 9, 11, 12]. The higher risk in collegiate players has been hypothesized to be likely due to the increased speed and size of the players, but also potentially influenced by the smaller total number of collegiate players in comparison to high school (effecting overall incidence risk), or even a structural/anatomical difference. Nyland et al. compared a cohort of 70 uninjured collegiate athletes to 119 high school athletes to find that the older athletes were more likely to have a greater flexed cervical resting posture, therefore placing the spine at greatest risk upon impact due to a greater loss of lordosis [17].

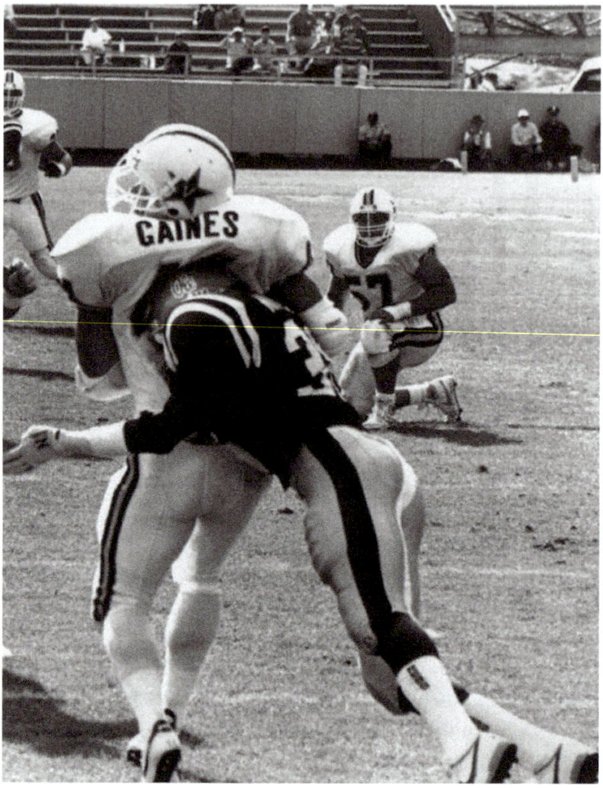

Fig. 8.2 Head-down contact poses significant risks of catastrophic cervical spine injury. This defensive back (dark jersey) sustained fractures of his fourth, fifth, and sixth cervical vertebrae. The hit resulted in quadriplegia. (With permission from Heck et al. [12])

Pathophysiology

The normal curvature of the cervical spine is roughly 40 ± 10° of lordosis [18]. When a force is applied across the crown of the head, the normal lordotic curvature allows transferring and dissipation of kinetic energy away from the axial skeleton and into the paraspinal muscles and associated ligaments within the cervical spine. When a player tackles with the top of their head, they affix their cervical spine in mild flexion, resulting in a straightening of the spine (Fig. 8.3). This loss of lordosis leads to the entirety of the force being applied along the axial spine, specifically the vertebral bodies and disc spaces. Once the compressive cushioning reserve of the disc spaces is reached, the cervical spine begins to buckle resulting in fractures, subluxation, dislocations, etc. (Fig. 8.4) [7, 13, 19, 20]. Though this is a simplified biomechanical view with an isolated vector, the additional rotational, flexion/extension, and even blunt forces that are applied during an actual tackle result in the heterogeneous mix of cervical injuries that occur to the vertebral bodies, facet joints, ligamentous structures, disc spaces, and associated cervical musculature. More importantly, violation of the integrity of the cervical spine's bony and ligamentous anatomy may result in injury to the neurological structures including the spinal cord and cervical spinal roots.

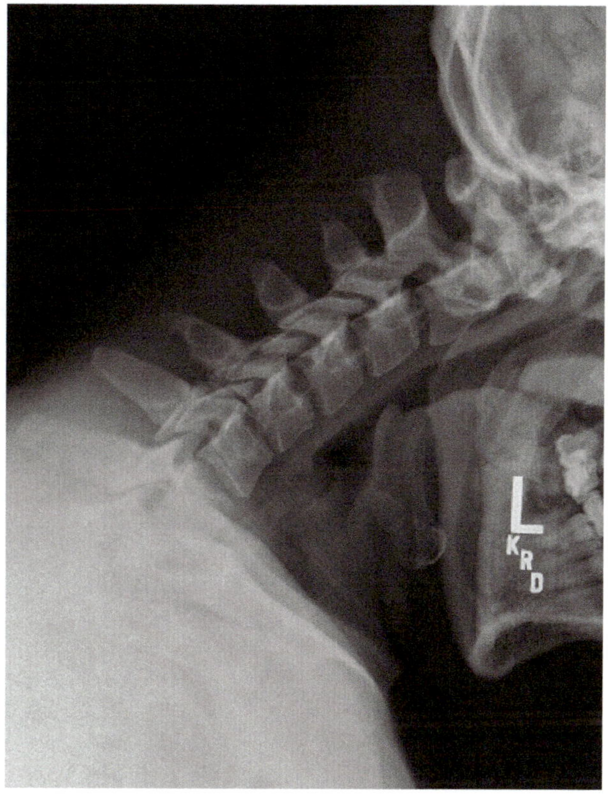

Fig. 8.3 Roughly 30° of flexion straightens the neck and removes the natural lordosis of the cervical spine. This eliminates muscular and ligamentous compensatory mechanisms to transfer force away from the axial skeleton

General Management of Cervical Spine Trauma

Pre-participation Preparation

Appropriate procedures of prehospital care for the spine-injured athlete should be discussed at a joint meeting and be documented in an emergency action plan (EAP). Key factors to consider including in the EAP are: roles of the medical team, methods to establish and control the scene, activation of emergency medical personnel to reduce redundency emergency medical service (EMS), directing EMS to the scene, assessment of the injured athlete, available equipment and its application, proper stabilization and restriction of unnecessary movement of the cervical spine, and where/how the athlete will be transported. Prior to the beginning of, and periodically throughout, any athletic season, the sports medicine team should review the EAP and perform hands-on practice sessions of the various steps included within the EAP, for example, removal of athletic equipment, spinal stabilization procedures, and spine boarding. If able, practice sessions should include both members of the on-field response team and also local EMS systems to ensure timely response and continuity of care for when an EAP is activated during a

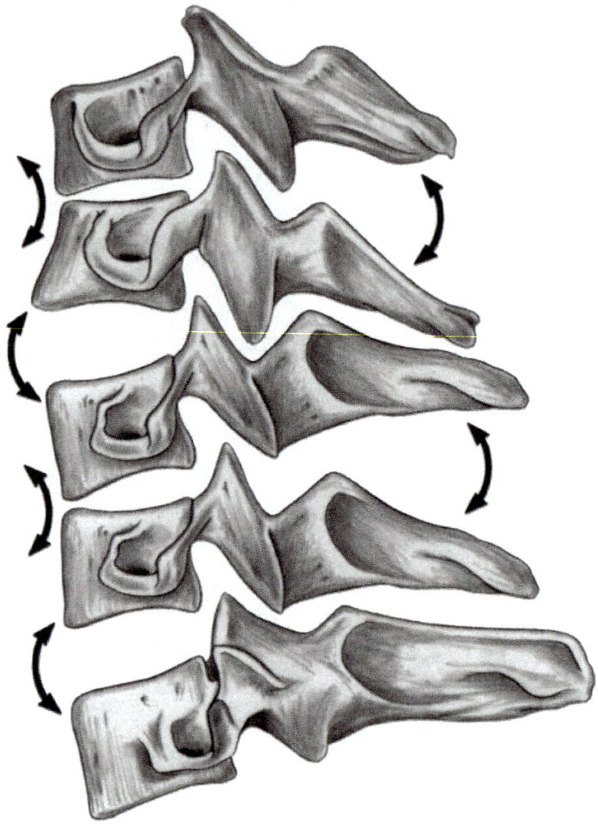

Fig. 8.4 Buckling effect in the cervical column under axial load. (With permission from Swartz et al. [19])

sporting event. Techniques currently used for transfer and transport during prehospital spine injury care are evolving as methods available for research have improved, providing additional information for appropriate care of these types of injuries. With these changes, EMS agencies throughout the country may follow different procedures and only have specific necessary equipment. It is therefore imperative that the medical staff meet with the local EMS to discuss details of the EAP. Lastly, prior to the start of any athletic competition, the medical teams from both institutions and the on-site EMS staff should meet to perform a "pregame medical time out," where the current EAP is reviewed [21, 22].

Further pre-event preparation must also include evaluation and inspection of the equipment needed for the care of the spine-injured athlete to ensure it is in excellent working condition. Inspection of the equipment should occur prior to the season and throughout the season. Standard equipment may include facemask removal devices (e.g., cordless screwdriver, cutting device), size-adjustable rigid cervical collar, long spine board, scoop stretcher, Kendrick extrication device (KED), and/or vacuum mattress [23, 24]. Additional supplies to enhance appropriate stabilization procedures include padding materials, head stabilization devices, and appropriate straps for the various transfer devices.

On-Field Primary Assessment

A cervical spine injury can occur following not only a collision between two players, but also from a player striking the ground or a stationary object. Upon approaching an athlete with concern for a cervical spine injury, a rapid and focused on-field primary evaluation should be performed by team personnel. This assessment includes evaluation of the player's alertness and cardiopulmonary status and a brief neurological assessment. This is essential in order to initiate a call to EMS, if necessary, as to not delay any needed transfer for a higher level of treatment. If the athlete is unresponsive, an assessment of their respiratory/cardiac function and initiation of the algorithm detailed by either the basic life support (BLS) or advanced cardiac life Support (ACLS) guidelines is appropriate [25, 26]. Since the pulmonary diaphragm receives its innervation from C3–C5 nerve roots, a high cervical injury can result in respiratory collapse requiring advanced life-saving airway techniques.

A player is likely receiving adequate respirations if he/she is communicative and without signs of respiratory distress (abnormal breathing patterns, rates, use of accessory respiratory muscles [demonstrated by suprasternal retractions], cyanotic color change of the lips, etc.). If aggressive airway techniques are required, initial management should begin with a "jaw thrust" rather than a "head-tilt, chin-lift." If unsuccessful in obtaining adequate respirations, the use of further advanced airway techniques is dependent on the expertise of the medical personnel present. Methods such as nasal fiber optic or video laryngoscopic intubation are preferred over direct laryngoscopy with attempted in-line cervical mobilization because this can cause significant motion of the cervical spine [27]. Following assessment of the "ABCs," a rapid motor and sensory exam of the upper and lower extremities should be performed on the athlete along with palpation of the cervical spine to assess for abnormalities (step-down) or discomfort/pain.

Spinal Stabilization and Movement of the Injured Athlete

Assessment of the scene and initiation of the primary survey is the first step prior to movement of the injured athlete. This assessment should provide information needed for the selection of the most appropriate procedure(s) to remove the athlete from the field/playing surface and what specific needs are required. An athlete suspected of sustaining a cervical spine injury should not be moved until the initial assessment has been completed. During the initial assessment, in-line stabilization of the cervical spine should be maintained to decrease the possibility of a secondary injury to the spinal cord. This should be performed by either the standard head-hold technique or the trap-squeeze technique. If the decision is made to use a form of spinal motion restriction following the initial assessment, the type of equipment and procedures for moving the athlete should be decided by the most experienced member of the sports medicine team. In most cases, a correctly sized rigid cervical collar may be placed on the athlete prior to transfer onto a stabilization device such as a long spine board, a scoop stretcher, a vacuum mattress, or a gurney. The efficacy of the rigid cervical collar has been questioned by several researchers due to its limitations on complete rigid cervical fixation [28–31]. However, at this time the application of a cervical collar is still recommended in most position statement documents. It is important to note that application of a cervical collar may not be appropriate in equipment-intensive sports (e.g., football), where application of the collar may result in increased motion of the cervical spine when the athlete is wearing a helmet and shoulder pads.

Once cervical spine in-line stabilization is in place, further assessment of the athlete is completed, EMS is contacted, and appropriate equipment to provide spinal motion restriction is brought on to the field. Recently, removal of football equipment on the field prior to transport has been gaining acceptance. Removal of equipment on the field provides direct access to the airway and chest if needed during transport to the hospital. Additionally, removal of equipment often makes placing and securing the athlete on the extrication device (e.g., long spine board, scoop stretcher, etc.) more efficient. The medical team must practice extensively to establish competence in all techniques of equipment removal and to be familiar with all the potentially different types of shoulder pads and helmets worn by the athletes on their team. While a set number of staff needed for removal of equipment has not been established, generally three to four trained medical team members are needed to safely remove football equipment from an athlete. If the football equipment is removed on the field, removal procedures can be started. In most cases, the helmet should be removed before the shoulder pads to prevent excessive forward flexion of the cervical spine. Additionally, the helmet may impede removal of the shoulder pads [32, 33].

It is not necessary to remove the facemask prior to removing the helmet but its removal should occur if the helmet is to remain. In the event the facemask cannot be removed, removal of the football helmet would be necessary to ensure access to the airway prior to transport. More than one type of equipment should be available for facemask removal if the first tool is not successful [34]. Former equipment removal protocols followed the all-or-none principle, suggesting the helmet and shoulder pads must be removed at the same time. However, more recent research has demonstrated that removal of the helmet followed by padding under the occiput maintains in-line stabilization of the cervical spine [33, 35, 36]. Removal of the helmet can be completed successfully by two trained individuals [34].

Shoulder pad removal begins with cutting the jersey and other structures of the shoulder pads. Cut the football jersey in a T-shaped method being sure to cut away from the face and neck region toward the abdomen and then toward the elbow of each arm. Cut any structures of the shoulder pads that would impede removal, such as side straps and laces. Shoulder pad removal is highly dependent on the type of shoulder pads the injured athlete is wearing. The medical staff should practice methods of shoulder pad removal that require the pads to go over the head using an elevated shoulder technique. A multi-person lift-and-slide technique, where the shoulder pads are removed when the athlete is raised to slide the long spine board under the athlete is another acceptable method. Videos of these shoulder pad removal techniques and others are available on the Internet and should be practiced by the medical team.

Numerous techniques are available to prepare the spine-injured athlete for transportation. Selection of the most appropriate technique is based on several factors including number and training of available medical staff, local protocols, status of the injured athlete, position and size of the athlete, and available equipment. The log roll was considered the standard of care procedure for placing an athlete on a long spine board. However, research over the past two decades has indicated that employing other procedures may decrease the amount of motion in an unstable spine.

For the supine-lying athlete, the multi-person lift-and-slide (previously described as the six-plus lift-and-slide) has been demonstrated to result in significantly less motion in the cervical spine when compared to the log roll [37–39]. Additionally, the use of a scoop stretcher for the supine injured athlete has been demonstrated to have significantly less motion than the log roll [40, 41]. When considering which technique to use for the supine athlete, one must take into account the number of trained medical staff available to lift or roll the athlete. If ample staff are available, the multi-person lift-and-slide may be considered the most efficacious technique. If a smaller number of staff are available, the use of the scoop stretcher should be considered, with the log roll technique being used only when necessary [40, 41].

The multi-person lift-and-slide typically requires eight trained staff; more staff members can be used if the athlete is very large. As with all spinal motion restriction methods, the lead person (i.e., one giving directions for moving the athlete) is the staff member providing in-line stabilization of the head. Three or more medical team members will be positioned on each side of the injured athlete and one person will be at the foot of the athlete ready to slide the long spine board under the athlete. On command of the lead staff member, those on the sides of the athlete will place their hands carefully under the athlete being sure not to cause any rough or unnecessary motions. Again, on command, the lead and side medical team members will lift the athlete from the ground only enough to slide the long spine board under the athlete. Then on command, the athlete is lowered to the long spine board.

The scoop stretcher can be used to transfer an injured athlete with as few as four trained medical staff. The lead staff member provides manual in-line stabilization. The two longitudinal halves of the scoop stretcher are separated and positioned on each side of the injured athlete. On command of the lead staff member, three medical team members (two at the shoulders and one at the feet) carefully slide the scoop stretcher halves beneath the athlete until the hinges at both ends are in close approximation. The latch at the head-end of the scoop stretcher is locked first followed by the latch at the feet.

The log roll is frequently completed with five trained staff members, but this number can change if needed based on the size of the athlete. The lead staff member will provide manual in-line stabilization of the head and be in charge of all commands when moving the injured athlete. Three medical team members position themselves along the side of the athlete. Typically, these team members are located at the level of the shoulders, another at the hips and pelvis, and the third at the thighs and knees. An additional team member carefully wedges the spine board beneath and along the back of the athlete. The injured athlete is then rolled to the supine position, at which point it is often necessary to make some minor adjustments to center the cadaver on the spine board [42].

For an athlete lying in the prone position, a log roll technique is required for placement onto the long spine board. The log roll push technique has been shown to produce less motion in the unstable cervical spine as compared to the log roll pull technique [35]. However, both techniques should be practiced to prepare the medical staff for unusual situations such as an athlete lying near a fence or goal post that prevents the use of the log roll push. Keep in mind every time an athlete with an unstable cervical spine is moved increases the potential for exacerbating the intial injury, leading to additional harm. Thus, when possible, log roll the athlete directly onto the stabilization device rather than log rolling supine on the field, and then needing to move the athlete a second time to place them on the stabilization device.

In some instances when the assessment of the injured athlete results in minimal concern for a cervical spine injury, placement of a cervical collar and requesting the athlete to move on their own cognition to the ambulance gurney may be considered appropriate care [43].

Lastly, the use of the long spine board has been questioned due to the associated morbidity with prolonged periods of immobilization, such as pulmonary function issues, increased occipital and sacral pressures, increased intracranial pressures, pain, and tissue breakdown.For this reason, immediate removal should be performed once the athlete has been cleared. Also, the use of other techniques and devices may reduce such risk. For example, if a long spine board is selected to transfer the athlete, the use of a padded long spine board could be considered. Finally, recent research has demonstrated that the use of the vacuum mattress provides cervical spine stabilization with decreased pressure on the athlete's torso, thus potentially decreasing the potential for systemic complications [44, 45]. Regardless of the technique selected to transfer the athlete from the field, ensuring the athlete is moved only as much as necessary will potentially decrease the likelihood of a secondary insult to the spine region [38].

Thus, use of spinal immobilization on the long spine board should be implemented only when appropriate and for the least amount of time as necessary for clearance. The presence of any of the following would indicate the possible need for use of a long spine board or other appropriate spinal stabilization procedures [46]:

- Blunt trauma and altered level of consciousness
- Spinal pain or tenderness
- Neurological complaint (e.g., numbness or motor weakness)
- Anatomic deformity of the spine
- High-energy mechanism of injury and any of the following:
  - Drug or alcohol intoxication
  - Inability to communicate
  - Distracting injury

Following placement of the athlete onto the stabilization device, it is important to secure the athlete in position prior to transport. The use of a seven-strap or spider-strap technique provides greater stabilization when compared to the three-strap technique. A head stabilization device should be used to maintain cervical spine alignment [47]. The straps securing the legs and torso are applied prior to securing the head within the head stabilization device. Once the athlete is fully secured, including the head, manual in-line stabilization may be stopped.

Detailed Secondary Assessment

Depending on the acuity of the athlete's cervical spine injury determined by the focused primary assessment and the training expertise of the available medical personnel, parts of the detailed secondary assessment may begin to occur on the field, during transportation, or upon arrival to a tertiary care center. Most importantly, at each phase of care, the athletes' examination should be repeated to assess for worsening or improving neurological complaints and deficits. This evaluation should include a detailed history including the nature of the impact, past medical history of the athlete (including history of previous spine injuries like cervical cord neuropraxia), current symptoms (paresthesia, pain, subjective weakness, brief periods of neurological symptoms, etc.), a thorough neurological assessment, and a detailed physical assessment to assess for things like midline tenderness, step-off, spinal deformities, or interspinous widening. The components of a complete neurological exam include the athlete's mental status, cranial nerve examination, motor strength testing (Table 8.1), sensation, deep tendon reflexes, pathological reflexes (i.e., Babinski's or Hoffman's sign), signs of spinal cord injury (e.g., priapism), and completeness of injury (perineal sensation, rectal contractility).

It is imperative to have a solid understanding of neuroanatomy, specifically upper cervical nerves and their associated myotomes (Table 8.2) and sensory dermatomes (Fig. 8.5), to be able to localize the specific lesion and to determine appropriate levels for imaging. Also, the extent of "completeness" of a spinal cord injury (absence of rectal contractility) in concordance with the American Spinal Injury Association (ASIA) Impairment Score influences the aggressiveness of surgical intervention because the likelihood of meaningful neurological recovery from a complete spinal cord injury is extremely minimal [48, 49].

Table 8.1 Clinical scale for motor strength testing (Medical Research Council System)

Grade	
5/5	Full strength
4/5	Moves extremity against some resistance, but not full strength
3/5	Able to move extremity full range of motion against gravity
2/5	Moves extremity full range of motion when gravity eliminated (parallel to floor)
1/5	Shows only muscle contractility
0/5	No movement

Table 8.2 Cervical nerve root myotomes

Cervical nerve root	Associated muscle
C5	Deltoid (arm abduction)
C5–6	Biceps (arm flexion)
C6	Brachioradialis (wrist extension)
C7	Triceps (arm extension)
C8	Flexor digitorum (grip)
T1	Hand intrinsics (finger abduction)

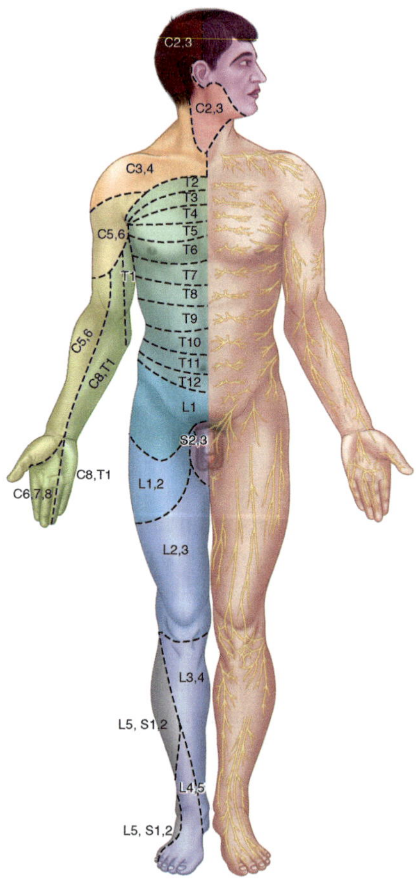

Fig. 8.5 Sensory dermatomes of the upper extremities, trunk, and lower extremities. (Mikael Häggström [100]. Public Domain)

Along with rectal contractility, it is imperative to assess for a bulbocavernosus reflex. This polysynaptic spinal cord reflex is mediated from S2–S4 and is elicited by tugging on a patient's foley catheter or stimulating the penis or vulva and evaluating for anal contraction. Testing this reflux ensures that the patient is not in spinal shock, which is a transient loss or reduction in neurological function below the level of injury. Therefore, a patient with absent rectal tone and no sensory or motor function below the level of injury would only be considered a complete SCI in the presence of an intact bulbocavernosus reflex. "Spinal shock" is frequently incorrectly used interchangeably with the term "neurogenic shock." Neurogenic shock is a form of distributive shock which involves trauma to the spinal cord, but specifically in the cervical to upper thoracic levels, leading to disruption of the descending sympathetic fibers resulting in systemic vasodilation and profound hypotension and paradoxical bradycardia. Clinically, neurogenic shock is appreciated in a patient who sustained a cervical/upper thoracic cord injury, is noted to have warm and flushed skin, and profound hypotension not responsive to fluid resuscitation. Therefore, to promote spinal cord perfusion in a patient in spinal shock, vasopressors should be used rather than crystalloid in order to prevent pulmonary edema and respiratory collapse.

Management Paradigms in Cervical Pathologies

Athletes are placed in an external cervical orthosis (cervical collar) by athletic trainers or emergency medical personnel following a suspected injury. After completing the thorough secondary assessment, the athlete is classified as one of three categories: asymptomatic, symptomatic (cervical neck pain) without neurological deficit, or symptomatic with a neurological deficit. Following a comprehensive neurological evaluation, experts should consider if cervical collar removal is safe/indicated. In efforts to reduce unnecessary imaging and radiation in patients with a low likelihood of cervical spine injury, multiple guidelines exist to assist clinicians in determining who requires cervical imaging following a trauma [50, 51]. In concordance with the most recent guidelines published by the Congress of Neurological Surgeons, radiographic imaging does not need to be obtained in an athlete following a traumatic event if he/she is asymptomatic (without neck pain or tenderness on midline posterior palpation), demonstrates a normal neurological examination, does not have a distracting injury, and is able to complete full cervical range of motion without symptoms [52]. For those athletes that meet this criteria, further imaging does not need to be obtained, and their cervical collar can be removed.

The second paradigm includes the athlete that is found to have cervical neck pain but has a normal neurological exam. These athletes should receive a high-quality computerized tomography scan (CT) of the cervical spine without contrast to evaluate for fractures and abnormal alignment [52]. If a fracture is present, the athlete should remain in the cervical collar with cervical spine precautions in place (bed rest with head of bed flat) until evaluated by a spine surgeon to determine the stability of the fracture and if further measures like traction or surgical intervention (decompression and/or fusion) are required. If the CT scan is negative, but the athlete has persistent pain, there are only Level-III guidelines to help assist the clinician due to a lack of strong evidence to support one specific recommendation. The determination of how to manage these athletes is dependent on multiple factors, for example, mechanism of injury, severity of pain, likelihood of returning for follow-up, level of play (high school versus professional), etc. Based on this, the clinician may decide to either attempt to clear the collar following a negative adequate flexion-extension radiograph, leave the collar on and have the athlete return in 1–2 weeks and obtain a flexion-extension film, or immediately obtain a magnetic resonance imaging (MRI) of the cervical spine [52]. Typically, following injury to the neck, significant paraspinal muscle spasms occur that restrict the athlete from performing an adequate range of flexion and extension, therefore limiting immediate evaluation by radiographs. Lastly, if an MRI is to be considered, this should be performed within 48 hours after injury to reduce false positive reads of ligamentous injury.

Lastly, any symptomatic athlete who is noted to have a neurological injury should remain in the cervical collar with strict spine precautions and receive a high-quality CT of the cervical spine, followed by consultation with a spine surgeon. Once a thorough neurological examination is performed by the treated surgeon to determine the level of injury, an MRI may be obtained. As this work-up is being performed, the athlete should be log rolled with strict in-line spine precautions to be removed from the backboard to prevent skin breakdown and admitted to the intensive care unit with serial hourly neurological exams. To promote spinal cord perfusion, an arterial line should be placed with a mean arterial pressure goal of 85–90 mmHg [53]. Once all of the imaging is obtained, the spine surgeon will assess the need for early surgical spinal decompression and possible fusion.

Controversies in Management of Cervical Spine Injuries

Acute traumatic spinal cord injuries have two pathophysiologic components: the initial traumatic insult to the spinal cord and the secondary injury elicited by inflammation and excitotoxicity of neurons. This section discusses various therapeutic modalities that have been studied in efforts at minimizing secondary injury of the spinal cord. Several pharmacologic agents (e.g., steroids) and physical treatments (e.g., hypothermia, cerebrospinal fluid [CSF] drainage) have been studied for their potential therapeutic role in neuroprotection with varied results.

Corticosteroids are potent anti-inflammatory agents and for this reason have been extensively studied in patients with acute spinal cord injuries. Several high-quality (class I) large, prospective multi-institutional studies as well as many lesser quality (class II, class III) studies have been published and have had conflicting conclusions regarding the therapeutic benefit of steroid use in acute spinal cord injury. The best quality studies are The National Acute SCI Study (NASCIS) and its follow-up studies, although interpretations of these studies have been controversial among experts.

NASCIS I was a prospective randomized controlled trial which evaluated the efficacy of steroid use in acute spinal cord injury [54]. Methylprednisolone was administered in either a high- or low-dose fashion to patients who had acute spinal cord injuries. This study found no benefit of a higher dose in terms of neurological function at 6 months follow-up, and the higher dose cohort of patients had three times greater rate of wound infection and death within 2 weeks. NASCIS II was a follow-up study designed as a prospective randomized clinical trial which evaluated the use of methylprednisolone and naloxone for spinal cord injury patients [55]. It also demonstrated no neuroprotective effect of either agent in primary analysis but did reveal higher rates of gastrointestinal hemorrhage, infection, and pulmonary embolus in patients who received steroids. A small benefit of motor function recovery was noted in a post-hoc analysis if steroids were administered within 8 hours of injury, but this finding is likely due to selection bias or random error rather than true benefit. Despite this, some experts insist that administration of methylprednisolone may benefit spinal cord recovery. NASCIS III was the third prospective randomized controlled trial which compared three treatments: administration of methylprednisolone for 24 hours, administration of methylprednisolone for 48 hours, or administration of a synthetically engineered "super steroid" tirilazad mesylate (designed to have better anti-oxidant properties than methylprednisolone) for 48 hours [56, 57]. Similar to NASCIS I and II, NASCIS III demonstrated that steroids had no class I evidence for benefit of neurological recovery and were associated with higher levels of medical complications and morbidity.

Upon review of these class I medical evidence studies and others, the Congress of Neurological Surgeons concluded in the spinal cord injury guidelines that methylprednisolone use for the treatment of spinal cord injury is not recommended [58]. No neurological benefit is obtained, and increased rates of harm are seen in patients treated with steroids for acute spinal cord injuries. Further, the Federal Drug Administration (FDA) has not approved steroids for use in spinal cord injury.

Nonpharmacologic treatments for acute spinal cord injury have not been as well studied as corticosteroid administration. Therapeutic hypothermia (32–34 °C core body temperature) is thought to serve a neuroprotective function by decreasing inflammatory reaction after injury and decreasing the basal metabolic rate of the central nervous system [59, 60]. Hypothermia has demonstrated benefit in patients with in-hospital cardiac arrest and is routine practice in major hospitals [59, 61]. Several preclinical and animal studies have demonstrated a protective effect of hypothermia for spinal cord injury with no increase in complications, and a larger phase II/III trial is planned to further investigate this hypothesis [62, 63].

Lastly, Cerebrospinal fluid (CSF) monitoring/drainage may be an additional tool to promote neurological recovery by reducing secondary injury following acute traumatic spinal cord injury. Recent studies have demonstrated that using sophisticated monitoring of spinal cord perfusion pressures through the use of invasive hemodynamic and intrathecal pressure monitors helps predict neurological outcomes [64]. This technique allows close monitoring of spinal cord perfusion pressure. It follows that lowering the intrathecal pressure in the spine, which allows more spinal cord perfusion, may be beneficial. A multicenter clinical trial evaluating CSF drainage in acute spinal cord injury is currently ongoing.

Although no currently studied pharmacologic therapies have demonstrated to improve neurological outcomes in spinal cord injury, ongoing research continues in hopes of finding treatments of this unfortunately common and devastating injury.

Specific Sports-Related Cervical Spine Injuries

As discussed earlier, axial loading resulting in cervical spine buckling is the primary biomechanical force that results in cervical spine trauma in football. Depending on the magnitude and duration of force coupled with other force vectors (axial rotation, flexion, and/or extension), various cervical pathologies can occur involving the cervical ligaments, disc spaces, bony structures (vertebral body, facets, lamina, spinous process, transverse process, etc.), or the spinal cord. The different types and combinations of cervical spine injuries a football player is prone to are innumerous and beyond the scope of this chapter; therefore, we will provide more detailed information only for a few common types of cervical spine injuries that could occur in football.

Cervical Sprain/Strain

Commonly confused terms: a sprain involves injury to a ligamentous structure while a strain involves a muscle, but clinically can occur in concert following a significant hyperflexion injury of the cervical spine. The athlete will complain of either midline or paraspinal pain that worsens with cervical motion. Importantly, a cervical sprain/strain will not result in any neurological deficits or symptoms in the extremities (radicular pain, paresthesias, etc.). The typical diagnostic sequence would involve a negative CT of the neck followed by either discharge in a cervical collar or obtaining an MRI which would demonstrate stir signal change within the cervical ligaments (nuchal, interspinous, etc.) or associated musculature (Fig. 8.6).

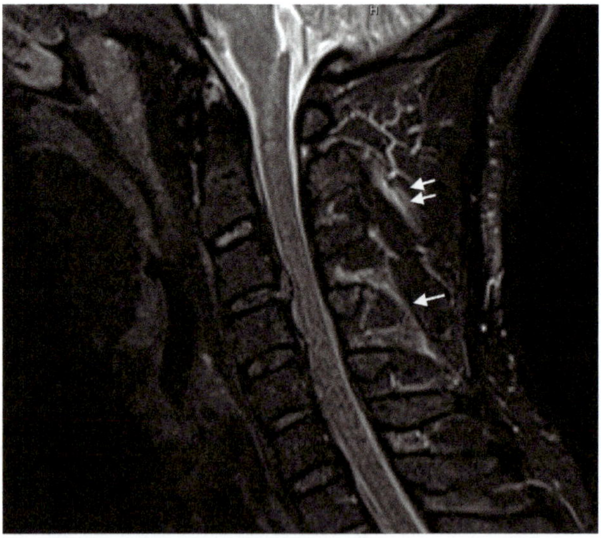

Fig. 8.6 Sagittal T2 stir sequence of the cervical spine demonstrating hyperintense stir signal in the paraspinal muscles at C2–3 (double arrow) and interspinous ligaments from C2 to C7 (single arrow) significant for a cervical ligamentous sprain and paraspinal strain

Typically in 2–4 weeks, an athlete that has suffered from a cervical sprain/strain should return for evaluation for collar clearance and consideration for return to play (RTP). The examiner should confirm that the athlete is without any symptoms, has undergone an intact neurological exam, and is able to perform a full range of motion of the cervical spine (flexion, extension, lateral rotation) without any symptoms. Once confirmed, a flexion-extension cervical x-ray should be performed to affirm absence of instability. If these criteria are met, the athlete may return to contact activities. If the athlete develops any "red flags" (weakness, radicular pain, paresthesias, etc.) or persistent pain, an MRI should be obtained.

Cervical Herniated Nucleus Pulposus

A retrospective review of spine injuries reported during 12 National Football league seasons (2000–2012) by Gray et al. demonstrated a total of 275 disc herniations (treated conservatively and surgically) accounting for roughly 13% of all spine injuries, and 23% of those disc herniations involved the cervical spine (most commonly at C3–4 and C5–6) [65]. The intervertebral disc is comprised of an outer tough anulus fibrosis which is composed of collagen and an inner soft nucleus pulposus. Either due to chronic degenerative forces or an acute traumatic event, the inner nucleus pulposus herniates through the annulus, compressing the associated exiting nerve root (Fig. 8.7). The athlete would complain of associated nerve root level radicular pain, paresthesias, or even associated nerve root myotome weakness. For example, a C6–7 left disc herniation would compress the exiting left C7 nerve root, causing radicular pain/paresthesias in the distribution of the 1st–3rd digits on the left hand and potentially triceps weakness on exam (Fig. 8.8).

Roughly 90% of cervical disc herniations will regress and improve without surgical intervention; therefore, unless a neurological deficit is present (associated weakness), the initial management of a cervical disc herniation should include various conservative therapy modalities such as non-steroidal anti-inflammatory medications, short course of tapered methylprednisolone, physical therapy, and/or injections [20, 66, 67]. Interestingly, a retrospective cohort review of 99 professional football players was performed by Hsu et al., which included at least a 2-year follow-up on 53 players treated operatively and 46 non-operatively for cervical disc herniations, and demonstrated a statically significant ($p < 0.04$) higher rate of return to play in those players treated operatively (72%) versus non operatively (46%) [68]. A long trial of conservative therapy until symptom resolution in a cervical disc herniation could be disadvantageous in a professional athlete whose career length is on average already quite diminutive.

If the athlete still has persistent symptoms (radicular pain, paresthesias) following a 6–8-week trial of conservative therapy or the athlete is noted to have an associated weakness on initial presentation, surgical intervention should be offered. Options include an anterior approach involving a discectomy and fusion or disc arthroplasty versus a posterior approach, including a non-fusion laminotomy/discectomy or a laminotomy foraminotomy and fusion. The benefits of anterior

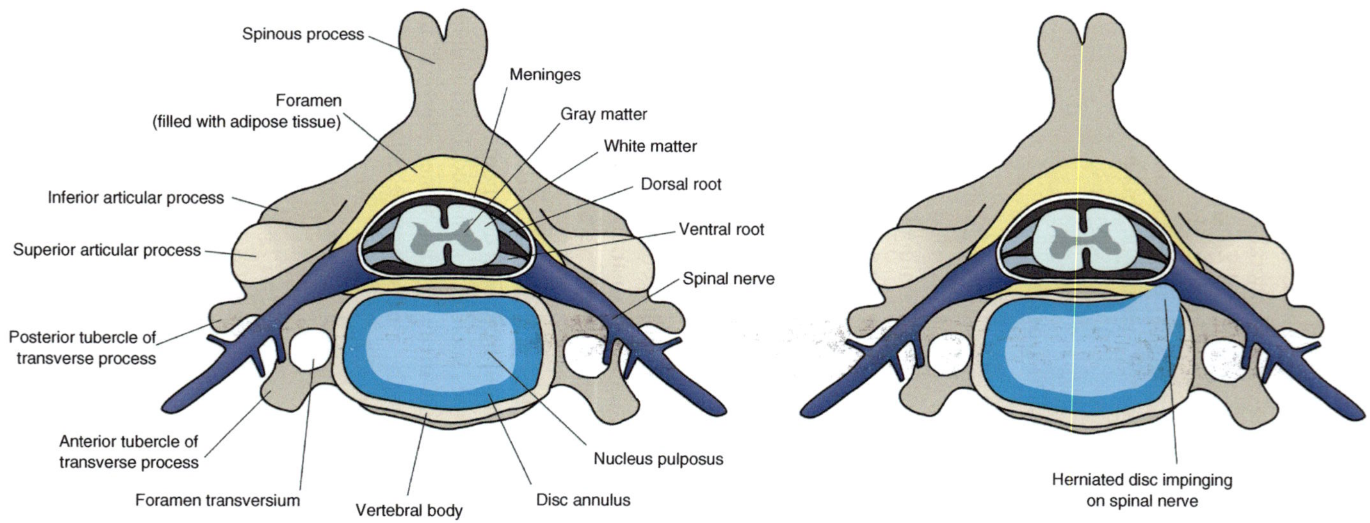

Fig. 8.7 Cartoon depiction of a cervical vertebra with associated labeled anatomy (Left) Herniation of the nucleus pulposus through the anulus fibrosis compressing the exiting nerve root (Right). (Used under the Creative Commons Attribution License, https://commons.wikimedia.org/wiki/File:ACDF_coronal_english.png)

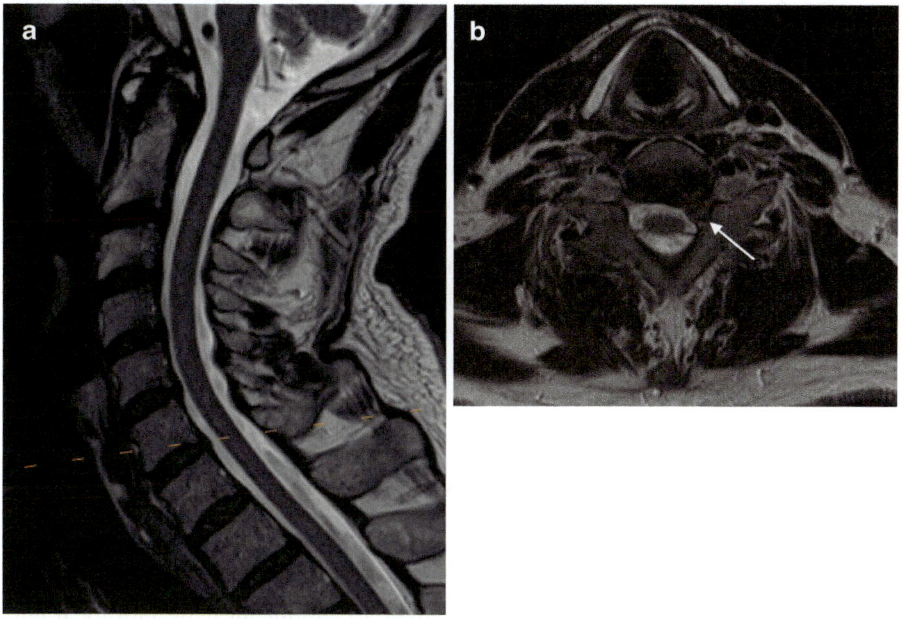

Fig. 8.8 MRI of the cervical spine with sagittal (**a**) and axial (**b**) slices demonstrating a large left-sided C6–7 disc herniation. The athlete presented with radicular pain in the hand and left triceps weakness

approach are less muscle dissection and possibly reduced postoperative pain but has an increased risk of postoperative swallowing dysfunction and 10% associated risk of adjacent segment disease in those requiring a fusion [69]. Alternatively, a posterior approach requires greater neck musculature dissection and possible worse pain but may not require a fusion. Limitations to successfully perform a posterior approach are dependent on the characteristics of the disc herniation: location, acuity, size, etc. Through limited and level III evidence, Mae et al. compared 101 professional athletes (of which 69 where NFL players) with a cervical disc herniation who received either a disc arthroplasty ($n = 2$), posterior foraminotomy ($n = 13$), or anterior discectomy and fusion ($n = 86$) with a mean follow-up of 13.5 years (range 2–34) to reveal a higher return to play in those who received a posterior foraminotomy, but these athletes were more likely to require a same level reoperation (46% vs. 6%, $p < 0.001$) [69, 70]. Though this study is limited by sample size and retrospective nature, it is important to consider when counseling an athlete prior to surgery. Lastly, with the advent of artificial discs, a disc arthroplasty can be offered in order to still perform an anterior approach and maintain motion at that segment; but at this time, there is limited evidence, specifically within a population of football players, to appreciate the long-term stability of these devices an athlete that is exposed to excessive axial loads [71].

Intervention type (operative vs. non-operative), presence of neurological deficit, and specific surgical approach will all influence RTP for an injured athlete. In general, a football player with a cervical disc herniation will RTP roughly between 1.5 and 3 months whether operative or nonoperative management occurs [9, 69]. Roughly three-fourths of football players will return to play following surgery, and those that receive operative intervention (anterior and posterior) for a single cervical disc herniation can be considered for RTP if they are without any significant neurological deficits, have a healed incision, have absence of symptoms with full range of motion, and with normal cervical alignment [20, 72, 73]. For those requiring a fusion, demonstration of bony fusion should be seen on lateral radiographs without evidence of instability prior to considering RTP [74]. Due to producing excessive strain at adjacent levels following a multilevel fusion creating a long segment lever arm, expert opinion considers 1–2 disc levels treated with a fusion as a relative contraindication and >2 levels to be an absolute contraindication to return to play in contact sports [71, 75–77].

Spinous Process/Transverse Process Fractures

Spinous process (Fig. 8.9) and transverse process (Fig. 8.10) fractures occur either due to direct blunt impact or excessive cervical extension or flexion. The symptoms can range from being completely asymptomatic to significant pain with focal tenderness and associated muscle spasms. A pure spinous process/transverse process fracture is a biomechanically and neurologically stable fracture that does not require any surgical intervention or cervical immobilization. The athlete can return to play once the fracture is healed, is symptom-free, and has full range of motion without

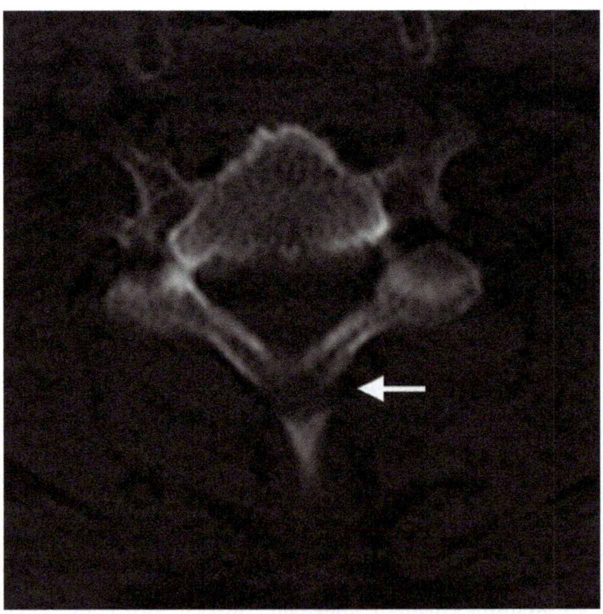

Fig. 8.9 A non-contrast CT of the cervical spine demonstrating a linear fracture through the spinous process of C5

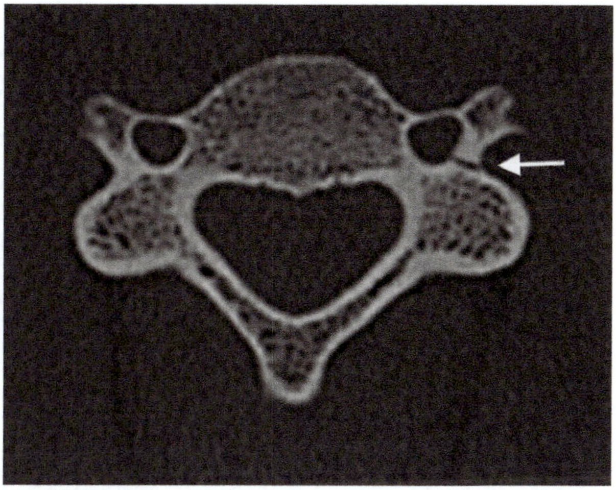

Fig. 8.10 A non-contrast CT of the cervical spine demonstrating a left C3 transverse process fracture involving the foramen transversarium. A follow-up CT angiography was negative for vertebral artery injury

pain. It is important to note that the vertebral artery travels through the foramen transversarium of the cervical transverse process from C1 to C6. Therefore, any athlete with a cervical transverse process fractures should receive a CT angiogram of the neck to assess for vertebral artery injury.

Cervical Compression/Burst Fractures

An axial load combined with flexion on the cervical spine can result in either a compression fracture or a burst fracture. A failure in the integrity of the anterior vertebral column results in a cervical compression fracture (Fig. 8.11), while further structural failure of the posterior column and potential retropulsion of bony fragments into the spinal canal results in a burst fracture (Fig. 8.12). Cervical compression fractures result in focal pain that does not cause a neurological deficit because the posterior vertebral column remains intact. Treatment involves the placement of a cervical collar for 6–8 weeks with return to play once the athlete's fracture is healed, with full range of motion without symptoms, and demonstrates normal alignment on upright cervical x-rays [20, 72]. A cervical burst fracture on the other hand is an unstable fracture that may require an anterior corpectomy for decompression of the spinal cord followed by posterior fusion depending on the extent of instability. Due to the likelihood of a neurological injury in the athlete, return to play following a cervical burst fracture is unlikely.

Cervical Facet Joint Pathologies

The facet joints of the cervical spine have a unique anatomy. They are oriented at 45° in the sagittal plane, and the facet capsule ligament has the strongest failure

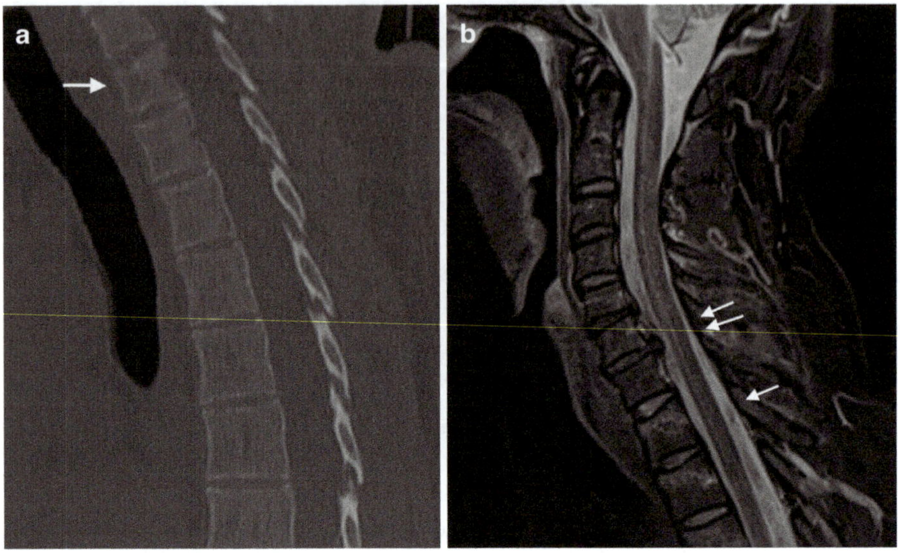

Fig. 8.11 (**a**) Non-contrast CT of the thoracic spine demonstrating T1 compression fracture (single arrow). (**b**) T2 stir cervical MRI sagittal view obtained in the same athlete demonstrating stir signal at the T1 compression fracture (single arrow) and adjacent superior endplate of T2. Also, with a clinically insignificant cervical disc herniation at C6–7 (double arrow)

strength of the spinal ligaments. Injury to the cervical facet joints can range from dislocation, disruption, and/or fractures requiring either external orthosis or even surgical intervention depending on the alignment, stability, and neurological exam of the patient. Significant axial load with hyperextension can result in unilateral or bilateral facet fractures (Fig. 8.13) while hyperflexion with axial rotation can lead to unilateral or bilateral perched/jumped facets (Fig. 8.14) or even cervical fracture dislocation. Only unilateral facet fractures in a neurologically intact athlete with minimal fracture displacement and good overall cervical alignment can be treated with a hard cervical collar for 6–10 weeks. Depending on the extent of fracture translation, repeat upright radiographs should be considered every 2–4 weeks to assess for stability of the fracture and overall cervical alignment. Once the fracture is healed, repeat radiographic imaging demonstrating normal alignment in an athlete with full cervical range of motion without symptoms is able to return to play [20, 72].

The treatment algorithm for determining management strategies in simple and complex facet injuries must involve a surgeon well versed in spinal trauma because even the decision on the timing of obtaining a cervical MRI depends on the clinical picture of the patient. The patient may require emergent closed reduction with weighted traction if a neurological deficit is noted in the awake athlete. The ability to reduce fractures will then determine the surgical intervention needed, whether it be an anterior, posterior, or combined approach.

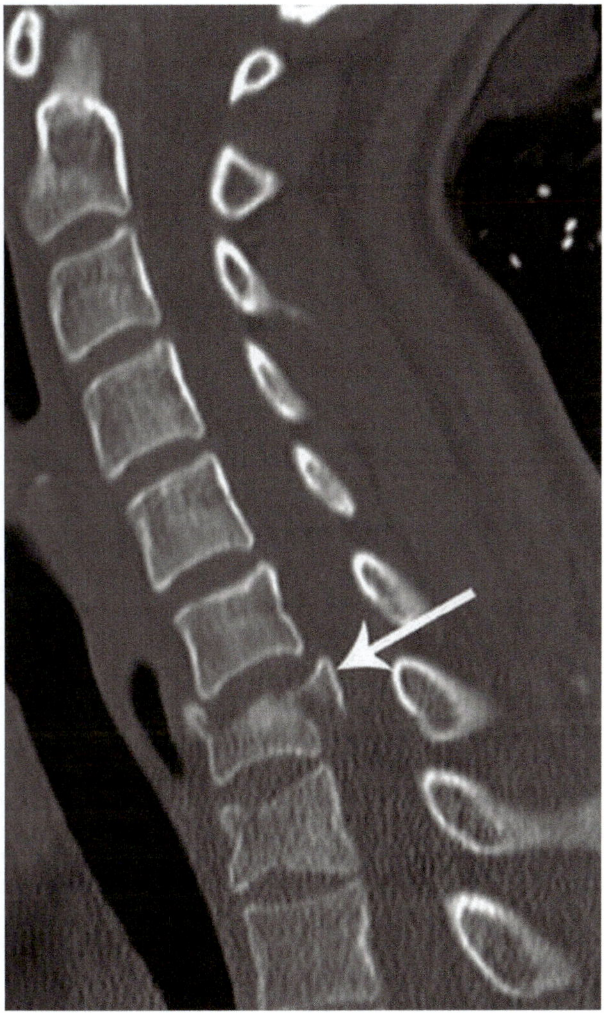

Fig. 8.12 Mid-sagittal CT image showing a comminuted fracture of C7 with nearly symmetrical loss of vertebral body height with extension of the fracture to the posterior cortex and retropulsion of fragment from the posterosuperior cortex of C7 (white arrow)—suggestive of a burst fracture. (Open Access and distributed under the Creative Commons Attribution License: Raniga et al. [101])

Cervical Cord Neuropraxia

Cervical cord neuropraxia (CCN), also termed "spinal cord concussion," "transient quadriplegia," or "commotio spinalis," is defined as an acute, transient neurological deficit that recovers in minutes to hours [77–80]. Sensory symptoms may include paresthesias, dysesthesias, burning/stinging, etc., and the motor deficits can range from paresis to even plegia. The presenting clinical neurological picture is determined by the extent and location of the cervical cord irritation. For example, a clinical entity known as "central cord" is a cervical cord injury in a spine with degenerative disease and stenosis that preferentially involves the central portion of

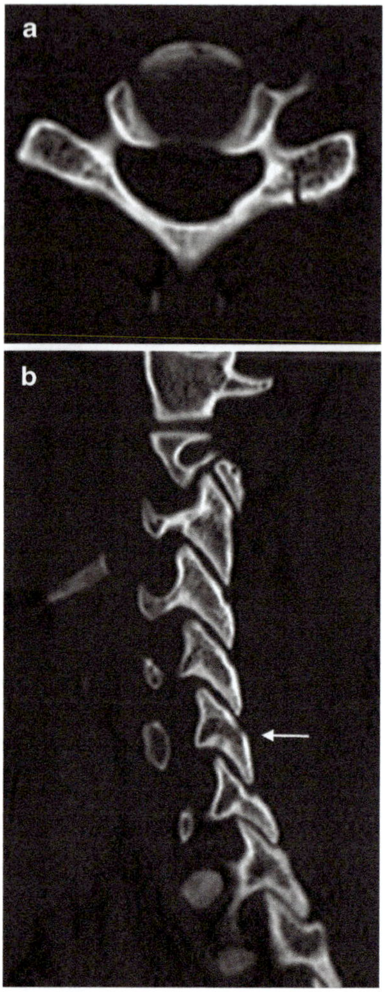

Fig. 8.13 A non-contrast CT of the neck demonstrating a non-displaced, linear fracture of the left C6 facet on (**a**) axial and (**b**) parasagittal images. The athlete's fracture was successfully treated conservatively with a hard collar for 8 weeks

the cervical cord possibly affecting the traversing central corticospinal and lateral spinothalamic tract. Therefore, involvement of the central corticospinal tract would cause weakness to the upper extremities and abnormal pain and temperature to the upper extremities if the lateral spinothalamic tract is also affected. More minor injuries with transient hand sensory symptoms has been termed "burning hands syndrome" [76, 81].

Grading of CCN is determined by the time required for the patient's symptoms to resolve: grade 1 is <15 minutes of symptoms, grade 2 is 15–24 minutes, and grade 3 is >24 hours [20, 82]. Boden et al. reported the details of recovery in 12 players with CCN with 42% of athletes having grade 1, 42% with grade 2, and 17% with grade 3 CCN [7]. A review of the National Center for Catastrophic Sports Injury Research from 1989 to 2002 demonstrated an incidence of CCN of 0.17 per 100,000 in high school and 2.05 per 100,000 in collegiate football players [7].

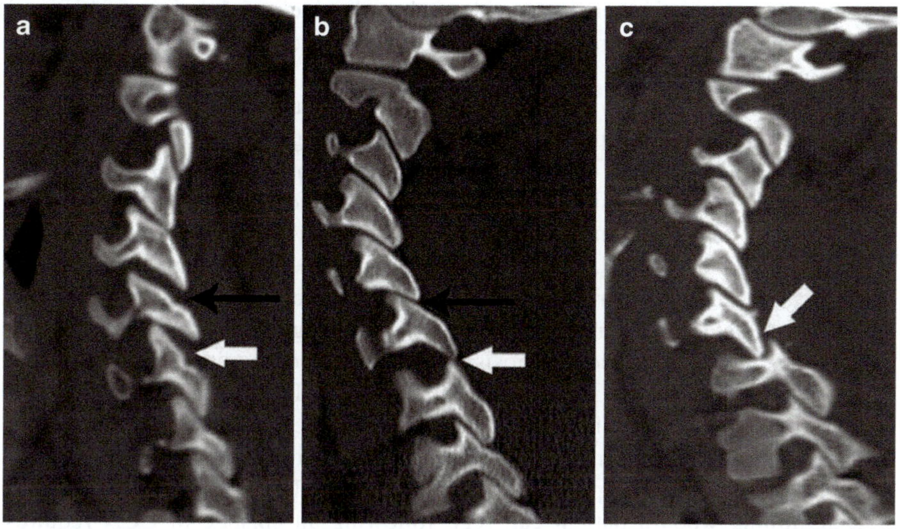

Fig. 8.14 Facet joint injury spectrum resulting from hyperflexion distraction. Parasagittal CT images. (**a**) The C4–5 facet joint shows diffuse widening-diastasis (black arrow), and the C5–6 facet joint shows focal anterior widening (white arrow), suggestive of distraction injury and partial disruption of facet joint capsule. Articular surfaces are congruent and no uncovering of the inferior articular process noted any of the injured levels. (**b**) C5–6 facet joint subluxation (black arrow) suggested by non-congruent articular surfaces of the facet joint with anterosuperior displacement of the inferior articular process of C5, resulting in partial uncovering of the superior articular surface of C6. However, some apposition of articular surface is still intact. C6–7 facet joint dislocation (white arrow) suggested by anterior and superior translation of inferior articular process of C6 resting on the top of the C7 articular facet. A facet joint injury as seen at C6–7 is also named as a "perched facet." (**c**) C6–7 facet joint dislocation with further anterior translation of the inferior articular process (white arrow), now resting anterior to the C7 articular pillar. This injury is also called a "locked" or "jumped facet." (Open Access and distributed under the Creative Commons Attribution License: Raniga et al. [101])

It is believed that CCN occurs due to an axial load and buckling of the cervical spine causing shear strain along the white matter tracts and/or direct compression of the spinal cord against the protruding ligamentum flavum and adjacent vertebral bodies [11]. For this reason, CCN is associated with cervical canal stenosis. First defined as canal diameter <14 mm on a lateral radiograph, critiques arose due to the varying sizes of cervical vertebra among different aged athletes. This was attempted to be corrected by the "Torg-Pavlov ratio method." The ratio was calculated by measuring the canal diameter on a lateral x-ray (from spinolaminar to posterior vertebral line) and dividing this by the length of the vertebral body. A ratio <0.8 was considered abnormal and the use of the ratio method allowed for variances in magnification, patient age, bone size, and reproducibility among different examiners [83]. This measurement was found to have high sensitivity but low specificity and has become an antiquated measurement in the advent of MR imaging [84–87]. Now with the use of MRI, the term "functional reserve" of the spinal cord is used to describe the CSF space that is separating the spinal cord from the surrounding bony anatomy [77]. Currently there is no evidence based guidelines defining an abnormal value of functional reserve but more so an absence or presence, and this to help risk stratify an athlete for return to play.

An athlete presenting with CCN and therefore neurological deficits on exam would receive both a CT of the neck, which would be negative for cervical fractures, followed by an MRI of the cervical spine without contrast. The MRI would likely demonstrate cervical stenosis with reduced functional reserve and may or may not show signs of cord myelomalacia or spinal cord injury (a T2 hyperintense lesion within the spinal cord) [82]. Surgical management varies depending on the source (anterior or posterior compression) and the number of cervical levels involved. An adolescent athlete with neurological deficits with imaging negative for fractures, ligamentous injury, or cervical stenosis would be diagnosed with "SCIWORA," or spinal cord injury without radiographic abnormality. This cervical SCI has been believed to occur secondarily to more lax ligaments seen in children and therefore management involves external orthosis for up to 2–3 months till asymptomatic followed by dynamic radiographs to assess for stability [71, 77, 88].

Determining when a patient can RTP following an episode of CCN requires expert evaluation through an individualized approach to the athlete by assessing the extent of initial injury (severity and duration of symptoms), history of previous CCN, current clinical evaluation, recent neuro-imaging, and level of athletic play (e.g., high school versus professional). For those athletes with minimal symptoms at time of injury, complete absence of symptoms and normal neurological exam, without previous episode of CCN, and normal cervical MR imaging (resolution or absence of cervical cord edema and good functional reserve), it is appropriate to consider return to competitive play following a discussion regarding the associated risks and appropriate tackling technique [11, 20, 72, 77, 80, 89]. Torg et al. reviewed 110 athletes following a CCN (in which 96 where football players) with an average follow-up of 3 years to report that none of the athletes demonstrated a permanent neurological deficit but of those that returned back to their sport, 56% had a recurrent episode [90]. Therefore, it is important to emphasize the potential recurrent risk of CCN following a return to football, but with an unknown but possible severe neurological sequalae following repeat episode. Absolute contraindications to RTP in an athlete that experienced a CCN would be: prior episode of CCN, persistent symptoms or prolonged symptoms (>24 hours), presence of neurological deficit, and/or significant CT or MRI findings (spear tackler's spine, poor functional reserve, cervical stenosis, persistent cervical cord myelomalacia, or anomalies such as Chiari or Klippel-Feil) [11, 13, 20, 72, 77, 80, 82, 85, 89].

Return to Play

Due to limited evidence, all RTP guidelines published for cervical spine pathologies are expert opinions; therefore, a physician well versed in managing spinal injuries is needed to thoroughly evaluate the athlete following such injury to determine when and if it is appropriate to return that player to football. Due to the limited evidence and guidance for RTP following cervical spine injuries, each athlete's medical clearance requires an individualized approach. This is determined by considering the initial injury, a subsequent follow-up history/physical exam, and evaluation of repeat cervical radiographs. Factors to be considered with the initial injury include presence, severity, duration, and history of neurological deficits; specific cervical pathology (strain, sprain, tear, fracture, etc.); and specific treatment modality used (surgical fusion versus external orthosis). These factors are all then used in summation to have a risk stratification discussion with the athlete, also taking into account their level of competitive play. As previously acknowledged in the RTP discussion for some of the specific cervical spine pathologies; generally, an athlete must be neurologically intact, without any symptoms, and have full range of motion of their cervical spine without pain prior to considering RTP. Automatic disqualifiers include [13, 72, 80, 82, 85]:

History: persistent symptoms (pain, extremity paresthesias, etc.), repeat occurrences

Physical Exam: neurological deficit, restricted cervical motion

Imaging: non-healed fracture, cervical instability/malalignment, significant cervical stenosis/absent functional reserve on MRI, spear tackler's spine, significant MRI abnormalities (edema, hemorrhage, contusion, etc.)

Treatment modality: multi-level (>3) fusion

Pre-participation Conditions

For various reasons, an athlete may receive a brain or cervical MRI demonstrating findings in the cervical spine such as stenosis, Klippel-Feil syndrome, and Chiari malformation. The absence of clinical signs or symptoms then presents the question: "Should this athlete still be allowed to participate in a contact sport, specifically football?" Due to the limited evidence regarding the incidence of associated catastrophic neurological injury for each of these pathologies, it becomes quite challenging in discussing the risk with both the athlete and potentially his/her parents. For this reason, referral to an expert in spine pathologies is required to thoroughly evaluate the athlete neurologically, assess for pertinent symptoms, review the appropriate imaging, and appropriately counsel the athlete about the risks associated with contact sports.

Cervical Stenosis

As discussed, cervical stenosis was first historically defined by canal diameter, which was then refined by the proposed ratio method during the pre-MRI era. Now, with the advent of MRI, evaluating for cervical stenosis by assessing the functional reserve or amount of CSF space surrounding the spinal cord has become more precise but more subjective. More severe stenosis is characterized on MRI by indentation of the cord or myelomalacia, which places the athlete at a considerably higher risk of developing cervical cord neuropraxia and/or catastrophic neurological injury.

Therefore, evaluation of a football player with cervical stenosis should involve a detailed history to identify symptoms of myelopathy (paresthesias, subjective weakness, gait imbalance, etc.), previous episodes of SCI (burning hands syndrome, CCN, etc.), full neurological exam paying close attention to signs of myelopathy (including evaluation for brisk reflexes and pathological reflexes), and degree of cervical stenosis on imaging. A truly asymptomatic, neurologically intact athlete with mild cervical stenosis can be allowed to participate in contact sports following a discussion and understanding of the associated potential risks of catastrophic neurological injury [89]. Those with either subjective symptoms, focal neurological deficits, significant cervical stenosis (moderate to severe, no CSF space around spinal cord, or cord myelomalacia), or evidence of spear tackler's spine should be educated about the associated risks and not allowed to participate in contact sports [13, 72, 82, 85, 89].

Klippel-Feil Syndrome

Klippel-Feil syndrome is a musculoskeletal condition that is due to the failure of segmentation of the vertebral body segments in the cervical spine resulting in a congenital fusion of multiple cervical segments (Fig. 8.15). More advanced cases may be associated with multiple fused levels and also coexisting conditions involving the heart and kidneys. If an athlete is noted to have Klippel-Feil on cervical radiographs, it is necessary to determine if further imaging, like an MRI, is needed to evaluate for adjacent segment degenerative pathology and/or stenosis. Therefore, a detailed history and neurological exam should be performed. Due to the fused segments, there is potential increased risk of degenerative stenosis at the adjacent levels or a lever arm phenomenon increasing the risk of traumatic pathologies. This risk is theoretically increased with the more levels that are fused. Published expert opinion recommendations are that Klippel-Feil syndrome is a relative contraindication for contact sports, and the athlete can still be considered to participate if there is only involvement of 2–3 vertebral segments in a neurologically intact patient without symptoms or restricted cervical motion. If there are multiple segments (>3) involved, this would be considered an absolute contraindication [72, 82, 91].

Chiari Malformation

Chiari malformation, or Type 1 "adult" Chiari, is a hindbrain abnormality resulting in cerebellar tonsillar herniation through the foramen magnum which leads to abnormal CSF flow (Fig. 8.16). Symptoms commonly associated with Chiari Type 1 malformation are occipital headaches or neck pain that are exacerbated by increased intracranial pressure (ICP) (Valsalva, coughing, sneezing, etc.), lower cranial nerve deficits (dysphagia), unsteady gait, extremity weakness or paresthesias, abnormal temperature sensation ("cape-like" distribution), or signs of myelopathy. Clinical symptomatology is due to direct tonsillar compression of the caudal

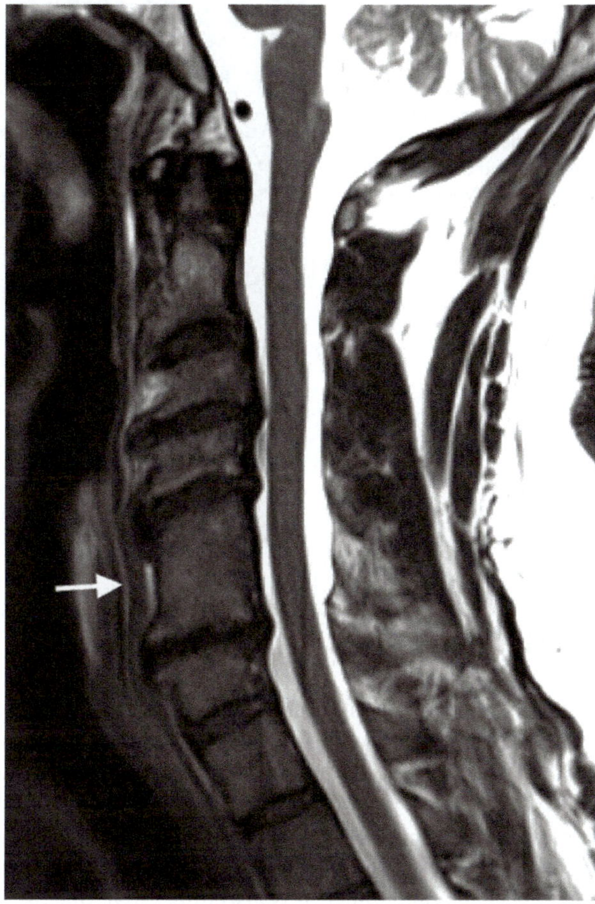

Fig. 8.15 Sagittal T2 weighted MRI of the cervical spine without contrast demonstrating Klippel-Feil syndrome with congenitally fused C5–6 vertebral body segments

brainstem or abnormal CSF migration and formation of a syrinx in the cervical or thoracic cord. For this reason, any athlete found to have a Chiari malformation should also receive cervical and possibly thoracic imaging to rule out presence of a syrinx depending on their symptomatology. Within the sports literature, there has been a handful of case reports of symptom exacerbation or development of neurological deficits (quadriparesis) in athletes with an undiagnosed Chiari malformation, but without any reports of catastrophic neurological injury aside from those reported secondarily to motor vehicle accidents [92–96]. Therefore, due to limited evidence, there only exists expert opinion regarding the player's eligibility for contact sports. A neurologically intact athlete with an asymptomatic Chiari malformation can participate in contact sports following a discussion of potential risks, if he/she is with minimal tonsillar herniation and adequate cervical cord functional reserve without a syrinx. A relative contraindication would be if the athlete is noted to have a syrinx and/or reduced functional reserve. An absolute contraindication would be if the athlete has significant symptoms, neurological deficits, and/or complete loss of functional reserve [93–95, 97–99].

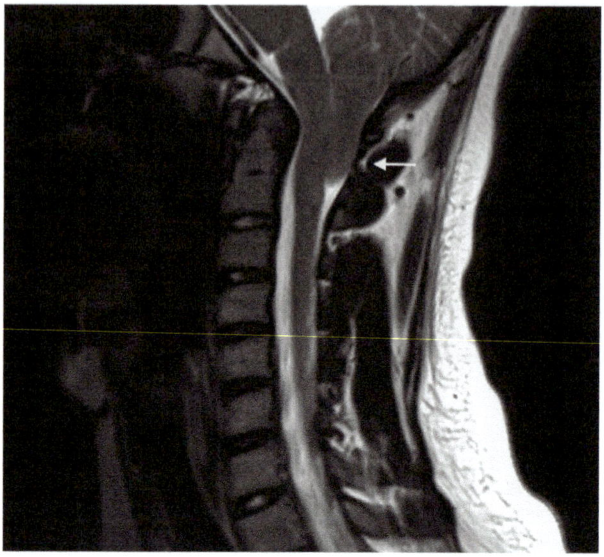

Fig. 8.16 A Chiari malformation in a 16-year-old with significant associated tonsillar decent below the level of the C1 ring demonstrated on a sagittal T2-weighted MRI of the cervical spine without contrast

Conclusion

Through the implementation of anti-spearing infractions imposed during football competition, the incidence of cervical spine injuries has reduced dramatically but it is not negligible. Therefore, it is necessary for all medical personnel working within the sport to have a general knowledge of the identification, management, and return to play recommendations for various cervical spine pathologies in order to make the sport safer. Since there is limited evidence regarding return to contact sport following a cervical spine injury, it is also imperative that all athletes receive a multidisciplinary approach specifically with the guidance from a surgeon well versed in the management of spinal trauma.

References

1. Center NSCIS. Facts and figures at a glance. Birmingham: University of Alabama at Birmingham; 2016.
2. Krueger H, Noonan VK, Trenaman LM, Joshi P, Rivers CS. The economic burden of traumatic spinal cord injury in Canada. Chronic Dis Inj Can. 2013;33(3):113–22.
3. Chan CW, Eng JJ, Tator CH, Krassioukov A. Epidemiology of sport-related spinal cord injuries: a systematic review. J Spinal Cord Med. 2016;39(3):255–64.
4. Babcock L, Olsen CS, Jaffe DM, Leonard JC. Cervical spine injuries in children associated with sports and recreational activities. Pediatr Emerg Care. 2018;34(10):677–86.
5. Meron A, McMullen C, Laker SR, Currie D, Comstock RD. Epidemiology of cervical spine injuries in high school athletes over a ten-year period. PM & R. 2018;10(4):365–72.
6. Cantu RC, Mueller FO. Catastrophic spine injuries in American football, 1977-2001. Neurosurgery. 2003;53(2):358–62; discussion 62–3.

7. Boden BP, Tacchetti RL, Cantu RC, Knowles SB, Mueller FO. Catastrophic cervical spine injuries in high school and college football players. Am J Sports Med. 2006;34(8):1223–32.
8. Delaney JS, Al-Kashmiri A. Neck injuries presenting to emergency departments in the United States from 1990 to 1999 for ice hockey, soccer, and American football. Br J Sports Med. 2005;39(4):e21.
9. Mall NA, Buchowski J, Zebala L, Brophy RH, Wright RW, Matava MJ. Spine and axial skeleton injuries in the National Football League. Am J Sports Med. 2012;40(8):1755–61.
10. Stone JL, Patel V, Bailes JE. The history of neurosurgical treatment of sports concussion. Neurosurgery. 2014;75(Suppl 4):S3–s23.
11. Rihn JA, Anderson DT, Lamb K, Deluca PF, Bata A, Marchetto PA, et al. Cervical spine injuries in American football. Sports Med. 2009;39(9):697–708.
12. Heck JF, Clarke KS, Peterson TR, Torg JS, Weis MP. National Athletic Trainers' Association position statement: head-down contact and spearing in tackle football. J Athl Train. 2004;39(1):101–11.
13. Chao S, Pacella MJ, Torg JS. The pathomechanics, pathophysiology and prevention of cervical spinal cord and brachial plexus injuries in athletics. Sports Med. 2010;40(1):59–75.
14. Torg J, Truex R Jr, Quedenfeld TC, Burstein A, Spealman A, Nichols C III. The National Football Head and Neck Injury Registry: report and conclusions. JAMA. 1978;(241):1477–9.
15. Boden BP, Breit I, Beachler JA, Williams A, Mueller FO. Fatalities in high school and college football players. Am J Sports Med. 2013;41(5):1108–16.
16. Hutton MJ, McGuire RA, Dunn R, Williams R, Robertson P, Twaddle B, et al. Catastrophic cervical spine injuries in contact sports. Global Spine J. 2016;6(7):721–34.
17. Nyland J, Johnson D. Collegiate football players display more active cervical spine mobility than high school football players. J Athl Train. 2004;39(2):146–50.
18. Hardacker JW, Shuford RF, Capicotto PN, Pryor PW. Radiographic standing cervical segmental alignment in adult volunteers without neck symptoms. Spine. 1997;22(13):1472–80; discussion 80.
19. Swartz EE, Floyd RT, Cendoma M. Cervical spine functional anatomy and the biomechanics of injury due to compressive loading. J Athl Train. 2005;40(3):155–61.
20. Boden BP, Jarvis CG. Spinal injuries in sports. Neurol Clin. 2008;26(1):63–78; viii.
21. Andersen J, Courson RW, Kleiner DM, McLoda TA. National Athletic Trainers' Association position statement: emergency planning in athletics. J Athl Train. 2002;37(1):99–104.
22. Scarneo SE, DiStefano LJ, Stearns RL, Register-Mihalik JK, Denegar CR, Casa DJ. Emergency action planning in secondary school athletics: a comprehensive evaluation of current adoption of best practice standards. J Athl Train. 2019;54(1):99–105.
23. Swartz EE, Norkus SA, Cappaert T, Decoster LC. Football equipment design affects face mask removal efficiency. Am J Sports Med. 2005;33(8):1210–9.
24. Sanchez AR 2nd, Sugalski MT, LaPrade RF. Field-side and prehospital management of the spine-injured athlete. Curr Sports Med Rep. 2005;4(1):50–5.
25. Chameides L, Samson R, Schexnayder S, Hazinski M. Pediatric advanced life support: provider manual. In: Association TAH, Pediatrics AAo, editors.: First American Heart Association Printing; 2011.
26. Sinz E, Navarro K. Advanced cardiovascular life support: provider manual. In: Association TAH, editor.: First American Heart Association; 2011.
27. Jung JY. Airway management of patients with traumatic brain injury/C-spine injury. Korean J Anesthesiol. 2015;68(3):213–9.
28. Del Rossi G, Heffernan TP, Horodyski M, Rechtine GR. The effectiveness of extrication collars tested during the execution of spine-board transfer techniques. Spine J. 2004;4(6):619–23.
29. Swartz EE, Boden BP, Courson RW, Decoster LC, Horodyski M, Norkus SA, et al. National athletic trainers' association position statement: acute management of the cervical spine-injured athlete. J Athl Train. 2009;44(3):306–31.
30. Horodyski M, DiPaola CP, Conrad BP, Rechtine GR 2nd. Cervical collars are insufficient for immobilizing an unstable cervical spine injury. J Emerg Med. 2011;41(5):513–9.

31. Correction to: Part 9: first aid: 2015 international consensus on first aid science with treatment recommendations. Circulation. 2017;135(24):e1143.
32. Dahl MC, Ananthakrishnan D, Nicandri G, Chapman JR, Ching RP. Helmet and shoulder pad removal in football players with unstable cervical spine injuries. J Appl Biomech. 2009;25(2):119–32.
33. Del Rossi G, Rechtine GR, Conrad BP, Horodyski M. Is sub-occipital padding necessary to maintain optimal alignment of the unstable spine in the prehospital setting? A preliminary report. J Emerg Med. 2013;45(3):366–71.
34. Copeland AJ, Decoster LC, Swartz EE, Gattie ER, Gale SD. Combined tool approach is 100% successful for emergency football face mask removal. Clin J Sport Med. 2007;17(6):452–7.
35. Conrad BP, Marchese DL, Rechtine GR, Prasarn M, Del Rossi G, Horodyski MH. Motion in the unstable cervical spine when transferring a patient positioned prone to a spine board. J Athl Train. 2013;48(6):797–803.
36. Decoster LC, Burns MF, Swartz EE, Murthi DS, Hernandez AE, Vailas JC, et al. Maintaining neutral sagittal cervical alignment after football helmet removal during emergency spine injury management. Spine. 2012;37(8):654–9.
37. Conrad BP, Horodyski M, Wright J, Ruetz P, Rechtine GR 2nd. Log-rolling technique producing unacceptable motion during body position changes in patients with traumatic spinal cord injury. J Neurosurg Spine. 2007;6(6):540–3.
38. Conrad BP, Rossi GD, Horodyski MB, Prasarn ML, Alemi Y, Rechtine GR. Eliminating log rolling as a spine trauma order. Surg Neurol Int. 2012;3(Suppl 3):S188–97.
39. Horodyski M, Conrad BP, Del Rossi G, DiPaola CP, Rechtine GR 2nd. Removing a patient from the spine board: is the lift and slide safer than the log roll? J Trauma. 2011;70(5):1282–5; discussion 5.
40. Del Rossi G, Rechtine GR, Conrad BP, Horodyski M. Are scoop stretchers suitable for use on spine-injured patients? Am J Emerg Med. 2010;28(7):751–6.
41. Del Rossi G, Horodyski MH, Conrad BP, Di Paola CP, Di Paola MJ, Rechtine GR. The 6-plus-person lift transfer technique compared with other methods of spine boarding. J Athl Train. 2008;43(1):6–13.
42. DuBose DN, Zdziarski LA, Scott N, Conrad B, Long A, Rechtine GR, et al. Horizontal slide creates less cervical motion when centering an injured patient on a spine board. J Emerg Med. 2016;50(5):728–33.
43. Swartz EE, Tucker WS, Nowak M, Roberto J, Hollingworth A, Decoster LC, et al. Prehospital cervical spine motion: immobilization versus spine motion restriction. Prehosp Emerg Care. 2018;22(5):630–6.
44. Prasarn ML, Hyldmo PK, Zdziarski LA, Loewy E, Dubose D, Horodyski M, et al. Comparison of the vacuum mattress versus the spine board alone for immobilization of the cervical spine injured patient: a biomechanical cadaveric study. Spine. 2017;42(24):E1398–E402.
45. Pernik MN, Seidel HH, Blalock RE, Burgess AR, Horodyski M, Rechtine GR, et al. Comparison of tissue-interface pressure in healthy subjects lying on two trauma splinting devices: the vacuum mattress splint and long spine board. Injury. 2016;47(8):1801–5.
46. White CC, Domeier RM, Millin MG, Standards, Clinical Practice Committee NAoEMSP. EMS spinal precautions and the use of the long backboard - resource document to the position statement of the National Association of EMS Physicians and the American College of Surgeons Committee on Trauma. Prehosp Emerg Care. 2014;18(2):306–14.
47. Peery CA, Brice J, White WD. Prehospital spinal immobilization and the backboard quality assessment study. Prehosp Emerg Care. 2007;11(3):293–7.
48. Internatinal standards for neurological classification of spinal cord injury, revised. Chicago: American Spinal Injury Association; 2000.
49. Hadley M, Walters B, Aarabi B, et al. Chapter 4. Clinical assessment following acute cervical spinal cord injury. Neurosurgery. 2013;72(3):40–53.
50. Hoffman JR, Mower WR, Wolfson AB, Todd KH, Zucker MI. Validity of a set of clinical criteria to rule out injury to the cervical spine in patients with blunt trauma. National Emergency X-Radiography Utilization Study Group. N Engl J Med. 2000;343(2):94–9.

51. Stiell I, Wells GA, Vandemheen KL, et al. The Canadian C-spine rule for radiography in alert and stable trauma patients. JAMA. 2001;286(15):1841–8.
52. Ryken T, Hadley MN, Walters BC, et al. Chapter 5. Radiographic assessment. Neurosurgery. 2013;72(3):54–72.
53. Ryken T, Hadley MN, Walters BC, et al. Chapter 7. The acute cardiopulmonary management of patients with cervical spinal cord injuries. Neurosurgery. 2013;72:84–92.
54. Young W. NASCIS. National Acute Spinal Cord Injury Study. J Neurotrauma. 1990;7(3): 113–4.
55. Bracken MB, Shepard MJ, Collins WF, Holford TR, Young W, Baskin DS, et al. A randomized, controlled trial of methylprednisolone or naloxone in the treatment of acute spinal-cord injury. Results of the Second National Acute Spinal Cord Injury Study. N Engl J Med. 1990;322(20):1405–11.
56. Bracken MB, Shepard MJ, Holford TR, Leo-Summers L, Aldrich EF, Fazl M, et al. Administration of methylprednisolone for 24 or 48 hours or tirilazad mesylate for 48 hours in the treatment of acute spinal cord injury. Results of the Third National Acute Spinal Cord Injury Randomized Controlled Trial. National Acute Spinal Cord Injury Study. JAMA. 1997;277(20):1597–604.
57. Bracken MB, Shepard MJ, Holford TR, Leo-Summers L, Aldrich EF, Fazl M, et al. Methylprednisolone or tirilazad mesylate administration after acute spinal cord injury: 1-year follow up. Results of the third National Acute Spinal Cord Injury randomized controlled trial. J Neurosurg. 1998;89(5):699–706.
58. Hurlbert RJ, Hadley MN, Walters BC, Aarabi B, Dhall SS, Gelb DE, et al. Pharmacological therapy for acute spinal cord injury. Neurosurgery. 2013;72(Suppl 2):93–105.
59. Kwon BK, Mann C, Sohn HM, Hilibrand AS, Phillips FM, Wang JC, et al. Hypothermia for spinal cord injury. Spine J. 2008;8(6):859–74.
60. Ahuja CS, Nori S, Tetreault L, Wilson J, Kwon B, Harrop J, et al. Traumatic spinal cord injury—repair and regeneration. Neurosurgery. 2017;80(3S):S9–S22.
61. Hypothermia after Cardiac Arrest Study Group. Mild therapeutic hypothermia to improve the neurologic outcome after cardiac arrest. N Engl J Med. 2002;346(8):549–56.
62. Levi AD, Green BA, Wang MY, Dietrich WD, Brindle T, Vanni S, et al. Clinical application of modest hypothermia after spinal cord injury. J Neurotrauma. 2009;26(3):407–15.
63. Lo TP Jr, Cho KS, Garg MS, Lynch MP, Marcillo AE, Koivisto DL, et al. Systemic hypothermia improves histological and functional outcome after cervical spinal cord contusion in rats. J Comp Neurol. 2009;514(5):433–48.
64. Squair JW, Belanger LM, Tsang A, Ritchie L, Mac-Thiong JM, Parent S, et al. Spinal cord perfusion pressure predicts neurologic recovery in acute spinal cord injury. Neurology. 2017;89(16):1660–7.
65. Gray BL, Buchowski JM, Bumpass DB, Lehman RA Jr, Mall NA, Matava MJ. Disc herniations in the National Football League. Spine. 2013;38(22):1934–8.
66. Meredith DS, Jones KJ, Barnes R, Rodeo SA, Cammisa FP, Warren RF. Operative and nonoperative treatment of cervical disc herniation in National Football League athletes. Am J Sports Med. 2013;41(9):2054–8.
67. Saal JS, Saal JA, Yurth EF. Nonoperative management of herniated cervical intervertebral disc with radiculopathy. Spine. 1996;21(16):1877–83.
68. Hsu WK. Outcomes following nonoperative and operative treatment for cervical disc herniations in National Football League athletes. Spine. 2011;36(10):800–5.
69. Mai HT, Burgmeier RJ, Mitchell SM, Hecht AC, Maroon JC, Nuber GW, et al. Does the level of cervical disc herniation surgery affect performance-based outcomes in National Football League athletes? Spine. 2016;41(23):1785–9.
70. Mai HT, Chun DS, Schneider AD, Hecht AC, Maroon JC, Hsu WK. The difference in clinical outcomes after anterior cervical fusion, disk replacement, and foraminotomy in professional athletes. Clin Spine Surg. 2018;31(1):E80–e4.
71. Brigham CD, Capo J. Cervical spinal cord contusion in professional athletes: a case series with implications for return to play. Spine. 2013;38(4):315–23.

72. Cantu RV, Cantu RC. Current thinking: return to play and transient quadriplegia. Curr Sports Med Rep. 2005;4(1):27–32.
73. Schroeder GD, Lynch TS, Gibbs DB, Chow I, LaBelle MW, Patel AA, et al. The impact of a cervical spine diagnosis on the careers of National Football League athletes. Spine. 2014;39(12):947–52.
74. Joaquim AF, Hsu WK, Patel AA. Cervical spine surgery in professional athletes: a systematic review. Neurosurg Focus. 2016;40(4):E10.
75. Torg JS. Cervical spine injuries and the return to football. Sports Health. 2009;1(5):376–83.
76. Maroon JC, El-Kadi H, Abla AA, Wecht DA, Bost J, Norwig J, et al. Cervical neurapraxia in elite athletes: evaluation and surgical treatment. Report of five cases. J Neurosurg Spine. 2007;6(4):356–63.
77. Bailes JE, Petschauer M, Guskiewicz KM, Marano G. Management of cervical spine injuries in athletes. J Athl Train. 2007;42(1):126–34.
78. Ladd AL, Scranton PE. Congenital cervical stenosis presenting as transient quadriplegia in athletes. Report of two cases. J Bone Joint Surg Am. 1986;68(9):1371–4.
79. Torg JS, Pavlov H, Genuario SE, Sennett B, Wisneski RJ, Robie BH, et al. Neurapraxia of the cervical spinal cord with transient quadriplegia. J Bone Joint Surg Am. 1986;68(9):1354–70.
80. Bailes JE, Hadley MN, Quigley MR, Sonntag VK, Cerullo LJ. Management of athletic injuries of the cervical spine and spinal cord. Neurosurgery. 1991;29(4):491–7.
81. Finnoff JT, Mildenberger D, Cassidy CD. Central cord syndrome in a football player with congenital spinal stenosis: a case report. Am J Sports Med. 2004;32(2):516–21.
82. Concannon LG, Harrast MA, Herring SA. Radiating upper limb pain in the contact sport athlete: an update on transient quadriparesis and stingers. Curr Sports Med Rep. 2012;11(1):28–34.
83. Pavlov H, Torg JS, Robie B, Jahre C. Cervical spinal stenosis: determination with vertebral body ratio method. Radiology. 1987;164(3):771–5.
84. Torg JS, Naranja RJ Jr, Pavlov H, Galinat BJ, Warren R, Stine RA. The relationship of developmental narrowing of the cervical spinal canal to reversible and irreversible injury of the cervical spinal cord in football players. J Bone Joint Surg Am. 1996;78(9):1308–14.
85. Torg JS. Cervical spinal stenosis with cord neurapraxia: evaluations and decisions regarding participation in athletics. Curr Sports Med Rep. 2002;1(1):43–6.
86. Herzog RJ, Wiens JJ, Dillingham MF, Sontag MJ. Normal cervical spine morphometry and cervical spinal stenosis in asymptomatic professional football players. Plain film radiography, multiplanar computed tomography, and magnetic resonance imaging. Spine. 1991;16(6 Suppl):S178–86.
87. Boockvar JA, Durham SR, Sun PP. Cervical spinal stenosis and sports-related cervical cord neurapraxia in children. Spine. 2001;26(24):2709–12; discussion 13.
88. Rozzelle C, Aarabi B, Dhall S, et al. Spinal cord injury without radiographic abnormality (SCIWORA). Neurosurgery. 2013;72(3):227–33.
89. Davis G, Ugokwe K, Roger EP, Benzel EC, Cantu RC, Rogers M, et al. Clinics in neurology and neurosurgery of sport: asymptomatic cervical canal stenosis and transient quadriparesis. Br J Sports Med. 2009;43(14):1154–8.
90. Torg J, Corcoran TA, Thibault LE, et al. Cervical cord neuropraxia: classification, pathomechnics, morbidity, and management guidelines. J Neurosurg. 1997;87(6):843–50.
91. Gupta SN, Piatt JH Jr, Belay B. Cervical spinal cord neurapraxia in the setting of Klippel-Feil anomaly: a diagnostic and therapeutic challenge. Spinal Cord. 2007;45(9):637–40.
92. Frogameni AD, Widoff BE, Jackson DW. Syringomyelia causing acute hemiparesis in a college football player. Orthopedics. 1994;17(6):552–3.
93. Callaway GH, O'Brien SJ, Tehrany AM. Chiari I malformation and spinal cord injury: cause for concern in contact athletes? Med Sci Sports Exerc. 1996;28(10):1218–20.
94. Harrell BR, Barootes BG. The type I Chiari malformation in a previously asymptomatic college athlete: addressing the issue of return to athletic participation. Clin J Sport Med. 2010;20(3):215–7.
95. Kirschen MP, Illes J. Ethical implications of an incidentally discovered asymptomatic Chiari malformation in a competitive athlete. Continuum. 2014;20(6 Sports Neurology):1683–7.

96. Meehan WP 3rd, Jordaan M, Prabhu SP, Carew L, Mannix RC, Proctor MR. Risk of athletes with Chiari malformations suffering catastrophic injuries during sports participation is low. Clin J Sport Med. 2015;25(2):133–7.
97. Schijman E, Steinbok P. International survey on the management of Chiari I malformation and syringomyelia. Childs Nerv Syst. 2004;20(5):341–8.
98. Miele VJ, Bailes JE, Martin NA. Participation in contact or collision sports in athletes with epilepsy, genetic risk factors, structural brain lesions, or history of craniotomy. Neurosurg Focus. 2006;21(4):E9.
99. Bailes JE, Cantu RC. Head injury in athletes. Neurosurgery. 2001;48(1):26–45; discussion -6.
100. Häggström M. Medical gallery of Mikael Häggström 2014. WikiJ Med. 2014;1(2) https://doi.org/10.15347/wjm/2014.008. ISSN 2002-4436.
101. Raniga SB, Menon V, Al Muzahmi KS, Butt S. MDCT of acute subaxial cervical spine trauma: a mechanism-based approach. Insights Imaging. 2014;5(3):321–38.

Pelvis and Hip Injuries/Core Injuries in Football

9

Ryan P. Roach, Terry Bradly Clay, and Benton A. Emblom

Introduction

The incidence of hip injuries has increased dramatically over the last decade, largely in part due to better recognition with improved diagnostic imaging and arthroscopy. Furthermore, the incidence of hip injuries in sports has been publicized in the media. With improved recognition and diagnosis, better treatment options with biologics, arthroscopy, and advanced rehabilitation have evolved.

Hip arthroscopy alone has allowed us to define numerous sources of disabling hip pain. Previously, athletes were resigned to living within the constraints of their symptoms. Among those athletes, 60% of intraarticular disorders were initially misdiagnosed as an extraarticular problem, such as a "strain." In those athletes, the average duration of treatment before arriving at an accurate diagnosis was 7 months [1].

Hip injuries in football are common and can range from a simple muscle strain to a career-ending hip dislocation with subsequent avascular necrosis. In this chapter, we will discuss common diagnoses that every sports medicine provider should be familiar with: hamstring strain and avulsion, hip dislocation, femoroacetabular impingement and labrum tears, and core muscle injury (aka "sports hernia"). We will also discuss the all too common hip pointer.

R. P. Roach
Sports Medicine and Hip Preservation, University of Florida, Gainesville, FL, USA

T. B. Clay
Sports Medicine and Hip Preservation, University of South Alabama, Mobile, AL, USA

B. A. Emblom (✉)
Sports Medicine and Hip Preservation, Andrews Sports Medicine & Orthopaedic Center, Birmingham, AL, USA
e-mail: Benton.emblom@andrewssm.com

K. W. Farmer (ed.), *Football Injuries*,
https://doi.org/10.1007/978-3-030-54875-9_9

Hamstring Injuries

The hamstring muscle group is important for football athletes, and injury is relatively common within this patient population. Rates in high school and collegiate football players range from 12% to 24% [2–5]. In the National Football League (NFL), 1716 hamstring strains were reported over a 10-year period. The majority of injuries occurred during the short preseason. Speed position players, such as the wide receiver, and defensive secondary, as well as players on the special teams' units, are at elevated risk for injury [6]. Feely et al. presented NFL data over 11 years and found that hamstring strain was the most common muscle strain and the second most common injury [7].

The hamstring complex occupies the posterior compartment of the thigh and includes the biceps femoris, semitendinosus and semimembranosus. The hamstring complex crosses both the hip and the knee and performs both eccentric and concentric contractions. This unique anatomy and important function undoubtedly contribute to the high rate of injury. Injuries can occur anywhere along the length of the muscle tendon complex and are generally grouped into proximal, midsubstance, and distal injuries (Fig. 9.1a). Pathology occurs on a spectrum from minor strains to complete tears. The injury mechanism is classically described as simultaneous eccentric load on a flexed hip and knee [8, 9]. In football, the injury mechanism is typically noncontact, rapid acceleration, and deceleration. Contact injuries can also occur with forced knee extension with a flexed hip. Treatment options are based on several factors and span the gamut from nonoperative physiotherapy, to oral medications and injections, to surgical intervention. Unfortunately, return to play is highly variable and recurrence is high.

History and Examination

Hamstring injuries sustained during football are highly variable. Simple strains may only present with pain, with or without weakness. Acute injuries are often associated with a "pop" sensation [10]. Sideline evaluation should be performed in the prone position. Tenderness is encountered in the area of injury, and the entirety of the posterior compartment should be examined, beginning at the ischial tuberosity and progressing to the knee. Pain and/or weakness can be elicited with active knee flexion in the prone position. Pain or weakness with running or walking can be encountered. More complex injuries may be associated with the development of posterior ecchymosis [11]. This ecchymosis can be extensive, often spanning the entire posterior thigh. Weakness is a common complaint in chronic injuries, but may also be noted in acute and subacute injuries. Paresthesia can be experienced due to irritation of the sciatic nerve from inflammation or hematoma.

Imaging

Athletes suspected for significant hamstring injury should be evaluated with imaging. Initial workup should include basic, orthogonal radiographs to rule out bony avulsion or injury. Advanced imaging is typically necessary to confirm and classify the injury. Magnetic resonance imaging (MRI) without contrast is preferred. Axial, sagittal, and coronal sequence should be thoroughly evaluated to define injury type and location. Different proximal tendon tear patterns can occur (Fig. 9.1a and b).

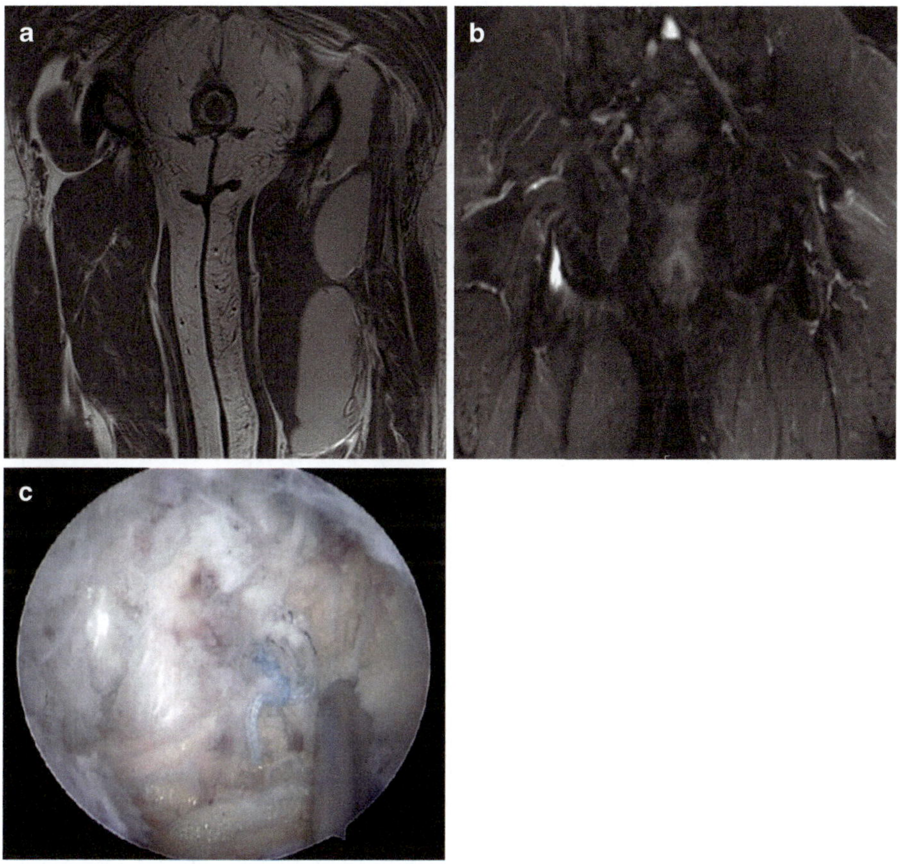

Fig. 9.1 (**a**) MRI demonstrating complete proximal hamstring three tendon avulsion. (**b**) MRI demonstrating partial hamstring avulsion. (**c**) Endoscopic visualization of the proximal hamstring repair with suture anchor

Complete tears should be evaluated for the number of tendons involved and the degree of retraction. Partial tears can be more difficult to discern. Thorough interrogation of available imaging and clinical correlation is often needed for accurate diagnosis. Musculotendinous and more distal injuries typically present with fluid collections in the area of injury. Ultrasound evaluation may be useful in certain instances, especially in situations when MRI is unavailable [12–14].

Treatment

Management depends on a number of factors. Surgical indications for the in-season athlete include complete tears with retraction, especially bony avulsions from the ischial tuberosity. The exact amount of retraction is debatable but is often quoted as 2 cm [11, 15, 16]. Refractory symptoms, despite nonoperative treatment, are another indication. Most other injuries are managed on a case-to-case basis, taking into account not only the type of injury but also the goals of the athlete. Nonoperative indications include strains, midsubstance partial tears, and partial proximal tears. A number of nonoperative modalities are available. All patients will require some degree of activity modification and physiotherapy. Physiotherapy should focus on stretching and strengthening of the hamstring muscle group. Eccentric-type exercises, such as the Nordic hamstring curls, are increasingly popular [11, 17]. Medications including nonsteroidal anti-inflammatory drugs (NSAIDs) and steroidal anti-inflammatories are important adjuvants. Biologic injections such as platelet-rich plasma (PRP) can be considered. Indications for biological-based injections are still being developed. Currently, the authors consider biologics for acute midsubstance injuries, partial proximal tendon tears, and chronic tendonopathy. Imaging guidance should be utilized to ensure accurate placement, often under ultrasound.

Operative treatment of proximal avulsions is performed through either open or arthroscopic approach. Arthroscopic techniques are evolving, affording increased utilization. Ryan and Emblom [18] defined pertinent portal site anatomy and biomechanical comparisons of the open and endoscopic technique. Arthroscopic repair of proximal tears is performed in the prone position. Two small incisions are utilized with accessory percutaneous portals established as needed. The sciatic nerve must be identified and protected. The footprint and tendon edge are debrided, and the tendon is directly repaired with use of suture anchors (Fig. 9.1c). In chronic cases, reconstruction with allograft may be necessary. Postoperatively, patients are placed in a hip brace that limits flexion, extension, and abduction. Weight bearing is limited for the first 2 weeks. Athletes begin a progressive rehabilitation schedule, beginning postoperative day 1. Return to sport after operative repair is often 6 months or greater, thus ending the current season.

Return-to-play criteria is nebulous. Generally, patients are considered cleared for return once asymptomatic. Fournier-Farley et al. [19] reported on determinants of return to play, following nonoperative treatment of hamstring injuries in athletes. A number of clinical factors were associated with prolonged recovery time, including stretching-type injuries, recreational-level sports, structural versus functional injuries, greater range of motion deficit with the hip flexed at 90°, time to first consultation >1 week, increased pain on the visual analog scale, and >1 day to be able to walk pain free after the injury. Rehabilitation approaches that included hamstring loading during extensive lengthening or four daily sessions of static hamstring stretching led to shorter rehabilitation times.

Outcomes

Outcomes of hamstring injuries in athletes are variable. Unfortunately, persistent weakness, pain, and reinjury are possible. Reinjury rates following hamstring strains are approximately 30%, which suggests, among other things, inadequate rehabilitation or premature return to play [20]. Much attention has been directed at determining the optimal rehabilitation program. Programs that incorporate trunk and agility rehabilitation in addition to progressive stretching and strengthening demonstrate quicker return [21] to play and lower reinjury rates [22]. Eccentric lengthening programs have similarly demonstrated quicker return to play compared with conventional rehabilitation [23, 24].

Few studies have investigated outcomes of corticosteroid (CS) injections, following hamstring injury in football players. Levine et al. reported on 58 NFL players with significant hamstring injury, treated with intramuscular CS injection. They concluded that the injection hastened return and lessened games missed [25]. Warren's group reported on a separate cohort of NFL players that received CS injections. They showed that proximal hamstring strains that received an injection missed an average of 3 games and 28 days [26]. The available literature for biologic injections is conflicting. PRP injections demonstrate efficacy in proximal injuries [27, 28], while midsubstance administrations show no clear benefit [29–31]. Anecdotally, both proximal and midsubstance administrations have led to quicker return to play without complication.

Results of nonoperative treatment of complete avulsions show persistent weakness, lower function, and lower return-to-play rates. Surgical outcomes are favorable. Bodendorfer et al. compared nonoperative to operative treatment of proximal hamstring avulsion and found superior outcomes in the surgical group [32]. Belk et al. reported on return to sport following hamstring repair and demonstrated a 93.8% return to sport with 83.5% returning to preinjury level on competition [33]. Only 12 were football players, and all surgeries were performed open.

Conclusion

Hamstring injuries are common among football players. Prompt, accurate diagnosis is key to optimizing healthy return to play. Rehabilitation is critical, and new, multimodal approaches are showing promising results. If indicated, surgical repair offers high patient satisfaction with high rates of return to play.

Hip Pointer

A hip pointer is a common injury in contact sport and results from contusion to the iliac crest or greater trochanter [34]. In football, this often occurs following a direct blow from an opponent or direct contact with the ground. This trauma leads to inflammation and bleeding into the surrounding musculature, including the sartorius, gluteus medius, tensor fascia lata, and abdominal muscles. Severity of these injuries varies, depending on the amount of energy imparted by the contact [35]. With severe contusions, a pelvis and lateral hip radiograph should be obtained to rule out a fracture. Treatment should include ice, nonsteroidal anti-inflammatory drugs (NSAIDs), and rest. An acute cortisone injection to the site of maximal tenderness immediately following the injury can help minimize the inflammatory response, with anecdotal evidence of earlier return to sport. An oral steroid taper can also help blunt the initial inflammatory response, but the pros and cons of such a medication should be discussed in detail with the athlete. Local injectable anesthetics like lidocaine can be used to ease symptoms. Extra padding over the injury site can provide protection from reinjury and help the athlete feel more comfortable. Recovery from hip pointers is variable and depends on the severity of the initial contusion and avoidance of any exacerbating factors. Myositis ossificans is a rare complication, following higher energy hip pointers [35].

Hip Dislocation

Given the hips' inherent stability, dislocations are an infrequent event, requiring considerable force (Fig. 9.2a). There are three types of traumatic hip dislocations: posterior, anterior, and inferior. The vast majority (90%) of hip dislocations are posterior and typically occur when the athlete falls onto a flexed knee with the hip in flexion and adduction. In football, this may occur when an athlete is on all four limbs in the

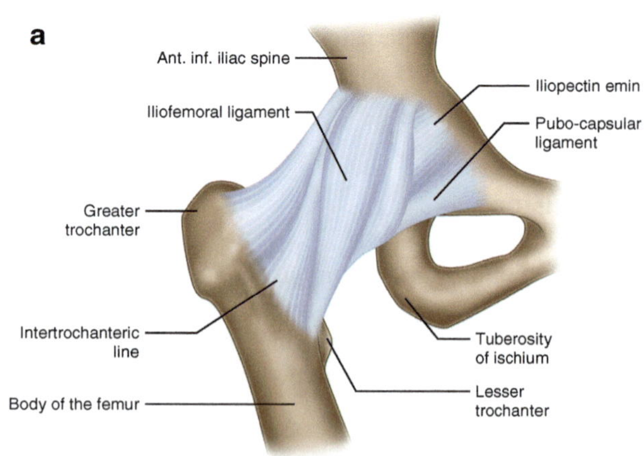

Fig. 9.2 (**a**) Osseous and ligament complex of the hip, noting specifically the size of the iliofemoral ligament. (**b**) Radiograph posterior hip dislocation. (**c**) Post-reduction CT imaging of the hip with incarcerated fragments. (**d**) MR image of the hip after dislocation with osteochondral impaction fracture and labral tear

Fig. 9.2 (continued)

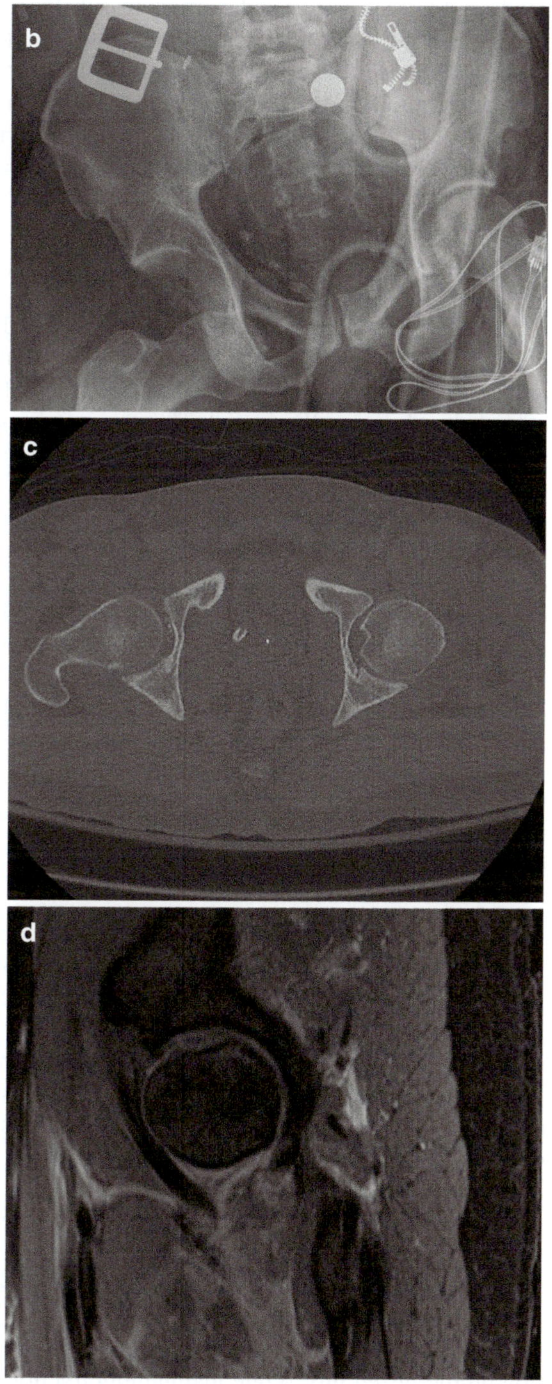

hands-and-knees position and is struck from behind. Hip dislocations can be classified as simple, if not associated with a fracture or complex, if a fracture of the femur and/or acetabulum is present. The degree of hip flexion and adduction at the time of dislocation determines the type of dislocation. The vast majority of hip dislocations occur following high-energy trauma situations, such as a motor vehicle accident, and only 2–5% of hip dislocations result from sports-related activity [36].

History and Examination

An athlete who sustains a typical posterior hip dislocation will present with the affected leg shortened, internally rotated, flexed at the knee, and flexed and adducted at the hip. In contrast, athletes with an anterior dislocation will present with the hip extended and externally rotated. The rare inferior dislocation will present with hip flexion, abduction, and external rotation. The athlete will be in significant pain and unable to move the affected limb or bear weight.

Urgent evaluation, diagnosis, and treatment are critical, as a delay in reduction can lead to increased pain, potential neurovascular compromise, and increased risk of avascular necrosis. A full examination of the patient should be performed to evaluate for concomitant injuries, as patients often have associated pathology. These include injury to the sciatic nerve as well as the ipsilateral intra-articular structures of the knee. A detailed neurovascular examination should be performed, and any deficits should be noted. The ipsilateral knee should be evaluated once the athlete's hip is reduced and stabilized. Neurovascular examination should again be performed, following reduction of the hip.

On-the-Field Management

If an experienced physician is available on the sideline, and the patient is otherwise stable without evidence of additional injury, a single attempt at closed reduction may be performed acutely. If successful, the athlete should be immediately transferred to the hospital for proper post-reduction imaging. If unsuccessful, or if a reduction attempt cannot be safely performed, the patient should be emergently transferred to the hospital for radiographs and closed reduction under anesthesia or sedation. The hip should be reduced as soon as safely possible, ideally within 6 hours of injury, as it has been shown that the incidence of avascular necrosis increases with delayed reduction [37].

There are numerous reduction methods described in the literature [38–43]. These maneuvers essentially pull in-line traction on the femur while flexing and adducting the hip to obtain reduction. The Allis maneuver [44] is considered the gold standard for posterior dislocations. This maneuver is best performed with two people: the assistant holds countertraction on the athlete's pelvis, while the provider pulls traction on the flexed hip. While maintaining traction, the hip is then gently internally rotated and adducted, obtaining satisfactory reduction of the hip.

Imaging

Radiographs should be taken upon arrival to the hospital, including anteroposterior (AP) pelvis as well as Judet views (Fig. 9.2b). Imaging should be scrutinized for evidence of concomitant acetabulum or proximal femur fracture or intra-articular fragments preventing reduction. Dislocations that are irreducible are often the result of a mechanical block such as buttonholing through the capsule or interposition of anatomic structures. If closed reduction is unsuccessful, open surgical management is necessary.

Post-reduction radiographs and fine-cut (2-mm sections) computed tomography (CT) scan should be obtained to confirm a concentric reduction and rule out any intra-articular fragments or subtle fractures (Fig. 9.2c). All sections should reveal a congruent relationship and any asymmetric widening should be critically assessed. Intra-articular fragments can lead to increased contact pressure in the hip and requires surgical intervention. MRI can be helpful in the athlete to assess for intra-articular injuries to the labrum and cartilage as well as monitor for evidence of avascular necrosis (Fig. 9.2d) [45, 46].

Treatment

As previously stated, prompt reduction is of critical importance. Post-reduction imaging (AP pelvis, Judet views, and fine-cut CT scan) is obtained to demonstrate concentric reduction. Once concentric reduction is confirmed, the athlete may begin physical therapy and rehabilitation. There has been much debate over the appropriate post-reduction management of hip dislocations, with little evidence in the literature. Typically, patients begin with protected weight bearing and gentle active and active-assisted range-of-motion exercises for 4–6 weeks. Following a posterior hip dislocation, athletes' flexion, adduction and internal rotation are generally limited and progressed over time. Hip bracing can be utilized to help restrict range of motion. Weight bearing and therapy are then progressed as symptoms allow. Once the athlete achieves full painless range of motion and weight bearing, strengthening exercises are initiated followed by endurance training. In general, athletes require 3 months before starting sports-specific training exercises and 6 months for return to play.

For nonconcentric reductions caused by entrapped intra-articular fragments or soft tissue interposition, removal of the interposed tissue is required. Traction should be considered in the interim to assist with pain control as well as prevent further articular cartilage injury as a result of the retained fragments. Surgical options include open or arthroscopic removal of the retained intra-articular tissue. Traditionally, an open approach was utilized and is still indicated for larger fragments. With the emergence of hip arthroscopy, arthroscopic management has become an option for removing smaller fragments [47, 48]. Concomitant fractures are treated with open reduction and internal fixation.

Outcomes and Complications

Given the infrequent occurrence of hip dislocations in athletes, there is a paucity of outcomes in this patient population. Rather, we use the available data in the trauma literature to guide our discussion of outcomes. Time to reduction appears to be the single most important factor with decreasing outcomes associated with delayed time to reduction [49–51]. In general, patients with simple dislocations have better outcomes than those associated with fractures. Complications from hip dislocations include avascular necrosis, post-traumatic arthritis, sciatic nerve injury, heterotopic ossification, and recurrent instability [52].

Conclusions

Hip dislocations are a rare injury in football athletes. Reduction of the dislocated hip should be performed as soon as possible. Plain radiographs and CT scan are required to evaluate for associated fractures as well as to prove a concentric reduction has been obtained. Athletes typically return to sport around 6 months post injury, but fractures may lead to longer return to sport.

Femoroacetabular Impingement and Labrum Tears

Femoroacetabular impingement (FAI) is a pathomechanical process that results in abnormal contact across the hip joint. Internal and external impingement can occur; however, internal impingement is more common. Internal impingement develops from abnormal acetabular and or femoral anatomy. Three forms of internal FAI exist: pincer, CAM, and combined. Pincer impingement is the term describing acetabular-based impingement while CAM impingement describes femoral-based impingement. Combined impingement occurs when both CAM and pincer lesions are present.

Pincer impingement results from abnormal bony prominence along the acetabulum. This typically occurs at the anterolateral portion of the acetabular rim and occurs either secondary to acetabular overgrowth or acetabular retroversion. With hip motion, abnormal contact between the femur and acetabulum results in labral injury. Pincer impingement occurs equally among males and females [53].

CAM impingement occurs with decreased femoral off-set, which results from asymmetric femoral overgrowth. This is often characterized as a "pistol-grip" deformity, although more subtle forms of CAM impingement are being recognized. Asymmetry in the femoral head-neck junction leads to abnormal contact between the femur and acetabulum through normal hip range of motion, thus leading to cartilage delamination and eventually labral pathology. Males are affected at higher rate, 3:1, compared with females [54].

Athletes are at higher risk of developing FAI. Nepple showed that male athletes are 1.8 to 8 times as likely to have proximal femoral deformity compared with male controls [55]. Frank et al. showed a similar increased rate of FAI among athletes

[56]. Blank characterized risk of FAI by sport participation and showed highest rates among NHL and lowest among NFL lineman.

History

Unfortunately, athletes with impingement present with variable symptoms and often these symptoms are subtle. This leads to either missed or delayed diagnosis. Hip joint disorders often go undetected for a protracted period. In one study of athletes, 60% were treated for an average of 7 months before appropriate hip diagnosis was made [1]. Pain may be the only presenting symptom. Impingement pain is typically localized to the groin. Though pain can also be localized to the lateral hip and posterior gluteal region. Athletes will often localize pain in an area between fingers of a cupped hand placed over lateral femur. This has been termed the "c-sign."[57] A precipitating event is not always present. Pain is typically exacerbated with activity. Twisting, cutting, planting, and other activities common to football athletes elicit symptoms. Deep flexion activities are also associated with pain provocation.

Examination

A thorough physical examination of the injured football hip should also include examination of the spine and gait. Pelvic inclination and leg lengths should also be assessed. Hip examination should be performed bilaterally as subtle findings may become more apparent with examination of the uninjured hip. We typically begin the hip examination with the athlete in a supine position. We assess symptoms with internal and external rotation log roll. Log roll test is most specific for intra-articular pathology [57]. Hip range of motion, specifically flexion and internal rotation and external rotation at 90° of hip flexion, are then tested. Patients with FAI often present with loss of internal rotation. Provocative testing includes: flexion, abduction, external rotation (FABER); flexion, adduction, internal rotation (FADIR); and anterior, superior, and posterior impingement tests.

Imaging

Athletes with a history and physical consistent with impingement should be evaluated with radiographs. High-quality imaging is necessary for radiographic assessment of FAI [58]. Standard impingement series included supine anteroposterior (AP) (Fig. 9.3a), frog lateral, 45° Dunn lateral (Fig. 9.3b), and standing false-profile views. Radiographs are critically analyzed for osseous abnormalities. Measurements are performed according to previous descriptions and include acetabular index, lateral center edge angle (LCEA), alpha angle, and anterior center edge angle (ACEA) [58].

Advanced imaging is often required in the workup of the injured athlete's hip. Soft tissue pathology is investigated best with magnetic resonance imaging (MRI). Arthrogram contrast-enhanced arthrography (MRI) is preferred and has been found

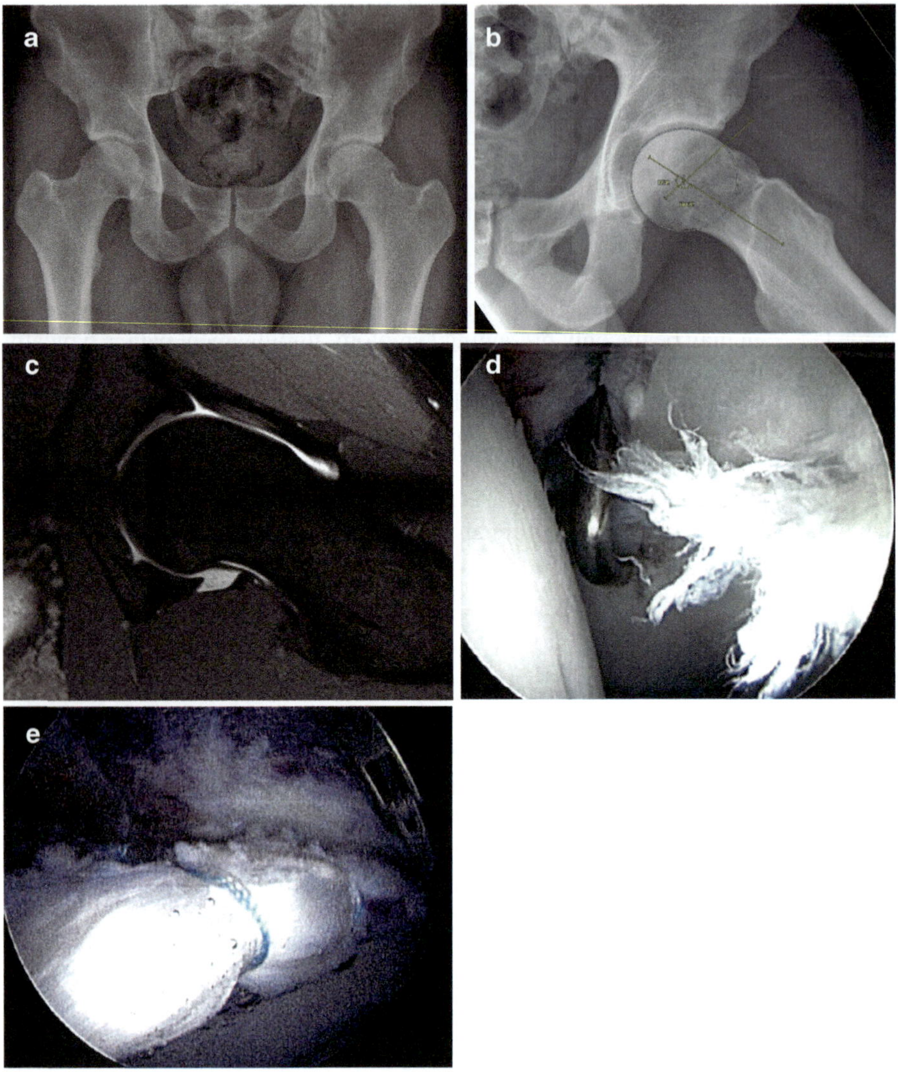

Fig. 9.3 (**a**) AP radiograph demonstrating CAM deformity. (**b**) A 45-degree Dunn lateral radiograph demonstrating CAM deformity. (**c**) MRI radial sequence demonstrating CAM deformity (**d**) Arthroscopic image of labral tear. (**e**) Arthroscopic image of labral repair

to be more sensitive for intra-articular pathology [59, 60]. Standard axial, coronal, and sagittal sequences are interrogated for evidence of pathologies, including labral tear, labral deficiencies, chondromalacia, and ligamentum teres tear. Newer radial sequences are helpful in identifying subtle femoral neck asymmetries and associated labral tears (Fig. 9.3c).

Radiographic evidence of FAI is common among football athletes. Nepple et al. reported on radiographic findings of FAI in National Football League (NFL) combine participants [61]. A high rate (94.3%) of players with hip pain had radiographic signs of FAI. Acetabular retroversion was the most common finding. Kapron et al. showed a similar high rate of acetabular retroversion among collegiate football players [62]. Both authors stressed the importance of prompt investigation of FAI in players with hip pain.

Treatment

Accurate and timely diagnosis is critical for determining the appropriate treatment plan. Management decisions should be based on the severity and chronicity of symptoms, as well as the athletic goals of the patient. Nonoperative treatment should be attempted in the appropriate athlete. Indications include acute, stable symptoms with no previous nonoperative treatment and the in-season athlete with minimal limitation. It is important to make athletes aware of the potential degenerative changes associated with FAI. Nonoperative management entails physical therapy, NSAIDs, and intra-articular injections. Oral steroid dose packs are sometimes considered, but risks should be discussed in detail. Intra-articular cortisone under ultrasound guidance is the usual first-line injection when trying to get an athlete through the season. Success is variable, and multiple injections should be avoided. Anecdotal reports of platelet-rich plasma and viscosupplementation have been mentioned, but little evidence or guidance exists to help physicians in using these modalities.

Operative management includes both open and arthroscopic procedures. Open procedures are reserved for athletes with dysplasia or severe deformity, while arthroscopic procedures are the mainstay for most injured football athletes. Arthroscopic treatment is determined partially by the preoperative workup and partially by intraoperative findings (Fig. 9.3d). Osseous abnormality is managed with acetabular and/or femoral osteoplasty. If labral injury is discovered, a repair is typically accomplished with use of suture anchors (Fig. 9.3e). Interrogation of labral integrity is key. If tissue is not amenable to repair, reconstruction or augmentation may be required. Capsular management is debated; however, the authors utilize an interportal capsulotomy and routinely repair the capsule at the conclusion of the arthroscopy.

Outcomes

The literature on FAI in football players is limited. No studies have reported on nonoperative treatment for football athletes with FAI. Outcomes following arthroscopic procedures in athletes have been reported.

Byrd el al. reported on 200 athletes that included 24 football players [63]. This cohort represented results of early surgical procedures, including the authors' learning curve. Although labral tears were noted, none were repaired. Despite this, 95% of professional and 85% of collegiate players were able to return to sport.

Nwachukwu et al. reported on 40 National Football League (NFL) players who underwent surgical intervention for FAI [64]. The cohort included 24 offensive and 16 defensive players. Eight patients underwent staged, bilateral procedures for a total of 48 hips. Labral tears were present in all hips and were repaired in 41. CAM impingement was present at a high rate, 87.5%. A total of 92.5% of patients were able to return to play at a mean time of 6 months from surgery.

Menge et al. reported on 51 NFL players that included 26 defensive, 17 offensive, and 8 position players [65]. Nine patients underwent bilateral procedures. Mixed-type impingement was most common. A total of 87% were able to return to play for an average of 3.2 seasons. Labral repair was performed in 45 hips, debridement in 11, and reconstruction in 4. Combined osteoplasty was performed in 47 hips. Five players required revision surgery with 4/5 returning to play. Linemen were least likely to return to play following hip arthroscopy.

Arthroscopic management of FAI demonstrates excellent results in terms of return to play. Unfortunately, data specific to football is limited to return to play, and studies evaluating validated pre- and post-outcome measures are not yet available. Despite this, arthroscopic procedures should be considered for the well-indicated athlete.

Conclusion

Rates of FAI among football athletes are high. Unfortunately, the diagnosis is not always apparent, which leads to delayed diagnosis and treatment. A high index of suspicion is needed for all football players with hip pain, and appropriate workup should be performed. Once the diagnosis is made, treatment options afford high rates of return to play.

Core Muscle Injury

Core muscle injury, commonly referred to as a sports hernia, and its treatment are a relatively new field of sports medicine, with an emergence and expansion of treatment options in the last decade. The injury is often misdiagnosed, and high index of suspicion is needed for athletes presenting with groin pain. Athletes sustain an injury at the confluence of the rectus abdominis and the adductor longus at its insertion and origin on the pubis, respectively. This confluence is commonly referred to as the conjoint tendon. Injury often occurs in athletes in their 20s who engage in repetitive hip flexion/abduction maneuvers such as football players [66, 67]. The differential diagnosis of football athletes presenting with groin pain is broad and includes core muscle injuries, intra-articular hip pathology, genitourinary issues, as well as lumbosacral pathology. Core muscle injury has been shown to be a common cause of groin pain in the National Football League (NFL) [68].

History and Examination

A detailed history and physical examination are required for the diagnosis of a core muscle injury and to rule out additional etiologies or concomitant pathologies. Athletes involved in pivoting, cutting, lateral motion, acceleration, and deceleration movements are at risk. Common complaints include activity-related lower abdominal and groin or proximal adductor pain. These symptoms typically resolve with rest. Exacerbating movements include trunk hyperextension and hip abduction.

The physical examination should not only focus on the conjoint tendon's insertion onto the pelvis but also on the surrounding structures that can often mimic a core muscle injury. The groin should be palpated to evaluate for a direct or indirect hernia. Intra-articular hip pathology often coincides with core muscle injuries in professional athletes [69], and thus an ipsilateral hip examination should be performed. Finally, the lumbar spine and paraspinal musculature should be examined as well.

Once the abovementioned organ systems have been evaluated, attention is turned to the core muscle examination. We begin by palpating the conjoint tendon, the confluence of the rectus and adductor tendon insertion onto the pubis, as well as their respective musculature. The patient will often have tenderness to palpation at this area. Provocative examination maneuvers include resisted hip adduction and resisted hemi-crunch. We have found that a combined resisted hip adduction/hemi-crunch test is the most sensitive finding for patients with core muscle injury. To perform this, you flex and adduct the patient's ipsilateral hip. You then place your hands on the ipsilateral knee and shoulder and ask the patient to adduct their hip and perform a crunch, while the evaluator provides resistance.

Imaging

Given the association of core muscle injury with concomitant femoroacetabular impingement (FAI), standard radiographs, including an anteroposterior (AP) pelvis as well as a modified Dunn and false profile views, are obtained. Measurements are performed to evaluate for evidence of FAI, dysplasia, or osteoarthritis. These views also assist in ruling out other causes of groin pain, including osteitis pubis, stress fractures, apophysitis, avulsion fractures, or heterotopic ossification, which can be indicative of chronic injuries.

A magnetic resonance imaging (MRI) is typically required to evaluate the tendon and its insertion onto the pubis. The patient is placed supine and undergoes a non-contrast core muscle injury MRI protocol. A systematic review of the MRI is performed and compared to the asymptomatic side. Evidence of degenerative changes, including subchondral sclerosis, subchondral cysts, and osseous erosions, should be identified and differentiated from a subentheseal pattern of bone marrow edema at the anteroinferior aspect of the superior pubic ramus more typical of a core muscle

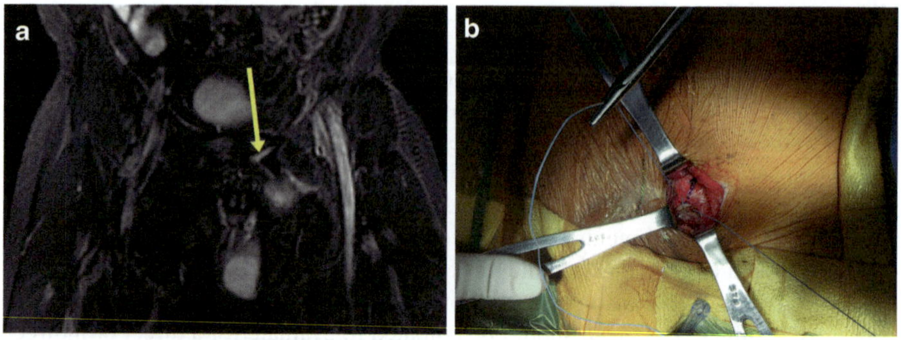

Fig. 9.4 (**a**) MRI demonstrating injury to the rectus abdominis–adductor longus aponeurosis. (**b**) Surgical photograph of the fractional lengthening of the adductor longus and subsequent turn-up flap reinforcement of the rectus abdominis

injury [70]. A cleft sign, a curvilinear increased T2 signal, representing disruption of the conjoint tendon insertion onto the pubis, often identifies the area of pain (Fig. 9.4a) [71].

Treatment

Numerous factors must be considered when determining the appropriate treatment algorithm for football athletes. These include clinical issues such as pain level and resulting disability, as well as the athletes' goal and athletic timeline. With that said, nonoperative management is generally first-line treatment. This includes activity modification, ice, analgesics, anti-inflammatories, physical therapy, and injections. Physical therapy should focus on core strengthening, stabilizing, and postural training. Both diagnostic and therapeutic injections can be attempted directly into the area of injury, utilizing corticosteroids, platelet-rich plasma (PRP), or local anesthetic, although there is a paucity of literature with regard to oies. There are anecdotal reports of PRP causing heterotopic ossification with this injury, and so physicians should keep that in mind when discussing options.

Typically, core muscle injuries will improve with rest and conservative therapy. However, symptoms often return upon resuming intense activities. If this occurs and the athlete is not able to perform at their expected level of competition, then surgical treatment is considered. Numerous surgical techniques have been described, including repair with or without the use of mesh [72–74] and with or without an adductor tenotomy [75–77]. Our preferred technique [77, 78] involves a fractional lengthening of the ipsilateral adductor longus tendon as well as a direct repair of the rectus abdominis tear. We typically place a dehydrated placental allograft over the adductor tenotomy site to inhibit scar tissue formation (Fig. 9.4b).

Outcomes

Regardless of the repair technique utilized, athletes are able to return to play at a rate of 80–100% [78–85]. Meyers et al. have the largest reported outcome studies in the literature on over 5460 open pelvic floor repairs, with a 95% return to play within 3 months [66, 67]. Brown et al. also demonstrated a 99% return to play, utilizing an open mesh repair technique [81]. Additional open repair techniques without the utilization of mesh [78, 82–85] have demonstrated excellent results as well ranging from 84% to 96% around 3–4 months postoperatively. Kluin et al. performed a prospective study on 17 hips treated with laparoscopic mesh repair, with a 93% return to play within 3 months [84]. Utilizing a similar repair technique, Genitsaris et al. demonstrated 100% return to play at 3 weeks in 131 athletes [85]. More recently, Emblom et al. described a fractional lengthening of the adductor longus and subsequent turn-up repair of the rectus abdominis insertion, with 96% return to play within 4 months [78]. Rossidis Ben-David and Farmer reported on 54 athletes who were able to return in 24 days, following laparoscopic sports hernia repair (range 21–28 days) [75].

Conclusion

Core muscle injuries can cause significant pain and dysfunction. Proper diagnosis is critical and often delayed as the diagnosis is not always straightforward. Conservative treatment can be attempted but often fails once full activities are reinitiated. For athletes that require surgical intervention, return to play ranges from 80% to 100% at 3–4 months postoperatively.

References

1. Byrd JW, Jones KS. Hip arthroscopy in athletes. Clin Sports Med. 2001;20(4):749–61.
2. Shankar PR, Fields SK, Collins CL, Dick RW, Comstock RD. Epidemiology of high school and collegiate football injuries in the United States, 2005-2006. Am J Sports Med. 2007;35(8):1295–303.
3. Powell JW, Barber-Foss KD. Injury patterns in selected high school sports: a review of the 1995-1997 seasons. J Athl Train. 1999;34(3):277–84.
4. Moretz A 3rd, Rashkin A, Grana WA. Oklahoma high school football injury study: a preliminary report. J Okla State Med Assoc. 1978;71(3):85–8.
5. Culpepper MI, Niemann KM. High school football injuries in Birmingham, Alabama. South Med J. 1983;76(7):873–5. 8
6. Elliott MC, Zarins B, Powell JW, Kenyon CD. Hamstring muscle strains in professional football players: a 10-year review. Am J Sports Med. 2011;39(4):843–50.
7. Feeley BT, Kennelly S, Barnes RP, Muller MS, Kelly BT, Rodeo SA, et al. Epidemiology of National Football League training camp injuries from 1998 to 2007. Am J Sports Med. 2008;36(8):1597–603.

8. Blasier RB, Morawa LG. Complete rupture of the hamstring origin from a water skiing injury. Am J Sports Med. 1990;18(4):435–7.
9. Sallay PI, Friedman RL, Coogan PG, Garrett WE. Hamstring muscle injuries among water skiers. Functional outcome and prevention. Am J Sports Med. 1996;24(2):130–6.
10. Sherry M. Examination and treatment of hamstring related injuries. Sports Health. 2012;4(2):107–14.
11. Arner JW, McClincy MP, Bradley JP. Hamstring injuries in athletes: evidence-based treatment. J Am Acad Orthop Surg. 2019;27(23):868–77.
12. Koulouris G, Connell D. Evaluation of the hamstring muscle complex following acute injury. Skelet Radiol. 2003;32(10):582–9.
13. Zissen MH, Wallace G, Stevens KJ, Fredericson M, Beaulieu CF. High hamstring tendinopathy: MRI and ultrasound imaging and therapeutic efficacy of percutaneous corticosteroid injection. AJR Am J Roentgenol. 2010;195(4):993–8.
14. Bengtzen RR, Ma OJ, Herzka A. Point-of-care ultrasound diagnosis of proximal hamstring rupture. J Emerg Med. 2018;54(2):225–8.
15. Wood DG, Packham I, Trikha SP, Linklater J. Avulsion of the proximal hamstring origin. J Bone Joint Surg Am. 2008;90(11):2365–74.
16. Piposar JR, Vinod AV, Olsen JR, Lacerte E, Miller SL. High-grade partial and retracted (<2 cm) proximal hamstring ruptures: nonsurgical treatment revisited. Orthop J Sports Med. 2017;5(2):2325967117692507.
17. van der Horst N, Smits DW, Petersen J, Goedhart EA, Backx FJ. The preventive effect of the Nordic hamstring exercise on hamstring injuries in amateur soccer players: a randomized controlled trial. Am J Sports Med. 2015;43(6):1316–23.
18. Ryan MK, Beason DP, Fleisig GS, Emblom BA. Portal placement and biomechanical performance of endoscopic proximal hamstring repair. Am J Sports Med. 2019;47(12):2985–92.
19. Fournier-Farley C, Lamontagne M, Gendron P, Gagnon DH. Determinants of return to play after the nonoperative management of hamstring injuries in athletes: a systematic review. Am J Sports Med. 2016;44(8):2166–72.
20. Erickson LN, Sherry MA. Rehabilitation and return to sport after hamstring strain injury. J Sport Health Sci. 2017;6(3):262–70.
21. Sherry MA, Best TM. A comparison of 2 rehabilitation programs in the treatment of acute hamstring strains. J Orthop Sports Phys Ther. 2004;34(3):116–25.
22. Silder A, Sherry MA, Sanfilippo J, Tuite MJ, Hetzel SJ, Heiderscheit BC. Clinical and morphological changes following 2 rehabilitation programs for acute hamstring strain injuries: a randomized clinical trial. J Orthop Sports Phys Ther. 2013;43(5):284–99.
23. Askling CM, Tengvar M, Thorstensson A. Acute hamstring injuries in Swedish elite football: a prospective randomised controlled clinical trial comparing two rehabilitation protocols. Br J Sports Med. 2013;47(15):953–9.
24. Askling CM, Tengvar M, Tarassova O, Thorstensson A. Acute hamstring injuries in Swedish elite sprinters and jumpers: a prospective randomised controlled clinical trial comparing two rehabilitation protocols. Br J Sports Med. 2014;48(7):532–9.
25. Levine WN, Bergfeld JA, Tessendorf W, Moorman CT 3rd. Intramuscular corticosteroid injection for hamstring injuries. A 13-year experience in the National Football League. Am J Sports Med. 2000;28(3):297–300.
26. Drakos M, Birmingham P, Delos D, Barnes R, Murphy C, Weiss L, et al. Corticosteroid and anesthetic injections for muscle strains and ligament sprains in the NFL. HSS J. 2014;10(2):136–42.
27. Fader RR, Mitchell JJ, Traub S, Nichols R, Roper M, Mei Dan O, et al. Platelet-rich plasma treatment improves outcomes for chronic proximal hamstring injuries in an athletic population. Muscles Ligaments Tendons J. 2014;4(4):461–6.
28. Park PYS, Cai C, Bawa P, Kumaravel M. Platelet-rich plasma vs. steroid injections for hamstring injury-is there really a choice? Skelet Radiol. 2019;48(4):577–82.
29. Hamid MS, Yusof A, Mohamed Ali MR. Platelet-rich plasma (PRP) for acute muscle injury: a systematic review. PLoS One. 2014;9(2):e90538.

30. Hamilton B, Tol JL, Almusa E, Boukarroum S, Eirale C, Farooq A, et al. Platelet-rich plasma does not enhance return to play in hamstring injuries: a randomised controlled trial. Br J Sports Med. 2015;49(14):943–50.
31. Reurink G, Goudswaard GJ, Moen MH, Weir A, Verhaar JA, Bierma-Zeinstra SM, et al. Rationale, secondary outcome scores and 1-year follow-up of a randomised trial of platelet-rich plasma injections in acute hamstring muscle injury: the Dutch Hamstring Injection Therapy study. Br J Sports Med. 2015;49(18):1206–12.
32. Bodendorfer BM, Curley AJ, Kotler JA, Ryan JM, Jejurikar NS, Kumar A, et al. Outcomes after operative and nonoperative treatment of proximal hamstring avulsions: a systematic review and meta-analysis. Am J Sports Med. 2018;46(11):2798–808.
33. Belk JW, Kraeutler MJ, Mei-Dan O, Houck DA, McCarty EC, Mulcahey MK. Return to sport after proximal hamstring tendon repair: a systematic review. Orthop J Sports Med. 2019;7(6):2325967119853218.
34. Hall M, Anderson J. Hip pointers. Clin Sports Med. 2013;32(2):325–30.
35. Varacallo M, Bordoni B. Hip pointer injuries (Iliac Crest Contusions). Treasure Island: StatPearls; 2020.
36. Chudik SC, Allen AA, Lopez V, Warren RF. Hip dislocations in athletes. Sports Med Arthrosc Rev. 2002;10(2):123–33.
37. Hougaard K, Thomsen PB. Traumatic posterior dislocation of the hip--prognostic factors influencing the incidence of avascular necrosis of the femoral head. Arch Orthop Trauma Surg. 1986;106(1):32–5.
38. Bassi JL, Ahuja SC, Singh H. A flexion adduction method for the reduction of posterior dislocation of the hip. J Bone Joint Surg Br. 1992;74(1):157–8.
39. Dahners LE, Hundley JD. Reduction of posterior hip dislocations in the lateral position using traction-countertraction: safer for the surgeon? J Orthop Trauma. 1999;13(5):373–4.
40. Herwig-Kempers A, Veraart BE. Reduction of posterior dislocation of the hip in the prone position. J Bone Joint Surg Br. 1993;75(2):328.
41. Lefkowitz M. A new method for reduction of hip dislocations. Orthop Rev. 1993;22(2):253–6.
42. Schafer SJ, Anglen JO. The East Baltimore Lift: a simple and effective method for reduction of posterior hip dislocations. J Orthop Trauma. 1999;13(1):56–7.
43. Sharma S, Kumar V, Dhillon MS. A new technique for closed reduction of traumatic posterior dislocations of the hip: the 'PGI technique'. Hip Int. 2014;24(4):394–8.
44. An inquiry into the difficulties encountered in the reduction of dislocations of the hip. Bristol Med Chir J (1883). 1897;15(55):66–7.
45. Stiris MG. MR imaging after sports-induced hip dislocations. Report of three cases. Acta Radiol. 2000;41(3):300–2.
46. Laorr A, Greenspan A, Anderson MW, Moehring HD, McKinley T. Traumatic hip dislocation: early MRI findings. Skelet Radiol. 1995;24(4):239–45.
47. Keene GS, Villar RN. Arthroscopic loose body retrieval following traumatic hip dislocation. Injury. 1994;25(8):507–10.
48. Begly JP, Robins B, Youm T. Arthroscopic treatment of traumatic hip dislocation. J Am Acad Orthop Surg. 2016;24(5):309–17.
49. Clegg TE, Roberts CS, Greene JW, Prather BA. Hip dislocations--epidemiology, treatment, and outcomes. Injury. 2010;41(4):329–34.
50. Dwyer AJ, John B, Singh SA, Mam MK. Complications after posterior dislocation of the hip. Int Orthop. 2006;30(4):224–7.
51. Kellam P, Ostrum RF. Systematic review and meta-analysis of avascular necrosis and post-traumatic arthritis after traumatic hip dislocation. J Orthop Trauma. 2016;30(1):10–6.
52. Sanders S, Tejwani N, Egol KA. Traumatic hip dislocation – a review. Bull NYU Hosp Jt Dis. 2010;68(2):91–6.
53. Byrd JW, Jones KS. Arthroscopic management of femoroacetabular impingement. Instr Course Lect. 2009;58:231–9.
54. Byrd JW, Jones KS. Arthroscopic femoroplasty in the management of cam-type femoroacetabular impingement. Clin Orthop Relat Res. 2009;467(3):739–46.

55. Nepple JJ, Vigdorchik JM, Clohisy JC. What is the association between sports participation and the development of proximal femoral cam deformity? A systematic review and meta-analysis. Am J Sports Med. 2015;43(11):2833–40.
56. Frank JM, Harris JD, Erickson BJ, Slikker W 3rd, Bush-Joseph CA, Salata MJ, et al. Prevalence of femoroacetabular impingement imaging findings in asymptomatic volunteers: a systematic review. Arthroscopy. 2015;31(6):1199–204.
57. Byrd JW. Evaluation of the hip: history and physical examination. N Am J Sports Phys Ther. 2007;2(4):231–40.
58. Clohisy JC, Carlisle JC, Beaule PE, Kim YJ, Trousdale RT, Sierra RJ, et al. A systematic approach to the plain radiographic evaluation of the young adult hip. J Bone Joint Surg Am. 2008;90(Suppl 4):47–66.
59. Sutter R, Zubler V, Hoffmann A, Mamisch-Saupe N, Dora C, Kalberer F, et al. Hip MRI: how useful is intraarticular contrast material for evaluating surgically proven lesions of the labrum and articular cartilage? AJR Am J Roentgenol. 2014;202(1):160–9.
60. Byrd JW, Jones KS. Diagnostic accuracy of clinical assessment, magnetic resonance imaging, magnetic resonance arthrography, and intra-articular injection in hip arthroscopy patients. Am J Sports Med. 2004;32(7):1668–74.
61. Nepple JJ, Clohisy JC. The dysplastic and unstable hip: a responsible balance of arthroscopic and open approaches. Sports Med Arthrosc Rev. 2015;23(4):180–6.
62. Kapron AL, Anderson AE, Peters CL, Phillips LG, Stoddard GJ, Petron DJ, et al. Hip internal rotation is correlated to radiographic findings of cam femoroacetabular impingement in collegiate football players. Arthroscopy. 2012;28(11):1661–70.
63. Byrd JW, Jones KS. Arthroscopic management of femoroacetabular impingement in athletes. Am J Sports Med. 2011 Jul;39(Suppl):7S–13S.
64. Nwachukwu BU, Bedi A, Premkumar A, Draovitch P, Kelly BT. Characteristics and outcomes of arthroscopic femoroacetabular impingement surgery in the National Football League. Am J Sports Med. 2018;46(1):144–8.
65. Menge TJ, Briggs KK, Dornan GJ, McNamara SC, Philippon MJ. Survivorship and outcomes 10 years following hip arthroscopy for femoroacetabular impingement: labral debridement compared with labral repair. J Bone Joint Surg Am. 2017;99(12):997–1004.
66. Meyers WC, Foley DP, Garrett WE, Lohnes JH, Mandlebaum BR. Management of severe lower abdominal or inguinal pain in high-performance athletes. PAIN (Performing Athletes with Abdominal or Inguinal Neuromuscular Pain Study Group). Am J Sports Med. 2000;28(1):2–8.
67. Meyers WC, McKechnie A, Philippon MJ, Horner MA, Zoga AC, Devon ON. Experience with "sports hernia" spanning two decades. Ann Surg. 2008;248(4):656–65.
68. Larson CM, Sikka RS, Sardelli MC, Byrd JW, Kelly BT, Jain RK, et al. Increasing alpha angle is predictive of athletic-related "hip" and "groin" pain in collegiate National Football League prospects. Arthroscopy. 2013;29(3):405–10.
69. Hammoud S, Bedi A, Magennis E, Meyers WC, Kelly BT. High incidence of athletic pubalgia symptoms in professional athletes with symptomatic femoroacetabular impingement. Arthroscopy. 2012;28(10):1388–95.
70. Mullens FE, Zoga AC, Morrison WB, Meyers WC. Review of MRI technique and imaging findings in athletic pubalgia and the "sports hernia". Eur J Radiol. 2012;81(12):3780–92.
71. Cunningham PM, Brennan D, O'Connell M, MacMahon P, O'Neill P, Eustace S. Patterns of bone and soft-tissue injury at the symphysis pubis in soccer players: observations at MRI. AJR Am J Roentgenol. 2007;188(3):W291–6.
72. Sheen AJ, Stephenson BM, Lloyd DM, Robinson P, Fevre D, Paajanen H, et al. 'Treatment of the sportsman's groin': British Hernia Society's 2014 position statement based on the Manchester Consensus Conference. Br J Sports Med. 2014;48(14):1079–87.
73. Kopelman D, Kaplan U, Hatoum OA, Abaya N, Karni D, Berber A, et al. The management of sportsman's groin hernia in professional and amateur soccer players: a revised concept. Hernia. 2016;20(1):69–75.
74. Paajanen H, Brinck T, Hermunen H, Airo I. Laparoscopic surgery for chronic groin pain in athletes is more effective than nonoperative treatment: a randomized clinical trial with

magnetic resonance imaging of 60 patients with sportsman's hernia (athletic pubalgia). Surgery. 2011;150(1):99–107.
75. Rossidis G, Perry A, Abbas H, Motamarry I, Lux T, Farmer K, et al. Laparoscopic hernia repair with adductor tenotomy for athletic pubalgia: an established procedure for an obscure entity. Surg Endosc. 2015;29(2):381–6.
76. Harr JN, Brody F. Sports hernia repair with adductor tenotomy. Hernia. 2017;21(1):139–47.
77. Scillia AJ, Pierce TP, Simone E, Novak RC, Emblom BA. Mini-open incision sports hernia repair: a surgical technique for core muscle injury. Arthrosc Tech. 2017;6(4):e1281–e4.
78. Emblom BA, Mathis T, Aune K. Athletic pubalgia secondary to rectus abdominis-adductor longus aponeurotic plate injury: diagnosis, management, and operative treatment of 100 competitive athletes. Orthop J Sports Med. 2018;6(9):2325967118798333.
79. Radic R, Annear P. Use of pubic symphysis curettage for treatment-resistant osteitis pubis in athletes. Am J Sports Med. 2008;36(1):122–8.
80. Jakoi A, O'Neill C, Damsgaard C, Fehring K, Tom J. Sports hernia in National Hockey League players: does surgery affect performance? Am J Sports Med. 2013 Jan;41(1):107–10.
81. Brown RA, Mascia A, Kinnear DG, Lacroix V, Feldman L, Mulder DS. An 18-year review of sports groin injuries in the elite hockey player: clinical presentation, new diagnostic imaging, treatment, and results. Clin J Sport Med. 2008;18(3):221–6.
82. Brannigan AE, Kerin MJ, McEntee GP. Gilmore's groin repair in athletes. J Orthop Sports Phys Ther. 2000;30(6):329–32.
83. Muschaweck U, Berger L. Minimal repair technique of sportsmen's groin: an innovative open-suture repair to treat chronic inguinal pain. Hernia. 2010;14(1):27–33.
84. Kluin J, den Hoed PT, van Linschoten R, IJzerman JC, van Steensel CJ. Endoscopic evaluation and treatment of groin pain in the athlete. Am J Sports Med. 2004;32(4):944–9.
85. Genitsaris M, Goulimaris I, Sikas N. Laparoscopic repair of groin pain in athletes. Am J Sports Med. 2004;32(5):1238–42.

Cartilage Injuries in Football

10

Adam Anz, Mark Callanan, Michael Goodlett, and James Andrews

Introduction and Incidence

Articular cartilage injury in football athletes is common and not always symptomatic [1]. Injury can manifest as a new cartilage lesion, as the result of an acute traumatic event, a symptomatic aggravation of a pre-existing asymptomatic chronic cartilage lesion, or a symptomatic exacerbation of a pre-existing asymptomatic chronic lesion. Articular cartilage lesions occur in up to 36% of athletes, which is almost twice the incidence of the general population [2]. A systematic review, involving both professional and nonprofessional athletes, found 14% of athletes diagnosed with a cartilage injury were asymptomatic [3]. When presented with symptoms of cartilage injury in season, thoroughly assess the exact extent and nature of the cartilage injury, determine what other collateral factors/injuries are associated with the cartilage lesion, and begin an initial management to treat the inflammatory response.

It is important to fully evaluate athletes with cartilage injuries because these injuries can have long-term consequences. A prevalence study in NFL combine participants found a full-thickness cartilage injury incidence of 20%, detected on screening MRI [4]. NFL performance studies have shown that articular cartilage injuries result in poorer overall performance, fewer games played, and an overall shorter career length versus matched controls [1, 5]. A prior meta-analysis looking at data from athletes determined that full-thickness cartilage lesions most commonly occurred on the patella (37%), followed closely by the femoral condyles

A. Anz (✉) · J. Andrews
Andrews Institute, Gulf Breeze, FL, USA

M. Callanan
The Orthopaedic Clinic, Shreveport, LA, USA

M. Goodlett
Auburn University, Auburn, AL, USA

K. W. Farmer (ed.), *Football Injuries*,
https://doi.org/10.1007/978-3-030-54875-9_10

(35%), and less frequently on the tibial plateaus (25%). When femoral condyles are involved, the medial femoral condyle is more commonly affected than the lateral femoral condyle (64% vs. 36%) [3].

Predisposing Factors

Predisposing factors are previous knee surgery, limb malalignment, ligamentous instability, patellar maltracking, and prior knee injury, including anterior cruciate ligament tear or meniscus tear [6]. It is important to consider the entire mechanical axis because limb malalignment has been associated with the progression of cartilage injuries to osteoarthritis (OA) [7]. Individuals with a BMI >30 have a higher prevalence of cartilage injuries compared to those with a lower ("normal") BMI [8, 9]. Prior meniscectomy has been shown to be associated with full-thickness cartilage injuries, and a study of NFL combine athletes determined that previous meniscectomy of 10% or more resulted in larger and more severe chondral injuries, resulting in overall decreased performance versus matched controls [6, 10]. Several studies have also shown that of all the football player positions, linemen have the highest incidence and predisposition to articular cartilage injury in the knee compared to other positions [5, 11]. Identifying athlete risk factors, as well as the proper evaluation and management of articular cartilage injuries in football players, is critical to the athlete returning to play at a competitive level, as well as developing prognostic recommendations for optimal long-term knee health.

Natural History

A study on the natural history of cartilage injury determined that approximately 1/3 of injuries will worsen, 1/3 will improve, and 1/3 will stay the same [8]. Overall, 50–66% of stable lesions have the potential to heal with nonoperative treatment [12–15]. Skeletally immature patients with open growth plates have the greatest potential to heal, but may require up to 6 months or more of nonoperative treatment before healing occurs. Larger-sized lesions, swelling, and presence of mechanical symptoms are all associated with a lower likelihood of healing [13–15]. A case-control study investigated the effect of cartilage injuries on outcomes after anterior cruciate ligament (ACL) reconstruction. When the cartilage injuries are not treated with a repair surgery, patients without a cartilage injury had significantly higher subjective scores than patients with a defect in the medial compartment (mean International Knee Documentation Committee Subjective Form (IKDC) score of 95.2 points versus 94.0 points; $p = 0.0451$), and those with a defect in the lateral compartment (mean IKDC scores of 95.9 points versus 92.8 points; $p = 0.0047$) [16]. A meta-analysis found that most studies have revealed poorer outcomes in patients undergoing ACL reconstruction, who are found to have a concurrent articular cartilage lesion at time of reconstruction [17, 18]. As such, the optimal treatment and management of cartilage injuries in athletes remains an ongoing debate, especially given the variability of outcomes in the literature.

Articular Cartilage Structure and Basic Science of Injury

Natural articular cartilage is typically 2–4 mm thick and made up of four distinct zones: the superficial (tangential) zone, intermediate zone, deep zone, and the tidemark (Fig. 10.1). A total of 65–80% of the overall mass of cartilage is water, and the remaining tissue is made up of collagen, predominantly type 2, proteoglycans, non-collagen proteins, and chondrocytes. Proteoglycans attract water to the cartilage and help resist compression. Chondrocytes, less than 2% by mass, produce the extracellular matrix, consisting predominantly of proteoglycans and collagen [19]. Cartilage is aneural and avascular, and the avascular nature is the proposed reason for its poor healing capacity after injury [19].

When a cartilage injury occurs, the balance between a reactive inflammatory cascade in the joint and the ability to re-achieve homeostasis ultimately determines which lesions may heal, and which will further progress to joint disease. When articular cartilage sustains an injury resulting in a full-thickness defect with penetration through the tidemark and into the subchondral bone, the body attempts a healing response and produces fibrocartilage (Fig. 10.2). Fibrocartilage is predominantly composed of type 1 cartilage as opposed to the type 2 collagen found in natural cartilage. Fibrocartilage also has a low overall proteoglycan content. While patients may symptomatically improve from the formation of fibrocartilage, the overall mechanical properties and wear characteristics are inferior to native hyaline

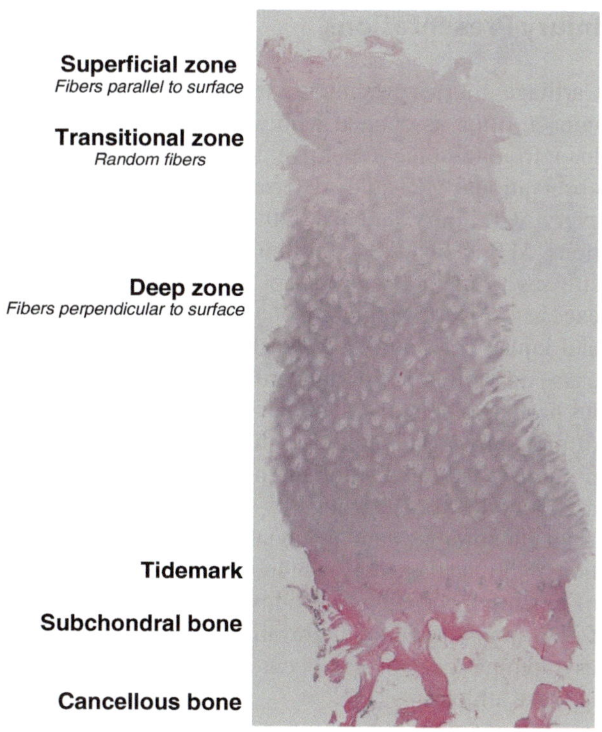

Fig. 10.1 The natural architecture of cartilage

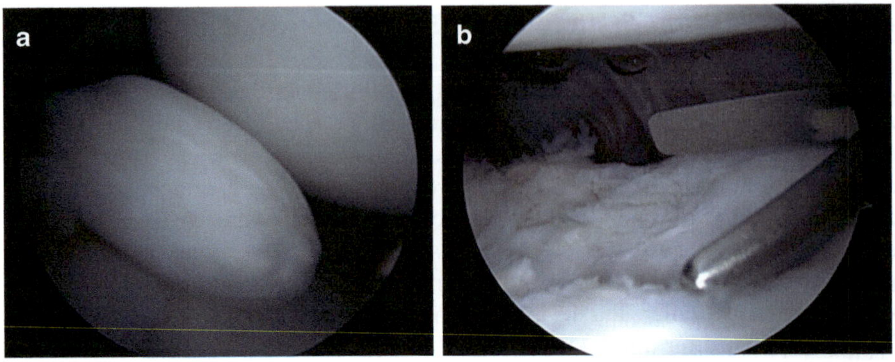

Fig. 10.2 Arthroscopic views of the knee in a young football athlete with dislodged Osteochondritis Dissecans (OCD) fragment, presenting as a symptomatic loose body (**a**). The source of the fragment had healed with fibrocartilage, which measured 12 mm × 10 mm (**b**)

cartilage that lines articular surfaces in the body [20]. An important consideration is the location of the cartilage injury and the activity demands of the athlete. Some areas of the knee may encounter load with deep knee flexion alone, such as the distal lateral trochlea. The prognosis of injuries that heal with fibrocartilage depends on the location of the lesion and the activity demands of the athlete, as subsequent compressive load on the area is dependent on both of these variables.

Injury Presentations

Cartilage injuries present as a result of two major mechanisms—acute injury from impact, often associated with acute ligament injury events and mechanical overload from chronic repetitive loading. Considering acute ligament injuries, an observational MRI study determined that some level of chondral injury occurs with every ACL injury, and this initial injury can lead to subsequent chondral degeneration [21]. Considering chronic overload, cartilage needs normal physiologic stresses to maintain normal proliferation; however, supraphysiologic loads from excessive repetitive loading of a joint surface may ultimately lead to cartilage wear and injury [22]. Studies have shown that impact forces greater than 24 MPa will cause disruption of normal cartilage structure, leading to injury [23]. Animal studies have also demonstrated that repetitive trauma will eventually cause breakdown of proteoglycans, which can ultimately lead to breakdown of cartilage [24]. After primary structural disruption, mechanical impact is also thought to cause a secondary breakdown of cartilage by an increase in the release of degradative proteins from chondrocytes and synovial cells, as well as a decrease in the natural production of the cartilage lubricant lubricin [25–30]. Linemen present a common scenario of repetitive chronic overload, which predisposes them to cartilage injury [5, 11]. Either a symptomatic aggravation or symptomatic exacerbation of a pre-existing asymptomatic lesion can occur during a period of intense training or performance in these athletes.

Clinical Evaluation

The history and clinical examination are an important part in the diagnosis of a cartilage injury. In the acute injury setting, knowing the exact mechanism by which the injury occurred can help with the overall diagnosis, the possibility of concomitant injury, and building a treatment strategy. The history will be notable for chief complaints including, but not limited to, pain, swelling, and stiffness. Aggravating factors will include increased pain when the cartilage surface is loaded and can include normal weight bearing or specific activities, such as squatting or stair ascending/descending. Associated symptoms may include catching, locking, and joint popping. On physical exams signs of an inflamed joint, that is, a joint effusion, warmth, and pain, may also be accompanied by joint crepitus. Physical examination should also include the presence and location of tenderness to palpation, range of motion, and a thorough ligamentous evaluation, including patellar stability tests.

Initial evaluation should also include a full-knee radiograph series, including a patellar sunrise/merchant view. Full-length standing films can be considered to evaluate for any mechanical axis deviations, which will aid with root cause analysis and prognostic determinations. There should be a low threshold for obtaining an MRI if there is clinical or radiographic concern of a cartilage injury (Fig. 10.3). Studies have shown MRI to have a high sensitivity and negative predictive value when evaluating smaller stable lesions [31]. However, the predictive value of MRI is lower when dealing with larger, more unstable lesions, and may overpredict instability in some cases [31, 32]. Ultimately, while MRI can be valuable in the assessment and evaluation of cartilage lesions, it should be used as a tool in conjunction with the overall clinical picture. In cases of patellar instability, CT scans or MRI scans may be employed to determine the tibial tubercle to trochlear groove distance (TT–TG distance) as well as femoral version.

After Diagnosis: What Now?

Once the diagnosis and circumstances associated with the cartilage injury are determined, the most important next step is communicating the exact diagnosis, prognosis, and treatment/rehabilitation plan with and coordinating the entire sports medicine team, including the athlete, family, coaches, physicians, athletic trainers, physical therapists, and strength-conditioning personnel team. This step is the art of sports medicine and relies on trust, relationship, and communication among all parts. The athlete's long-term health is the most important consideration, while considering short-term athletic return-to-play goals and role for the team secondary. A treatment plan must be created and implemented as a team, in order for it to be successful, and the athlete must feel that his/her welfare is the pinnacle of consideration.

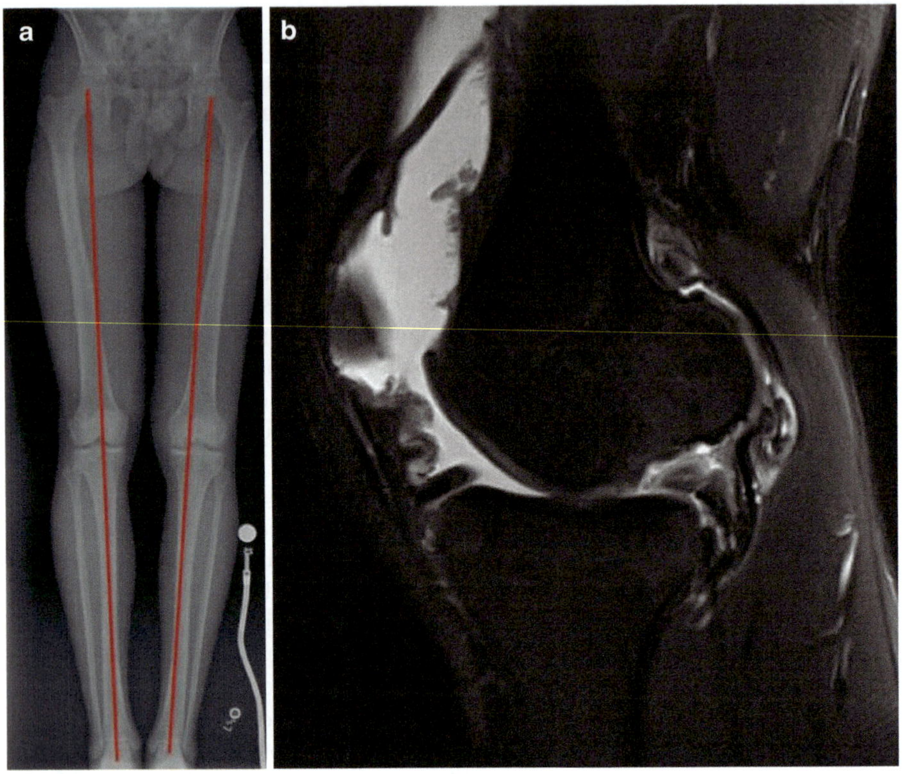

Fig. 10.3 Long-leg radiograph (**a**) and associated MRI (**b**) of a 17-year-old football athlete with activity-related swelling and mechanical symptoms of the left knee. Mechanical axes have been drawn in red and note the medial mechanical axis on the left knee

Treating the Inflammatory Response: Rest and Reducing Joint Inflammation

The first steps in management are to remove the offending agent, that is, whatever activity caused the injury presentation, and decrease the inflammatory response, including a period of rest, joint modalities, and oral/systemic anti-inflammatory medication. If the cartilage injury is associated with a cruciate or collateral ligament injury, the treatment plan for the ligament injury will determine next steps. If the cartilage injury is associated with overloading activities, the period of rest will be combined with methods to re-establish joint homeostasis and ways to mitigate the deforming force associated with the cartilage injury. In episodes where a period of overtraining is associated with the inflammatory event, rest combined with restoring joint homeostasis and altering the training regimen may be sufficient treatment. Joint treatments to eliminate effusion may include elevation, cold/compression therapy, unloaded motion, and other soft-tissue treatments. The implementation of a short-term oral steroid dose pack in an effort to reduce the acute effusion should also be considered.

Joint aspiration and injection can also be considered, based upon the timing of presentation, as well as expectations/requirements for performance. Injections require a period of at least 3 days before returning to participation. The goal of all injection treatments is to treat inflammation and restore joint homeostasis. Steroid injections have been around for decades and have a role when used in the correct setting. The authors have found that when a quick inflammatory event needs a quick response, joint aspiration and steroid injection can fit this bill. It is important to have a period of rest after a steroid injection and not use these injections too close to participation. If oral steroids or a steroid joint injection are utilized, their effect on any coexistent medical conditions must be considered.

Other injections, including viscosupplementation and biologic injections, require a longer period to have an effect on joint inflammation and should be considered when a longer period of time is available for the rest and rehabilitation period. A combination of corticosteroid and viscosupplementation can have a role for both immediate (corticosteroid) and longer (viscosupplementation) effect. While viscosupplementation has been around for a long time, sports medicine and the public have recently turned greater attention to biologic injections, and a thorough understanding of the current status of development and regulation in this space is important.

Biologic Injections

Biologic injections can be useful to treat the inflammatory response of the joint and aid in the joint's re-establishment of homeostasis. While claims of cartilage regeneration are sometimes made, in the setting of injection alone, the claims currently are unsubstantiated. Platelet-rich plasma, bone marrow aspirate concentrate, processed lipoaspirate, incubated blood products, and processed placental products are all available at some level to the clinician and athlete. All of these products have developmental and regulatory considerations that should be contemplated. The authors currently utilize leukocyte-poor platelet-rich plasma most often when a biologic injection fits the treatment plan because there is a strong evidence base for this recommendation, and a series of three at 1-week intervals when time permits is preferred. Recent animal data suggests a greater long-term effect on the joint with a three-injection series when compared to one injection alone [33].

Platelet-rich plasma has built a pyramid of evidence for the indication of osteoarthritis, and this can be applied to the treatment of inflammatory events associated with cartilage injury. The base of the pyramid is animal and benchtop studies, developing a clear mechanism of action to improve the catabolic and inflammatory environment of cartilage injury. Benchtop studies have shown that platelet-rich plasma stimulates proliferation of chondrocytes in culture, decreases production of matrix metalloproteinases by synovial cells, and decreased inflammatory gene expression in an OA model [34–41]. Case series, comparative cohort studies, and randomized controlled trials illustrating safety and efficacy have continued to support platelet-rich plasma, and systematic reviews and meta-analysis of comparative clinical trials have confirmed reproducible efficacy. No other biologic injection has as clear a body of work to guide clinical application [42–45].

Regulatory concerns are present for adipose-based injections, placenta-derived injections, and incubated blood products, and at this time, these products require further developmental progress before they can be fully advocated [46–48]. Bone marrow aspirate concentrate, while a more cellular product, has yet to outperform platelet-rich plasma, and the authors have recently completed a randomized controlled trial between these two biologic products with similar results in each group [49–51]. Regardless of a lack of clear superiority, at times, bone marrow aspirate concentrate is still chosen as the biologic injection for treatment by the authors at times, primarily due to compositional studies on bone marrow aspirate, suggesting that it should be more effective [50].

Traditional Rehabilitation Options: Braces and Physical Therapy

Braces have a role in certain scenarios, as they can provide mechanical support, improve an athlete's symptoms, and partially remove a deforming force. Application depends on the specific location of the cartilage injury, as well as other concurrent injuries. Patellofemoral braces may be used to aid in proper patellar tracking. Varus and valgus unloader braces may be employed for injuries that occur on the medial or lateral compartments of the knee, as a way to offload and protect the site of injury during the recovery period, as well as during the return to performance.

A physical therapist or certified athletic trainer should be used to help monitor and rehabilitate any athlete that has sustained a cartilage injury. During the immediate phase after injury presentation, weight-bearing restrictions should be considered, based upon the extent of the inflammatory response and nature/location of the cartilage injury. However, studies have demonstrated that sub-physiologic loading of articular cartilage following impact injury helps maintain the viability of the chondrocytes, thus touch down weight bearing should be considered as opposed to full non–weight bearing [52]. The ultimate goal of therapy in the acute period following injury should be to reduce the joint effusion, restore joint homeostasis, maintain an athlete's range of motion and flexibility, and work on core and extremity strengthening. The overall goal during this phase is to optimize the biomechanical forces across the injured joint and restore joint homeostasis.

After restoring joint homeostasis and removing the joint effusion, rehabilitation can focus on optimizing the athlete's kinetics in light of the injury. Range of motion and flexibility should be maintained, as well as strengthening muscle groups that would improve the clinical situation. For example, in cases of lateral patella compression syndrome, improving hip abductor and vastus medialis strength may improve the kinetics of motion and decrease lateral patellar overload. Progressing with strengthening of the injured extremity as well as progressing to full loading of the joint should be the focus. After successful return to full weight bearing, maintenance of range of motion and flexibility, and progression in weight training without any clinically detrimental symptoms, the patient may then be advanced further. The patient should continue to maintain limb flexibility and range of motion, while gradually increasing the loading forces across the joint, progressing to unilateral exercises across the injured joint.

After a sufficient period of time and successful progression through each phase of therapy to full weight bearing and advancement of their strengthening exercises from bilateral to unilateral, the athlete can then progress their rehab to a final return to participation phase. A focused return to football rehabilitation protocol that is tailored to the specific needs based on the player's position should be employed. The goal of this final phase of rehabilitation would be to maintain joint flexibility and range of motion, and gradually increase joint loading until the player is able to return to full running and football-specific drills [53].

Throughout the entire rehabilitation phase and return to play protocol, it is of utmost importance for the athlete, the entire sports medicine and strength-conditionings teams, as well as the coaching staff and family to all have a clear understanding of the plan and progression status. Feedback from the athlete during all phases of the rehabilitation is critical and must be continually communicated to all involved parties.

Emerging Rehabilitation Options: Blood Flow Restriction Therapy and Alternate Strengthening Regimens

An emerging field of interest in the rehabilitation of athletes is the use of blood flow restriction (BFR) therapy. Blood flow restriction therapy involves weight-lifting activities with a tourniquet-style device on the limb of focus. The device occludes venous outflow from the limb, which builds up higher levels of lactic acid within the occluded limb than standard exercise. A spike of lactic acid on the endocrine system is associated with the release of beneficial chemokines, as well as a systemic cellular response. Blood flow restriction therapy is quickly gaining popularity in orthopedic rehabilitation, showing promise in muscle recovery, limb salvage after injury, and postoperatively, following orthopedic surgery procedures [54–58]. Blood flow restriction therapy even at low-resistance loads can result in increases in the size and strength of muscles, even in proximal muscle groups that are not directly occluded. This suggests a strong systemic effect resulting from the training [59]. Even in well-trained athletes, blood flow restriction therapy has demonstrated increases in strength and hypertrophy, using submaximal loads that were not otherwise found compared to controls [60–64]. The authors have recently completed a controlled laboratory study, demonstrating increases in both platelets and hematopoietic pluripotent stem cells in the peripheral circulation following blood flow restriction exercise, a possible explanation for the systemic efficacy noted following use.

Blood flow restriction is especially useful in patients with cartilage injury. For example, if a patellofemoral lesion presents in a lineman, blood flow restriction with altered weight-room practices can maintain muscle volume and strength within the extremity, while avoiding weight-room practices that may directly load the patellofemoral joint, such as traditional squats and lunges. This application could be particularly important during the acute phase following injury or surgery, where decreasing inflammation, promoting a healing environment, and stimulating a systemic training response while respecting weight-bearing restrictions are beneficial (Fig. 10.4). Given the strong supportive literature and great potential benefits with minimal athlete risk, we recommend the application of blood flow restriction therapy as an adjunct in the recovery of a cartilage injury when available.

Alternative weight-room practices should be pursued for patients with cartilage injuries with and without blood flow restriction to maintain the strength that the athlete requires while considering the area of cartilage injury. Strengthening decisions should be based on the lesion location, size, and symptoms of the patient. Close observation and collaboration of the physician, athletic trainer, physical therapist, and strength/conditioning coaches are important to monitor an athlete's symptoms, as well as ensure appropriate milestones are being met. Many injuries require tailored weight-room protocols during and after recovery. The authors have found that grouping athletes from multiple injuries, together with alternative

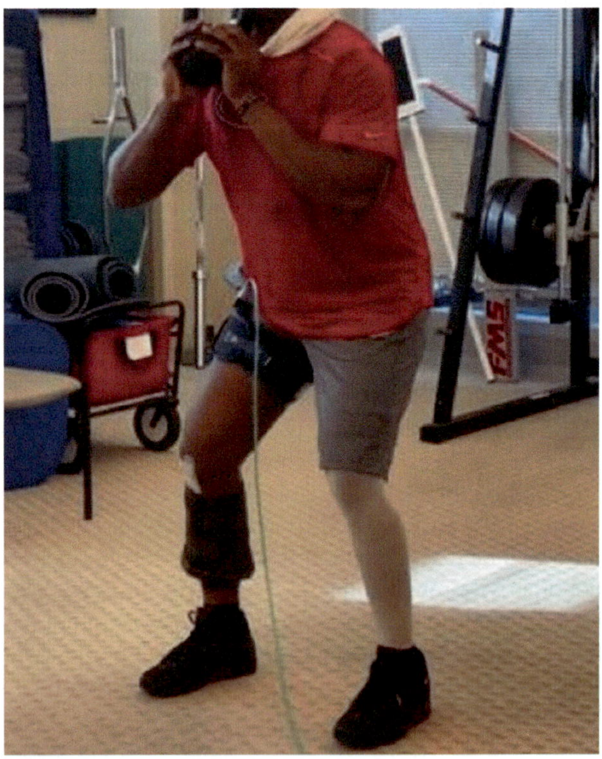

Fig. 10.4 Strengthening with blood flow restriction therapy after a surgery

strengthening regimens, can help maintain moral and team unity. The importance of coordination of the entire sports medicine team during these periods cannot be overstated. A specific example involves athletes with patellofemoral cartilage lesions. In these athletes, traditional quadriceps strengthening activities in the weight room may continue to exacerbate the pathology. Blood flow restriction therapy may aid maintenance of muscle strength and volume with less weight and nontraditional methods. Having athletes grouped together who are pursuing weight-training methods aids buy-in of the entire team, while still fostering the team moral.

Surgical Treatment Options

In patients who have large or unstable lesions or have failed a trial of nonoperative management, surgical options are available for cartilage repair. Multiple cartilage repair options are available, and consensus on optimal methods is not clear. There is not one surgical method for all lesions, and algorithms to fit a cartilage lesion are typically based on lesion size and have "multiple arrows in the quiver" (Fig. 10.5). Considerations of malalignment, joint instability, or maltracking of the patella should be considered on an individual athlete basis, as well as the lesion size and location.

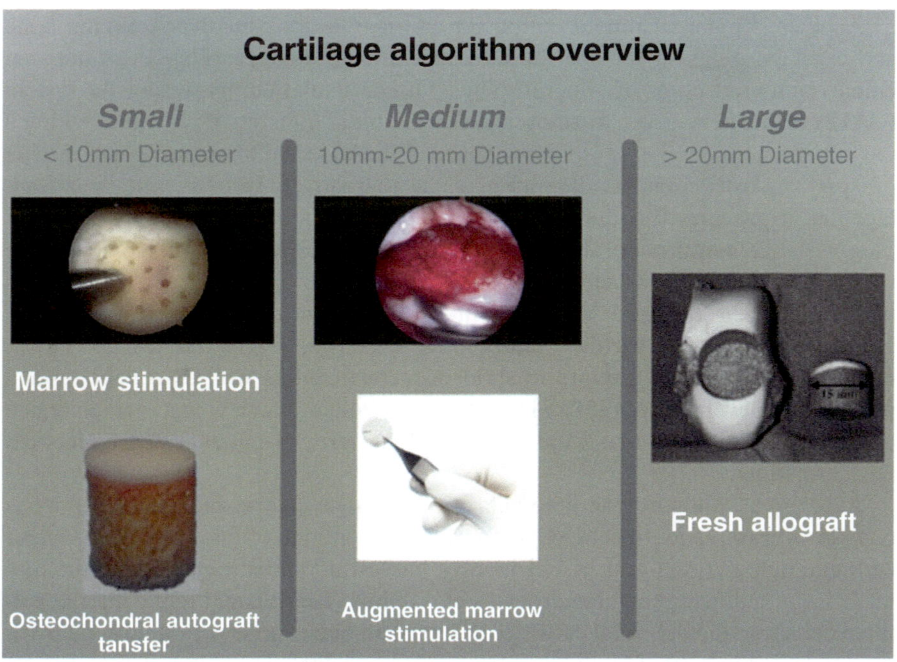

Fig. 10.5 The authors' current cartilage repair algorithm. Cartilage repair technologies continue to evolve and subsequent algorithms as well

In small lesions that measure less than 10 mm, surgical treatment options include direct fixation of a loose osteochondral fragment, marrow stimulation techniques (including microfracture, subchondral drilling, and abrasion chondroplasty), and replacement of the lesion with an osteochondral plug. Direct fixation of the injured fragment is most common in younger patients with unstable osteochondral dissecans lesion or in acute osteochondral lesions associated with ligament injury. Marrow stimulation techniques remain the most common cartilage repair technique in the United States. Abrasion chondroplasty involves burring to an underlying bleeding bed to stimulate healing by the release of bone marrow factors. To create a conduit from the bone to the marrow, an awl (microfracture) or a drill (subchondral drilling) can be combined with abrasion chondroplasty, and authors theorize that this further improves access of the cartilage lesion to progenitor cells from the bone marrow. The recovery time and return to play with marrow stimulation techniques are often shorter compared to other cartilage treatment options. Literature has shown that in smaller lesions, in younger athletes, microfracture offers improved outcomes and return to athletics [65, 66]. However, a recent systematic review and meta-analysis found that while microfracture had clinical improvements in short- and mid-term follow-up, the clinical improvement was not sustained long term [67]. A study of NFL athletes determined that only 67% returned to play after arthroscopic treatment of cartilage lesions, including chondroplasty, with even lower odds of return with players who underwent microfracture [68]. This was independent of lesion, size, grade, or player position.

Another popular treatment option for cartilage lesions involves utilizing bone and cartilage plugs to replace the area of cartilage damage. This technique can employ autograft plugs or allograft plugs. Osteoarticular autograft transfer system (OATS) is the name given to autograft osteochondral transfer and involves taking a plug from a peripheral non-articulating area of the knee and transferring it to the site of injury. An osteochondral allograft plug can alternatively be used, with the advantage that it provides less donor-site morbidity by negating the harvest of a donor plug. Osteochondral allograft is also advantageous for larger cartilage lesions. A recent systematic review determined a 75–82% range of return to sport and general improvement in reported outcomes in athletes who underwent osteochondral allograft transplant for cartilage injury in the knee [69]. OATS has also been demonstrated to have a high return to sport in recreational as well as collegiate- and professional-level athletes [70, 71]. A recent systematic review also demonstrated clinical improvements that were sustained long term in patients that underwent OATS treatment [67].

Autologous chondrocyte implantation (ACI) or matrix-induced autologous chondrocyte implantation (MACI) are treatment options often reserved for larger cartilage defects. ACI and MACI involve harvesting chondrocytes from the athlete's knee, culturing the chondrocytes at a remote facility, and replacing the cultured cells into the debrided cartilage defect in an open surgery. In traditional ACI, a periosteal membrane is sewn over the top of the defect, and cultured chondrocyte cells are injected under the periosteal flap. MACI is the recent evolution of the technique and involves loading the cultured cells onto a porcine collagen bilayer scaffold. The scaffold is secured in place with fibrin glue, negating the need for a periosteal layer to hold the cells in place. Studies have shown similar outcomes between ACI/MACI [72–74]. Multiple studies have also shown long-term durability of outcome improvements with ACI [75, 76]. Both techniques have also been found to be efficacious in the treatment of adolescent cartilage injuries [75, 77, 78]. The cost of ACI and MACI has proven prohibitive to widespread clinical application.

Multiple studies ultimately demonstrated that at intermediate follow-up, there are similar outcome improvements between marrow stimulation, OATS, and ACI procedures [67, 79–81]. Two recent meta-analysis determined around a 76% return-to-sport rate in athletes when accounting for all techniques, with the highest return to sport noted after OATS procedure, and the lowest return to sport occurring in patients who underwent microfracture [82, 83]. Another recent meta-analysis determined that even with literature showing improved clinical outcomes, it should be noted that almost all studies still have patients that failed surgical intervention, regardless of the treatment [84]. Ultimately, while some studies have shown inferior outcomes in athletes using microfracture, all of the aforementioned cartilage repair techniques have literature demonstrating their efficacy [67, 68, 79, 80, 85]. The choice of surgical intervention ultimately depends on specific athlete factors, goals, lesion size, and location. These options should be thoroughly discussed between the athlete and the surgeon prior to undergoing any procedure.

Future Cartilage Repair Direction

It is clear that future cartilage repair techniques will involve stem cell technologies. One developing technique for chondral defects is currently under an FDA clinical trial at the authors' institution. The technique involves augmenting arthroscopic marrow stimulation with postoperative injections of autologous peripheral blood stem cells. The technique leverages the same stem cell source that is used in bone marrow transplant. Individuals with cartilage defects are treated with arthroscopic subchondral drilling and postoperatively given doses of filgrastim, a synthetic form of granulocyte colony–stimulating factor, a glycoprotein that stimulates the bone marrow to produce stem cells and release them into the bloodstream. After 3 days of dosing with filgrastim, peripheral blood stem cells are harvested from the peripheral circulation by apheresis, a blood collection process developed for bone marrow transplant. This produces a large yield of stem cells, which are aliquoted and cryopreserved. Multiple postsurgical injections of the stem cells into the knee are performed, seeding the maturing cartilage as it heals (Fig. 10.6). Early clinical studies are promising, including healing of the large chondral defects with histological samples suggesting a cartilage repair more consistent with natural cartilage as opposed to fibrocartilage [86–89]. This may provide a very viable option for athletes in the near future.

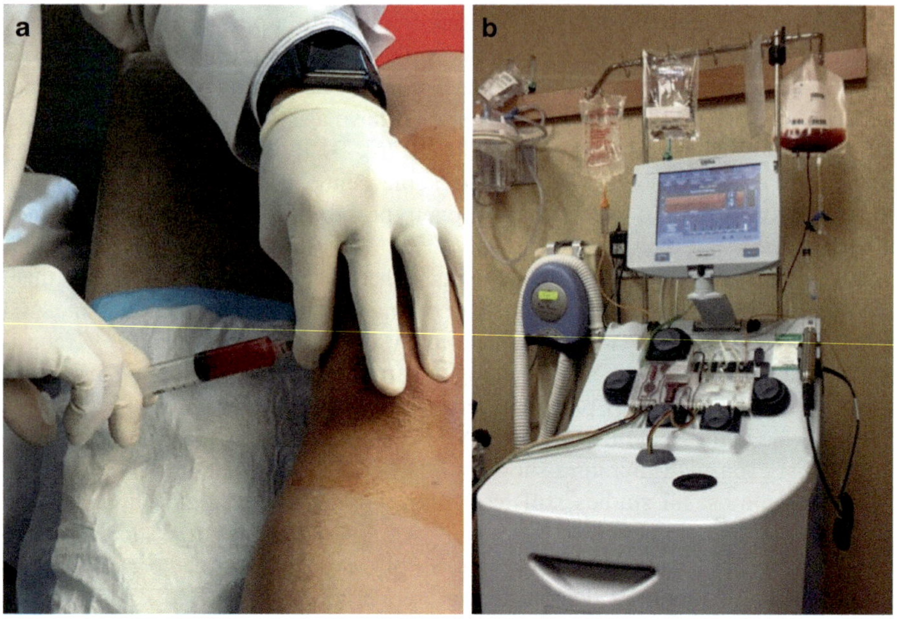

Fig. 10.6 As part of a clinical trial at the Andrews Institute, patients undergo knee injections (**a**) of autologous filgrastim-mobilized peripheral blood stem cells, harvested with apheresis (**b**), after arthroscopic subchondral drilling

Summary

The proper evaluation and management of cartilage injuries in football players is essential to maximize the short-term and long-term athletic career, but more importantly long-term joint health. Thorough physical examination and appropriate imaging should be undertaken in players with the suspicion of articular cartilage injury. Nonoperative management is almost always the first-line treatment, with consideration for the use of braces, biologics, and BFR therapy, in conjunction with a goal-directed rehabilitation program. In cases where an athlete has failed nonoperative management or sustains an injury not conducive to nonoperative treatment, a sized-based algorithm is available to fit the best surgical option to the clinical scenario. There are ever-evolving operative and nonoperative treatment options for articular cartilage injuries, as well as continued development and application of biologics. Providers involved in the care of athletes should work to stay current with literature regarding these treatment options and biologic applications to ensure they are giving the athlete the best chance of success, both short and long term.

References

1. Wang D, Weiss LJ, Abrams M, et al. Athletes with musculoskeletal injuries identified at the NFL scouting combine and prediction of outcomes in the NFL: a systematic review. Orthop J Sports Med. 2018;6(12):2325967118813083.
2. Steinwachs MR, Engebretsen L, Brophy RH. Scientific evidence base for cartilage injury and repair in the athlete. Cartilage. 2012;3(1 Suppl):11S–7S.
3. Flanigan DC, Harris JD, Trinh TQ, Siston RA, Brophy RH. Prevalence of chondral defects in athletes' knees: a systematic review. Med Sci Sports Exerc. 2010;42(10):1795–801.
4. Hirshorn KC, Cates T, Gillogly S. Magnetic resonance imaging-documented chondral injuries about the knee in college football players: 3-year National Football League Combine data. Arthroscopy. 2010;26(9):1237–40.
5. Provencher MT, Chahla J, Cinque ME, et al. Symptomatic focal knee chondral injuries in National Football League combine players are Associated with poorer performance and less volume of play. Arthroscopy. 2018;34(3):671–7.
6. Nepple JJ, Wright RW, Matava MJ, Brophy RH. Full-thickness knee articular cartilage defects in national football league combine athletes undergoing magnetic resonance imaging: prevalence, location, and association with previous surgery. Arthroscopy. 2012;28(6):798–806.
7. Tanamas S, Hanna FS, Cicuttini FM, Wluka AE, Berry P, Urquhart DM. Does knee malalignment increase the risk of development and progression of knee osteoarthritis? A systematic review. Arthritis Rheum. 2009;61(4):459–67.
8. Ding C, Cicuttini F, Scott F, Cooley H, Boon C, Jones G. Natural history of knee cartilage defects and factors affecting change. Arch Intern Med. 2006;166(6):651–8.
9. Keng A, Sayre EC, Guermazi A, et al. Association of body mass index with knee cartilage damage in an asymptomatic population-based study. BMC Musculoskelet Disord. 2017;18(1):517.
10. Chahla J, Cinque ME, Godin JA, et al. Meniscectomy and resultant articular cartilage lesions of the knee among prospective National Football League Players: an imaging and performance analysis. Am J Sports Med. 2018;46(1):200–7.
11. Brophy RH, Rodeo SA, Barnes RP, Powell JW, Warren RF. Knee articular cartilage injuries in the National Football League: epidemiology and treatment approach by team physicians. J Knee Surg. 2009;22(4):331–8.
12. Eismann EA, Pettit RJ, Wall EJ, Myer GD. Management strategies for osteochondritis dissecans of the knee in the skeletally immature athlete. J Orthop Sports Phys Ther. 2014;44(9):665–79.
13. Krause M, Hapfelmeier A, Moller M, Amling M, Bohndorf K, Meenen NM. Healing predictors of stable juvenile osteochondritis dissecans knee lesions after 6 and 12 months of nonoperative treatment. Am J Sports Med. 2013;41(10):2384–91.
14. Wall EJ, Vourazeris J, Myer GD, et al. The healing potential of stable juvenile osteochondritis dissecans knee lesions. J Bone Joint Surg Am. 2008;90(12):2655–64.
15. Yang JS, Bogunovic L, Wright RW. Nonoperative treatment of osteochondritis dissecans of the knee. Clin Sports Med. 2014;33(2):295–304.
16. Shelbourne KD, Jari S, Gray T. Outcome of untreated traumatic articular cartilage defects of the knee: a natural history study. J Bone Joint Surg Am. 2003;85-A(Suppl 2):8–16.
17. Cinque ME, Chahla J, Mitchell JJ, et al. Influence of meniscal and chondral lesions on patient-reported outcomes after primary anterior cruciate ligament reconstruction at 2-year follow-up. Orthop J Sports Med. 2018;6(2):2325967117754189.
18. Filardo G, de Caro F, Andriolo L, Kon E, Zaffagnini S, Marcacci M. Do cartilage lesions affect the clinical outcome of anterior cruciate ligament reconstruction? A systematic review. Knee Surg Sports Traumatol Arthrosc. 2017;25(10):3061–75.
19. Sophia Fox AJ, Bedi A, Rodeo SA. The basic science of articular cartilage: structure, composition, and function. Sports Health. 2009;1(6):461–8.
20. Pickett AM, Hensley DT Jr. Knee cell-based cartilage restoration. J Knee Surg. 2019;32(2):127–33.

21. Potter HG, Jain SK, Ma Y, Black BR, Fung S, Lyman S. Cartilage injury after acute, isolated anterior cruciate ligament tear: immediate and longitudinal effect with clinical/MRI follow-up. Am J Sports Med. 2012;40(2):276–85.
22. Wei F, Golenberg N, Kepich ET, Haut RC. Effect of intermittent cyclic preloads on the response of articular cartilage explants to an excessive level of unconfined compression. J Orthop Res. 2008;26(12):1636–42.
23. Kurz B, Jin M, Patwari P, Cheng DM, Lark MW, Grodzinsky AJ. Biosynthetic response and mechanical properties of articular cartilage after injurious compression. J Orthop Res. 2001;19(6):1140–6.
24. Arokoski J, Kiviranta I, Jurvelin J, Tammi M, Helminen HJ. Long-distance running causes site-dependent decrease of cartilage glycosaminoglycan content in the knee joints of beagle dogs. Arthritis Rheum. 1993;36(10):1451–9.
25. Bonnevie ED, Delco ML, Galesso D, Secchieri C, Fortier LA, Bonassar LJ. Sub-critical impact inhibits the lubricating mechanisms of articular cartilage. J Biomech. 2017;53:64–70.
26. Carter DR, Beaupre GS, Wong M, Smith RL, Andriacchi TP, Schurman DJ. The mechanobiology of articular cartilage development and degeneration. Clin Orthop Relat Res. 2004;(427 Suppl):S69–77.
27. Ding L, Heying E, Nicholson N, et al. Mechanical impact induces cartilage degradation via mitogen activated protein kinases. Osteoarthr Cartil. 2010;18(11):1509–17.
28. McAdams TR, Mithoefer K, Scopp JM, Mandelbaum BR. Articular cartilage injury in athletes. Cartilage. 2010;1(3):165–79.
29. Santos S, Emery N, Neu CP, Pierce DM. Propagation of microcracks in collagen networks of cartilage under mechanical loads. Osteoarthritis Cartilage. 2019;27(9):1392–402.
30. Wong M, Carter DR. Articular cartilage functional histomorphology and mechanobiology: a research perspective. Bone. 2003;33(1):1–13.
31. Samora WP, Chevillet J, Adler B, Young GS, Klingele KE. Juvenile osteochondritis dissecans of the knee: predictors of lesion stability. J Pediatr Orthop. 2012;32(1):1–4.
32. Heywood CS, Benke MT, Brindle K, Fine KM. Correlation of magnetic resonance imaging to arthroscopic findings of stability in juvenile osteochondritis dissecans. Arthroscopy. 2011;27(2):194–9.
33. Chouhan DK, Dhillon MS, Patel S, Bansai T, Bhatia A. Kanwat. Multiple platelet-rich plasma injections versus single platelet-rich plasma injection in early osteoarthritis of the knee: an experimental study in Guinea pig model of early knee osteoarthritis. Am J Sports Med. 2019;47(10):2300–7.
34. Cavallo C, Filardo G, Mariani E, et al. Comparison of platelet-rich plasma formulations for cartilage healing: an in vitro study. J Bone Joint Surg Am. 2014;96(5):423–9.
35. Kennedy MI, Whitney K, Evans T, LaPrade RF. Platelet-rich plasma and cartilage repair. Curr Rev Musculoskelet Med. 2018;11(4):573–82.
36. Khatab S, van Buul GM, Kops N, et al. Intra-articular injections of platelet-rich plasma releasate reduce pain and synovial inflammation in a mouse model of osteoarthritis. Am J Sports Med. 2018;46(4):977–86.
37. Osterman C, McCarthy MB, Cote MP, et al. Platelet-rich plasma increases anti-inflammatory markers in a human Coculture model for osteoarthritis. Am J Sports Med. 2015;43(6):1474–84.
38. Saito M, Takahashi KA, Arai Y, et al. Intraarticular administration of platelet-rich plasma with biodegradable gelatin hydrogel microspheres prevents osteoarthritis progression in the rabbit knee. Clin Exp Rheumatol. 2009;27(2):201–7.
39. Sakata R, Reddi AH. Platelet-rich plasma modulates actions on articular cartilage lubrication and regeneration. Tissue Eng Part B Rev. 2016;22(5):408–19.
40. Yin WJ, Xu HT, Sheng JG, et al. Advantages of pure platelet-rich plasma compared with leukocyte- and platelet-rich plasma in treating rabbit knee osteoarthritis. Med Sci Monit. 2016;22:1280–90.
41. Zhou Q, Xu C, Cheng X, et al. Platelets promote cartilage repair and chondrocyte proliferation via ADP in a rodent model of osteoarthritis. Platelets. 2016;27(3):212–22.

42. Campbell KA, Saltzman BM, Mascarenhas R, et al. Does intra-articular platelet-rich plasma injection provide clinically superior outcomes compared with other therapies in the treatment of knee osteoarthritis? A systematic review of overlapping meta-analyses. Arthroscopy. 2015;31(11):2213–21.
43. Dai WL, Zhou AG, Zhang H, Zhang J. Efficacy of platelet-rich plasma in the treatment of knee osteoarthritis: a meta-analysis of randomized controlled trials. Arthroscopy. 2017;33(3):659–70. e651.
44. Khoshbin A, Leroux T, Wasserstein D, et al. The efficacy of platelet-rich plasma in the treatment of symptomatic knee osteoarthritis: a systematic review with quantitative synthesis. Arthroscopy. 2013;29(12):2037–48.
45. Meheux CJ, McCulloch PC, Lintner DM, Varner KE, Harris JD. Efficacy of intra-articular platelet-rich plasma injections in knee osteoarthritis: a systematic review. Arthroscopy. 2016;32(3):495–505.
46. Regulatory considerations for human cells, tissues, and cellular and tissue- based products: minimal manipulation and homologous use. Food and Drug Administration. November 2017. Available at: https://www.fda.gov/regulatory-information/search-fda-guidance-documents/regulatory-considerations-human-cells-tissues-and-cellular-and-tissue-based-products-minimal. Accessed 16 Apr 2020.
47. Chu CR, Rodeo S, Bhutani N, et al. Optimizing clinical use of biologics in orthopaedic surgery: consensus recommendations from the 2018 AAOS/NIH U-13 conference. J Am Acad Orthop Surg. 2019;27(2):e50–63.
48. Lamplot JD, Rodeo SA, Brophy RH. A practical guide for the current use of biologic therapies in sports medicine. Am J Sports Med. 2020;48(2):488–503.
49. Anz AW, Hubbard R, Rendos NK, Everts PA, Andrews JR, Hackel JG. Bone marrow aspirate concentrate is equivalent to platelet-rich plasma for the treatment of knee osteoarthritis at 1 year: a prospective, randomized trial. Orthop J Sports Med. 2020;8(2):2325967119900958.
50. Cassano JM, Kennedy JG, Ross KA, Fraser EJ, Goodale MB, Fortier LA. Bone marrow concentrate and platelet-rich plasma differ in cell distribution and interleukin 1 receptor antagonist protein concentration. Knee Surg Sports Traumatol Arthrosc. 2018;26(1):333–42.
51. Shapiro SA, Kazmerchak SE, Heckman MG, Zubair AC, O'Connor MI. A prospective, single-blind, placebo-controlled trial of bone marrow aspirate concentrate for knee osteoarthritis. Am J Sports Med. 2017;45(1):82–90.
52. Vernon L, Abadin A, Wilensky D, Huang CY, Kaplan L. Subphysiological compressive loading reduces apoptosis following acute impact injury in a porcine cartilage model. Sports Health. 2014;6(1):81–8.
53. Wilk KE, Briem K, Reinold MM, Devine KM, Dugas J, Andrews JR. Rehabilitation of articular lesions in the athlete's knee. J Orthop Sports Phys Ther. 2006;36(10):815–27.
54. Day B. Personalized blood flow restriction therapy: how, when and where can it accelerate rehabilitation after surgery? Arthroscopy. 2018;34(8):2511–3.
55. Hylden C, Burns T, Stinner D, Owens J. Blood flow restriction rehabilitation for extremity weakness: a case series. J Spec Oper Med. 2015;15(1):50–6.
56. Takarada Y, Takazawa H, Ishii N. Applications of vascular occlusion diminish disuse atrophy of knee extensor muscles. Med Sci Sports Exerc. 2000;32(12):2035–9.
57. Takarada Y, Takazawa H, Sato Y, Takebayashi S, Tanaka Y, Ishii N. Effects of resistance exercise combined with moderate vascular occlusion on muscular function in humans. J Appl Physiol (1985). 2000;88(6):2097–106.
58. Vechin FC, Libardi CA, Conceicao MS, et al. Comparisons between low-intensity resistance training with blood flow restriction and high-intensity resistance training on quadriceps muscle mass and strength in elderly. J Strength Cond Res. 2015;29(4):1071–6.
59. Dankel SJ, Jessee MB, Abe T, Loenneke JP. The effects of blood flow restriction on upper-body musculature located distal and proximal to applied pressure. Sports Med. 2016;46(1):23–33.
60. Kim D, Singh H, Loenneke JP, et al. Comparative effects of vigorous-intensity and low-intensity blood flow restricted cycle training and detraining on muscle mass, strength, and aerobic capacity. J Strength Cond Res. 2016;30(5):1453–61.

61. Pope ZK, Willardson JM, Schoenfeld BJ. Exercise and blood flow restriction. J Strength Cond Res. 2013;27(10):2914–26.
62. Scott BR, Loenneke JP, Slattery KM, Dascombe BJ. Blood flow restricted exercise for athletes: a review of available evidence. J Sci Med Sport. 2016;19(5):360–7.
63. Slysz J, Stultz J, Burr JF. The efficacy of blood flow restricted exercise: a systematic review & meta-analysis. J Sci Med Sport. 2016;19(8):669–75.
64. Yasuda T, Fujita S, Ogasawara R, Sato Y, Abe T. Effects of low-intensity bench press training with restricted arm muscle blood flow on chest muscle hypertrophy: a pilot study. Clin Physiol Funct Imaging. 2010;30(5):338–43.
65. Mithoefer K, Gill TJ, Cole BJ, Williams RJ, Mandelbaum BR. Clinical outcome and return to competition after microfracture in the athlete's knee: an evidence-based systematic review. Cartilage. 2010;1(2):113–20.
66. Mithoefer K, Williams RJ 3rd, Warren RF, Wickiewicz TL, Marx RG. High-impact athletics after knee articular cartilage repair: a prospective evaluation of the microfracture technique. Am J Sports Med. 2006;34(9):1413–8.
67. Jones KJ, Kelley BV, Arshi A, McAllister DR, Fabricant PD. Comparative effectiveness of cartilage repair with respect to the minimal clinically important difference. Am J Sports Med. 2019;47(13):3284–93. https://doi.org/10.1177/0363546518824552.
68. Scillia AJ, Aune KT, Andrachuk JS, et al. Return to play after chondroplasty of the knee in National Football League athletes. Am J Sports Med. 2015;43(3):663–8.
69. Crawford ZT, Schumaier AP, Glogovac G, Grawe BM. Return to sport and sports-specific outcomes after osteochondral allograft transplantation in the knee: a systematic review of studies with at least 2 years' mean follow-up. Arthroscopy. 2019;35(6):1880–9.
70. Balazs GC, Wang D, Burge AJ, Sinatro AL, Wong AC, Williams RJ 3rd. Return to play among elite basketball players after osteochondral allograft transplantation of full-thickness cartilage lesions. Orthop J Sports Med. 2018;6(7):2325967118786941.
71. Nielsen ES, McCauley JC, Pulido PA, Bugbee WD. Return to sport and recreational activity after osteochondral allograft transplantation in the knee. Am J Sports Med. 2017;45(7):1608–14.
72. Bartlett W, Skinner JA, Gooding CR, et al. Autologous chondrocyte implantation versus matrix-induced autologous chondrocyte implantation for osteochondral defects of the knee: a prospective, randomised study. J Bone Joint Surg Br. 2005;87(5):640–5.
73. Gomoll AH, Ambra LF, Phan A, Mastrocola M, Shah N. Cell-seeded autologous chondrocyte implantation: a simplified implantation technique that maintains high clinical outcomes. Am J Sports Med. 2017;45(5):1028–36.
74. Zeifang F, Oberle D, Nierhoff C, Richter W, Moradi B, Schmitt H. Autologous chondrocyte implantation using the original periosteum-cover technique versus matrix-associated autologous chondrocyte implantation: a randomized clinical trial. Am J Sports Med. 2010;38(5):924–33.
75. Hoburg A, Loer I, Korsmeier K, et al. Matrix-associated autologous chondrocyte implantation is an effective treatment at midterm follow-up in adolescents and young adults. Orthop J Sports Med. 2019;7(4):2325967119841077.
76. Peterson L, Vasiliadis HS, Brittberg M, Lindahl A. Autologous chondrocyte implantation: a long-term follow-up. Am J Sports Med. 2010;38(6):1117–24.
77. Beck JJ, Sugimoto D, Micheli L. Sustained results in long-term follow-up of autologous chondrocyte implantation (ACI) for distal femur juvenile osteochondritis dissecans (JOCD). Adv Orthop. 2018;2018:7912975.
78. DiBartola AC, Wright BM, Magnussen RA, Flanigan DC. Clinical outcomes after autologous chondrocyte implantation in adolescents' knees: a systematic review. Arthroscopy. 2016;32(9):1905–16.
79. Mundi R, Bedi A, Chow L, et al. Cartilage restoration of the knee: a systematic review and meta-analysis of level 1 studies. Am J Sports Med. 2016;44(7):1888–95.
80. Ossendorff R, Franke K, Erdle B, Uhl M, Sudkamp NP, Salzmann GM. Clinical and radiographical ten years long-term outcome of microfracture vs. autologous chondrocyte implantation: a matched-pair analysis. Int Orthop. 2019;43(3):553–9.

81. Schrock JB, Kraeutler MJ, Houck DA, McQueen MB, McCarty EC. A cost-effectiveness analysis of surgical treatment modalities for chondral lesions of the knee: microfracture, osteochondral autograft transplantation, and autologous chondrocyte implantation. Orthop J Sports ed. 2017;5(5):2325967117704634.
82. Campbell AB, Pineda M, Harris JD, Flanigan DC. Return to sport after articular cartilage repair in athletes' knees: a systematic review. Arthroscopy. 2016;32(4):651–68. e651
83. Krych AJ, Pareek A, King AH, Johnson NR, Stuart MJ, Williams RJ 3rd. Return to sport after the surgical management of articular cartilage lesions in the knee: a meta-analysis. Knee Surg Sports Traumatol Arthrosc. 2017;25(10):3186–96.
84. Gracitelli GC, Moraes VY, Franciozi CE, Luzo MV, Belloti JC. Surgical interventions (microfracture, drilling, mosaicplasty, and allograft transplantation) for treating isolated cartilage defects of the knee in adults. Cochrane Database Syst Rev. 2016;9:CD010675.
85. Kraeutler MJ, Belk JW, Purcell JM, McCarty EC. Microfracture versus autologous chondrocyte implantation for articular cartilage lesions in the knee: a systematic review of 5-year outcomes. Am J Sports Med. 2018;46(4):995–9.
86. Saw KY, Anz A, Jee CS, Ng RC, Mohtarrudin N, Ragavanaidu K. High tibial osteotomy in combination with chondrogenesis after stem cell therapy: a report of 8 cases. Arthroscopy. 2015;31(10):1909–20.
87. Saw KY, Anz A, Merican S, et al. Articular cartilage regeneration with autologous peripheral blood progenitor cells and hyaluronic acid after arthroscopic subchondral drilling: a report of 5 cases with histology. Arthroscopy. 2011;27(4):493–506.
88. Saw KY, Anz A, Siew-Yoke Jee C, et al. Articular cartilage regeneration with autologous peripheral blood stem cells versus hyaluronic acid: a randomized controlled trial. Arthroscopy. 2013;29(4):684–94.
89. Saw KY, Hussin P, Loke SC, et al. Articular cartilage regeneration with autologous marrow aspirate and hyaluronic acid: an experimental study in a goat model. Arthroscopy. 2009;25(12):1391–400.

Considerations for the Young Football Player

11

Jeremy S. Frank and Jennifer Kurowicki

Introduction

Tackle football has historically been linked to significantly greater injury risks in comparison to other sports [1]. The sport alone accounts for approximately 44% of all youth sport–related emergency room visits per year [2], and several studies have demonstrated that while other sports decrease injury rates, tackle football continues to rise [1, 3]. From 2010 to 2014, fractures of the lower extremity were reported the most common injury in tackle football [4]. Furthermore, lower extremity fractures account for more than two-thirds of all football-associated fractures [5].

As a youth athlete, injury patterns are specific to the developing musculoskeletal system and pose a clinical challenge to the treating physician. During the adolescent growth spurt, there is a temporary decline in coordination and associated muscle imbalance [6]. The open physes and growing cartilage where the musculotendinous unit and ligamentous attachments insert are more susceptible to injury during this phase [7]. It is during this same period that there tends to be an exponential rise in youth sports participation, thus predisposing youth athletes to physeal and avulsion injuries, particularly in the lower extremity in football [8]. In this chapter, we will discuss common lower extremity avulsion and physeal fractures seen in the adolescent football athlete.

J. S. Frank (✉)
Department of Pediatric Orthopaedic Surgery, Joe DiMaggio Children's Hospital, [U18] Sports Medicine, Hollywood, FL, USA
e-mail: jefrank@mhs.net

J. Kurowicki
Department of Orthopaedic Surgery, St. Joseph's University Medical Center, Seton Hall University, Paterson, NJ, USA

K. W. Farmer (ed.), *Football Injuries*,
https://doi.org/10.1007/978-3-030-54875-9_11

Hip and Pelvis

Apophyseal avulsion fractures of the hip and pelvis are injuries that occur almost exclusively in the adolescent athlete due to failure of the secondary ossification centers [9]. During puberty, hormonal shifts promote strengthening of the muscles and growth at the cartilaginous apophyses, resulting in a stronger musculotendinous unit. Consequently, when the athlete experiences sudden, explosive concentric muscle contraction as seen in football movements such as sprinting, jumping or kicking, this imbalance causes the musculotendinous unit to avulse from its origin [9–11].

Without a firm understanding of the developmental stages of each secondary ossification center and relevant anatomy, appropriate diagnosis of these pediatric lower extremity avulsion fractures may be missed. Apophyseal avulsion fractures can be seen at the insertion of the hamstrings at the ischial tuberosity (IT), the sartorius insertion at the anterior superior iliac spine (ASIS), rectus femoris at the anterior inferior iliac spine (AIIS), and less commonly at the iliopsoas insertion on the lesser trochanter (LT). The secondary ossification center of the AIIS appears between 13 and15 years and fuses at 16 years of age, while the ASIS appears between ages 15 and 17 years and fuses between 19 and 25 years of age [12]. Athletes are at highest susceptibility to these injuries prior to fusion of the secondary ossification centers between 13 and 16 years of age; however, they can present into an athlete's mid-20s due to the late closure of the ASIS [13]. Several studies have demonstrated that males account for the majority of these injuries, with reports between 76% and 87% [9, 11, 13, 14].

It is important to recognize that the fracture site is a result of the mechanism of trauma, patient age, and physiologic development with each fracture site demonstrating slight nuances, which will be highlighted in this chapter (Table 11.1). In a review of 228 avulsion fractures, Schuett et al. found the most common location for these injures to be the AIIS (49%), followed by the ASIS (30%), and ischial tuberosity (IT) (11%) [14]. In contrast, Rossi and Dragoni found that in a series of 203 avulsion fractures, the IT was the most common (54%), followed by AIIS (22%) and ASIS (19%) [11]. Nonetheless, a meta-analysis encompassing 596 patients demonstrated the most common site to be AIIS (33.2%), IT (29.7%), ASIS (27.9%), and LT (1.8%) [15]. The same study went on to demonstrate "ball sports" were a predisposing factor to 70% of AIIS, 45% of IT, 46% of ASIS, and 67% of LT avulsion fractures [15].

On initial presentation, patients will report a discrete, usually noncontact, event during activity that resulted in sudden onset of pain. Additionally, the patient may describe a cracking or popping sensation in the pelvic region. These injuries can be considered the "great mimicker" in the pelvis, often misdiagnosed as muscle strain or apophysitis. It is crucial to maintain high clinical suspicion in adolescent athletes for avulsion fractures, particularly if pain persists, patients are younger, or there is inability to return to sport [12]. Missed or misdiagnosis can result in more extensive surgery and higher rates of postoperative complications [16]. Physical examination may vary depending on fracture location, but in general patients have pain with

Table 11.1 Pelvic avulsion fractures

	Anterior superior iliac spine	Anterior inferior iliac spine	Ischial tuberosity	Lesser trochanter
Muscle attachment	Sartorius and tensor fasciae lata	Straight head of the rectus femoris	Hamstring complex: long head of the biceps femoris, semitendinosus, and semimembranosus	Iliopsoas
Mechanism of injury	Sudden, forceful twisting	Forceful hip hyperextension + knee flexion	Forced flexion of the hip + knee in extension	
Physical exam findings	Weakness of hip flexion and extension +/− weakness in hip abduction	Weakness in hip flexion + knee extension	Weakness of knee flexion and hip extension	Weakness on hip flexion
Imaging	Fragment displaces lateral and distal	Fragment displaces anterior lateral Best observed on frog lateral view	Fragment seen on AP radiograph	
Complications	Meralgia paresthetica secondary to lateral femoral cutaneous nerve	Sup-spine impingement	Hamstring syndrome	Non-union

passive stretch, localized tenderness, ecchymosis, and decreased range of motion (ROM) compared to the contralateral side.

All adolescent athletes presenting with acute hip pain following a sport injury should obtain a plain anteroposterior (AP) of the pelvis and frog lateral hip radiograph [14, 17, 18] to confirm diagnosis and assess size and displacement of fragment. IT avulsions are generally observed on AP pelvis, while AIIS avulsions are better appreciated on the frog lateral view due to the anterolateral displacement of the avulsed fragment [19] (Fig. 11.1).

Advanced imaging such as CT or MRI has not demonstrated added utility in the majority of cases. Plain radiographs have been shown to be sufficient for accurate identification of avulsion fragment, as demonstrated in a series of 228 avulsion fractures in which only 0.9% required a CT or MRI for diagnosis. Furthermore, when compared to CT or MRI images in 31 cases, radiographs accurately identified fracture displacement and size in 90% and 97%, respectively [14]. In regard to MRI, in very young patients in whom secondary ossification centers have not yet formed, this scan may be useful in diagnosing cartilaginous avulsions [20].

Historically, pelvic avulsion fractures have primarily been treated conservatively, particularly for non-displaced to minimally displaced fractures. A five-stage guided therapy protocol over the course of 2 months has demonstrated successful outcomes [10]. The proposed five-stage therapy protocol can be seen in Table 11.2. To help guide operative treatment, McKinney et al. expanded the original pelvic classification system set forth by Torode and Zieg to better establish treatment for avulsion

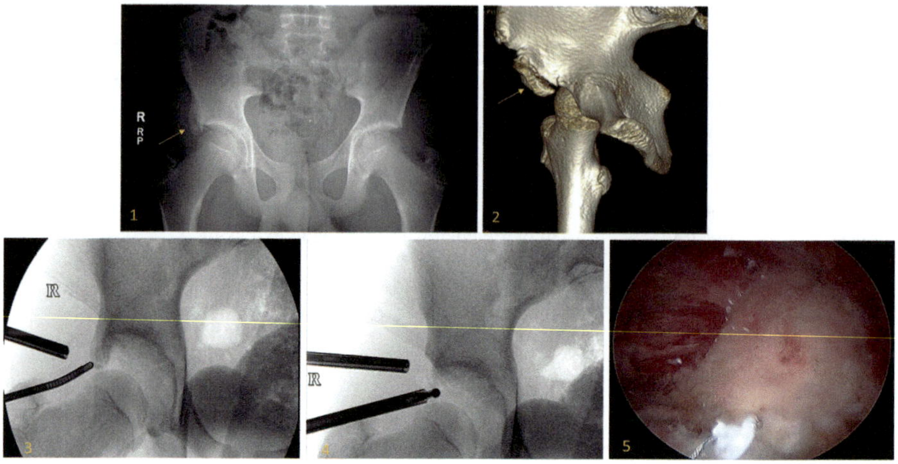

Fig. 11.1 (1) AP pelvis X-ray demonstrating malunion of right AIIS avulsion fracture (*arrow*). (2) 3D CT depicting AIIS malunion (*arrow*). (3) Intra-operative fluoroscopy outlining bony landmarks for subspine decompression. (4) Intra-operative fluoroscopy after decompression of AIIS malunion with arthroscopic burr. (5) Arthroscopic image of recessed subspine impingement

Table 11.2 Five phase non-operative protocol

Physical therapy protocol [2]							
Phase	Postinjury (d)	Subjective pain	Palpation tenderness	ROM	Muscle strength	Activity level	Radiographic appearance
I	0–7	Moderate	Moderate-severe	Very limited	Poor	None, protected WB	Osseous separation
II	7 to 14–20	Minimal	Moderate	Improving with guided exercise	Fair	Protected WB, guided exercise	Osseous separation
III	14–20 to 30	Minimal with stress	Moderate	Improving with gentle stress	Good	Guided exercise, resistance	Early callus
IV	30–60	None	Minimal	Normal	Good-normal	Limited athletic participation	Maturing callus
V	60 to return	None	None	Normal	Normal	Full activity	Maturing callus

Taken from Metzmaker et al. [10]
Abbreviations: *ROM* range of motion, *WB* weight bearing

fractures of the pelvis [9, 21]. The McKinney classification of apophyseal avulsion fractures defines: Type I, nondisplaced fractures; Type II, displacement ≤2 cm; Type III, displacement >2 cm; and Type IV, symptomatic nonunion or painful exostosis [9].

McKinney et al. established that Type II/III ischial tuberosity avulsion fractures with associated neurologic symptoms or any Type IV was indicated for surgery. Furthermore, relative indications included Type III in professional/collegiate level athletes or ASIS, AIIS, or IT Type III avulsion fractures that have failed conservative treatment. However, literature supports operative management of fragments displaced >2 cm due to increased risks of nonunion and muscle shortening if treated nonoperatively [9]. When considering treatment options, it is important to consider the amount of fracture displacement, site of the fracture, and the physical demands of the athlete [12, 17, 22].

Ischial Tuberosity

Ischial tuberosity avulsions are frequently observed in younger patients compared to avulsions at other anatomic sites within the pelvis, with up to 15% occurring prior to closure of the triradiate cartilage [14, 22] and most commonly are injured during sprinting and falls [14]. Avulsions are easily seen on AP radiographs, since fragments are typically the largest and more displaced compared to ASIS, AIIS, or iliac crest [14]. Nonoperative management is the mainstay of treatment; however, for patients in which surgical management is an indication, several small case series have described techniques, including plate fixation, cancellous screws, and suture anchors [16, 22–25]. Recent biomechanical studies demonstrate that five small suture anchors most closely replicate the intact tendon strength; thus, the introduction of suture bridge techniques for proximal hamstring avulsions have been recently explored [26, 27]. Surgery is performed in the prone position with fragment reduction best achieved with hip extension and knee flexion. Approach through the gluteal crease is popular; however, sub-gluteal and Kocher-Langenbeck have been described [16, 22–25, 27]. Due to the strong hamstring contraction, postoperative recovery is longest among IT avulsion fracture patients, in order to allow complete healing with return to full play at 6 months [12, 23].

In patients with delayed presentation of IT avulsion fractures or those who failed conservative management, common complications include pseudarthrosis and hamstring syndrome. Up to 50% of patients with greater than 15 mm of displacement treated nonoperatively will develop pseudarthrosis [22]. Patients with hamstring syndrome present with symptoms consistent with irritation of the sciatic nerve. The most common complaint is posterior leg pain with prolonged sitting, and neurolysis may be indicated [28].

Anterior Superior Iliac Spine

White et al. have described avulsions of the ASIS into two categories—Type I occurring at the sartorius and Type II occurring at the tensor fasciae lata—in order to account for the two tendinous attachments [8]. The majority of patients with this fracture pattern are older, with up to 84% classified as Risser 4 [14]. Nonoperative management with NSAIDs and 2 months of protected weightbearing is the preferred treatment for ASIS avulsions. However, in patients who meet the criteria, surgical options include open reduction internal fixation (ORIF) with lag screw, utilizing a direct incision over anterior aspect of iliac crest with the patient supine.

Other surgical options include a double-row suture bridge technique with anchors [29]. The majority of the literature supporting surgical management is comprised of small case series. Kautzner et al. performed a retrospective case-control study, comparing operatively managed versus conservative cases in 23 patients (13 operative, 10 nonoperative) with ASIS avulsions [30]. They concluded that there were no long-term differences in terms of range of motion or pain scores; however, operative patients were able to return to sport earlier. Postoperative rehabilitation includes 1 week of non-weightbearing followed by 3–6 weeks of progressive physical therapy with full return to sport ranging between 4 weeks and 6 weeks, depending on radiographic healing [31].

Misdiagnosis of ASIS avulsion fractures is not uncommon. On plain radiographs, the avulsed fragment displaces laterally and distally, making it easy to be mistaken for an AIIS avulsion [12]. Frog lateral radiographs can provide needed clarity. However, in the event that the initial diagnosis is missed, these patients may present to the clinic with tingling, numbness, or burning in the distribution of the lateral femoral cutaneous nerve [17]. This is termed meralgia paresthetica, and entrapment of the nerve may occur in large, displaced fracture fragments. Additionally, these avulsions are associated with large hematoma formation, which aids in further compression of the nerve or misdiagnosis for a tumor or infection [10].

Anterior Inferior Iliac Spine

AIIS avulsions are among the most common pelvic avulsion fractures and also carry the highest long-term morbidity. The AIIS is the first secondary ossification center to form and is the origin of the straight head of the rectus femoris. These fractures have a high prevalence in young athletic males, with 85% of AIIS fractures observed in Risser 0 patients and those with incompletely closed triradiate cartilage [14]. Opposite to ischial tuberosity avulsions, AIIS avulsion fragments are typically small in size and minimally displaced [14]. This contributes to the difficulty in diagnosis of these fracture on normal AP pelvic radiographs, oftentimes requiring additional views and a high index of suspicion in an adolescent athlete with groin pain (AIIS sub-spine).

The relatively small size and minimal displacement of these fragments make operative management in the acute setting rare. Only one case report exists, describing open reduction with internal fixation utilizing a 6.5-mm screw and washer in the acute setting [32]. The patient in this case was pain free and engaging in full sport participation at 1-year postoperatively. Nonoperative treatment in accordance with the previously described progressive rehabilitation protocol has demonstrated satisfactory outcomes with return to sport reported as early as 3 weeks, but the majority of athletes should expect full recovery by 3 months [9, 33]. However, patients managed nonoperatively are 4.5 times more likely to have persistent hip pain, with 22% of patients reporting continued pain 3 or months after the initial injury [14, 34].

Factors that contribute to persistent hip pain include concomitant anterosuperior labrum injury or development of sub-spine impingement due to missed diagnosis, malunion of a displaced fragment, or partial avulsion with repetitive traction,

Table 11.3 Diagnostic pearls consistent with AIIS impingement

History and physical examination
Anterior/groin pain with straight hip flexion
Anterior pain with prolonged hip flexion
Limited hip flexion range of motion on physical examination
Tenderness to palpation over AIIS that re-creates typical pain
Partial pain relief and persistent hip flexion limitations after intra-articular anesthetic hip injection
Imaging studies
Plain radiographs
Evidence for prior AIIS avulsion
Calcific deposits within rectus femoris origin
Extension of AIIS below acetabular sourcil on anteroposterior pelvis radiograph
Excessive anterior and distal extension of AIIS on false-profile radiograph
Acetabular retroversion with increased anterior rim sclerosis
Impingement cysts located at distal femoral neck
Three-dimensional computed tomography
Deformity of AIIS from prior AIIS avulsion
Excessive anterior extension of AIIS
Extension of AIIS to or below anterior acetabular rim
Intraoperative findings
Focal synovitis anteriorly at level of AIIS
Focal peripheral labral ecchymosis anteriorly at level of AIIS
Focal bony buildup of anterior acetabular rim representing inferior extension of AIIS
Calcific deposits within proximal rectus femoris

causing hypertrophy and exostosis formation at the apophysis. Sub-spine impingement is characterized by a decrease in hip flexion and internal rotation, secondary to a prominent AIIS abutting the distal aspect of the femoral neck. It is recognized as an extra-articular cause of femoroacetabular impingement (FAI). Diagnostic pearls were first described by Larson et al. in 2011 (Table 11.3). Both intra- and extra-articular pathology is often present in these patients. Carton et al. classified sub-spine impingement into four categories (Fig. 11.2) and found that the incidence of labrum bruising increased with worsening degrees of sub-spine impingement [35].

It is the development of sub-spine impingement months to years later that necessitates surgical intervention in these patients. Arthroscopic decompression of the sub-spine space is the preferred modality, allowing for management of intra- and extra-articular pathology and providing superior exposure. Mostly case reports demonstrate successful arthroscopic decompression and dissection of heterotopic bone fragments [36, 37]. Arthroscopic decompression of fragments as large as 3.5 cm have been reported; however, overly aggressive resection with subsequent avulsion of the rectus femoris, following sub-spine impingement surgery, has been reported [36, 38]. Open surgery utilizing a modified Smith-Peterson approach has been described in a 13-year-old football player with full return to football participation at 6 months [39]. Four to six weeks of prophylactic indomethacin or naproxen after injury or arthroscopy could be considered to prevent formation of excessive heterotopic ossification [40].

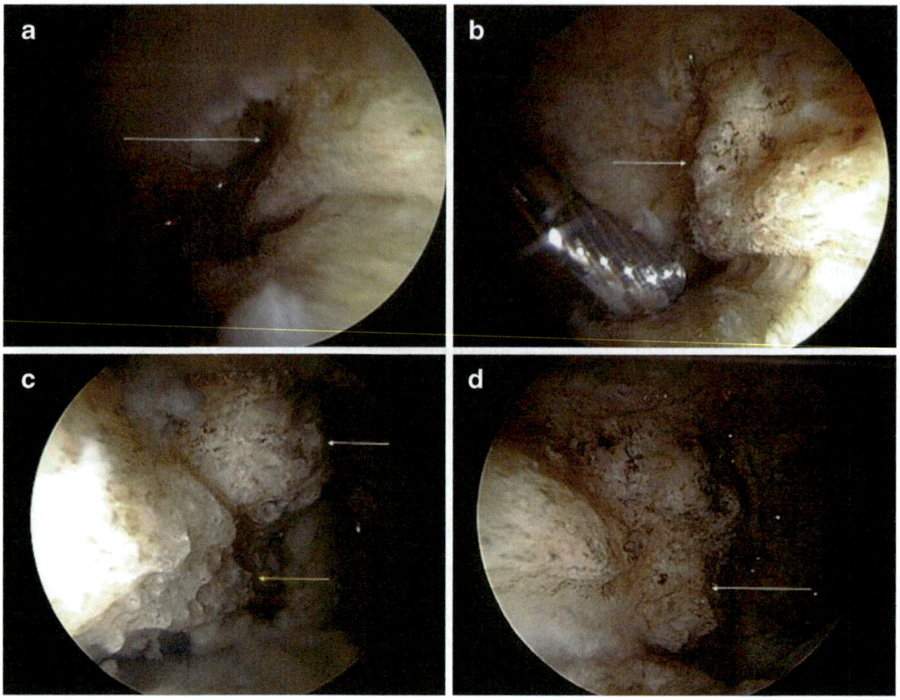

Fig. 11.2 (**a–d**) Arthroscopic classification of subspine hypertrophy: (**a**) Type 1: Normal concave recess extending from acetabular rim (white arrow); (**b**) Type 2: Convex bony prominence in continuity with rim (white arrow); (**c**) Type 3: Subspine prominence (white arrow) distinct from acetabular rim (yellow arrow); (**d**) Type 4: Sub-articular extension of the deformity beneath the acetabular rim (white arrow)

Lesser Trochanter

Avulsions of the LT are rare. These occur as a result of sudden contraction of the iliopsoas muscle. Ruffing et al. reported in a retrospective, multicenter study looking at LT avulsion fractures and found that these fractures occur between 13 and 15 years of age predominantly in males. Only Type II and Type III fractures were observed, and all were treated successfully with nonoperative management [41]. Operative management should only be attempted in Type IV fractures. Traditionally, excision of fragment with reattachment of iliopsoas can be performed, although development of a new retrograde fixation using a mini-open anterior approach has been described with excellent outcomes [42].

Distal Femur Fractures

Injuries to the distal femoral physis are rare fractures, comprising 2–5% of all physeal injuries [43, 44]. While these injuries may be rare, a case series of 49 pediatric athletes identified 50% of distal femoral fractures were attributed to football-related injuries [45]. Furthermore, these injuries carry severe consequences due to the contribution of the distal femoral physis to overall growth. Leg length growth on average continues until age 14 years in girls and 16 years in boys, with the distal femoral physis contributing approximately 40% of longitudinal growth or 9 mm per year [46]. Injury to this physis has been associated with poor prognosis and growth disturbance.

Up to 60% of these injuries are sports related, with tackling during football the most common mechanism [47]. Typically, these injuries are a result of valgus-type load applied across the knee, causing the periosteum on the tension side of the physis to fail, coronal displacement of the fracture, and a fragment of the metaphysis on the opposing side [44, 48]. Other mechanisms of injury include a hyperextension force, resulting in an anteriorly displaced fracture fragment, direct blow while the knee is in flexion producing a posterior displaced fragment, or a varus-type load with subsequent lateral fragment displacement and complete displacement of the epiphysis off the physis [44, 46, 48, 49].

Athletes may present with obvious deformity to the lower extremity with pain, hemarthrosis, and inability to weight bear. Hamstring spasm may cause the knee to maintain a flexed position. In patients with non-displaced fractures, initial presentation may often be similar to knee ligamentous injuries, with focal knee pain. While concomitant ligamentous or meniscal injury may be present in up to 12% of cases, distal femur physeal fractures occur in patients with open growth plates at a 6:1 predominance for males, so it is important for the evaluating physician to maintain a high clinical suspicion in an athlete with acute knee pain and swelling [45, 47]. Due to the close anatomical relationship to the popliteal artery, tibial, and peroneal nerve, a thorough neurovascular examination is critical.

Initial diagnostic imaging includes AP and lateral views of the knee, evaluating for physeal widening and obvious signs of fracture. If initial radiographs fail to demonstrate obvious fracture but suspicion remains high, stress radiograph or advanced imaging such as MRI or CT scan may be performed. Caution should be used while performing stress-view radiographs, as they may cause increased disruption to the physis and discomfort to the patient. CT scans are more useful to delineate the amount of articular displacement, while MRI may be useful in identifying concomitant ligamentous injury or edema within the bone [44]. In patients with posterior metaphyseal fragments, displacement in the sagittal plane, and/or diminished pulses, a femoral angiogram to rule out vascular injury may be indicated.

These fractures have classically been classified, utilizing the Salter-Harris (SH) classification system (Fig. 11.3). This classification system correlates to likelihood of growth arrest, with a meta-analysis demonstrating 58% of Type II fractures, result in growth disturbance [50]. The most common fracture pattern is an SH II fracture, in which there is failure of the physis on the tension side and a metaphyseal fragment on the compressive side, creating a Thurston-Holland fragment. The remainder of this section will focus primarily on the treatment of SH II fractures.

Management of distal femoral physeal fractures is dependent on the type of fracture pattern observed coupled with patient factors. In SH I and SH II fractures, which are non-displaced or stable following closed reduction, athletes can be

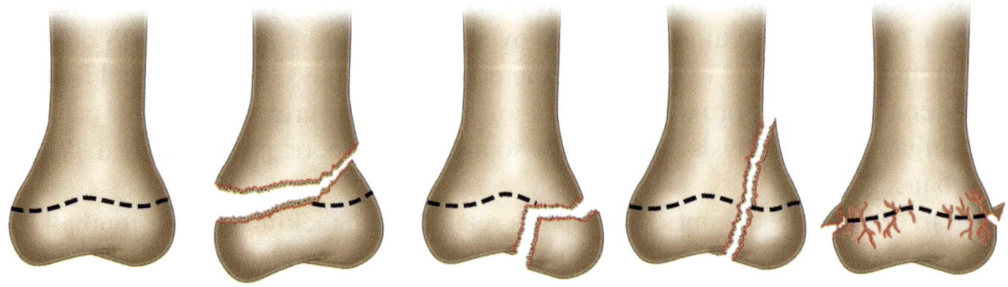

Fig. 11.3 Classification of epiphyseal fractures according to the Salter-Harris system [5]. In type I fractures, the fracture line traverses the physis, staying entirely within it. In type II injuries, the fracture line traverses the growth plate for a variable length and then exits obliquely through the metaphysis. Type III fractures also begin in the physis but exit through the epiphysis toward the joint. Type IV fractures involve a vertical split of the epiphysis, physis, and metaphysis. Type V fractures are crush injuries to the physeal plate

non-weightbearing with immobilization in a long leg cast. Closed reduction should be achieved under adequate relaxation with more traction than manipulation. Multiple closed reductions should not be avoided to prevent additional risk of injury to the physis and surrounding neurovascular structures. Adequate closed reduction is defined as less than 2 mm of physeal displacement and <5° of coronal plane angulation. Fracture displacement influences casting positioning. Immobilization in full extension is indicated for posteriorly displaced factures, and anteriorly displaced fractures should be placed in 30 degrees of flexion [48]. It is important to take patient factors into account when placing immobilization. Football athletes with a muscular thigh or obese, hip spica casts have great efficacy [51]. Nonetheless, loss of positioning, following closed reduction and casting, has been reported as high as 30% [51]. Thus, patients placed in a long leg bivalved cast for 4–6 weeks require close radiographic follow-up with weekly radiographs is mandatory to ensure maintenance of alignment.

Irreducible and displaced fractures that have been successfully closed and reduced but are unstable require two percutaneous crossed transphyseal smooth pins for maintenance of reduction. In fracture patterns with a large Thurston-Holland fragments, fixation can be achieved with lag screws in the metaphysis. A postoperative bivalved bent knee long leg casts is applied under anesthesia with removal of the cast and K-wires at 4–6 weeks postoperatively.

Outcomes following distal femoral physeal fractures have not been favorable, with 46% patients having SH Type II fractures reporting poor outcomes [47]. The Salter Harris classification has been correlated with growth disturbance, noting that 58% of SH II fractures have a resulting limb-length discrepancy or angular deformity [50]. Inadequate reduction with displacement greater than half the shaft diameter, inability to maintain reduction, and younger age thus greater growth potential have been identified as risk factors for growth disturbance [52]. Patient should be followed until skeletal maturity, with serial radiographs to assess for physeal arrest. Limb-length discrepancy of less than 2 mm can be managed with shoe modification, while larger discrepancies indicate an epiphysiodesis of contralateral femur. Angular deformity may result from malunion, inadequate reduction, or fractures involving less than 50% of the physis. In patients that develop an angular deformity and have a minimum of 2 years or 2.5 cm of growth remaining, a physeal bridge excision may be indicated [51–53]. Neurovascular injuries including peroneal nerve palsy and compartment syndrome have been reported. Peroneal nerve palsy can be observed in up to 7% of cases but have been known to resolve within 3 months of the injury [47]. Vascular compromise is rare, but a high index of suspicion must be maintained in hyperextension, posteriorly displaced fractures.

Tibial Tubercle

Tibial tubercle avulsion fractures (TTAF) account for less than 1% of pediatric fractures [54, 55]. The patella tendon inserts onto the secondary ossification center of the tibial tubercle apophysis, which appears between 8 and 12 years old in girls and between 9 and 14 years old in boys [56]. The unique fusion pattern of the tibial tubercle apophysis from posterior to anterior and proximal to distal leaves it susceptible to injury during forceful contraction of the quadriceps [57]. During activities such as football where the athlete is jumping or sprinting, there is an explosive contraction of the quadriceps during active knee extension, which translates energy through the patellar tendon to the vulnerable fusing tibial tubercle apophysis [12]. When this unique fusion pattern is exposed to these forces, it may avulse and fracture up to exit through the epiphysis into the joint. As a result, TTAFs are predominately seen in boys nearing the end of skeletal growth around the age of 12–16 years.

Following the initiation of sprinting and/or jumping, the athlete will experience sudden onset of pain, with immediate inability to ambulate. The knee will appear swollen with possible hemarthrosis if the fracture extends intra-articularly, with focal tenderness over the tibial tuberosity. Spasms of the hamstring may cause the knee to be in slight flexion, and there will be pain with extension of the knee. It is important to recognize that flexion of the knee >30° indicates that there is avulsion of both tibial tubercle and proximal tibial epiphysis [58]. It is important for the evaluating physician to perform a neurovascular exam for possible anterior compartment syndrome as a result of injury to the recurrent anterior tibial artery. This is a potentially devastating complication, causing the compression of the anterior tibial artery and deep peroneal nerve within the anterior compartment. Thus, serial exams should be performed and compartments thoroughly evaluated with a low threshold to perform urgent anterior compartment fasciotomy.

Initial diagnostic imaging should include an AP and lateral radiograph of the leg. In younger, skeletally immature patients, contralateral leg films should be obtained for comparison. In a retrospective review of 41 TTAF, Pandya et al. found that plain radiographs underestimated fracture severity in half of the patients and advocated the utility of CT scans to accurately assess intra-articular and metaphyseal involvement [57]. Additionally, while isolated TTAF can occur up to 16% of the time, there is an associated lateral meniscal tear, osteochondral defect, collateral or cruciate

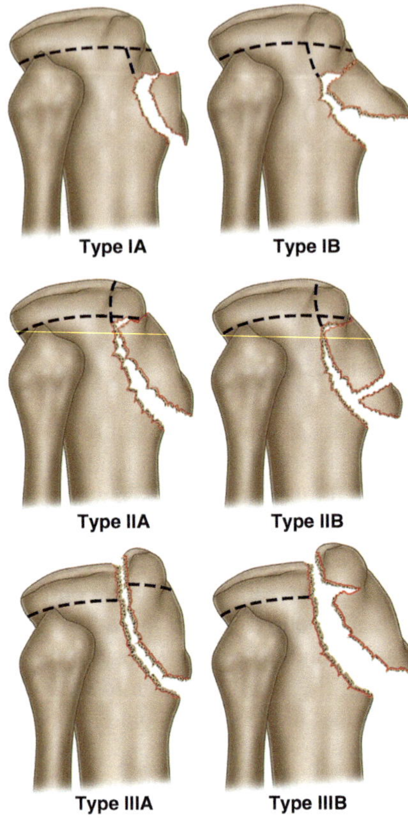

Fig. 11.4 Ogden modification of the Watson-Jones classification of tibial tubercle fractures. Type IA fractures are distal to the junction between the proximal tibia and the apophysis and are nondisplaced or minimally displaced, whereas type IB fractures are hinged in this location. Type IIA fractures are at the junction of the proximal tibia and tubercle, and type IIB fractures are comminuted with anterior translation of the distal fragment. Type IIIA fractures extend into the articular surface, and type IIIB fractures are intra-articular and comminuted. (Adapted from Edwards, Jr. and Grana [48])

ligament tear, patellar tendon rupture, or quadricep tendon rupture [58]. MRI may be used as an adjunct to evaluate for these associated intra-articular pathologies but provide less utility in evaluation of fracture pattern than 3D CT.

The Ogden classification system, which was later modified by Watson-Jones, Ryu–Debenham, and McKoy, is utilized to dictate treatment and counsel patients on expected outcomes [56, 59, 60] (Fig. 11.4). Type 1 fractures occur near the insertion of the patellar tendon; Type II occur at the junction of proximal tibia and tubercle; and Type III extend into the articular surface. Nondisplaced fractures are denoted with an "A" modifier, while displaced/comminuted fractures have a "B" modifier. Ryu et al. described a Type IV pattern, which extends out the posterior aspect of the tibia, and McKoy et al. introduced the Type V fracture in which a "Y" configuration is formed as a combination of a Type IIIB and Type IV [56, 59]. Pandya proposed a classification system that corresponds to the phase of development, with Type A as open physis and Type D as closure of the physis [57].

Goals of treatment include anatomic reduction, which can be achieved via hyperextension of the knee and thus restoration of extensor mechanism and joint line congruency [60, 61]. Non-weightbearing in a long leg extension cast for 4–6 weeks followed by weightbearing in a cylinder cast or range-of-motion brace is indicated for fractures with <5 mm of displacement (Type IA/B, IIA). Close radiographic follow-up should be obtained weekly to assess for displacement or nonunion. Nonoperatively managed TTAF typically return to full range of motion at 8 weeks [62]. Type IIB, IIIA/B, IV, and V fracture or those with >5 mm of residual displacement require open reduction and internal fixation with cannulated, partially threaded screws. Arkader et al. demonstrated no difference in outcomes between unicortical and bicortical fixation in consecutive series of 90 TTAF [63]. Type III fractures are often associated with meniscal or capsular pathology. In patients with intra-articular extension, it is imperative that the articular extension of the fracture is anatomically reduced with all epiphyseal fixation. Postoperatively, patients remain partial-weightbearing in a long leg cast for 3–4 weeks, followed by progressive range of motion and quadriceps strengthening in a hinged knee brace [64, 65]. Resistance training and full weightbearing may begin at 9 weeks postoperatively with full return to play at 2–3 months for Type I/II and 3–6 months for severe fractures [62, 65].

Outcomes following TTAF have been successful, with union rates reported up to 99% [58, 66]. Complications including tenderness to palpation at the tibial tubercle, refracture, wound infection, and limb-length discrepancy have been reported. Serial neurovascular compartment checks should be performed pre- and postoperatively, as it is estimated that the incidence of compartment syndrome ranges from 2% to 20% [67]. While uncommon, growth arrest anteriorly may result in genu recurvatum and a decreased tibial slope. One of the most common complications is implant prominence, which is seen in up to 55% of cases and may require return to the operating room for hardware removal.

Pediatric Ankle Fractures

Pediatric physeal ankle injuries are among the most common injuries seen in children aged 10–15 years of age [68]. As the second most common type of fracture seen in children, they account for 9–18% of all physeal injuries [69, 70]. Of particular concern in the football athlete are transitional fractures (Tillaux and Triplane ankle fractures), which occur during the approximately 18-month period where the physis of the ankle begins to close.

Closure of the distal tibial physis occurs at approximately 16 years of age in boys and 14 years of age in girls. Over an 18-month period, the distal tibial physis begins to close, starting centrally and sequentially closing anteromedially to posteromedial, with the lateral aspect fusing last [71]. Stability to the ankle is provided via ligamentous restraint medially from the deltoid ligament; laterally from the posterior talofibular, calcaneofibular, and anterior talofibular ligaments; and distally from the posterior tibiofibular and anterior tibiofibular ligaments. These ligaments are stronger than the growing physis to which they are attached, leaving the ankle, particularly the lateral aspect of the epiphysis, vulnerable during the adolescent growth spurt.

Tillaux Fracture

Tillaux fractures account for 3–5% of pediatric ankle fractures [72]. A Tillaux fracture is the traumatic avulsion of the anterior inferior tibiofibular ligament, resulting in SH-III fracture of the anterolateral aspect of the distal tibia epiphysis. Salter-Harris III fracture is characterized as extending horizontally through the physis, vertically through the epiphysis, and exiting intra-articularly. These fractures are commonly seen in athletes by everting a supinated foot.

Upon presentation, the patient is typically too sore to bear weight. Physical examination will reveal swelling and ecchymosis on the anterior ankle, with point tenderness at the anterolateral distal tibial epiphysis. Diagnostic imaging, including AP, lateral, and mortise radiographs should be obtained. Mortise view radiographs are best utilized to see the fracture line; however, due to osseous overlap, true delineation of displacement may be difficult to assess on plain X-rays. 3D CT scans may be indicated to help better visualize the fracture pattern [68].

Fractures with <2 mm of displacement can be treated nonoperatively in a non-weightbearing long leg cast for 3–4 weeks controlling for rotational component of the injury. Additional immobilization for 2–4 weeks in a short-leg weightbearing cast or walking boot with range-of-motion exercises should follow. Patients must be followed closely during initial casting treatment with radiographs to verify maintenance of adequate alignment. Fractures that have >2 mm of displacement are not amenable to nonoperative treatment. Open reduction and internal fixation can be performed via and anterolateral approach, using cancellous screws or K-wires. Residual step-off or displacement may lead to early degenerative changes; however, growth arrest is of low concern in these patients, as they are near the end of their distal tibial physeal growth potential [68].

Triplane Fracture

Triplane fractures account for 5–15% of pediatric ankle fractures and are predominately seen in males with a mean age of 13 years. The triplane fracture is a traumatic injury, resulting in a Salter-Harris III injury pattern on the AP radiograph and SH-II fracture pattern on the lateral x-ray creating an injury component in all three planes: sagittal, axial, and coronal. Lateral triplane fractures are the most common and occur when a supinated foot is subjected to external rotation forces. This results in epiphyseal fracture in sagittal, metaphyseal fracture in coronal, and physeal fracture in the axial plane. Medial triplane fractures are a result of an adduction injury, resulting in epiphyseal fracture in the coronal, metaphyseal fracture in the sagittal, and physeal fracture in the axial plane [68].

AP, lateral, and mortise ankle views are imperative for initial diagnosis; however, CT is necessary for surgical planning. In a survey of surgeons, Jones et al. reported that 100% of surgeons changed their surgical plan after reviewing the CT scan [73]. Eismann et al. classified 25 triplane fractures on radiograph and then CT scan finding that the degree of displacement went from <2 mm to >2 mm in 39% of cases [74]. Degree of fracture displacement drives management of triplane fractures. For non-displaced or minimally displaced (<2 mm) fractures, a long leg bent knee non-weightbearing cast with the foot in internal rotation may be utilized for 4–6 weeks, followed by a short-leg weightbearing cast or walking boot for 2–3 weeks thereafter. Post-reduction CT scans must be obtained to confirm maintenance of alignment, and weekly radiographs should be obtained [75].

In any fracture in which there is >2 mm of displacement or anatomic reduction is unobtainable, surgical management is indicated. Early operative intervention with ORIF or closed reduction and percutaneous pinning (CRPP) traditionally yield good fixation and restoration of anatomic alignment, while avoiding early degenerative changes and persistent pain. Common postoperative complications include transient neuropathy and hardware irritation. However, growth arrest is of the utmost concern for physeal fractures. It is recommended that patients with more than 2 years of expected growth remaining, pronation–abduction injuries and residual step-off should be followed closely until physeal closure [75].

References

1. Radelet MA, Lephart SM, Rubinstein EN, Myers JB. Survey of the injury rate for children in community sports. Pediatrics. 2002;110:e28.
2. Mello MJ, Myers R, Christian JB, Palmisciano L, Linakis JG. Injuries in youth football: national emergency department visits during 2001-2005 for young and adolescent players. Acad Emerg Med. 2009;16:243–8.
3. Nation AD, Nelson NG, Yard EE, Comstock RD, McKenzie LB. Football-related injuries among 6- to 17-year-olds treated in US emergency departments, 1990-2007. Clin Pediatr (Phila). 2011;50:200–7.
4. Smith PJ, Hollins AM, Sawyer JR, Spence DD, Outlaw S, Kelly DM. Characterization of American football injuries in children and adolescents. J Pediatr Orthop. 2018;38:e57–60.
5. Montgomery C, Porter A 3rd, Parks C, Sachleben B, Blasier RD, Rabenhorst B. Football-related pediatric extremity fractures and dislocations: size matters. Orthopedics. 2018;41:216–21.
6. Hawkins D, Metheny J. Overuse injuries in youth sports: biomechanical considerations. Med Sci Sports Exerc. 2001;33:1701–7.
7. Kovacevic D, Mariscalco M, Goodwin RC. Injuries about the hip in the adolescent athlete. Sports Med Arthrosc Rev. 2011;19:64–74.
8. White KK, Williams SK, Mubarak SJ. Definition of two types of anterior superior iliac spine avulsion fractures. J Pediatr Orthop. 2002;22:578–82.
9. McKinney BI, Nelson C, Carrion W. Apophyseal avulsion fractures of the hip and pelvis. Orthopedics. 2009;32:42.
10. Metzmaker JN, Pappas AM. Avulsion fractures of the pelvis. Am J Sports Med. 1985;13:349–58.
11. Rossi F, Dragoni S. Acute avulsion fractures of the pelvis in adolescent competitive athletes: prevalence, location and sports distribution of 203 cases collected. Skelet Radiol. 2001;30:127–31.
12. Schiller J, DeFroda S, Blood T. Lower extremity avulsion fractures in the pediatric and adolescent athlete. J Am Acad Orthop Surg. 2017;25:251–9.
13. Fernbach SK, Wilkinson RH. Avulsion injuries of the pelvis and proximal femur. AJR Am J Roentgenol. 1981;137:581–4.
14. Schuett DJ, Bomar JD, Pennock AT. Pelvic apophyseal avulsion fractures: a retrospective review of 228 cases. J Pediatr Orthop. 2015;35:617–23.
15. Eberbach H, Hohloch L, Feucht MJ, Konstantinidis L, Sudkamp NP, Zwingmann J. Operative versus conservative treatment of apophyseal avulsion fractures of the pelvis in the adolescents: a systematical review with meta-analysis of clinical outcome and return to sports. BMC Musculoskelet Disord. 2017;18:162.

16. Gidwani S, Bircher MD. Avulsion injuries of the hamstring origin - a series of 12 patients and management algorithm. Ann R Coll Surg Engl. 2007;89:394–9.
17. Singer G, Eberl R, Wegmann H, Marterer R, Kraus T, Sorantin E. Diagnosis and treatment of apophyseal injuries of the pelvis in adolescents. Semin Musculoskelet Radiol. 2014;18:498–504.
18. Nguyen JC, Sheehan SE, Davis KW, Gill KG. Sports and the growing musculoskeletal system: sports imaging series. Radiology. 2017;284:25–42.
19. Ali E, Khanduja V. Adolescent avulsion injuries of the pelvis: a case study and review of the literature. Orthop Nurs. 2015;34:21–6, quiz 27–28.
20. Meyers AB, Laor T, Zbojniewicz AM, Anton CG. MRI of radiographically occult ischial apophyseal avulsions. Pediatr Radiol. 2012;42:1357–63.
21. Torode I, Zieg D. Pelvic fractures in children. J Pediatr Orthop. 1985;5:76–84.
22. Ferlic PW, Sadoghi P, Singer G, Kraus T, Eberl R. Treatment for ischial tuberosity avulsion fractures in adolescent athletes. Knee Surg Sports Traumatol Arthrosc. 2014;22:893–7.
23. Biedert RM. Surgical management of traumatic avulsion of the ischial tuberosity in young athletes. Clin J Sport Med. 2015;25:67–72.
24. Buckley PS, Dodson CC. Repair of a proximal hamstring rupture in a 14-year-old patient: a case report. HSS J. 2018;14:302–6.
25. Kaneyama S, Yoshida K, Matsushima S, Wakami T, Tsunoda M, Doita M. A surgical approach for an avulsion fracture of the ischial tuberosity: a case report. J Orthop Trauma. 2006;20:363–5.
26. Hamming MG, Philippon MJ, Rasmussen MT, et al. Structural properties of the intact proximal hamstring origin and evaluation of varying avulsion repair techniques: an in vitro biomechanical analysis. Am J Sports Med. 2015;43:721–8.
27. Tetsunaga T, Endo H, Tetsunaga T, Yamada K, Furumatsu T, Ozaki T. Avulsion fracture of the ischial tuberosity treated with the suture bridge technique: a case report. BMC Musculoskelet Disord. 2019;20:9.
28. Spinner RJ, Atkinson JL, Wenger DE, Stuart MJ. Tardy sciatic nerve palsy following apophyseal avulsion fracture of the ischial tuberosity. Case report. J Neurosurg. 1998;89:819–21.
29. Willinger L, Schanda JE, Lorenz S, Imhoff AB, Buchmann S. Surgical treatment of two adolescent athletes with dislocated avulsion fracture of the anterior superior iliac spine (ASIS). Arch Orthop Trauma Surg. 2017;137:173–7.
30. Kautzner J, Trc T, Havlas V. Comparison of conservative against surgical treatment of anterior-superior iliac spine avulsion fractures in children and adolescents. Int Orthop. 2014;38:1495–8.
31. Veselko M, Smrkolj V. Avulsion of the anterior-superior iliac spine in athletes: case reports. J Trauma. 1994;36:444–6.
32. Rajasekhar C, Kumar KS, Bhamra MS. Avulsion fractures of the anterior inferior iliac spine: the case for surgical intervention. Int Orthop. 2001;24:364–5.
33. Uzun M, Alpan B, Ozger H. Avulsion fractures involving the straight and reflected heads of the rectus femoris. Hip Int. 2014;24:206–9.
34. Foote CJ, Maizlin ZV, Shrouder J, Grant MM, Bedi A, Ayeni OR. The association between avulsions of the reflected head of the rectus femoris and labral tears: a retrospective study. J Pediatr Orthop. 2013;33:227–31.
35. Carton P, Filan D. Anterior inferior iliac spine (AIIS) and subspine hip impingement. Muscles Ligaments Tendons J. 2016;6:324–36.
36. Nakano N, Lisenda L, Khanduja V. Arthroscopic excision of heterotopic ossification in the rectus femoris muscle causing extra-articular anterior hip impingement. SICOT J. 2018;4:41.
37. Larson CM, Kelly BT, Stone RM. Making a case for anterior inferior iliac spine/subspine hip impingement: three representative case reports and proposed concept. Arthroscopy. 2011;27:1732–7.
38. Devitt BM, Smith B, Stapf R, O'Donnell JM. Avulsion of the direct head of rectus femoris following arthroscopic subspine impingement resection: a case report. J Hip Preserv Surg. 2016;3:56–60.

39. Novais EN, Riederer MF, Provance AJ. Anterior inferior iliac spine deformity as a cause for extra-articular hip impingement in Young athletes after an avulsion fracture: a case report. Sports Health. 2018;10:272–6.
40. Beckmann JT, Wylie JD, Potter MQ, Maak TG, Greene TH, Aoki SK. Effect of naproxen prophylaxis on heterotopic ossification following hip arthroscopy: a double-blind randomized placebo-controlled trial. J Bone Joint Surg Am. 2015;97:2032–7.
41. Ruffing T, Ruckauer T, Bludau F, Hofmann A, Muhm M, Suda AJ. Avulsion fracture of the lesser trochanter in adolescents. Injury. 2018;49(7):1278–81.
42. Otto A, Banke IJ, Mehl J, Beitzel K, Imhoff AB, Scheiderer B. Retrograde fixation of the lesser trochanter in the adolescent: new surgical technique and clinical results of two cases. Arch Orthop Trauma Surg. 2019;139:537–45.
43. Garrett BR, Hoffman EB, Carrara H. The effect of percutaneous pin fixation in the treatment of distal femoral physeal fractures. J Bone Joint Surg. 2011;93:689–94.
44. Mayer S, Albright JC, Stoneback JW. Pediatric knee dislocations and physeal fractures about the knee. J Am Acad Orthop Surg. 2015;23:571–80.
45. Pennock AT, Ellis HB, Willimon SC, et al. Intra-articular physeal fractures of the distal femur: a frequently missed diagnosis in adolescent athletes. Orthop J Sports Med. 2017;5:2325967117731567.
46. Little RM, Milewski MD. Physeal fractures about the knee. Curr Rev Musculoskelet Med. 2016;9:478–86.
47. Eid AM, Hafez MA. Traumatic injuries of the distal femoral physis. Retrospective study on 151 cases. Injury. 2002;33:251–5.
48. Edwards PH Jr, Grana WA. Physeal fractures about the knee. J Am Acad Orthop Surg. 1995;3:63–9.
49. Young EY, Stans AA. Distal femoral physeal fractures. J Knee Surg. 2018;31:486–9.
50. Basener CJ, Mehlman CT, DiPasquale TG. Growth disturbance after distal femoral growth plate fractures in children: a meta-analysis. J Orthop Trauma. 2009;23:663–7.
51. Riseborough EJ, Barrett IR, Shapiro F. Growth disturbances following distal femoral physeal fracture-separations. J Bone Joint Surg Am. 1983;65:885–93.
52. Lombardo SJ, Harvey JP Jr. Fractures of the distal femoral epiphyses. Factors influencing prognosis: a review of thirty-four cases. J Bone Joint Surg Am. 1977;59:742–51.
53. Stephens DC, Louis E, Louis DS. Traumatic separation of the distal femoral epiphyseal cartilage plate. J Bone Joint Surg Am. 1974;56:1383–90.
54. Bolesta MJ, Fitch RD. Tibial tubercle avulsions. J Pediatr Orthop. 1986;6:186–92.
55. Hamilton SW, Gibson PH. Simultaneous bilateral avulsion fractures of the tibial tuberosity in adolescence: a case report and review of over 50 years of literature. Knee. 2006;13:404–7.
56. McKoy BE, Stanitski CL. Acute tibial tubercle avulsion fractures. Orthop Clin North Am. 2003;34:397–403.
57. Pandya NK, Edmonds EW, Roocroft JH, Mubarak SJ. Tibial tubercle fractures: complications, classification, and the need for intra-articular assessment. J Pediatr Orthop. 2012;32:749–59.
58. Pretell-Mazzini J, Kelly DM, Sawyer JR, et al. Outcomes and complications of tibial tubercle fractures in pediatric patients: a systematic review of the literature. J Pediatr Orthop. 2016;36:440–6.
59. Ryu RK, Debenham JO. An unusual avulsion fracture of the proximal tibial epiphysis. Case report and proposed addition to the Watson-Jones classification. Clin Orthop Relat Res. 1985;(194):181–4.
60. Ogden JA, Tross RB, Murphy MJ. Fractures of the tibial tuberosity in adolescents. J Bone Joint Surg Am. 1980;62:205–15.
61. Agarwalla A, Puzzitiello R, Stone AV, Forsythe B. Tibial tubercle avulsion fracture with multiple concomitant injuries in an adolescent male athlete. Case Rep Orthop. 2018;2018:1070628.
62. Cole WW 3rd, Brown SM, Vopat B, Heard WMR, Mulcahey MK. Epidemiology, diagnosis, and management of tibial tubercle avulsion fractures in adolescents. JBJS Rev. 2020;8:e0186.

63. Arkader A, Schur M, Refakis C, Capraro A, Woon R, Choi P. Unicortical fixation is sufficient for surgical treatment of tibial tubercle avulsion fractures in children. J Pediatr Orthop. 2019;39:e18–22.
64. Howarth WR, Gottschalk HP, Hosalkar HS. Tibial tubercle fractures in children with intra-articular involvement: surgical tips for technical ease. J Child Orthop. 2011;5:465–70.
65. Nicolini AP, Carvalho RT, Ferretti M, Cohen M. Simultaneous bilateral tibial tubercle avulsion fracture in a male teenager: case report and literature review. J Pediatr Orthop B. 2018;27:40–6.
66. Zrig M, Annabi H, Ammari T, Trabelsi M, Mbarek M, Ben Hassine H. Acute tibial tubercle avulsion fractures in the sporting adolescent. Arch Orthop Trauma Surg. 2008;128:1437–42.
67. Frey S, Hosalkar H, Cameron DB, Heath A, David Horn B, Ganley TJ. Tibial tuberosity fractures in adolescents. J Child Orthop. 2008;2:469–74.
68. Wuerz TH, Gurd DP. Pediatric physeal ankle fracture. J Am Acad Orthop Surg. 2013;21:234–44.
69. King J, Diefendorf D, Apthorp J, Negrete VF, Carlson M. Analysis of 429 fractures in 189 battered children. J Pediatr Orthop. 1988;8:585–9.
70. Mann DC, Rajmaira S. Distribution of physeal and nonphyseal fractures in 2,650 long-bone fractures in children aged 0-16 years. J Pediatr Orthop. 1990;10:713–6.
71. Johnson EW Jr, Fahl JC. Fractures involving the distal epiphysis of the tibia and fibula in children. Am J Surg. 1957;93:778–81.
72. Caterini R, Farsetti P, Ippolito E. Long-term followup of physeal injury to the ankle. Foot Ankle. 1991;11:372–83.
73. Jones S, Phillips N, Ali F, Fernandes JA, Flowers MJ, Smith TW. Triplane fractures of the distal tibia requiring open reduction and internal fixation. Pre-operative planning using computed tomography. Injury. 2003;34:293–8.
74. Eismann EA, Stephan ZA, Mehlman CT, et al. Pediatric triplane ankle fractures: impact of radiographs and computed tomography on fracture classification and treatment planning. J Bone Joint Surg Am. 2015;97:995–1002.
75. Olgun ZD, Maestre S. Management of pediatric ankle fractures. Curr Rev Musculoskelet Med. 2018;11:475–84.

Platelet-Rich Plasma in Football

12

David A. Ajibade, Corey S. Cook, and Patrick A. Smith

Introduction

Platelet-rich plasma (PRP) was first used in maxillofacial surgery with more recent and increasing use in orthopedic surgery [1]. PRP is formulated by centrifuging autologous blood from the patient to obtain a preparation of platelets at least twice the concentration of whole blood. Cellular content includes red blood cells (RBC) and white blood cells (WBCs), the latter consisting of both leukocytes and neutrophils. The alpha granules of platelets have been shown to contain the critical growth factors [2].

Despite the rising interest of PRP research and application, there is no consensus for standardized concentration of constituents or method of preparation. There are differences in blood volume, centrifuge rate and time, PRP volume, WBC and RBC counts, platelet and growth factor concentration, delivery method, and activating agent use. Most systems utilize single-spin or double-spin sequences. Single-spin sequences are typically slower and shorter, yielding products that are two to three times baseline platelet concentration while excluding WBCs (leukocyte poor; LP-PRP). Double-spin sequences can yield greater platelet concentrations and commonly include WBCs in the yielded preparations (leukocyte rich; LR-PRP). There is also a flow cytometry option, which allows for more customizable ratios of platelets and white blood cells [3].

D. A. Ajibade
Department of Orthopaedic Surgery, University of Missouri, Columbia, MO, USA
e-mail: ajibaded@health.missouri.edu

C. S. Cook
Columbia Orthopaedic Group, Columbia, MO, USA

P. A. Smith (✉)
Department of Orthopaedic Surgery, University of Missouri, Columbia, MO, USA

Columbia Orthopaedic Group, Columbia, MO, USA

K. W. Farmer (ed.), *Football Injuries*,
https://doi.org/10.1007/978-3-030-54875-9_12

Commercially available PRP preparation systems utilize either the single-spin or dual-spin methods; dual-spin methods are more time consuming to prepare [4, 5]. LR-PRP has up to three times the number of neutrophils, which contain catabolic enzymes that can degrade collagen and can cause direct injury to muscle via metalloproteinases and reactive oxygen species [6]. Platelets include important growth factors such as insulin-like growth factor 1 (IGF-1) that can affect tissue modulation. PRP enhances proliferation of myoblasts, chondrocytes, and osteoblasts in culture [7]. Platelets can also recruit stem cells in vitro [8]. There can be daily variation in platelet growth factors, serum WBCs, and serum platelets, compromising standardization in study populations. Heterogeneity of preparation and delivery methods can also make results reported in the literature difficult to access and compare clinically [9, 10].

Authors' Preference for Platelet-Rich Plasma Preparation

LR-PRP generally has higher overall concentrations of platelet-derived growth factor (PDGF), transforming growth factor beta (TGF-β), epidermal growth factor (EGF), vascular endothelial growth factor (VEGF), and soluble CD40 ligand [11]. This suggests that LR-PRP may be more beneficial in clinical scenarios that involve areas of hypovascularity, such as tendinopathy in more anatomically susceptible or watershed areas of relative hypovascularity, where stimulation of a vascular response and healing is a priority [12].

However, a 2019 Level I randomized controlled trial in athletes with ultrasound-confirmed patellar tendinopathy treated with an exercise-based rehabilitation program combined with LR-PRP, LP-PRP, or saline showed no significant difference between the groups in outcome measures, including pain scores at 6 weeks, 12 weeks, 6 months, and 12 months [13]. A meta-analysis of 18 randomized controlled clinical trials for treatment of tendinopathy published in 2016 found that patients treated with LR-PRP had a stronger positive effect with changes in pain intensity as a primary outcome measure, when compared with the LP-PRP patients [14]. However, both treatments had an overall positive benefit over placebo, regardless of the leukocyte concentration.

Our preference for PRP preparation is Autologous Conditioned Plasma (ACP, Arthrex, Naples, FL), a plasma-based leukocyte-poor preparation. It is a simple and fast preparation technique that is advantageous when dealing with an athletic population. A total of 15 cc of blood is drawn in a special double syringe (Arthrex, Inc) and centrifuged for a single 5-min spin at 1500 revolutions per minute with the upper yellow plasma layer containing platelets separated from the lower, higher-density red and white blood cell layer (Fig. 12.1). Utilizing the inner syringe, this plasma layer is easily extracted for injection. The platelet count for ACP is 2.40 times normal blood concentration on average. The typical white blood cell count is a mean of 1.3×10^9/L. Generally, 4–6 cc of LP-PRP is obtained from the process. No anticoagulant (like ACD-A in double-spin systems) has to be added to ACP after the single spin, as it is ready for injection after just 5 minutes. This has the potential

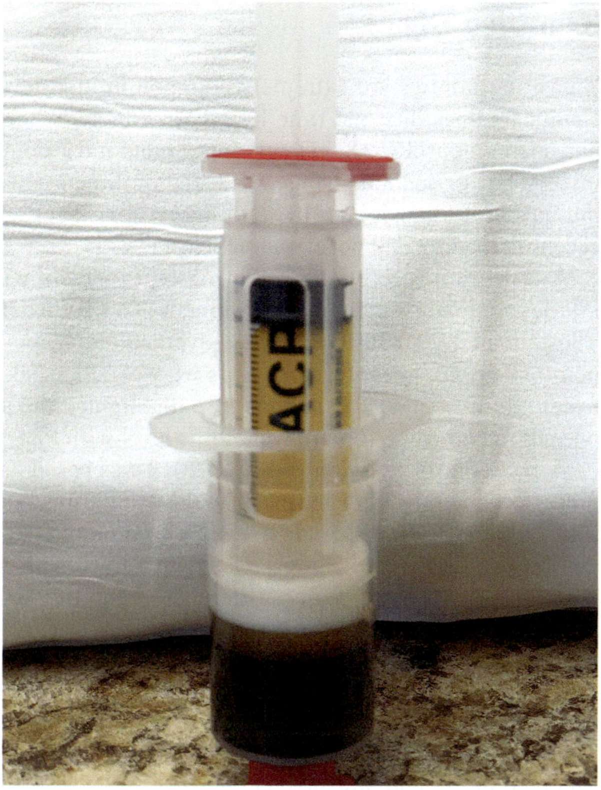

Fig. 12.1 An autologous conditioned plasma (ACP) vial, with the leukocyte-poor, platelet-rich plasma separated from the red blood cells.

for reduced pain after the injection, since the low pH of 5 for ACD-A could contribute to increased pain with a soft tissue injection [15]. No activating agents are added; the platelets are activated by the tissue thromboplastin method [16].

Use of Platelet-Rich Plasma in the Treatment of Specific Football Injuries

Platelet-rich plasma has numerous specific applications in football, including treatment for both acute and chronic muscle strain and tendon injuries, as well as inflammatory joint conditions. We have utilized LP-PRP exclusively when appropriate for the treatment of specific football injuries in our Division I program. This is in combination with a comprehensive post-injection protocol, incorporating other treatment modalities to control inflammation and promote mobility to enhance the healing process. Rehabilitation, with a focus on eccentric exercises, is instituted early on in the process. A return-to-play progression plan is customized to each individual athlete based on injury, position, and functional assessment by training staff and team physicians.

Hamstring Strains

Hamstring injuries are extremely common in high-level athletes and can result in significant disability and time loss. Furthermore, recurrence of hamstring strain is not uncommon [17, 18]. Hamstring strains most commonly occur in sports that involve fast or sudden changes in speed or direction. Given the fact the hamstring muscles cross two joints, they are more at risk for strain injury, especially with eccentric loading and deceleration [19–21].

A 2019 retrospective review of 61 NFL players with acute grade 2 hamstring injuries compared outcomes of treatment of a LP-PRP injection versus no injection. Those treated with PRP missed an average of 1.7 games versus 2.7 games in the non-PRP group. Notably, no re-tears were experienced by the PRP group, despite a faster return to play. The authors also highlighted the potential financial benefit of one additional game for a player at this level with PRP treatment [20, 22].

A case control study published in 2013 was based on only ten NFL players with grade 2 hamstring injury, treated with a single injection of LR-PRP under ultrasound guidance. Rettig et al. showed a mean return to play of 20 days in the PRP group and 17 days in the non-PRP group treated with rehabilitation and functional progression alone. A major difference from the Arner study was the use of LR-PRP [23].

In a randomized controlled trial, Hamid et al. demonstrated statistically significant earlier return to play after full recovery and lower pain severity scores in 28 patients treated with a single injection of LR-PRP combined with a rehabilitation program versus a rehabilitation program alone in acute grade 2 hamstring injuries. The PRP group patients also had lower pain interference scores (interference with daily activities, such as general activity, walking, work, mood, enjoyment of life, relations with others, and sleep), but no statistical difference was found [24].

In a more recent LR-PRP study on grade 2 hamstring strain in soccer players, return to play averaged 36.76 days with a reinjury rate of 12%. Although there was no control group, the authors found no difference in their outcomes from untreated hamstring strain patients based on the literature [25].

Our preferred approach for hamstring strains is to offer an ultrasound-guided LP-PRP ACP injection, which is generally administered approximately 24 hours after injury. In many cases, a magnetic resonance imaging (MRI) is done for injury grading purposes. We first discuss the potential advantages of PRP treatment with the athlete, based on the evidence and our experience, along with the risks and complications of this treatment. Therefore, the athlete is better equipped to make an informed decision. In many cases, athletes will request PRP based on discussion with teammates who have undergone the procedure for a hamstring strain with a good outcome. The injection is performed under sterile technique with betadine skin preparation followed by alcohol. The ultrasound is performed with use of sterile ultrasound gel and is used to localize the injection site. After the injection, the affected area is thoroughly massaged to enhance tissue activation. Again, since the ACP injection is easily prepared and administered in under 30 minutes without the use of an anticoagulant, potentially lessening local injection site pain. In severe grade 2 strains with a large area of involvement or grade 3 injuries, the ACP injection is repeated in 5–7 days. Direct cryotherapy is followed with various training modalities and graduated advancement to full painless knee flexion and hip extension. This is followed initially with concentric and then eccentric light strengthening exercises, focusing on the knee and hip. Fortunately, we have not seen any adverse reactions or consequences to this ACP treatment approach.

From 2009 to 2019, we treated 41 Division I football players with 44 total hamstring injuries with LP-PRP injected in the zone of injury. The average age was 20.36 years with an average of 10.5 days (SD 4.37) to full return to play from date of treatment. There were 10 Grade 1 injuries with average of 9 days (SD 4.69) to full return to play from date of treatment, 29 Grade 2 injuries with average of 11.25 days (SD 4.4) to return to play from date of treatment, and 5 Grade 3 injuries with an average of 16.80 days (SD 6.14 days) to return to play from date of treatment. The increased time to full return to play with increased severity of the injury is expected. Our average return to play of 10.5 days is within the lower ranges what has been reported for hamstring strains [26, 27]. LR-PRP with a graduated rehabilitation and return-to-play protocol has been utilized at our institution for over a decade with excellent results.

Inflammatory Knee Conditions

Inflammation in the knee can have a multitude of etiologies. In football, it is not uncommon to have generalized knee inflammation while adjusting to workload changes, learning a new position, recovering from a previous injury, or rehabilitating from surgery. Intra-articular injections can be part of the treatment armamentarium for such knee inflammation issues, but it should be emphasized that any intra-articular joint injection for in-season management can lead to suboptimal results if the underlying causative disease process is not addressed by other means.

Corticosteroids are commonly used to treat pain and inflammation in the knee. They recently have been implicated in promoting cartilage volume loss in the treatment of knee osteoarthritis, although the clinical relevance of this finding for other joint conditions is unclear [28]. Certainly, in a young athletic population from a joint injection standpoint, an "arthroprotective" injection is desired. Hyaluronic acid (HA) viscosupplementation would be a potential option if knee osteoarthritis is the underlying problem in an athlete.

PRP, particularly LP-PRP, has been well documented in multiple level 1 studies to be efficacious and safe when treating knee osteoarthritis, which does affect young football players due to chondral injury [29, 30]. Furthermore, in head-to-head studies, LP-PRP has outperformed HA [31–36]. However, based on mechanism of action, PRP has the advantage of also reducing joint inflammation even when osteoarthritis is not the primary etiology. Specifically, PRP helps to stimulate chondrocyte proliferation and inhibit pro-inflammatory cytokines through growth factor mediation [37–41]. Additionally, LP-PRP ACP when compared to LR-PRP has been shown in a laboratory study to decrease metalloproteinases (MMP-9) and interleukin-1β (IL-1β), which are powerful cytokines that promote inflammation and matrix degradation [42]. Also, an in vitro tissue model study showed ACP actually increased endogenous HA production from synoviocytes compared to HA itself (SYNVISC; Sanofi-Aventis, Paris, France), as well as decreased MMP-13 production, which is a known powerful cytokine for knee arthritis [43]. Finally, a laboratory study showed ACP significantly stimulated secretion of superficial zone protein or lubricin from articular cartilage and synovium, which is a very important substance for joint health and lubrication [44]. From the clinical standpoint, Smith showed both the safety and efficacy of knee joint ACP injections for osteoarthritis [29].

ACP has been very helpful in our experience in managing a number of inflammatory knee conditions in football players, and we feel it is both safer and more efficacious than corticosteroids, given the above documented scientific evidence. For instance, ACP has helped reduce reactive joint swelling in players returning to play after anterior cruciate ligament (ACL) reconstruction or meniscal surgery. Also, ACP has also been helpful in athletes who sustain isolated traumatic bone contusions with associated swelling. Our approach is to decompress the joint with an aspiration prior to the ACP injection. Compression and icing are utilized along with an early emphasis on isometric quadriceps exercises. In some cases, a second ACP treatment is administered 5–7 days later if needed.

Patellar and Achilles Tendinopathy

PRP and its growth factors can stimulate angiogenesis, cell migration, collagen synthesis, and matrix formation. These attributes seemingly make PRP ideal for use in the treatment of tendinopathy conditions, given these are areas generally with limited blood supply and slow cell turnover. Controversy exists over the WBC content of the preparation that is preferred, along with number and timing of injections. WBCs promote inflammation, and an argument could be made that an inflammatory response is what is needed to stimulate healing in a chronically avascular and degenerative tendon [45]. In a meta-analysis of randomized controlled trials of PRP in the treatment of tendinopathy, Fitzpatrick et al. found that the most significant reductions in pain were found in patients treated with leukocyte-rich PRP injections [14]. However, studies involving both leukocyte-rich and leukocyte-poor PRP injections have shown promise in the setting of tendinopathy [45–49].

Patellar tendinopathy is a common problem in American football players, possibly related to heavy squatting and eccentric overload. When symptoms persist despite standard conservative treatment measures, which include eccentric quadriceps strengthening exercises, PRP can be helpful.

Charousset et al. published results on a case series of professional and semiprofessional athletes treated with three consecutive ultrasound-guided LP-PRP injections for the treatment of chronic patellar tendinopathy (jumper's knee). At 2-year follow-up, 75% (21 out of 28) were able to return to pre-symptom sporting level at a mean of 3 months, and 57% had healing and return of normal structural integrity of the tendon demonstrated on follow-up MRI at 3 months. These athletes were in a variety of sports that involved explosive movements, such as high jump, basketball, soccer, gymnastics, volleyball, judo, tennis, and badminton. They were permitted to return to sport as tolerated at 8 weeks from the last injection following a rehabilitation program that included eccentric exercises on a board. Three patients eventually underwent surgical intervention. This series shows the potential for clinical benefit from a series of LP-PRP injections for patellar tendinopathy in athletes [50].

Vetranoet et al. published a study utilizing two injections of LP-PRP versus extracorporeal shock wave therapy for patellar tendinopathy and found LP-PRP was significantly better at both 6 months and 12 months with PRP based on the Victorian Institute of Sports Assessment (VISA) validated outcome questionnaire [46].

In a double-blind randomized control trial with 23 patients who had failed previous nonoperative treatment, Dragoo et al. demonstrated improvement in VISA outcome scores in the treatment of patellar tendinopathy with a one-time LR-PRP injection (GPS III, Biomet Inc., Warsaw, IN, USA) compared with a dry needling group, who also received an injection of bupivacaine. All patients in the study were also given instructions on a standardized eccentric exercise program coordinated by physical therapists [47].

Our approach for refractory patellar tendinopathy includes an MRI to confirm that the diseased patellar tendon involves at least 50% of the posterior half of the tendon. Frequently, there is associated increased signal in the fat pad and sometimes bone edema with the inferior pole of the patella (Fig. 12.2). Ultrasound guidance for optimal needle placement is routinely done under sterile conditions with skin preparation with betadine and alcohol and then use of sterile ultrasound gel. After the ACP injection, the area is massaged thoroughly. Generally, two injections are given, typically 5–7 days apart. Rehabilitation progresses from isometric to eccentric quadriceps strengthening.

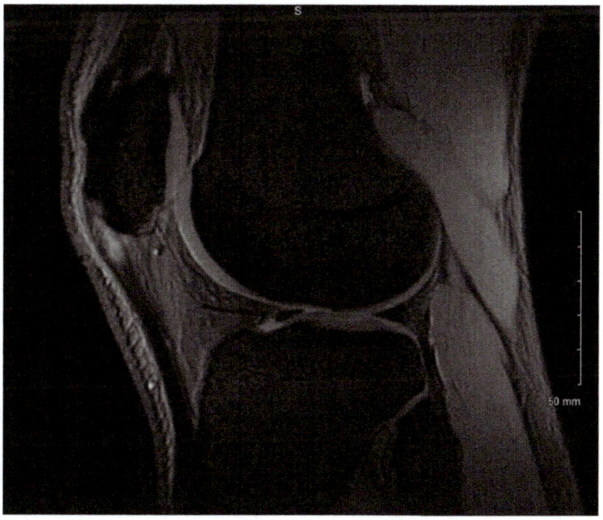

Fig. 12.2 A sagittal MRI demonstrating high-grade patellar tendinosis and partial-thickness tearing

Achilles tendinopathy is also seen in American football players. Gaweda, in 2010, reported significant improvement in both clinical scores and ultrasound with LP-PRP treatment [51]. In 2010, DeVos also reported no difference between the use of LR-PRP and saline injections in a group of 54 randomized patients with Achilles tendinopathy [52].

In a case series of 30 patients who had failed conservative management for at least 6 months with noninvasive measures for Achilles tendinosis, Monto found an increase in American Orthopedic Foot and Ankle (AOFAS) score at both 6 months and 24 months after injection of LR-PRP; patients also had resolution of pre-treatment imaging pathology noted on MRI and ultrasound in 93% of patients [53].

Acute Ankle Injuries

We have found PRP particularly useful in the treatment of acute low-grade syndesmotic injuries and lateral ankle sprains for reducing initial injury pain and swelling to enhance rehabilitation efforts. The results in the literature have shown some benefit, but results are not conclusive as studies include a low number of patients, thus increasing the chance of not detecting significant changes with small effect sizes [54].

In a cohort-controlled pilot study of ten rugby players, Samra et al. demonstrated that the time to return to play from acute syndesmotic injury was significantly less in the group that had a single ultrasound-guided LR-PRP injection into the anterior inferior tibifibular ligament (ATFL). The intervention group also demonstrated a higher vertical jump than the nonintervention group. However, in a double-blind, randomized controlled study of LR-PRP use in 37 patients for ankle sprains in the emergency department, Rowden et al. demonstrated no difference in pain scores or validated outcomes (Lower Extremity Functional Scale) over placebo [55].

Conclusion

Platelet-rich plasma can be an effective adjunctive treatment measure along with training room modalities and a comprehensive rehabilitation program for football injuries. The value of returning to play even a few days earlier after injury can have significant implications for each athlete that can be difficult to quantify. The science behind PRP continues to evolve as more research is performed, and clearly the current clinical use and application of PRP is ahead of high-level data for many injury patterns. There is still uncertainty related to whether LR versus LP-PRP preparations are preferred for certain conditions. Our preference for LP-PRP, and specifically ACP, is based on the available basic science, in combination with published clinical studies and our own anecdotal evidence. In this chapter, we have reviewed the current literature for use of PRP in some of the more common injuries seen in college football players. We have provided our clinical data on ACP treatment for hamstring strains, which is our most common use, and has represented a paradigm shift in our treatment of this very common football injury. Unfortunately, we do not have a control group for comparison, but that may not be a practical or realistic approach with a Division I football team. Nonetheless, PRP has been a safe treatment intervention with no known complications in the ACP injections that we have performed to date. Above all, our primary goals with PRP treatment are minimizing overall injury time and facilitating return to play, while doing so safely.

References

1. Marx RE. Platelet-rich plasma: evidence to support its use. J Oral Maxillofac Surg. 2004;62(4):489–96.
2. Blair P, Flaumenhaft R. Platelet α-granules: basic biology and clinical correlates. Blood Rev. 2009;23(4):177–89.
3. The Angel® cPRP System for Customized Cellular Concentrations of Platelet-Rich Plasma for Customized Cellular Concentrations of Platelet-Rich Plasma, Arthrex, Naples, FL, 2019., Available from: www.arthrex.com.
4. Mazzocca AD, McCarthy MB, Chowaniec DM, Cote MP, Romeo AA, Bradley JP, Arciero RA, Beitzel K. Platelet-rich plasma differs according to preparation method and human variability. JBJS. 2012;94(4):308–16.
5. Oudelaar BW, Peerbooms JC, Huis in 't Veld R, Vochteloo AJ. Concentrations of blood components in commercial platelet-rich plasma separation systems: a review of the literature. Am J Sports Med. 2019;47(2):479–87.
6. Schneider BS, Tiidus PM. Neutrophil infiltration in exercise-injured skeletal muscle. Sports Med. 2007;37(10):837–56.
7. Cole BJ, Seroyer ST, Filardo G, Bajaj S, Fortier LA. Platelet-rich plasma: where are we now and where are we going? Sports health. 2010;2(3):203–10.
8. Holmes HL, Wilson B, Goerger JP, Silverberg JL, Cohen I, Zipfel WR, Fortier LA. Facilitated recruitment of mesenchymal stromal cells by bone marrow concentrate and platelet rich plasma. PLoS One. 2018;13(3):e0194567.
9. Opper C, Weiner N, Xü F, Adam W, Fruhstorfer H, Wesemann W. Daily variations of functional parameters and density distribution in human blood platelets. Chronobiol Int. 1994;11(5):309–19.
10. Chahla J, Cinque ME, Piuzzi NS, Mannava S, Geeslin AG, Murray IR, Dornan GJ, Muschler GF, LaPrade RF. A call for standardization in platelet-rich plasma preparation protocols and composition reporting: a systematic review of the clinical orthopaedic literature. JBJS. 2017;99(20):1769–79.
11. Ziegler CG, Van Sloun R, Gonzalez S, Whitney KE, DePhillipo NN, Kennedy MI, Dornan GJ, Evans TA, Huard J, LaPrade RF. Characterization of growth factors, cytokines, and chemokines in bone marrow concentrate and platelet-rich plasma: a prospective analysis. Am J Sports Med. 2019;47(9):2174–87.
12. Braun HJ, Kim HJ, Chu CR, Dragoo JL. The effect of platelet-rich plasma formulations and blood products on human synoviocytes: implications for intra-articular injury and therapy. Am J Sports Med. 2014;42(5):1204–10.
13. Scott A, LaPrade RF, Harmon KG, Filardo G, Kon E, Della Villa S, Bahr R, Moksnes H, Torgalsen T, Lee J, Dragoo JL. Platelet-rich plasma for patellar tendinopathy: a randomized controlled trial of leukocyte-rich PRP or leukocyte-poor PRP versus saline. Am J Sports Med. 2019;47(7):1654–61.
14. Fitzpatrick J, Bulsara M, Zheng MH. The effectiveness of platelet-rich plasma in the treatment of tendinopathy: a meta-analysis of randomized controlled clinical trials. Am J Sports Med. 2017;45(1):226–33.
15. CitraLabs, Complete Instructions for Risk/Use Information, Available from: http://www.citralabs.com/fileLibrary/FL9350-ACD-A.pdf
16. Fufa D, Shealy B, Jacobson M, Kevy S, Murray MM. Activation of platelet-rich plasma using soluble type I collagen. J Oral Maxillofac Surg. 2008;66(4):684–90.

17. Malliaropoulos N, Isinkaye T, Tsitas K, Maffulli N. Reinjury after acute posterior thigh muscle injuries in elite track and field athletes. Am J Sports Med. 2011;39(2):304–10.
18. Elliott MC, Zarins B, Powell JW, Kenyon CD. Hamstring muscle strains in professional football players: a 10-year review. Am J Sports Med. 2011;39(4):843–50.
19. Setayesh K, Villarreal A, Gottschalk A, Tokish JM, Choate WS. Treatment of muscle injuries with platelet-rich plasma: a review of the literature. Curr Rev Musculoskelet Med. 2018;11(4):635–42.
20. Arner JW, McClincy MP, Bradley JP. Hamstring injuries in athletes: evidence-based treatment. J Am Acad Orthop Surg. 2019;23:868–77.
21. Ahmad CS, Redler LH, Ciccotti MG, Maffulli N, Longo UG, Bradley J. Evaluation and management of hamstring injuries. Am J Sports Med. 2013;41(12):2933–47.
22. Arner JW, Lawyer TJ, Mauro CS, Bradley JP. Platelet-rich plasma (PRP) shortens return to play in National Football League (NFL) players with acute hamstring injuries. Orthop J Sports Med. 2019;7(7_suppl5):2325967119S00425.
23. Rettig AC, Meyer S, Bhadra AK. Platelet-rich plasma in addition to rehabilitation for acute hamstring injuries in NFL players: clinical effects and time to return to play. Orthop J Sports Med. 2013 Jun 24;1(1):2325967113494354.
24. Hamid MS, Mohamed Ali MR, Yusof A, George J, Lee LP. Platelet-rich plasma injections for the treatment of hamstring injuries: a randomized controlled trial. Am J Sports Med. 2014;42(10):2410–8.
25. Zanon G, Combi F, Combi A, Perticarini L, Sammarchi L, Benazzo F. Platelet-rich plasma in the treatment of acute hamstring injuries in professional football players. Joints. 2016;4(01):017–23.
26. Moen MH, Reurink G, Weir A, Tol JL, Maas M, Goudswaard GJ. Predicting return to play after hamstring injuries. Br J Sports Med. 2014;48(18):1358–63.
27. Erickson LN, Sherry MA. Rehabilitation and return to sport after hamstring strain injury. J Sport Health Sci. 2017;6(3):262–70.
28. Levy DM, Petersen KA, Vaught MS, Christian DR, Cole BJ. Injections for knee osteoarthritis: corticosteroids, Viscosupplementation, platelet-rich plasma, and autologous stem cells. Arthrosc J Arthrosc Related Surg. 2018;34(5):1730–43.
29. Smith PA. Intra-articular autologous conditioned plasma injections provide safe and efficacious treatment for knee osteoarthritis: an FDA-sanctioned, randomized, double-blind, placebo-controlled clinical trial. Am J Sports Med. 2016;44(4):884–91.
30. Patel S, Dhillon MS, Aggarwal S, Marwaha N, Jain A. Treatment with platelet-rich plasma is more effective than placebo for knee osteoarthritis: a prospective, double-blind, randomized trial. Am J Sports Med. 2013;41(2):356–64.
31. Cole BJ, Karas V, Hussey K, Merkow DB, Pilz K, Fortier LA. Hyaluronic acid versus platelet-rich plasma: a prospective, double-blind randomized controlled trial comparing clinical outcomes and effects on intra-articular biology for the treatment of knee osteoarthritis. Am J Sports Med. 2017;45(2):339–46.
32. Cerza F, Carnì S, Carcangiu A, Di Vavo I, Schiavilla V, Pecora A, De Biasi G, Ciuffreda M. Comparison between hyaluronic acid and platelet-rich plasma, intra-articular infiltration in the treatment of gonarthrosis. Am J Sports Med. 2012;40(12):2822–7.
33. Vaquerizo V, Plasencia MÁ, Arribas I, Seijas R, Padilla S, Orive G, Anitua E. Comparison of intra-articular injections of plasma rich in growth factors (PRGF-Endoret) versus Durolane hyaluronic acid in the treatment of patients with symptomatic osteoarthritis: a randomized controlled trial. Arthrosc J Arthrosc Relat Surg. 2013;29(10):1635–43.
34. Montañez-Heredia E, Irízar S, Huertas P, Otero E, del Valle M, Prat I, Díaz-Gallardo M, Perán M, Marchal J, Hernandez-Lamas M. Intra-articular injections of platelet-rich plasma versus hyaluronic acid in the treatment of osteoarthritic knee pain: a randomized clinical trial in the context of the Spanish National Health Care System. Int J Mol Sci. 2016;17(7):1064.
35. Sánchez M, Fiz N, Azofra J, Usabiaga J, Recalde EA, Gutierrez AG, Albillos J, Gárate R, Aguirre JJ, Padilla S, Orive G. A randomized clinical trial evaluating plasma rich in growth

factors (PRGF-Endoret) versus hyaluronic acid in the short-term treatment of symptomatic knee osteoarthritis. J Arthrosc Relat Surg. 2012;28(8):1070–8.
36. Cook CS, Smith PA. Clinical update: why PRP should be your first choice for injection therapy in treating osteoarthritis of the knee. Curr Rev Musculoskelet Med. 2018;11(4):583–92.
37. Zhu Y, Yuan M, Meng HY, Wang AY, Guo QY, Wang Y, Peng J. Basic science and clinical application of platelet-rich plasma for cartilage defects and osteoarthritis: a review. Osteoarthr Cartil. 2013;21(11):1627–37.
38. Nasi S, Ea HK, So A, Busso N. Revisiting the role of interleukin-1 pathway in osteoarthritis: interleukin-1α and-1β, and NLRP3 inflammasome are not involved in the pathological features of the murine menisectomy model of osteoarthritis. Front Pharmacol. 2017;8:282.
39. Schmidt MB, Chen EH, Lynch SE. A review of the effects of insulin-like growth factor and platelet derived growth factor on in vivo cartilage healing and repair. Osteoarthr Cartil. 2006;14(5):403–12.
40. Yin WJ, Xu HT, Sheng JG, An ZQ, Guo SC, Xie XT, Zhang CQ. Advantages of pure platelet-rich plasma compared with leukocyte-and platelet-rich plasma in treating rabbit knee osteoarthritis. Med Sci Monitor. 2016;22:1280.
41. Khoshbin A, Leroux T, Wasserstein D, Marks P, Theodoropoulos J, Ogilvie-Harris D, Gandhi R, Takhar K, Lum G, Chahal J. The efficacy of platelet-rich plasma in the treatment of symptomatic knee osteoarthritis: a systematic review with quantitative synthesis. J Arthroscop Relat Surg. 2013;29(12):2037–48.
42. Sundman EA, Cole BJ, Fortier LA. Growth factor and catabolic cytokine concentrations are influenced by the cellular composition of platelet-rich plasma. Am J Sports Med. 2011;39(10):2135–40.
43. Sundman EA, Cole BJ, Karas V, Della Valle C, Tetreault MW, Mohammed HO, Fortier LA. The anti-inflammatory and matrix restorative mechanisms of platelet-rich plasma in osteoarthritis. Am J Sports Med. 2014;42(1):35–41.
44. Sakata R, McNary SM, Miyatake K, Lee CA, Van den Bogaerde JM, Marder RA, Reddi AH. Stimulation of the superficial zone protein and lubrication in the articular cartilage by human platelet-rich plasma. Am J Sports Med. 2015;43(6):1467–73.
45. Wasterlain AS, Braun HJ, Dragoo JL. Platelet-rich plasma as a treatment for patellar tendinopathy: a double-blind randomized controlled trial (SS-60). Arthroscopy. 2012;28(6):e31–2.
46. Vulpiani MC, Vetrano M, Savoia V, Di Pangrazio E, Trischitta D, Ferretti A. Jumper's knee treatment with extracorporeal shock wave therapy: a long-term follow-up observational study. J Sports Med Phys Fitness. 2007;47(3):323.
47. Dragoo JL, Wasterlain AS, Braun HJ, Nead KT. Platelet-rich plasma as a treatment for patellar tendinopathy: a double-blind, randomized controlled trial. Am J Sports Med. 2014;42(3):610–8.
48. Gosens T, Den Oudsten BL, Fievez E, van't pijker P, Fievez A. Pain and activity levels before and after platelet-rich plasma injection treatment of patellar tendinopathy: a prospective cohort study and the influence of previous treatments. Int Orthop. 2012;36(9):1941–6.
49. Kon E, Filardo G, Delcogliano M, Presti ML, Russo A, Bondi A, Di Martino A, Cenacchi A, Fornasari PM, Marcacci M. Platelet-rich plasma: new clinical application: a pilot study for treatment of jumper's knee. Injury. 2009;40(6):598–603.
50. Charousset C, Zaoui A, Bellaiche L, Bouyer B. Are multiple platelet-rich plasma injections useful for treatment of chronic patellar tendinopathy in athletes? A prospective study. Am J Sports Med. 2014;42(4):906–11.
51. Gaweda K, Tarczynska M, Krzyzanowski W. Treatment of Achilles tendinopathy with platelet-rich plasma. Int J Sports Med. 2010;31(08):577–83.
52. de Vos RJ, Weir A, Tol JL, Verhaar JA, Weinans H, Van Schie HT. No effects of PRP on ultrasonographic tendon structure and neovascularisation in chronic midportion Achilles tendinopathy. Br J Sports Med. 2011;45(5):387–92.
53. Monto RR. Platelet rich plasma treatment for chronic Achilles tendinosis. Foot Ankle Int. 2012;33(5):379–85.

54. Rowden A, Dominici P, D'Orazio J, Manur R, Deitch K, Simpson S, Kowalski MJ, Salzman M, Ngu D. Double-blind, randomized, placebo-controlled study evaluating the use of platelet-rich plasma therapy (PRP) for acute ankle sprains in the emergency department. J Emerg Med. 2015;49(4):546–51.
55. Samra DJ, Sman AD, Rae K, Linklater J, Refshauge KM, Hiller CE. Effectiveness of a single platelet-rich plasma injection to promote recovery in rugby players with ankle syndesmosis injury. BMJ Open Sport Exerc Med. 2015;1(1):e000033.

Part II

Medical Topics

Associate Editor
James R. Clugston

Emergency Action Plans in Football

13

Ron Courson, Fred Reifsteck, and Samantha E. Scarneo-Miller

Although most injuries in athletics are relatively minor, life-threatening injuries are unpredictable and can occur without warning. Because of the relatively low incidence rate of catastrophic injuries, health care providers may develop a false sense of security. However, *catastrophic injuries or illnesses* can occur during any physical activity and at any level of participation, which demands plans to be in place to react to a potential catastrophic event. Between the fall of 1982 through spring of 2017, there were 372 fatalities in football at the secondary school and collegiate levels [1]. An *Emergency Action Plan* (EAP) is a vital part to a successful sports medicine program to improve the health and safety of athletes [2]. EAPs are necessary to have written information on how to react to an emergency situation. These plans incorporate step-by-step guides on what to do, who to call, when to call, where equipment is located, address and venue information, and documentation of approvals of the plan, among other items. Planning for athletics emergencies is very similar to that of school-based emergency operations planning. They require time, dedication, and specifics to ensure the best possible outcomes are met.

The most common causes of sudden death in athletics are cardiac events (see Chap. 16), head (Chap. 16) and spinal cord injuries (Chap. 9), exertional heat illness (Chap. 15), asthma, and sickle cell crisis (exertional sickling) (Chap. 17). There is often a heightened public awareness associated with the nature and management of these events. Medico-legal interests may lead to questions regarding the qualifications of the personnel involved, the preparedness of the organization, and the actions taken. Proper management of emergencies in athletics is critical. Emergencies should be handled by trained medical and allied health personnel. Preparation should include

R. Courson (✉) · F. Reifsteck
University of Georgia Athletic Association, Athens, GA, USA
e-mail: rcourson@sports.uga.edu

S. E. Scarneo-Miller
West Virginia University, Division of Athletic Training, Health Sciences South, Morgantown, WV, USA

K. W. Farmer (ed.), *Football Injuries*,
https://doi.org/10.1007/978-3-030-54875-9_13

education and training, maintenance of emergency equipment, and supplies, appropriate use of personnel, and formation and implementation of an EAP [2–6].

Emergency action plans allow for deliberate, thorough planning for management of a catastrophic injury in football. Though not an everyday occurrence, catastrophic injury in football must be considered, and appropriate personnel must be trained on the appropriate response for various types of injuries. For example, if an athlete suffers from a cardiac arrest (indirect injury) on the field, personnel must be able to identify the steps of action for activating emergency medical services (EMS), accessing an automated external defibrillator (AED) as soon as possible, and begin cardiopulmonary resuscitation (CPR) on the athlete. Fatal football injuries account for 88.8% and 88.2% of indirect injuries in high school and collegiate sports, respectively [1]. If an athlete suffers from a cervical spine injury following a tackle (direct injury), the personnel must be able to quickly identify the nature of the injury and carry out the steps for managing a potential spinal cord injury. Of the direct injuries reported to the National Center for Catastrophic Sport Injury in Research, 44.2% are nonfatal (permanent, severe functional disability) in high school sport, and 70.4% are serious (no permanent functional disability, but a severe injury) in collegiate sport [1]. Based on current numbers, it is estimated that approximately 16 athletes will die in high school sports per year from indirect injuries [1]. Regardless of the type of injury, prompt recognition and treatment is imperative to improve patient outcomes.

The Need for an Emergency Action Plan

Emergencies are rarely predictable, and they call for a rapid, controlled response. An EAP should include all necessary contingencies, even the worst-case scenario. Health care providers should take lessons from past emergencies: experience is a great teacher. The National Athletic Trainers' Association (NATA) position statement "Emergency Planning in Athletics" provides guidelines for the development and implementation of an EAP [2].

Athletic health care providers may be responsible for the care of others in addition to athletes, such as coaches, officials, and spectators. All personnel involved with the organization or sponsorship of athletic activities share a professional and legal responsibility to provide for the emergency care of an injured person and a legal duty to develop, implement, and evaluate an emergency plan for all sponsored athletic activities. A written EAP document defines the *standard of care*. The absence of an EAP frequently is a basis for claims and suits based on negligence. Thus, each institution or organization that sponsors athletic activities should have a written emergency plan. The EAP should be comprehensive and practical, and flexible enough to adapt to any emergency situation. The EAP should be developed in consultation with local emergency medical services (EMS) personnel, and the written document should be approved and signed by the medical director for the athletic organization. The EAP should be distributed to attending physicians, athletic trainers and athletic training students, institutional and organizational safety personnel and administrators, coaches, and strength and conditioning staff.

Legal Basis for an Emergency Plan

The existence of an emergency plan for athletics is an accepted standard of care. Sports medicine providers have a duty to provide reasonable and prudent care in a timely manner. Sports medicine providers additionally have a duty to foresee the possibility of emergency situations in athletics and to develop a plan to address such situations. Court cases in recent years have addressed or alluded to emergency care and the emergency plan. In a landmark legal case in 1993 regarding emergency action planning, *Kleinknecht v. Gettysburg College* [7], the parents of a college lacrosse player who suffered sudden cardiac arrest during lacrosse practice brought a negligence action against the college. The Court of Appeals held that the college owed the player a duty of care as well as a duty to take reasonable precautions against the risk of reasonably foreseeable life-threatening injuries during participation in athletic events [7]. Adequate planning includes expediting emergency vehicles to the site of an accident and ensuring the availability of medical personnel qualified to care for the injured athlete.

Medical Time Out

Sports medicine teams should conduct a "Medical Time Out" before each athletic event. As miscommunication may lead to potentially catastrophic errors, information sharing, team training, and collaborative skill development among the emergency medical providers are critical components of emergency medical care and the obligation of the host institution/organization. The "Time Out" should include a review of items such as medically qualified personnel on-site, equipment available, management protocols for all types of catastrophic injuries, medical professional in charge of the response, signals and communication, contact numbers to local facilities, transport procedures, and local hospital trauma management plans. Additionally, a review of the equipment to be used will prevent the inadvertent use of equipment that may not fit into the transport vehicle. It is incumbent on the host to coordinate with the visiting team and medical personnel to plan the emergency response, which will help to ensure that a coordinated emergency approach is in place for all athletic medical care team members. This information is important to prepare in advance of the event, particularly for those events hosted at neutral sites for which neither team is familiar with the venue or local medical facilities [8].

Scene Control: "Calm is Contagious"

Former Navy SEAL Commander, Rorke Denver, advocates the axiom "calm is contagious." It is critical that the emergency scene be controlled, calm, and orderly to facilitate the best medical care. Bystanders may be well intentioned but may cause distractions and interfere with the delivery of care. As a part of the Medical Time Out prior to competition, the sports medicine team should review with the game officials their role with an injury. Keeping the players away from the emergency scene allows adequate space for the sports medicine team to work and position emergency equipment, carts, and ambulances. Coaches and chaplains, if available, can assist in this role as well [9].

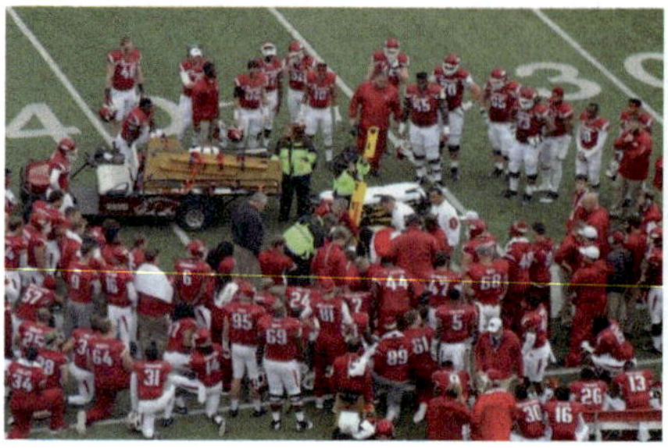

This emergency scene does not allow adequate space for rescuers to work

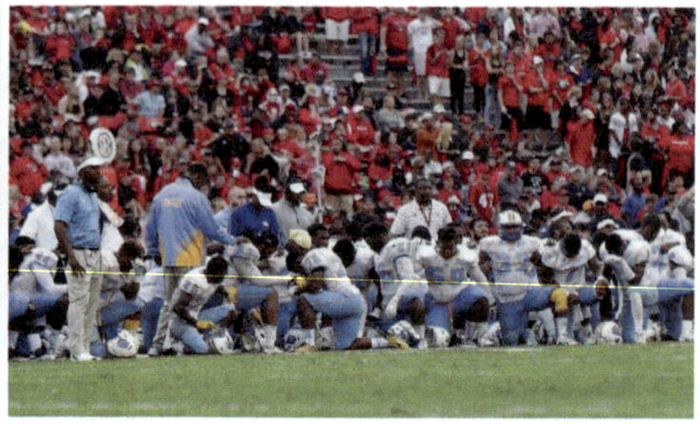

By bringing players over to the sideline, the game officials, coaches, and chaplain have helped control the scene for the sports medicine team.

Emergency Action Plan Case Study

During the Georgia vs. Southern football game in 2015, Devon Gales from Southern sustained a cervical spine injury. While blocking on a kick-off, he lowered his head immediately prior to contact and had an axial load mechanism of injury, striking his opponent in the chest with the crown of his helmet. His body immediately went limp, and he fell to the ground supine with no motor or sensation from the shoulders down. The injury happened in front of the Georgia bench, and their sports medicine staff responded first. Recognizing the seriousness of the injury, they activated the emergency action plan (EAP). The Georgia and Southern sports medical team members worked together to evaluate Gales on the field, carefully remove his helmet and shoulder pads, and immobilize him on a spinal restriction device for transport by ambulance to the trauma center in Athens, Georgia. Diagnostic testing revealed an incomplete C5–C6 spinal cord injury. He underwent emergency surgery by the Georgia team neurosurgeon to stabilize his spinal column and was transferred 3 days post injury to the Shepherd Center, a neurological rehabilitation hospital in Atlanta, Georgia.

Prior to the kick-off, the Georgia sports medicine staff conducted a Medical Time Out, where they met with the Southern sports medicine staff along with EMS and conducted a pre-athletic event checklist, reviewing the venue's emergency action plan. They introduced all of the medical staff members and discussed their role and location; established how communication would occur; explained where ambulance, EMS, emergency cart, and x-ray were located within the stadium and how to access, where the designated hospital was in location to the stadium, what emergency equipment was available on-site, and reviewed the c-spine injury protocol.

A critical incident review was conducted the following day. Everyone involved felt that the Medical Time Out played a critical role in having a coordinated emergency response and outcome. Effective communication with all relevant parties is critical to ensure the injured athlete receives the best care when an emergency arises. This case study demonstrates the effectiveness of an emergency plan.

The Sports Medicine Team Concept

The goal of the sports medicine team is the delivery of the highest possible quality health care to the athlete. An athletic emergency situation may involve certified and student athletic trainers, emergency medical technicians, physicians, and coaches working together. Just as with an athletic team, the sports medicine team must work together as an efficient unit, in order to accomplish its goals. In an emergency situation, the team concept becomes even more critical because seconds may mean the difference between life or death or permanent disability. The sharing of information, training, and skills among the various emergency medical providers help to reach the goal of the delivery of the highest-quality emergency health care to the athlete.

Components of the Emergency Plan

The EAP should be specific to each individual athletic venue and encompass the following subjects:

1. Emergency personnel
2. Emergency communication
3. Emergency equipment
4. Medical emergency transportation
5. Venue directions with map

Emergency Personnel

For athletic practices and competitions, the *first responder* to an emergency situation is typically a member of the sports medicine staff—most commonly a certified athletic trainer—or EMS personnel. A team physician may not always be present at every organized practice or competition. The type and degree of sports medicine coverage for an athletic event may vary widely, based on such factors as the sport or activity, the setting, and the type of training or competition. The first responder in some instances may be a coach, strength and conditioning staff, or other institutional personnel. Certification in CPR and *first aid*, knowledge concerning the prevention of disease transmission, and review of the existing EAP should be required for all athletic personnel associated with practices, competitions, skills instruction, and strength and conditioning; copies of training certificates or cards should be maintained.

The development of an EAP cannot be complete without the formation of an emergency team. The emergency team may consist of a number of health care providers, including physicians, emergency medical technicians, certified athletic trainers, athletic training students, coaches, equipment managers, and, possibly, bystanders. For example, game officials may play a critical role in the emergency plan by keeping the field clear of others when an emergency arises, allowing the health care providers room to work. The roles of these individuals within the emergency team may vary, depending on factors such as the number of members of the team, the athletic venue itself, or the preference of the head athletic trainer.

There are four basic roles within the emergency team. The first and most important role is establishing the safety of the scene and providing immediate care of the athlete. Acute care in an emergency situation should be provided by the most qualified individual on the scene. Individuals with lesser qualification should yield to those with more appropriate training. The second role, EMS activation, may be necessary in situations in which emergency transportation is not already present at the sporting event. This should be done as soon as the situation is deemed an emergency or a life-threatening event. Time is the most critical factor under emergency conditions. Activating the EMS system may be done by anyone on the team. However, the person chosen for this duty should be someone who is calm under pressure and who communicates well over the telephone. This person should also be familiar with the specific location and address of the sporting event.

The third role, equipment retrieval, may be done by anyone on the emergency team who is familiar with the types and location of the specific equipment needed. Athletic training students, equipment managers, and coaches are good choices for this role. The fourth role of the emergency team is that of directing EMS personnel to the scene. One member of the team should be responsible for meeting emergency medical personnel, as they arrive at the site of the emergency. Depending on ease of access, this person should have keys to any locked gates or doors that may slow the arrival of medical personnel. An athletic training student, equipment manager, or coach may be appropriate for this role.

When forming the emergency team, it is important to adapt the team to each situation or sport. It may also be advantageous to have more than one individual assigned to each role. This allows the emergency team to function even though certain members may not always be present. Preparation is the key to emergency response. The health care team should regularly review the EAP and rehearse emergency simulations to work effectively as a team.

Sports medicine staff may pursue specialized in-service training in required skill areas or advanced training such as CPR/first aid instructor, emergency medical technician (EMT) or paramedic, pre-hospital trauma life support, or advanced cardiac life support. Sports medicine staff may additionally develop standardized emergency protocols in areas such as automated external defibrillators (AEDs), oxygen/airway adjuncts, head and cervical spine management, and so forth. Figure 13.1 is an example of a spine injury protocol.

University of Georgia Sports Medicine Spine Injury Management Protocol
July 23, 2019

General Guidelines

Any athlete suspected of having a spinal injury should initially not be moved and should be managed as though a spinal injury exists. C-spine in-line stabilization should be maintained.

The primary acute treatment goals are to ensure that the cervical spine is immobilized in a neutral position and vital life functions are accessible. The athlete's airway, breathing, circulation, level of consciousness (AVPU), and neurological status should be assessed. If airway is impaired, maintain c-spine in-line stabilization simultaneously with airway, using a modified jaw thrust maneuver. If the athlete's breathing is inadequate, assist ventilations with bag-valve-mask, airway adjuncts as appropriate, and supplemental oxygen.

During initial assessment, the presence of any of the following, alone or in combination, requires the initiation of the spine injury management protocol: unconsciousness or altered level of consciousness, bilateral neurological findings or complaints, significant midline spine pain with or without palpation, or obvious spinal column deformity.

EMS should be activated.

The athlete should not be moved until immobilized unless absolutely essential to maintain airway, breathing, and circulation. If the athlete must be moved, the athlete should be placed in a supine position, while maintaining spinal immobilization.

In a situation where it may not be appropriate for on-site medical personnel to transfer the athlete to a long spine board prior to EMS arrival (lack of enough qualified help or other factors), the rescuer(s) should maintain in-line stabilization, place a rigid cervical collar on (if possible), support ABCs, and continue to monitor baseline vital signs and complete secondary evaluation while awaiting EMS.

Spine Immobilization

If the spine is not in a neutral position, rescuers should realign the c-spine to minimize secondary injury to the spinal cord and to allow for optimal airway management. However, the presence or development of any of the following, alone or in combination, represents a contraindication for moving the c-spine to neutral position:

Movement causes increased pain, neurological symptoms, muscle spasm, or airway compromise;

Resistance is encountered during the attempt at realignment; or

The athlete expresses apprehension.

If possible, a correctly sized rigid cervical collar should be placed on athlete prior to moving.

When moving a suspected spine-injured athlete, the head and trunk should be moved as a unit by securing the athlete to a rigid immobilization device (i.e., long spine board, scoop stretcher, KED, or full-body vacuum mattress). Either the multi-person lift, one of the various log-roll maneuvers, or scoop stretcher should be used to place the athlete on the rigid immobilization device. It is ideal that at minimum three (3) rescuers with preferably five to six (5–6) be in place to perform the log-roll procedure and that at minimum eight (8) rescuers be in place to perform the multi-person lift. Rescuers should select the most appropriate transfer techniques, which best fits the individual circumstances associated with each athlete (i.e., position: supine or prone, number of rescuers available, space available, etc.).

Fig. 13.1 University of georgia sports medicine spine injury management protocol

The rescuer controlling c-spine stabilization will be in command of multi-person lift or log-roll maneuvers and transfer to rigid immobilization device.

Once positioned onto long spine board, the athlete's torso and legs should first be secured, using spider straps or speed clips (if speed clips are used, ideally seven straps should be applied: two crossing chest from shoulder to opposite axilla, one across chest under axilla, one across the abdomen, one across the pelvis, one across the mid thighs and one across the mid tibias). Athlete's arms should be left free from long spine board straps to facilitate vital sign monitoring and IV access. The athlete's wrists may be secured together in front of the body with Velcro strap or tape once secured to the rigid immobilization device. Padding may be used between the patient and straps to help secure them tightly.

Once torso and legs are secured, the head should be secured last. If necessary, padding should be applied under the athlete's head to fill any voids and maintain neutral in-line position. The head should be secured with lateral restraint pads and then secured to board with tape over forehead and at chin.

Following securing athlete to board, neurological status should be reassessed.

The secondary survey should be completed with baseline vital signs (reassessed regularly), head-to-toe survey, and SAMPLE history.

Athlete should be transported to the most appropriate emergency medical facility and head team physician, and appropriate subspecialist(s) notified.

A member of the University of Georgia medical staff should accompany the athlete in the ambulance.

Additional Guidelines for Care of Spine-Injured Football Athlete

In an emergency situation with equipment-intensive sports, the *protective equipment may be removed prior to ambulance transport to the hospital*. The rationale for consideration of equipment removal on the field is based upon four concepts:

Advances in equipment technology: Changes in helmet and shoulder pad design have helped to facilitate equipment removal.

Equipment removal should be performed by those with highest level of training: On the field of play, there may be multiple individuals (athletic trainers, emergency medical technicians, physicians) with knowledge of equipment removal versus the hospital emergency department (ED).

Better packaging: With both the helmet and shoulder pads removed, the athlete is in a spine-neutral position. A cervical collar may be applied. Packaging straps are closer to body with equipment removed.

Expedited care in ED: With equipment removed prior to arrival in ED, physician evaluation and diagnostic tests may be expedited

Factors to consider in equipment removal include the nature of the injury, type of protective equipment worn (helmet, shoulder pads, neck roll, rib pads, etc.), the number of rescuers on-site, and the level of training of rescuers in equipment removal. Protective equipment left in place, following a spine injury may, impede the evaluation and treatment process, while inappropriately removed protective equipment may cause spinal movement, potentially causing harm. As protective equipment varies by sport and types of equipment differ, rescuers should be familiar with both the types of equipment and removal techniques.

Equipment removal should be done by at least three rescuers trained and experienced with equipment removal at the earliest possible time. If fewer than three people are present, the equipment should be removed at the earliest possible time after enough trained individuals arrive. Rescuers should utilize a medical time out pre-activity session to plan out the options with the personnel available for that practice/game. Clinical judgment in each situation may recommend something different than this best practices recommendation (i.e., changes in clinical status, equipment failure, space barriers, etc.). Rescuers should be able to recognize when is it NOT appropriate to remove equipment on field of play and have a plan to best manage the patient.

Fig. 13.1 (continued)

General Principles of Helmet and Shoulder Pad Removal

The helmet should be removed first, followed by the shoulder pads. Once the shoulder pads are removed, rescuers should properly fit and apply a cervical collar. The athlete should then be secured to a rigid immobilization device (i.e., spine board, scoop stretcher, KED, or full-body vacuum mattress).

Helmet removal technique:

Rescuer 1 stabilizes c-spine.

Rescuer 2 cuts chin strap (do not unbuckle) and removes it.

Rescuer 2 assumes c-spine control from front, allowing Rescuer 1 to release: "I have c-spine control; you can release."

Rescuer 1 removes helmet; then again assumes c-spine control, allowing Rescuer 2 to release: "I have c-spine control; you can release"

Shoulder pad removal techniques:

Several techniques exist to remove shoulder pads (*following helmet removal*). Rescuers should select the techniques which best fit the individual circumstances associated with each athlete.

Supine athlete:

Multi-Person Lift: Rescuer 1 stabilizes c-spine; jersey, and shoulder pads cut in front; Rescuers 2–7 (three on each side) lift athlete 12" on command (to allow shoulder pad clearance for removal); Rescuer 8 slides board in; Rescuer 9 carefully removes shoulder pads without interfering with Rescuer 1's c-spine control. Once Rescuer 9 communicates "shoulder pads are clear," the athlete is lowered to board on command.

Tilt Technique (also known as *elevated torso*): Rescuer 1 reaches inside shoulder pads and stabilizes c-spine from front. Rescuers 2 and 3 tilt athlete to 50 degrees at waist, similar to motion of a "sit-up". Rescuer 4 removes shoulder pads from over top of head. Rescuer 4 then grasps both sides of head and assists Rescuer 1 with c-spine stabilization as the athlete is lowered down. Note that the tilt should not be utilized as a shoulder pad removal technique with suspected concomitant thoracic and/or lumbar injury.

Straddle technique (also known as *lift and slide*): This technique may be utilized with small athletes. Rescuer 1 stabilizes c-spine; jersey and shoulder pads cut in front; Rescuers 2–4 standing over straddling the athlete lift athlete 12" on command (to allow shoulder pad clearance for removal); Rescuer 5 slides board in; Rescuer 6 carefully removes shoulder pads without interfering with Rescuer 1's c-spine control. Once Rescuer 6 communicates "shoulder pads are clear," the athlete is lowered to board on command

Flat Torso Technique: Jersey and shoulder pads are cut in front. Rescuer 1 reaches inside shoulder pads and stabilizes c-spine from front. Rescuers 2 and 3 grasp shoulder pads from either side of athlete and slide pads out in an axial direction.

Log-Roll Technique: A standard log-roll technique is utilized. Rescuer 1 stabilizes c-spine. Rescuers 2–4 perform supine log roll, pausing at the top of the roll. Rescuer 5 cuts the jersey and shoulder pads in the back, then positions spine board, and athlete is lowered down onto board. The jersey and shoulder pads are then cut in the front, and the bivalved shoulder pads are removed from each side by Rescuers 2 and 3, while Rescuer 1 continues to stabilize c-spine.

Quick Release Shoulder Pads: One shoulder pad manufacturer currently makes a quick-release shoulder pad. Rescuer 1 stabilizes c-spine. The jersey and shoulder pads are cut in front. Rescuer 2 cuts the emergency quick-release tab and pulls a cable, which releases the shoulder pads in back. The bivalved shoulder pads are removed from each side by Rescuers 2 and 3, while Rescuer 1 continues to stabilize c-spine.

Prone athlete: The prone athlete must be log rolled as the eight-person lift and scoop stretcher techniques may only be utilized on supine athletes. Rescuers should select either the log roll–push or log roll–pull technique based upon the individual circumstances associated with each athlete.

Fig. 13.1 (continued)

Rescuer 1 stabilizes c-spine. Prior to initiating the log roll, Rescuer 2 cuts the jersey and shoulder pads in back, then positions spine board, and the athlete is lowered down onto board by Rescuers 3–5. The jersey and shoulder pads cut in front by Rescuer 2 and the bivalved shoulder pads are removed from each side by Rescuers 2 and 3.

At a minimum, access to the face for airway should be managed prior to transportation, regardless of current respiratory status. This is accomplished by either helmet or face-mask removal, based upon the individual situation. Tools for face-mask removal (power screwdriver, FM Extractor, Anvil Pruners, or ratcheting PVC pipe cutter) should be readily accessible. If possible, consideration should be given to the use of quick-release face-mask clips to facilitate face-mask removal.

Procedures for Training in Spine Immobilization:

On at least an annual basis, personnel should review signs and symptoms of spine injury and complete a training session each year with in-line stabilization, rigid cervical collar application, log-roll maneuver (supine and prone), eight-person lift maneuver, equipment removal techniques, and rigid immobilization device packaging. Additionally, personnel providing football medical coverage should review face-mask removal with appropriate tools, helmet removal, and shoulder pad removal.

Approved by: ______________________ **Date:** ____________
Fred Reifsteck, M.D.

Approved by: ______________________ **Date:** ____________
Kim Walpert, M.D.

Approved by: ______________________ **Date:** ____________
Ron Courson, ATC, PT, NRAEMT, CSCS

Approved by: ______________________ **Date:** ____________
Glenn Henry, MA, EMT-P

Approved by: ______________________ **Date:** ____________
Anna Randa, MEd, ATC, NREMT

Refs. [16–27]

Fig. 13.1 (continued)

Emergency Communication

Communication is the critical piece in determining success or failure in many aspects of Sports Medicine, and the EAP is no different. The communication needs to be open, honest, and two way. Harsh, condescending, and authoritative words and language do nothing to improve team dynamics or create a good EAP. Communication consists of both spoken word and written documentation. As the saying goes, "if it is not documented it didn't happen."

Communication starts when the Sports Medicine team provides the Administration with the clear need for the EAP. The communication continues with the development of the plan, especially the resources needed to have the equipment that will be used. Expert opinions, especially those with football experience, should be sought out and followed as the plan is brought together. Learning and following best practices may help eliminate some of the problems or issues encountered when starting to put a plan together. The decisions made should be a team effort, especially utilizing the opinions of the stakeholders who have to carry out the EAP.

The plan itself needs to be reviewed at least annually, as many aspects can change from personnel to facilities to equipment. Football offers many clinical scenarios that can be reviewed and practiced on a yearly basis. Any changes made based on these practice scenarios need to be clearly communicated to all stakeholders, especially those that may not take part in the practice scenarios. In some cases, transport personnel and emergency room personnel may not be up to date on the latest clinical guidelines. This has especially been seen in the area of equipment removal (Chap. 9). The hope is that the scenarios will never have to be performed, but the team needs to be ready for them.

Communication is critical in creating the safest environment possible for athletic competitions. A well-thought-out, and well-executed plan can improve the chances at achieving the best clinical outcomes.

Communication Equipment

Access to a working telephone or other telecommunications device, whether fixed or mobile, should be ensured. The communication system should be checked prior to each practice or competition to ensure it is in proper working order. A back-up communication plan should be in effect should there be a failure of the primary communication system. At any athletic venue, whether home or away, it is important to know the location of a functioning telephone. Prearranged access to the phone should be established if it is not easily accessible.

Other considerations include:

- What number do you call?
- Is 911 available in your venue's location?
- Do you have to dial a prefix number (such as "9") to get off campus?
- Are 911 calls screened by the campus or venue operator before they go out?
- Do security personnel/police/sheriff have radio contact with "public service access points" or dispatch centers to get EMS activated?

A copy of the EAP should be posted by the telephone. When activating EMS, the following information should be provided:

- Name and telephone number of the caller and the address to which to respond
- Number of athletes affected
- Condition of athlete(s)
- First-aid treatment initiated
- Specific directions
- Other information as requested by the dispatcher

Emergency Equipment

All necessary emergency equipment should be at the site and quickly accessible. Personnel should be familiar with the function and operation of each type of emergency equipment. Equipment should be in good operating condition, and personnel must be trained in advance to use it properly. Emergency equipment should be checked on a regular basis and its use rehearsed by emergency personnel. The emergency equipment available should be appropriate for the level of training of the emergency medical providers.

The creation of an equipment inspection log book for continued inspection is strongly recommended. A few members of the emergency team should be trained and responsible for the care of the equipment. It is also important to know the proper way to care for and store the equipment. Equipment should be stored in a clean and environmentally controlled area. It should be readily available when emergency situations arise.

The equipment available should be based on the type of event being covered and the possible emergency scenarios anticipated. For example, when covering an outdoor event with the possibility of exertional heat illness, such as a distance road race, health care providers should have ready in advance an ice-water immersion tub, a rectal thermometer, IV fluids, and other necessary equipment. Health care providers covering an event in which sickle cell trait athletes are participating should have oxygen and IV fluids available. Figure 13.2 provides a sample trauma bag checklist, detailing basic emergency equipment for athletics, and Table 13.1 lists recommended emergency equipment for athletic venues.

Emergency Transportation

Emphasis should be placed on having an ambulance on site at high-risk sporting events. EMS response time should be factored in when determining whether on-site ambulance coverage is warranted.

Emergency Action Plan Tip: EMS Response Time

It is beneficial to know the average EMS response time for your region. This information is available through your local EMS agency. The length of your region's EMS response time may factor into your emergency plan. For example, a metropolitan high school with a local fire/rescue station two blocks away will generally have a quicker response time than a rural high school with the closest station 15 miles away. If a longer response time is anticipated, it may be prudent for care providers to have the necessary equipment to provide extended emergency care until EMS arrives. When reviewing EMS response, factor in both horizontal and vertical response times. Horizontal response time is measured from the time the EMS call goes out until the dispatched unit arrives on scene. Once the unit arrives, time is required to remove emergency equipment from the unit and travel to the site of the patient. Vertical response time is measured from the time the dispatched unit arrives on scene until patient treatment begins.

Trauma Bag Inventory

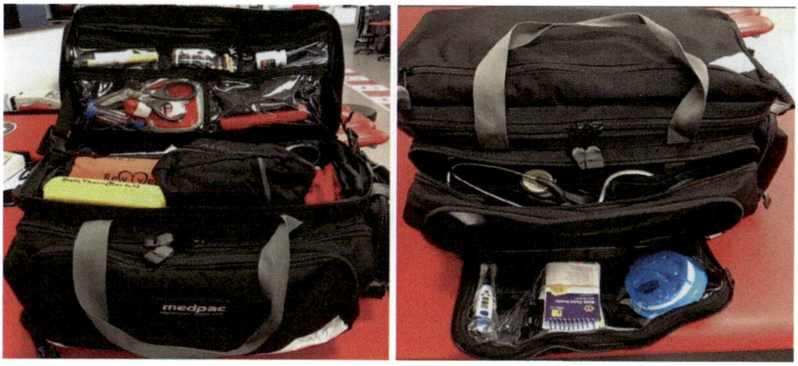

Top Pocket
- Weather cover for trauma kit
- Biohazard spill clean-up kit

Main Compartment:
- ReviveR AED with two sets of adult electrodes and one set of pediatric electrodes
- AED accessory kit with trauma shears, towel, stick anti-perspirant, razor, pocket mask
- **Airway kit**: bag-valve-mask, OP airway set, NP airway set, lubricant, three King LT airways (sizes 3,4,5), oxygen tubing, non-rebreather mask, tape
- DataTherm rectal thermometer, two temp probes pre-marked at 6", lubricant, tape
- **Hemorrhage control kit** : gloves, trauma shears, tourniquet, hemostatic gauze, trauma wound dressing, Quik Clot sponge
- Oxygen tank with regulator
- V-Vac manual suction (with adapter tip/catheter tube and extra canister)
- Sterile saline spray
- Gauze (variety of sizes, including trauma dressings and sterile roll gauze)

Inside Pocket: Top Lid:
- Medications: Albuterol inhaler/spacer, chewable aspirin(81 mg.), Epi-Pen (adult), Glucose gel, Glucagon emergency injection kit, Narcan nasal spray
- Paramedic shears
- Glucose monitoring kit: glucometer, strips, lancets
- Emergency blanket
- Spare batteries

1st Front Pocket:
- Digital oral thermometer with sheaths
- Penlight
- Pulse oximeter
- Emesis bags (2)
- EMS Field Guide
- Vital signs notebook and notepad
- Pen
- Sharpie

2nd Front Pocket:
- Stethoscope
- Blood pressure cuffs (1 nml, 1thigh)

Right Side Pocket
- BBP PPE: gown, gloves, mask, eye protection
- Trauma dressings & Kerlix roll gauze (sterile)

Back Pocket:
- King Vision video laryngoscope with 2 blades(size 3)
- Endotracheal tubes (one 18 mm and one 17.5 mm)
- 12 cc syringe
- Rusch Quick Trach Kit

Note: items highlighted in red should be regularly checked for expiration dates, battery life, etc...

Fig. 13.2 University of Georgia trauma bag checklist

Spine/EHI Kit Inventories

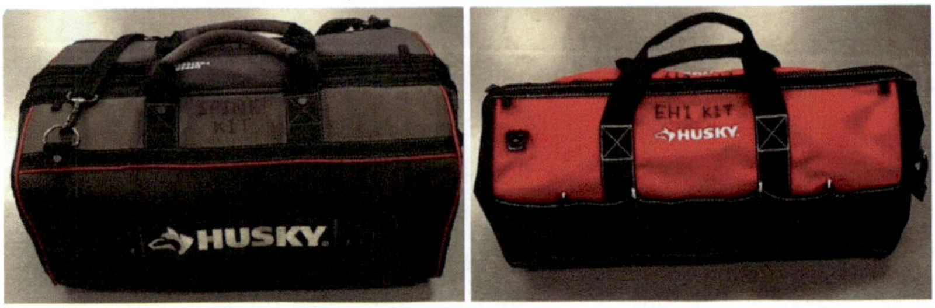

Spine Kit

- Trauma shears
- Facemask removal tools:
  - Two cordless screwdrivers (battery must be kept charged)
  - Screwdriver
  - Facemask clip cutting tools (FM extractor, pruning shears)
- Speed clips (Two complete sets plus back-ups)
- Spider strap set
- X-strap set
- Foam head blocks
- Towels (fill-in space)
- Duct tape (to secure head to board)
- Powerflex tape (to secure wrists together)

Exertional Heat Illness Kit

"Cool first, then transport!"

- Rubbermaid tub for cold water immersion, located immediately adjacent to water supply and ice source, and pre-filled with water when athletes participating in an environment conducive to possibility of EHI
- Quick litter
- DataTherm electronic rectal thermometer with 6' disposable probes pre-marked at 6"
- KY jelly
- Waterproof tape
- Sheet or strap to place under axilla to support athlete in water
- Infrared thermometer to monitor temperature of cold waterimmersion tub
- Small paddle for water agitation
- Heavy duty tarp (for "Taco" method of whole body cooling)
- *Access to trauma kit*

Note: items highlighted in red should be regularly checked for expiration dates, battery life, etc…

Fig. 13.2 (continued)

Consideration should be given to the capabilities of the transportation service available (i.e., basic life support or advanced life support), and the equipment and level of trained personnel on board the ambulance. In the event that an ambulance is on-site, it should be in a designated location with rapid access to the site and a cleared route for entering and exiting the venue.

In the medical emergency evaluation, the primary survey assists the emergency care provider in identifying emergencies requiring critical intervention and in determining transport decisions. In an emergency situation, the athlete should be transported by ambulance, where the necessary staff and equipment are available to deliver appropriate care. Emergency care providers should refrain from transporting unstable athletes in inappropriate vehicles. Care must be taken to ensure that the

Table 13.1 Recommended emergency equipment for athletic venues

Automated external defibrillator (AED)
Airway management supplies (oropharyngeal and nasopharyngeal airways)
Oxygen delivery system and pulse oximeter
Suction device (manual, battery, or oxygen powered)
Body substance isolation equipment (per OSHA guidelines)
Wound care supplies
Vital signs assessment: blood pressure cuff, stethoscope, penlight
Emergency shears
CPR pocket mask
Bag-valve-mask
Rigid cervical collar
Long spine board, strapping system, cervical/head immobilization device
Extremity splints
Face mask removal tools if the sport involves use of a helmet with face mask

CPR cardiopulmonary resuscitation, *OSHA* Occupational Safety and Health Administration

activity areas are supervised should the emergency care provider leave the site to transport the athlete. Any emergency situations in which there is impairment in level of consciousness or in airway, breathing, or circulation (ABCs) or there is neurovascular compromise should be considered a "load and go" situation, and emphasis should be placed on rapid evaluation, treatment, and transportation.

Venue Directions with Map

The EAP should include specific directions to the venue, including the exact street address, cross streets, and any landmarks that may make the site easier for EMS to locate (Fig. 13.3). Ideally, prior to the start of the athletic season, a meeting should be held at the athletic venue site with sports medicine staff members and EMS personnel to familiarize everyone with the exact location and discuss emergency management issues. Plans should be made for ambulance ingress and egress to the site in terms of gates, stadium portals, and so forth. If helicopter transport is a viable option, a landing site should be designated and its GPS coordinates included in the EAP. Host providers should orient visiting health care providers to the venue and discuss emergency procedures prior to the competition. Visiting health care providers should explore the issue of emergency care prior to arrival.

Emergency Care Facilities

In designing the EAP, incorporate the emergency care facilities to which injured individuals will be taken. It is helpful, if possible, to notify emergency receiving facilities in advance of scheduled events and contests. Factors to consider in the selection of the appropriate emergency care facilities include location with respect to venue and level of capabilities. Reviewing the plan with facility staff is helpful. Additionally, in-service training of emergency department physicians and nurses

Emergency Action Plan (EAP): Football Facility and Practice Fields

Revised 7/9/19

Address: 1 Selig Circle Athens, GA 30602 *(cross Streets: Pinecrest & Rutherford)* **GPS Coordinates:** 33.942541,-83.380231

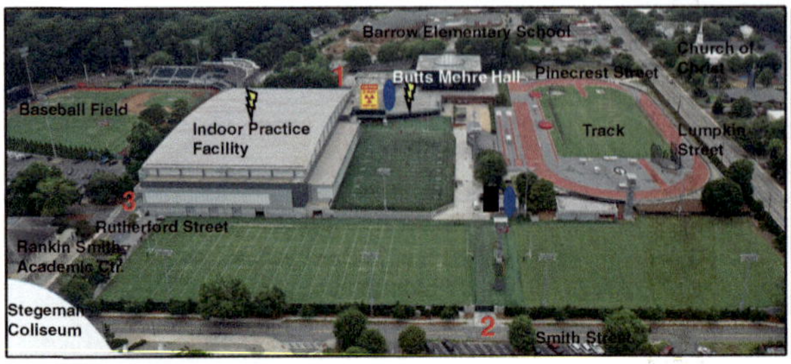

Emergency Action Plan Key

EMS/Flatbed Carts

X-Ray

Cold Immersion Tub

Lightning/Tornado Shelter

Emergency Signal: clenched fist held overhead

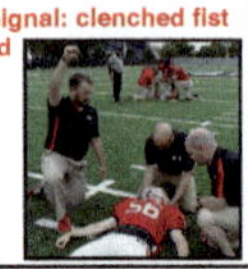

Role of First Responders

1. Immediate care of the injured or ill athlete
2. Activate EMS
   a. Designate individual to call 911
   b. Provide pertinent information: name, location, telephone number, number of injured individuals, condition of the injured, first aid rendered, specific directions, and other information as requested
   c. Notify campus police at (706) 542-2200
3. Retrieve emergency equipment
4. Direct EMS to scene
5. Scene control

Venue Directions

a. **Position 1:** *Butts-Mehre Side Entrance:* designate an individual to open the side door and wait for EMS at **position 1**. If outside of normal business hours, use **911-OK,9111-OK emergency access code**
b. **Position 2:** *Smith Street Gate:* designate an individual to open the gate and wait for EMS to direct to exact location
c. **Position 3:** *Rutherford Gate:* designate individual to the gate on and wait for EMS to direct to exact location

Emergency Personnel

Certified athletic trainers and athletic training student(s) onsite for practice and workouts; physician(s) may be onsite for practice on limited basis

Ron Courson 706-255-7690
Chris Blaszka 908-619-7446
David Jack 801-707-6839
Connor Norman 678-12-1790
Liz Smart 801-682-6047
Drew Willson 269-598-1758
Butts-Mehre athletic training room 706-542-9060

Emergency Equipment

AED, trauma kit, splint bag, and oversized spine board maintained on a motorized cart parked under practice shed during outdoor practices (may be relocated with practice in indoor practice facility). A flatbed cart is additionally available to transport injured athlete(s) from the field if needed. Additional equipment as well as x-ray is accessible in the Butts-Mehre athletic training room. If exertional heat illness is expected, there is an emergency cooling tub and equipment located under practice shed. Emergency cooling may also be performed in the athletic training room hydrotherapy area.

Medical Facilities: Ambulance transports will go to Piedmont Athens Regional Medical Center, a Level II Trauma Center located at 1199 Prince Avenue (main switchboard: 706-475-7000; ED 706-475-3304).

Medical Time Out: A meeting should be conducted with medical staff prior to start of athletic events to go through a pre-athletic checklist reviewing the venue EAP, staff members (roles and locations), discuss communication, location of ambulance and EMS cart, emergency equipment (type and location), designated transport facility, emergency protocols, and any issues that could potentially impact the EAP (i.e. crowd flow, weather, construction.

Fig. 13.3 Venue-specific emergency action plans for both football practice and football game

Emergency Action Plan (EAP): Sanford stadium-football game

Revised 7/9/19

Address: 100 Sanford Drive,Athens, GA30602 **GPS Coordinates:** 33.949937, -83.373388

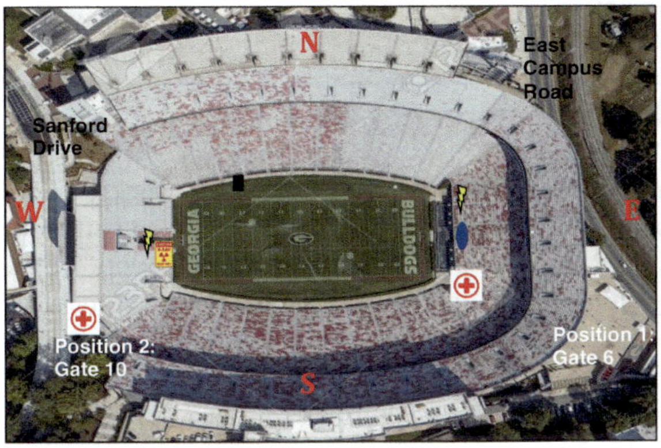

Emergency Action Plan Key

Ambulance

EMS/Flatbed Carts

X-Ray

Cold Immersion Tub

Lightning/Tornado Shelter

Emergency Signal: clenched fist held overhead

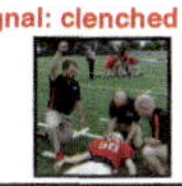

Role of First Responders

1. Immediate care of the injured/ill athlete(s)
2. ActivateEMS(paramedics on both sidelines)
3. retrieve emergency equipment
4. control scene

Venue Directions: Sanford Stadium is located between East Campus Road and Sanford Drive. A dedicated EMSunit for athletics is on site for competition.Two gates provide access to the field.From the Players'Gate (**position 1**) located off of East Campus Road on the southeast side of the stadium, enter through the gate and follow the ramp down to field level. For emergencyaccess when stadium is closed, the **gateaccesscode**is**911-OK,9111-OK**. From Gate 10 (**position 2**) located on the southwest side of the stadium, enter the Tate Student Center parking lot from Lumpkin Street and continue under the Sanford Drive Bridge to fieldevel.

Emergency Personnel

Certifiedathletic trainers, athletic training students, physicians (primary care, orthopedic, internal medicine, vascula neurosurgeon, optometrist), paramedics, and radiological techniciansare on the home sideline. Physician and certifiedathletic trainers are stationed on the visiting sideline. Dentist and maxillofacial surgeon are available on call:

Ron Courson
Chris Blaszka
David Jack
Liz Smart
Drew Willson
Connor Norman
Fred Reifsteck, MD (head team physician)
Glenn Henry (EMS director)
Lovie Tabron (host athletic trainer)
Steve Bryant (host athletic trainer)
Ron Elliott, MD (host physician)

Emergency Equipment: A fully equipped motorized EMS cart with gurney is located on the visitor's sideline. It has an AED, trauma kit, splint bag, and oversized spine board. Additional equipment is accessible from a dedicated National EMS ambulance located in the southeast tunnel. A flatbed cart is additionally available to transport an injured athlete from the field if needed. X-ray is located in the west end zone sports medicine complex. If exertional heat illness is expected, there is an emergency cooling tub and equipmentlocated in the east end zone adjacent to the visiting team locker room.

Medical Facilities: Ambulance transportswill go to Piedmont Athens Regional Medical Center, a Level II Trauma Center locatedat 1199 Prince Avenue (main switchboard: 706-475-7000; ED 706-475-3304).

Medical Time Out: A meeting will be conducted on the field with both medicals staffs prior to start of athletic event to go through a pre-athletic checklist reviewing the venue EAP, introducing staff members (rolesand locations), discuss communication, locationof ambulance and EMS cart, emergency equipment (type and location), designated transport facility, emergency protocols, and any issues that could potentially impact the EAP (i.e. crowd flow, weather, construction).

Fig. 13.3 (continued)

may be beneficial. For example, reviewing emergency football equipment removal on an annual basis prior to the start of football season may help to facilitate proper removal of helmet and shoulder pads in the management of a head or cervical spine injury in the emergency department.

Emergency Action Plan Pocket Emergency Card

Sports medicine health care professionals should consider preparing pocket emergency cards. This index card-sized item can be laminated and carried on person in the event of an emergency. The EAP cards should include the emergency action plan with written directions and highlighted map on one side and the pertinent medical information of participating athletes, such as medical conditions, allergies, and medications, on the other side. Table 13.2 provides an example of pertinent medical information that can be printed on a pocket emergency card.

Table 13.2 Sports medicine: pertinent medical conditions

Athlete A	hx concussion
Athlete B	sickle cell trait
Athlete C	allergic to Septra (sulfa drugs), yellow jackets
Athlete D	hx asthma, hx concussion
Athlete E	hx concussion with LOC, amnesia
Athlete F	hx concussion, catheter ablation, PSVT
Athlete G	heart murmur, concussion
Athlete H	hx concussion, hx heat cramps
Athlete I	hx heat cramps, exertional headaches
Athlete J	allergic to PCN, hx severe heat cramps, hx concussion, endocarditis prophylaxis, heat syncope
Athlete K	sickle cell trait
Athlete L	hx concussion, hx HTN
Athlete M	hx concussion
Athlete N	hx concussion, EIB, endocarditis prophylaxis, hx stingers
Athlete O	hx asthma
Athlete P	hx concussion
Athlete Q	hx asthma
Athlete R	hx concussion
Athlete S	hx heat cramps
Athlete T	allergic to PCN
Athlete U	family hx cardiomyopathy
Athlete V	craniotomy age 10 (blood clot)
Athlete W	exercise-induced headaches, hx heat illness
Athlete X	allergic to sulfa and Ceclor, hx concussion
Athlete Y	hx of heat syncope, hx of concussion, exertional headaches
Athlete Z	hx hypertension, allergic to penicillin, hx concussion, Norvasc, lisinopril

EIB exercise-induced bronchoconstriction, *HTN* hypertension, *hx* history, *LOC* loss of consciousness, *PCN* penicillin, *PSVT* paroxysmal supraventricular tachycardia

Emergency Documentation

A written emergency plan should be reviewed and approved by the team members and institutions involved. If multiple facilities or sites are used, each will require a separate plan. Documentation should encompass the following:

- Who is responsible for documenting the events of the emergency situation
- Follow-up documentation on evaluation of the response to the emergency situation, such as time of injury, treatment start, EMS call, arrival, treatment provided, and departure
- Documentation of periodic rehearsal of the emergency plan
- Documentation of institutional personnel training

When an athletic emergency occurs, post-episode documentation is an important component and should not be neglected. Reasons for documentation include the medico-legal record, continuity of care, quality assurance, organization of thought processes, and research and statistical review. Written documentation of all actions taken during treatment and transport can be very useful in situations in which liability is an issue. It should also be noted that consent is implied during most athletic emergencies.

Rehearsal

Rehearsal of the emergency action plan is an imperative component to improve skills of those involved with carrying out the plan. The rehearsal should attempt to expose deficiencies, so that they can be corrected, and include resources both internal and external to the institution. Literature on memory recall, which involves the searching of the memory stores, suggests that when we recall we produce something learned earlier if it is constantly practiced compared to retrieval cues without constant rehearsal [10, 11]. In brief, continued practice is needed as knowledge quickly deteriorates if not used or updated regularly [10]. This theory can be demonstrated through CPR re-training literature, which suggests there is decay in knowledge as soon as 2 weeks after training up to 18 months, which describes why CPR re-training must be conducted every 2 years [12–14]. The need for this is most easily explained with the well-known school fire drill requirements. Fire drills are strategic plans developed to quickly evacuate a school or building in case of fire or emergency. Fire drills are often conducted once every 1–3 months in schools to ensure that all students and staff know their evacuation routes and assembly points. If you ask people in an organization where their fire drill assembly points are, you will get different results 3 months after a fire drill compared to the day after the fire drill [15].

Catastrophic Incident Guidelines

Catastrophic incident guidelines should be developed in the event of a sudden death or of an injury that results in disability or an alteration of quality of life of a student-athlete, coach, or staff member. A catastrophic incident management team should be developed, along with a checklist of chain of command responsibilities. Although there are many types of catastrophic incidents, not all will require activation of the emergency plan. However, a catastrophic injury/incident plan can be considered a companion document to the emergency plan. This written plan should include both direct and indirect catastrophic athletic injuries and incidents.

Depending on the sport sponsor, sport venue, and nature of the emergency, certain notifications may need to be made; these should be described in the emergency plan. Obviously, in the high school setting, a minor athlete's parents will need to be notified. Depending on the school or system size, the athletic coordinator, principal, and possibly the district superintendent may also need to be notified of the incident.

Notifications at the collegiate level might include the athletic director, one or more deans or vice-presidents, and, in the event of a catastrophic event, possibly the president or CEO of the college or university. The parents, spouse, or other family members of the injured student-athlete may also need to be notified. Travel plans for the parents or spouse of the injured athlete should be considered if distance is a factor. Counseling may need to be made available for students, team members, and the sports medicine team. When there is considerable media interest, the sports information director or other institutional media relations personnel should be included to handle media inquiries. The institutional insurance carrier, risk management office, legal counsel, or a combination of these should also be notified.

The catastrophic injury plan should include the formation of a catastrophic injury team. Obvious members of this team would include the organization's athletic director or coordinator, the head athletic trainer, sports information or media relations personnel, senior administrators, the team physician, and organizational legal counsel. This team will direct all aspects of crisis management, including providing appropriate counseling (athlete, family, and team), releasing information to the media, and documenting the incident. Figure 13.4 provides an example of a catastrophic incident guideline card and emergency contact information card.

Conclusion

It is critically important to properly prepare for athletic emergencies. An athlete's survival may hinge on how well trained and prepared athletic health care providers are. Organizations sponsoring athletic activities invest "ownership" in an EAP by involving athletic administration personnel, sport coaches, and sports medicine personnel. It is important to review the EAP yearly with all athletic personnel, including CPR and first-aid refresher training. Through development and implementation of an emergency action plan, health-care providers help to ensure that athletes will have the best care provided when an emergency situation does arise.

Emergency contact information card

Emer. contact	Department/area	Office	Cell/pager	*After hours*
Jere Morehead	University President			
Teresa Houle	UGAA Travel Coordinator			
Anna Randa	Assoc. AD Sports Medicine			
Will Lawler	Ex. Assoc. AD: Compliance			
Victor Wilson	VP for Student Affairs			
Bill McDonald	Dean of Students			
Ron Courson	Sr. Assoc. AD - Spts Med.			
Stephanie Ransom	Deputy Athletic Dir.			
Claude Felton	Sr. Assoc. AD / SID			
Greg McGarity	Director of Athletics			
Thomas Settles	Chaplain			
Karri Hobson-Pape	University Spokesperson			
Jack Hu	Provost			
Heather Jordaneat	Dir. Of Student Services			
Fred Reifsteck,MD	Head Team Physician			
Charlotte Warren	Counselor			
Michael Raeber	University Legal Affairs			
David Shipley	Faculty Athletics Rep.			
Jeanne Vaughn	UGAA Insurance Coord.			
Amy Thomas	Human Resources Director			
Darrice Griffin	Deputy Director of Athletics			
Dan Silk	Chief of Police			

Crisis management guidelines

Contact Ron Courson/Anna Randa; Fred Reifsteck, MD
- **Work with medical specialists assisting athlete**

Contact UGAAA/UGA administration
- **Greg McGarity, notifiesJere Morehead, Michael Raeber**
- **Darrice Griffin and Will Lawler**
- **Claude Felton, notifies Karri Hobson-Pape**

Designate athletic administrator point person
Contact/update sport staff if not yet familiar with situation
Contact family by appropriate individual (assist as needed):
- **Teresa Houle: travel**
- **Air Med International**

Assign athletic staff member to be with family at all times upon arrival; assist family as needed; protect from outside persons
Involve appropriate counseling/ministerial support
Coordinated media plan
- **No contact with media/comments from athletic training staff, hospital staff or med. personnel except through SID**

Meeting with athletes to discuss situation
- **No outside discussion of meeting with media**

Contact catastrophic/malpractice insurance providers
- **Mercer (Zach Cardoza)**
- **Chartis**
- **NCAA: American Specialty:**
- **Seabury & Smith (malpractice):**

Complete documentation of events from everyone involved in incident
Collect and secure all equipment/materials involved
Construct detailed time line of events related to the incident
Catastrophic incident stress management as necessary for individuals involved in incident

Fig. 13.4 Emergency contact information card

Resources

1. National Athletic Trainers' Association position statement: emergency planning in athletics. Available at: http://www.nata.org/statements/position/emergency-planning.pdf.
2. Inter-Association Task Force recommendations on emergency preparedness and management of sudden cardiac arrest in high school and college athletic programs: a consensus statement. Available at: http://www.nata.org/statements/consensus/SCA_statement.pdf.

References

1. Catastrohpic sports injury research - thirty-fifth annual report (Fall 1982–Spring 2017); 2018.
2. Andersen J, Courson RW, Kleiner DM, McLoda TA. National Athletic Trainers' Association position statement: emergency planning in athletics. J Athl Train. 2002;37:99–104.
3. Assembly FEM. Guide for developing high-quality school emergency operations plans. Philadelphia; 2013.
4. Barishansky RM, O'Connor KE. Best practices in emergency medical services. Clinical response planning–syndromic surveillance. Emerg Med Serv. 2005;34:84–6.
5. Drezner JA, Rao AL, Heistand J, Bloomingdale MK, Harmon KG. Effectiveness of emergency response planning for sudden cardiac arrest in United States high schools with automated external defibrillators. Circulation. 2009;120:518–25.
6. Johnson ST, Norcross MF, Bovbjerg VE, Hoffman MA, Chang E, Koester MC. Sports-related emergency preparedness in Oregon High Schools. Sports Health. 2017;37:1941738116686782–184.
7. Kleinknecht v Gettysburg College, 786 F. Supp. 449 (M.D. Pa. 1992); 1992.
8. National Athletic Trainers' Association official statement on athletic health care provider "time outs" before athletic events; 2012.
9. Denver R Calm is Contagious. https://www.businessinsider.com/former-navy-seal-rorke-denver-leadership-lesson-2017-2.
10. Broomfield R. A quasi-experimental research to investigate the retention of basic cardiopulmonary resuscitation skills and knowledge hy qualified nurses following a course in professional development. J Adv Nurs. 2006;23:1–9.
11. Gross RD. The science of mind and behaviour. Psychology. 1991;29:381–2.
12. Hamilton R. Nurses' knowledge and skill retention following cardiopulmonary resuscitation training: a review of the literature. J Adv Nurs. 2005;51:288–97.
13. Sullivan N. An integrative review: instructional strategies to improve nurses' retention of cardiopulmonary resuscitation priorities. Int J Nurs Educ Scholarsh;12. https://doi.org/10.1515/ijnes-2014-0012.
14. Kaye W, Mancini ME. Retention of cardiopulmonary resuscitation skills by physicians, registered nurses, and the general public. Crit Care Med. 1986;14:620–2.
15. Boyle T. Health and safety: risk management. New York, NY and Abingdon, Oxon: Routledge; 2015.
16. Morrissey J. Research suggests time for change in prehospital spinal immobilization. J Emerg Med Serv. Published on jems.com March 19, 2013. https://www.jems.com/2013/03/19/research-suggests-time-change-prehospita/.
17. Position Statement: EMS spinal precautions and the use of the long backboard. National Association of EMS Physicians and American College of Surgeons Committee on Trauma. Prehosp Emerg Care. 2014;18(2):392.

18. White CC, Domeier RM, Millin MG. Resource document: EMS spinal precautions and the use of the long backboard – resource document to the position statement of the National Association of EMS Physicians and American College of Surgeons Committee on Trauma. Prehosp Emerg Care. 2014;18(2):306–14.
19. Zahir U, Ludwig SC. Sports-related cervical spine injuries: On Field Assessment and Managment. Seminars in Spine Surgery. 2010;22(4):173-180. https://doi.org/10.1053/j.semss.2010.06.012.
20. Hauswald M. A re-conceptualisation of acute spinal care. Emerg Med J. 2013;230(9):720–3.
21. Bailes JE, et al. Management of cervical spine injuries in athletes. J Athl Train. 2007;42(1):126–34.
22. Waninger KN. Management of the helmeted athlete with suspected cervical spine injury. Am J Sports Med. 2004;32(5):1331–50.
23. Kleiner DM et al. Prehospital care of the spine-injured athlete. A document from the Inter-Association Task Force for appropriate care of the spine-injured athlete. National Athletic Trainers' Association; 1998
24. Dahl MC, et al. Helmet and shoulder pad removal in football players with unstable cervical spine injuries. J Appl Biomech. 2009;25:119–32.
25. Official statement: EMS changes to pre-hospital care of the athlete with acute cervical spine injury. National Athletic Trainers' Association; 2014.
26. Ellis J, Courson R, Daniels B. Spinal trauma: on field management of sports injuries. Curr Rev Musculoskelet Med. 2014;7(4):381–6.
27. Swartz EE, et al. National athletic trainers' association position statement: acute management of the cervical spine-injured athlete. J Athl Train. 2009;44(3):306–11.

Heat Illness in Football

14

Michael Seth Smith, Douglas Casa, Rebecca Stearns, Erica Filep, and Brad Endres

Epidemiology of Exertional Heat Illnesses in Football

Exertional heat illnesses (EHIs) include multiple types of heat-related injuries including exercise-associated muscle cramps, heat syncope, heat exhaustion, and exertional heat stroke (EHS), the most severe of the EHIs [1]. EHIs are common among athletes, laborers, and warfighters. Regarding football, EHI occurs across all levels of sport. EHI rates for youth, high school, and collegiate football were 1.82, 0.57, and 1.67 per 10,000 athlete-exposures (AE) (i.e., one student-athlete participating in one practice or one competition), respectively [2]. Across all levels of football, rates were highest during the preseason (youth: 2.76; high school: 1.47; college: 3.66 per 10,000 AE) [2]. Further research has shown that collegiate football student-athletes are nearly six times more likely to experience an EHI during preseason practice than all other time periods [3]. When compared to other sports, football has been shown to have the highest rate of EHI at the high school and collegiate levels [4]. In the high school setting, football has an overall EHI incidence rate of 4.42 per 100,000 AE, which is 11.4 times that in all other sports combined [5]. In the collegiate setting, football has an overall EHI incidence rate of 1.55 per 10,000 AE during the 2009–2010 through 2014–2015 academic years [3]. Regarding EHS in football, four cases were reported at the high school and collegiate levels in the United States during the 2016–2017 academic year, and three of these were fatal [6].

M. S. Smith (✉)
University of Florida, Department of Orthopedics/Rehabilitation, Division of Sports Medicine, Gainesville, FL, USA
e-mail: smithms@ortho.ufl.edu

D. Casa · R. Stearns · E. Filep · B. Endres
Korey Stringer Institute, University of Connecticut, Storrs, CT, USA

K. W. Farmer (ed.), *Football Injuries*,
https://doi.org/10.1007/978-3-030-54875-9_14

Prevention of EHI

When highlighting the ways in which to prevent EHI, it is prudent to first discuss the predisposing factors that can lead to EHI. These predisposing factors have long been established in the literature. As early as the 1960s, Minard suggested a paradigm to describe the predisposing factors of EHS [7]. These factors were divided into three groups: (1) host factors, (2) environmental factors, and (3) organizational factors [7, 8]. Host factors include physiologic limiting factors such as recent illness, inadequate physical fitness, improper acclimatization to the surrounding environment, and lack of sleep. Environmental factors include the environmental heat load at the place of activity. Environmental heat load is comprised of ambient temperature, humidity, and solar radiation. These environmental factors are described in the following heat balance equation [1]:

$$S = M(\pm \text{work}) - E \pm R \pm C \pm K,$$

where S is the amount of stored heat, M is the heat produced via metabolism, E is the heat loss due to evaporation, R is the heat gained or lost via radiation, C is the heat gained or lost via convection, and K is the heat gained or lost via conduction. Metabolic heat produced by the body at rest (basal metabolic rate) is approximately 60 kcal/hour to 70 kcal/hour in the average adult [9]. During exercise, metabolic heat produced may approach 1000 kcal/hour [9]. Organizational factors include regulations regarding work-rest cycles, rehydration regimens, exercise intensity, and training schedules. Further research has expanded the understanding of the predisposing factors of EHI and EHS into non-modifiable and modifiable intrinsic or extrinsic factors. Figure 14.1 displays the predisposing factors of EHI and EHS on a Cartesian coordinate graph [10].

As evident from the Fig. 14.1, some factors are "flexible" to a certain degree. For example, individuals can affect their levels of hydration by the amount of water they plan to drink (intrinsic factor), but they may not have the ability to do so if a water source is not available due to an organizational policy or procedure (extrinsic factor). Furthermore, some of these factors are flexible in the amount they can be modified. For example, clothing, equipment, and training intensity can all be modified by the individual if they are allowed to do so. However, in some settings, organizational policies or procedures are established in a manner that limits the extent to which these factors may be modified during sports participation, occupational work, or military training.

In order to decrease the incidence of EHI and EHS, governing bodies of athletic institutions have sought to implement activity modification policies and procedures that would address these risk factors. In 2003, the National Collegiate Athletic Association (NCAA) mandated that member schools utilize heat acclimatization guidelines during all preseason, August football practices. Prior to the 2003 guidelines, an average of 1–2 NCAA football student-athletes died each year due to EHS [11]. Since the policy, only one August EHS-related death has been reported in NCAA football [12]. A similar trend has occurred after 2009 in the high school

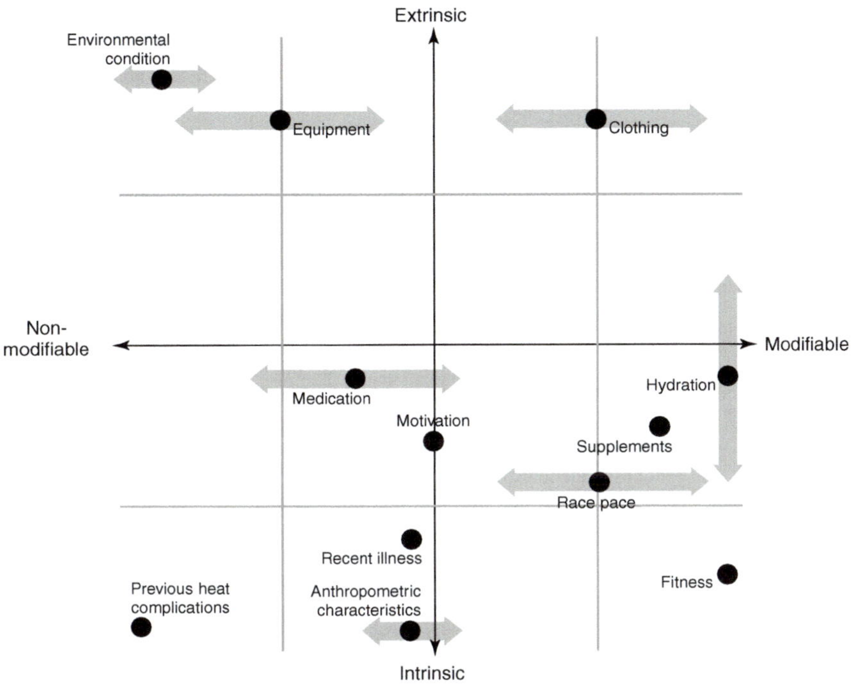

Fig. 14.1 Predisposing factors of exertional heat illness (EHI) and exertional heat stroke (EHS). Horizontal axis weighs whether the factor is modifiable (+) or non-modifiable (−). Vertical axis weighs whether the factor is influenced by an extrinsic (+) or an intrinsic variable (−). Gray band indicates the flexibility of the factor

setting. In 15 states whose high school athletic associations adopted 2009 preseason heat acclimatization guidelines for high school football, no student-athletes died from EHS when the mandated guidelines were followed [12, 13]. More recent evidence suggests that the implementation of best practice heat safety policies in preseason football practice has been associated with a 55% reduction in EHI rates [14]. Table 14.1 compares the NCAA and high school preseason heat acclimatization policies. Clearly, organizational policies and procedures aimed at improving the safety of athletes do have an effect on decreasing the incidence of EHI and EHS.

EHI Recognition and Treatment

As previously stated, EHI is a broad term that describes a group of clinical conditions including exercise-associated muscle cramps (EAMCs), heat syncope, heat exhaustion, and EHS [1, 3, 15] (Table 14.2). While not strictly defined as a type of exertional heat illness, exercise-associated hyponatremia (EAH) can occur with excessive hydration and has signs and symptoms that may be confused with EHI and must remain on the differential diagnosis when considering EHI [16]. EHS is

Table 14.1 Comparison of NCAA and high school heat acclimatization policies

	NCAA (2003)	High school (2009)
Length of acclimatization period	5-day acclimatization period	14-day acclimatization period
Equipment allowed during acclimatization	Days 1 & 2: Helmets only Days 3 & 4: Helmets and shoulder pads Days 5+: All equipment	Days 1 & 2: Helmets only Days 3–5: Helmets and shoulder pads Days 6+: All equipment
Single-practice days	Practice time should not exceed 3 hours	Practice time should not exceed 3 hours A 1-hour walkthrough is allowed if practice is separated by at least 3 hours
Double-practice days	May have a 1-hour testing session and a 2-hour practice on one of the 5 days 3 hours of recovery must separate the two sessions	Only on days 6+ Must be followed by a single-practice day Must be separated by 3 hours of rest Neither practice should be longer than 3 hours Total practice time should not be longer than 5 hours
Missed day policy	All athletes must complete the heat acclimatization period regardless of arrival to preseason practice	Days on which athletes do not practice, either individually or team-wide, do not count to the 14 days
Drills allowed during practice		Football may use tackling dummies and blocking sleds on days 3+ Live contact drills may begin on days 6+
Medical coverage		Athletic trainer recommended to be on site

the most severe type of EHI and will be discussed in a separate section, while the recognition and treatment of the less severe forms of EHI and EAH will be discussed here.

Exercise-Associated Muscle Cramps

Exercise-associated muscle cramps (EAMCs) are acute, painful, involuntary contractions of skeletal muscles that are associated with exercise and are the most common form of EHI that occurs in athletes [15, 17]. While exercise-associated muscle cramps are classified as an exertional heat illness, they are not directly related to an

Table 14.2 Exertional heat illnesses/exercise-associated hyponatremia [1, 15, 23]

Condition	Definition, signs, and symptoms
Exercise-associated muscle cramps (EAMCs)	Present as acute, painful, involuntary muscle contractions Patient is usually hypohydrated, thirsty, sweating, fatigued Thought to be caused by fluid losses, electrolyte imbalances, fatigue, or a combination of these factors Treatment includes rest, passive stretching, ice and massage to affected muscle, and rehydration
Heat syncope	Orthostatic dizziness associated with peripheral vasodilation, postural blood pooling, diminished venous return, decreased cardiac output, and cerebral ischemia Occurs during periods of acclimatization (before plasma volume expansion) Presents immediately after stopping activity and standing (i.e., breaking immediately after a sprint) Patient is usually hypohydrated, fatigued, and has diminished pulse Patient will complain of tunnel vision, lightheadedness, or will faint/collapse with immediate response Treatment includes moving the athlete to a shaded area, elevating the legs above heart level, and rehydration
Exertional heat exhaustion	Usually occurs in hot, humid conditions when a patient experiences heavy sweating, hypohydration, sodium losses, and energy losses Difficult to differentiate with exertional heat stroke without assessing rectal temperature, in that the patient may present with early onset of altered mental status May present with weakness, fainting, dizziness, headache, hyperventilation, nausea, diarrhea, intestinal cramping or persistent muscle cramping, decreased urine output, and mild hyperthermia (range = 36 °C [97 °F] to 40.5 °C [105 °F]) Treatment consists of removal of excess equipment/clothing, initiation of cooling, rehydration, and close monitoring of vital signs

(continued)

Table 14.2 (continued)

Condition	Definition, signs, and symptoms
Exertional heat stroke Usually occurs in hot, humid conditions and presents with elevated core body temperature (usually >40 °C [104 °F]) and altered mental status Results from excessive heat production or inhibited heat loss Presents with tachycardia, hypohydration, hypotension, sweating, hyperventilation, vomiting, diarrhea, dizziness, drowsiness, irrational behavior, confusion, irritability, emotional instability, hysteria, apathy, aggressiveness, delirium, disorientation, staggering, seizures, loss of consciousness, and coma Results in organ system failure when immediate whole body cooling is not used to return core temperature to near normal temperatures	Usually occurs in hot, humid conditions and presents with elevated core body temperature obtained rectally (>40.5 °C [105 °F]) and CNS dysfunction Results from excessive heat production or inhibited heat loss Presents with tachycardia, hypohydration, hypotension, sweating, hyperventilation, vomiting, diarrhea, dizziness, drowsiness, irrational behavior, confusion, irritability, emotional instability, hysteria, apathy, aggressiveness, delirium, disorientation, staggering, seizures, loss of consciousness, and coma Results in organ system failure when immediate whole body cooling is not used to return core temperature to near normal temperatures
Exercise-associated hyponatremia (EAH)	May present similarly to EHI with lightheadedness, dizziness, nausea and vomiting, and mental status changes Serum sodium level of less than 135 mg/dL. Typically seen when athletes drink beyond sweat losses Can lead to coma and death if not recognized and treated promptly Treatment consists of fluid restriction and salt-containing foods for mild cases and intravenous hypertonic saline and emergency transport for severe cases

Adapted from: Tripp et al. [15]. Copyright © 2015 The Authors. Reprinted by permission of SAGE Publications, Inc

elevated body temperature but likely due to multiple factors including loss of sodium and/or potassium, neuromuscular fatigue, and dehydration [1, 18]. The signs and symptoms initially begin as muscle twitches, tics, or contractions and then progress to more widespread muscle spasms often affecting the lower extremities more than the upper extremities. Treatment of EAMCs should always include rest and passive stretching of the cramping muscle until pain improves [1, 19]. Ice and massage of the affected muscles can also be considered. Rehydration is encouraged including replacement of sodium that may have been lost due to heavy sweating. It should be noted that oral hydration is the recommended form of rehydration unless oral fluids cannot be tolerated or fluid-electrolyte losses exceed intake of fluids [16]. It is important to note that other medical conditions, particularly sickle cell trait in athletes, can present with similar symptoms and should be considered when treating athletes with presumed EAMCs.

Heat Syncope

Heat syncope is a syncopal event or near-syncopal event that can be associated with lightheadedness, dizziness, or tunnel vision that occurs with prolonged standing in the heat or immediately after completing a significant workout [15, 20]. This happens due to an abrupt decrease in venous return associated with peripheral vasodilation and postural blood pooling in the extremities [21]. Heat syncope typically is seen during the acclimatization period before plasma volume expansion and cardiovascular adaptations have occurred [15]. It is imperative that other more emergent conditions (cardiac etiologies, hypoglycemia, etc.) with similar signs and symptoms be ruled out first as heat syncope is a diagnosis of exclusion [20]. After heat syncope has been appropriately diagnosed, treatment includes moving the athlete to a shaded area, elevating the legs above heart level to facilitate venous return, and rehydrating the athlete. If athletes with heat syncope do not recover within 20 minutes, emergent evaluation should occur promptly [21].

Exertional Heat Exhaustion

Exertional heat exhaustion is the inability to continue physical activity in the heat due to a combination of factors including inappropriate cardiac output, hypotension, and lack of energy [1, 18]. Signs and symptoms of heat exhaustion include visible difficulties with exercise, weakness, fainting, dizziness, nausea, and muscle cramping [15]. Athletes with heat exhaustion have an elevated core body temperature but it does not exceed 40.5 °C (105 °F) [1]. Furthermore, significant central nervous system (CNS) dysfunction (combativeness, confusion, altered consciousness, seizures) and signs/symptoms of end organ damage (renal or hepatic injury, rhabdomyolysis) should not be present [1, 15]. Risk factors for heat exhaustion are similar to those for other EHIs and include dehydration, lack of acclimatization, excess clothing/equipment, and increased body mass index [22]. Treatment begins by removing any equipment and extra clothing to enhance evaporative cooling while moving the athlete to a shaded/cooler area. Rehydration and cooling should be started immediately and vital signs, including a rectal temperature to evaluate for EHS, should be obtained. If EHS is not diagnosed on initial assessment, cooling should continue but aggressive methods such as cold water immersion or tarp-assisted cooling with oscillation (TACO) are not required unless the athlete's clinical picture worsens and EHS is more likely [19]. Athletes with heat exhaustion should be continuously monitored and re-evaluated until complete recovery. Emergency medical services (EMS) should be activated immediately if resolution has not occurred within 30 minutes of initiation of treatment or the athlete decompensates during appropriate treatment [1].

Exercise-Associated Hyponatremia

Exercise-associated hyponatremia (EAH) is a potentially fatal condition that is defined by a serum sodium level of less than 135 mg/dL [19]. EAH typically occurs in athletes who drink beyond sweat losses [19, 23]. Signs and symptoms of EAH are similar to those of EHI and can include lightheadedness, dizziness, nausea and vomiting, headache, confusion, and mental status changes [23]. EAH should be considered in any athlete who develops mental status changes, particularly those who have been exercising for a prolonged amount of time or endurance athletes, as failure to recognize and treat can possibly lead to coma and death [23]. Mild symptoms may be treated with fluid restriction and salt-containing foods while more severe symptoms require intravenous administration of a hypertonic saline solution and emergent hospital transport [19, 23].

Return to Play Following EHI/EAH (Excluding EHS)

Validated return to play guidelines for EHI do not currently exist. Therefore, decisions for guiding return to play (RTP) after an athlete has suffered an EHI should be individualized on a case-by-case basis assuring that the athlete's safety is the top priority [24]. Return to play activities should occur under the direct supervision of a sports medicine provider (i.e., athletic trainer (AT), sports medicine physician). "Common sense" recommendations for returning any athlete back to activity after suffering an EHI include ensuring that the athlete is asymptomatic with all laboratory and radiological studies returning to normal [25]. After other similar conditions have been ruled out and EAMCs have been appropriately diagnosed, athletes should be closely monitored until the signs and symptoms resolve. Once this occurs, most athletes can return to activities on the same day as symptoms allow [20]. Athletes who have experienced heat syncope can also return to activities as tolerated once other more critical causes of syncope have been excluded [1, 20]. Unlike EAMCs and heat syncope, current recommendations suggest that athletes who have been diagnosed with heat exhaustion should not return to play on the same day [1]. It is believed that an athlete's vulnerability to heat stress is increased when exposure to high wet bulb globe temperatures (WBGTs) occurred on the previous day and that being treated for heat exhaustion potentially increases one's risk of suffering EHS on the following day [20, 26]. Given these concerns, a thorough evaluation of any potential risk factors for exertional heat exhaustion should occur and the athlete should be allowed to gradually return to activities as tolerated under appropriate supervision by a sports medicine provider [27]. Return to play recommendations after EAH should focus on identifying risk factors, providing athlete education including appropriate hydration, confirming normalization of laboratory values, and ensuring that the patient is asymptomatic prior to providing clearance to return to athletics [20].

Exertional Heat Stroke

Exertional heat stroke (EHS) is defined by central nervous system (CNS) dysfunction and core body temperature of 40.5 °C (105 °F) [1]. Not to be confused with classic heat stroke, the onset of EHS is related to high-intensity or long-duration physical activity [1]. Physical environment, fitness level of an individual, previous history of EHS, type of intensity, and physical activity are factors that can contribute to EHS [1, 28]. Increased body mass index, lack of heat acclimation, and recent illnesses can predispose an individual to EHS [1]. The appearance of signs and symptoms of EHS should initiate the following three steps: (1) rapid recognition of EHS, (2) quick and effective cooling, and (3) advanced medical care.

Rapid Recognition

EHS is completely survivable with no long-term complications with proper recognition and treatment [1, 29, 30]. Quick recognition of the signs and symptoms of EHS is critically important to the survival of an athlete (Table 14.3). Misdiagnosis or failure to provide care within the first 30 minutes of an EHS event can prove fatal [1, 28, 30, 31]. CNS dysfunction (described above) and elevated core body temperature above 40.5 °C (105 °F) are the two hallmark diagnostic criteria for EHS. Environmental factors such as wet bulb globe temperature (WBGT) above 30 °C and increased relative humidity reduce the body's ability to dissipate heat and evaporate sweat [1]. This imbalance of heat production can be dangerous and affect individuals who have risk factors for EHS.

Quick and Effective Cooling

It is critical to cool the athlete prior to transferring care to the emergency department (ED). While emergency medical services should be initiated according to one's emergency action plan (EAP), it is vital to keep cooling the athlete on-site prior to transfer to the hospital. Cooling interventions that have a cooling rate between 0.10 °C/min and 0.35 °C/min are preferred when treating EHS [32, 33]. Cold-water immersion (CWI) is the gold standard of treatment for EHS cases. In a case series with 274 patients, the average cooling rate using CWI was 0.22°C/min [34]. CWI cooling rates have also been documented up to 0.38°C/min and can be achieved via low-cost methods by utilizing stock tanks, commercial tubs, and inflatable pools [35]. Ice towels with air circulation and ice bag massage with continuous water dousing can provide decent cooling (cooling rate of 0.14°C/min) if CWI is not available [36, 37]. Another inexpensive option is a tarp from a local home improvement store. For football programs located in a rural area or areas with diminished access to EMS, tarps can also provide adequate cooling in an EHS emergency.

Table 14.3 Recognition and treatment of exertional heat stroke [1, 29, 38, 40]

Recognition	Treatment
Central nervous system dysfunction Collapse, syncope Unresponsiveness Rapid change in demeanor Combative Emotional Slurring words Inability to follow directions Loss of balance Possible lucid interval Rapid deterioration of symptoms	Activate emergency action plan for environmental stress Remove athlete from direct sun and prepare cooling intervention Activate emergency medical services Obtain core body temperature with a valid device Utilize coaches and other athletes to assist in lifting the athlete into the cooling modality Direct other personnel to obtain emergency contact information for the athlete
Valid core temperature assessment devices Rectal thermistor Gastrointestinal (GI) transmitter Esophageal thermistor (laboratory use)	Cold-water immersion Covering torso as much as possible with water circulation Water circulation introduces cooler water to the skin while moving water already warmed by the body Tarp-assisted cooling with oscillation (TACO) method [38] Ice towels with air circulation Ice bag massage with water dousing [33, 37]
Core body temperature diagnostic criteria At or above 40.5 °C (105 °F)	During treatment Reduce core body temperature to 39 °C (102 °F) within 30 minutes of collapse [1, 28] Monitor core body temperature throughout duration of treatment Record other vital signs such as pulse and blood pressure
Heat acclimation and hydration Wet bulb globe temperature (WBGT) conditions Increased relative humidity % Previous exposure to environment Urine specific gravity above 1.020 or dark-colored urine	Post-treatment/transfer to emergency department Cooling procedures completed on-site and before transfer to emergency department Communication with EMS and follow-up with the athlete post event
Previous medical history Recent illness Influenza/cold, fever, infection Previous EHS episode Medications affecting metabolic rate or medications for ADHD	

Ten-gallon coolers filled with ice and water, a tarp, and/or the use of a golf cart type vehicle with a flatbed can effectively cool someone experiencing EHS. The tarp-assisted cooling with oscillation (TACO) method has documented cooling rates of 0.14–0.17 °C/min in hyperthermic individuals [38]. Access to ice and water, tub, tarp, and ice towels can help efficiently treat an athlete in an EHS event.

Advanced Medical Care

Access to advanced medical care should be established in the athletics EAP. Once the athlete has been properly cooled to 38.5 °C (102 °F), transfer to ED should take place. Fatalities and complications from EHS occur due to delayed treatment and cooling [1, 28]. Liver and kidney function are heavily affected by hyperthermia [1]. The longer an individual is hyperthermic, the greater the damage to these organs [39]. The majority of ambulances and EDs do not have the space to utilize CWI nor a tub in which to perform CWI [29]. This is an important factor when designing an EAP for EHS. If the athlete has not been properly cooled before arrival to the ED, their core body temperature will remain hyperthermic and they will most likely suffer secondary injuries or death from EHS.

Implications for Practice in the Athletic Setting

It is not enough to know the signs and symptoms of EHS. Proper recognition, quick reduction in core body temperature, and access to advanced medical care are vital in an EHS emergency. All athletics personnel should be educated on EHS, plan and design an area to cool an athlete, and refer to the ED once cooling has ceased. If all three of these steps are followed, EHS is 100% survivable [1] (Fig. 14.2).

Return to Play Following Exertional Heat Stroke

The successful treatment of EHS has been clearly outlined and supported by substantial, high-quality research studies. However, the process of returning individuals who have survived EHS to play is much more ambiguous. A gap in evidence that outlines the best approach exists due to the inability to systematically research this topic in a human population. Additionally, the relatively low occurrence of EHS compared to other catastrophic injuries limits the cases available for evaluation.

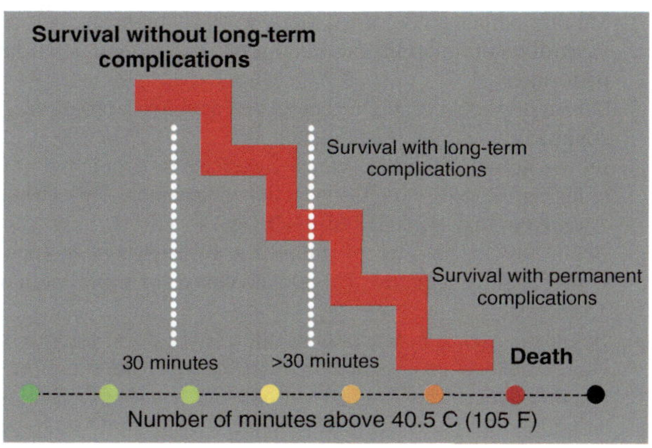

Fig. 14.2 Survival outcomes and length of time with elevated core body temperature

However, recovery and therefore return decisions are vastly less complicated when appropriate and immediate care is provided. The return to activity and recovery process becomes extremely varied for EHS cases when CWI is not promptly utilized, allowing a greater exposure to body temperatures above the critical threshold for cell damage.

Immediately following an EHS, blood markers should be used to monitor organ function and are viewed as functional indicators of recovery status. Unfortunately, today's current biomarkers are not diagnostic tools and therefore remain as supporting values to aid in determining progression back to activity. Traditional markers include those related to liver function (aspartate aminotransferase [AST], alanine aminotransferase [ALT], kidney function (blood urea nitrogen [BUN]) and muscle damage, most notably creatine kinase (CK). It is important to note that these markers are not necessarily specific to EHS as they may also be altered by a variety of conditions or factors [41]. Current recommendations call for these biomarkers to return to normal values, followed by a progressive return to activity [41]. It is important to highlight that throughout this recovery period, an athlete is being evaluated for his or her potential to continue forward in the recovery progression or whether additional time/re-evaluation is needed. Only once the athlete has demonstrated the ability to perform high-intensity exercise under stressful conditions similar to those that they are expected to perform in, should a final decision regarding their clearance to return to activity be made. Currently, consensus remains that the progression outlined in Table 14.4 is the best approach for the assessment of an individual's ability to return to activity following EHS [1, 22, 42].

Ideally, body temperature (either via rectal or gastrointestinal temperature) should be monitored during the initial return to exercise and during the initial 7–14 exposures to exercise in warm to hot environments. This allows complete confirmation that the athlete is participating within safe limits of their body temperature. Progression may be halted due to an inability to thermoregulate (specifically if body temperature approaches 105 °F, especially during non-strenuous exercise), reoccurrence of symptoms, and/or an inability to recover from a previous day's training

Table 14.4 Return to activity progression following an exertional heat stroke

1. Monitor athlete until normal blood work is obtained
2. Regardless of timeframe needed for #1, wait at least 7–21 days before any activity is performed
3. Obtain physician clearance before any activity or progression for return to activity starts in conjunction with the first two bullets
4. Initiate activity with low-intensity exercise in a cool environment to progressively increase to higher intensity exercise in a cool environment This should consist of a minimum of 1 week but may typically take 1–3 weeks
5. Begin exercise progression within a warm environment once exercise in a cool environment is successfully achieved. This should consist of a minimum of 1 week but may take 1–3 weeks
6. Begin a period of heat acclimatization (7–14 days) prior to full return to activity
7. Have a medical professional monitor for signs and symptoms of exertional heat illness or whether athlete may need a heat tolerance test (HTT). Stall or halt progression if the athlete struggles or expresses difficulty in recovering from exercise sessions

All timeframes are approximate and can vary greatly depending on the individual's case session. Providing the athlete more time or slowing the rate of exercise progression should be done to determine if the athlete simply needs additional recovery time or further evaluation. In an ideal scenario, the most optimal outcome from EHS would result in an athlete beginning their return to play (RTP) progression about 2 weeks after the initial EHS insult with full return to activity about 4–6 weeks after the EHS. However, many cases, especially those that are not treated aggressively or appropriately, may have an elongated return time of up to several months to 1–2 years.

If an athlete fails to progress, has symptoms of heat illness, is unable to regulate body temperature and maintain it below 105 °F, or is struggling to handle a slow reintroduction of exercise sessions, a heat tolerance test (HTT) should be considered. Two other circumstances exist where a HTT should be automatically performed as part of the RTP process. First, if the individual has not received the standard of care for EHS (if the individual was not completely cooled to a rectal temperature of 102 °F or lower within 30 minutes of the onset of EHS), a HTT should be performed prior to any exercise with heat exposure. Second, a HTT should also be performed when the person has had a previous episode of EHS as this could suggest incomplete recovery from the previous EHS or other underlying pathology (i.e., malignant hyperthermia) [43, 44].

The HTT has been a highly successful tool that was originally developed within the Israeli Defense Force military to determine if a soldier is prepared to return to duty [45, 46] (Table 14.5).

Table 14.5 Israeli Defense Force Heat Tolerance Test Protocol with suggested athlete-specific considerations—if applicable

Israeli Defense Force HTT	Athlete-specific alterations
Individual's core (rectal) temperature must be below 37.5 °C (99.5 °F) to start	None
Walks on treadmill for 120 minutes at 5 km/h with 2% incline	None
Environment is controlled to maintain 40 °C (104 °F) and 40% relative humidity	None
Individuals are instructed to avoid tobacco, alcohol, and caffeine prior to the test	None
Individuals are instructed to sleep at least 7 hours the night before and drink 0.5 L of water the hour before the test	None
Heat intolerance is determined when core body temperature elevates above 38.5 °C (101.3 °F), heart rate elevates above 150 bpm, or when either does not plateau. (8) Core temperature plateau is defined as an increase no more than 0.45 °C during the second hour of the test [47]	Suggest prioritizing body temperature above heart rate measures due to great variability in athlete demographics
If response is abnormal, soldier is scheduled for a second test 1–3 months later	If test results are abnormal, consider modifiable factors that can be safely addressed over 1–3 months (i.e., fitness in cool weather) and consider retesting at that time

HTT heat tolerance test, *BPM* beats per minute

Table 14.6 Potential risk factors for recovering heat stroke victims that should be considered for determining future participation in sport and when interpreting heat tolerance test results

Modifiable risk factors	Non-modifiable risk factors
Fitness/aerobic capacity[a]	History of exertional heat stroke
Acclimatization status[a]	Potential genetic risk factors (i.e., malignant hyperthermia)
Body fat[a]	Diabetes mellitus
Concurrent infectious disease	Age
Dehydration	
Fatigue and or sleep deprivation	
Drugs/dietary supplements	

[a]Indicates that these have been shown to be significant predictors in heat tolerance testing success [45, 47, 49–55]

If the second test is abnormal, the soldier is defined as heat-intolerant and cannot continue combat military service, but may serve in other capacities.

Recently, a publication by Shermann [48] demonstrated that HTT had a specificity of 77.7%, suggesting that a negative test is a strong indicator for successful return to the military without further EHS incidents. A successful HTT should be a tool that is incorporated into a larger decision-making process that considers other factors impacting an individual's ability to return to a pre-EHS lifestyle (Table 14.6).

The HTT does not account for modifiable factors such as aerobic capacity, training, acclimatization status, or body fat, which have all been demonstrated as significant predictors of HTT outcomes [49, 50]. Therefore, the status of each of these items must be assessed at the time of the HTT to determine if further improvement may be possible via these modifiable factors. This also provides justification for allowing the athlete time to gain back an aerobic fitness base in cooler environments prior to attempting the HTT.

While there is no sport-specific HTT, standard HTT does serve as a functional test to assess a person's ability to handle low-intensity exercise in the heat within that given moment. Standard HTT still provides a good starting point within the athletic population for early identification of individuals who undoubtedly should not return to sport if they are unable to pass the HTT. These individuals should also be assessed for modifiable risk factors (fitness, acclimatization status, and body fat) to determine if there is room for improvement via one of these factors. If so, a second test may be deemed appropriate in ~2–3 months after the athlete has had time to address these modifiable risk factors. While there is no guarantee for athletes who pass the HTT, they should continue their progression forward with close monitoring by the medical staff until they are able to demonstrate appropriate physiological responses to the demands of their sport. As noted above, athletes should be monitored during the initial weeks of returning to activity and demonstrate a successful full return to normal practices before tapering active medical monitoring.

When determining an individual's ability to return to activity, it will be important to determine the cause and prognosis of an individual who has had an EHS. Unfortunately, at this point, it is not clear which particular biological markers can be used to identify recovery or future risk for EHS, and the same holds true with regard to the diagnostic feasibility of the HTT. Data to assess future risk for subsequent heat illness are still emerging and no evidence can definitively outline one's risk following EHS. However, current best practices combine the use of blood biomarkers, overall clinical picture, results of an HTT, and ability to successfully complete a progressive return protocol to determine if an athlete should return to play.

References

1. Casa DJ, DeMartini JK, Bergeron MF, et al. National Athletic Trainers' Association position statement: exertional heat illnesses. J Athl Train. 2015;50(9):986–1000.
2. Yeargin SW, Kerr ZY, Casa DJ, et al. Epidemiology of exertional heat illnesses in youth, high school, and college football. Med Sci Sports Exerc. 2016;48(8):1523–9.
3. Yeargin SW, Dompier TP, Casa DJ, et al. Epidemiology of exertional heat illnesses in National Collegiate Athletic Association athletes during the 2009-2010 through 2014-2015 academic years. J Athl Train. 2019;54(1):55–63.
4. Yard EE, Gilchrist J, Haileyesus T, et al. Heat illness among high school athletes – United States, 2005-2009. J Saf Res. 2010;41:471–4.
5. Kerr ZY, Casa DJ, Marshall SW. Epidemiology of exertional heat illness among U.S. high school athletes. Am J Prev Med. 2013;44(1):8–14.
6. Yau RK, Kucera KL, Cox-Thomas L, et al. National Center for Catastrophic Sport Injury Research: Thirty-fifth annual report Fall 1982-Spring 2017. National Center for Catastrophic Sport Injury Research, Chapel Hill, NC. 2018.
7. Minard D. Prevention of heat casualties in Marine Corps recruits. Period of 1955-1960, with comparative incidence rates and climatic heat stresses in other training categories. Mil Med. 1961;126:261–72.
8. Rav Acha M. Fatal exertional heat stroke: a case series. Am J Med Sci. 2004;328(2):84–7.
9. Armstrong LE. Exertional heat illnesses. Champaign: Human Kinetics; 2003.
10. Hosokawa Y. Physiological, behavorial, and knowledge assessment of Runner's readiness to perform in the heat. Doctoral Dissertations. 2016.
11. Boden BP, Breit I, Beachler JA, et al. Fatalities in high school and college football players. Am J Sports Med. 2013;41:1108–16.
12. Adams WM, Casa DJ, Drezner JA. Sport safety policy changes: saving lives and protecting athletes. J Athl Train. 2016;51:358–60.
13. Casa DJ, Csillan D. Preseason heat-acclimatization guidelines for secondary school athletics. J Athl Train. 2009;44(3):332–3.
14. Kerr ZY, Register-Mihalik JK, Pryor RR, et al. The association between mandated preseason heat acclimatization guidelines and exertional heat illness during preseason high school American football practices. Environ Health Perspect. 2019;127(4):1–6.
15. Tripp BL, Eberman LE, Smith MS. Exertional heat illnesses and environmental conditions during high school football practices. Am J Sports Med. 2015;43(10):2490–5. https://doi.org/10.1177/0363546515593947.
16. McDermott BP, Anderson SA, Armstrong LE, et al. National Athletic Trainer's Association position statement: fluid replacement for the physically active. J Athl Train. 2017;52(9):877–95.
17. Bergeron MF. Muscle cramps during exercise - is it fatigue or electrolyte deficit? Curr Sports Med Rep. 2008;7(4):S50–5.
18. Smith MS, Prine BR, Smith KB. Current concepts in the management of exertional heat stroke in athletes. Curr Orthop Pract. 2015;26(3):287–90.
19. Nichols AW. Heat-related illness in sports and exercise. Curr Rev Musculoskelet Med. 2014;7:355–65.
20. Pryor RR, Roth RN, Suyama J, et al. Exertional heat illness: emerging concepts and advances in prehospital care. Prehosp Disaster Med. 2015;30(3):297–305.

21. Asplund CA, O'Connor FG, Noakes TD. Exercise-associated collapse: an evidence-based review and primer for clinicians. Br J Sports Med. 2011;45(14):1157–62.
22. Armstrong LE, Casa DJ, Millard-Stafford M, et al. American College of Sports Medicine position stand: exertional heat illness during training and competition. Med Sci Sports Exerc. 2007;39(3):556–72.
23. Hew-Butler T, Rosner MH, Fowkes-Godek S, et al. Statement of the third international exercise-associated hyponatremia consensus development conference. Clin J Sport Med. 2015;25(4):303–20.
24. Asplund AC, O'Connor FG. Challenging return to play decisions: heat stroke, exertional rhabdomyolysis, and exertional collapse associated with sickle cell trait. Sports Health. 2015;8(2):117–25.
25. O'Connor FG, Casa DJ, Bergeron MF. American College of Sports Medicine roundtable on exertional heat stroke – return to duty/return to play: conference proceedings. Curr Sports Med Rep. 2010;9(5):314–21.
26. Grundstein AJ, Hosokawa Y, Casa DJ. Fatal exertional heat stroke and American football players: the need for regional heat-safety guidelines. J Athl Train. 2018;53(1):43–50.
27. Lopez RM, Jardine JF. Exertional heat illnesses. In: Casa DJ, editor. Sport and physical activity in the heat. Cham: Springer International Publishing; 2018. p. 313–29.
28. Casa DJ, et al. Exertional heat stroke: new concepts regarding cause and care. Curr Sports Med Rep. 2012;11(3):115–23.
29. Belval LN, Casa DJ, Adams WM, et al. Consensus statement – prehospital care of exertional heat stroke. Prehosp Emerg Care. 2018;22(3):392–7.
30. Kerr ZY, Marshall SW, Comstock RD, et al. Exertional heat stroke management strategies in American high school football. Am J Sports Med. 2013;42(1):70–7.
31. Adams WM, Hosokawa Y, Casa DJ. The timing of exertional heat stroke survival starts prior to collapse. Curr Sports Med Rep. 2015;14(4):273–4.
32. Casa DJ, McDermott BP, Lee EC, et al. Cold water immersion: the gold standard for exertional heatstroke treatment. Exerc Sport Sci Rev. 2007;35(3):141–9.
33. McDermott BP, Casa DJ, Ganio MS, et al. Acute whole-body cooling for exercise-induced hyperthermia: a systematic review. J Athl Train. 2009;44(1):84–93.
34. DeMartini JK, Casa DJ, Stearns R, et al. Effectiveness of CWI in the treatment of EHS at the Falmouth Road Race. Med Sci Sports Exerc. 2015;47(2):240–5.
35. Proulx CI, Ducharme MB, Kenny GP. Effect of water temperature on cooling efficiency during hyperthermia in humans. J Appl Phys. 2003;94(4):1317–23.
36. Armstrong LE, et al. Whole-body cooling of hyperthermic runners: comparison of two field therapies. Am J Emerg Med. 1996;14(4):355–8.
37. McDermott BP, et al. Cold-water dousing with ice massage and to treat exertional heat stroke: a case series. Aviat Space Environ Med. 2009;80(8):720–2.
38. Hosokawa Y, Adams WM, Belval LN, et al. Tarp-assisted cooling as a method of whole-body cooling in hyperthemic individuals. Ann Emerg Med. 2017;69(3):347–52.
39. Costrini A. Emergency treatment of exertional heatstroke and comparison of whole body cooling techniques. Med Sci Sports Exerc. 1990;22(1):15–8.
40. Lopez RM, et al. Exertional heat stroke in athletic setting: a review of the literature. Athl Train Sports Health Care. 2011;3(4):189–200.
41. Goddard CJ, Warnes TW. Raised liver enzymes in asymptomatic patients; investigation and outcome. Dig Dis. 1992;10(4):218–26.
42. Casa DJ, Guskiewicz KM, Anderson SA, et al. National athletic trainers' position statement: preventing sudden death in sports. J Athl Train. 2012;47(1):96–118.
43. Poussel M, Guerci P, Kaminsky P, et al. Exertional heat stroke and susceptibility to malignant hyperthermia in an athlete: evidence for a link? J Athl Train. 2015;50(11):1212–4.
44. Sagui E, Montigon C, Abriat A, et al. Is there a link between exertional heat stroke and susceptibility to malignant hyperthermia? PLoS One. 2015;10(8):e0135496.
45. Epstein Y. Heat intolerance: predisposing factor or residual injury? Med Sci Sports Exerc. 1990;22(1):29–35.

46. Moran DS, Erlich T, Epstein Y. The heat tolerance test: an efficient screening tool for evaluating susceptibility to heat. J Sport Rehabil. 2007;16(3):215–21.
47. Druyan A, Ketko I, Yanovich R, Epstein Y, Heled Y. Refining the distinction between heat tolerant and intolerant individuals during a heat tolerance test. J Therm Biol. 2013;8(38):539–42.
48. Schermann H, Heled Y, Fleischmann C, Ketko I, Schiffmann N, Epstein Y, et al. The validity of the heat tolerance test in prediction of recurrent exertional heat illness events. J Sci Med Sport. 2018;21(6):549–52.
49. Druyan A, Amit D, Makranz C, Moran D, Yanovich R, Epstein Y, et al. Heat tolerance in women – reconsidering the criteria. Aviat Space Environ Med. 2012;83(1):58–60.
50. Lisman P, Kazman JB, O'Connor FG, Heled Y, Deuster PA. Heat tolerance testing: association between heat intolerance and anthropometric and fitness measurements. Mil Med. 2014;179(11):1339–46.
51. Hursel R, Westerterp-Plantenga MS. Thermogenic ingredients and body weight regulation. Int J Obes. 2010;34(4):659–69.
52. Lyons J, Allsopp A, Bilzon J. Influences of body composition upon the relative metabolic and cardiovascular demands of load-carriage. Occup Med (Lond). 2005;55(5):380–4.
53. Ricciardi R, Deuster PA, Talbot LA. Metabolic demands of body armor on physical performance in simulated conditions. Mil Med. 2008;173(9):817–24.
54. Vaughan RA, Conn CA, Mermier CM. Effects of commercially available dietary supplements on resting energy expenditure: a brief report. ISRN Nutr. 2014;2014:650264.
55. Kazman JB, Heled Y, Lisman PJ, Druyan A, Deuster PA, O'Connor FG. Exertional heat illness: the role of heat tolerance testing. Curr Sports Med Rep. 2013;12(2):101–5.

Cardiac Issues in Football

15

Katherine M. Edenfield and Kimberly G. Harmon

Epidemiology

Incidence of Sudden Cardiac Death

Sudden cardiac death (SCD) in athletes is tragic, affecting not only the victim and their families but also teammates, schools, and entire communities. It is often portrayed as a rare, but tragic event; however, SCD is the most common medical cause of death in athletes, including football athletes.

The reported incidence of SCD varies widely depending on study methodology. In order to calculate a precise incidence of SCD, an accurate numerator (number of cases) and denominator (the population at risk) are needed. There is no mandatory reporting of SCD in the United States and deaths are often identified via media report or insurance claim information. Media reports will miss SCDs, particularly those in "lower profile" athletes or those that occur away from the field. In NCAA athletes, media reports identified only 70% of SCDs, with deaths that occurred in lower divisions less likely to be reported [1]. In competitive Danish athletes, media reports identified only 4–20% of the sports-related deaths [2, 3]. Likewise, insurance claims do not identify the vast majority of SCDs in athletes. In a study of Minnesota high school athletes, insurance claims identified only 14% of the SCDs and in National Collegiate Athletic Association (NCAA) athletes, insurance claims identified only 10% [4].

K. M. Edenfield (✉)
Department of Community Health and Family Medicine, University of Florida, Gainesville, FL, USA
e-mail: kedenfield@ufl.edu

K. G. Harmon
Departments of Family Medicine and Orthopedics and Sports Medicine, University of Washington, Seattle, WA, USA
e-mail: kharmon@uw.edu

K. W. Farmer (ed.), *Football Injuries*,
https://doi.org/10.1007/978-3-030-54875-9_15

Denominators are often estimated based on generalized sport participation numbers or activity surveys, which are then extrapolated to the population, leading to compounded error. Populations of similar risk should be grouped together. For incidence calculations, populations where the sex, race/ethnicity and sport played are known provide the most precise estimation, however this level of detail is rare. Risk of cardiovascular disease varies significantly with age, especially after the age of 25 where coronary artery disease (CAD) becomes a more common cause of death; thus, inclusion of wide age ranges decreases accuracy. Only age groups of similar risk should be pooled. Inaccuracy in numerator, denominator, or both can lead to wildly varied estimates. Methodology must be carefully scrutinized when considering estimates of SCD.

Another source of inaccuracy is reporting only SCD cases occurring with exertion, sometimes referred to as "exertional death" or "sports-related SCD," or those occurring only during official team activities. This approach will miss many deaths and underrepresent the true burden of SCD. In one study of NCAA athletes, 42% of deaths did not occur during exertion [1]. Sports-related SCD *is not the same* as SCD in athletes and is a critical distinction. The incidence of SCD in athletes, occurring at any time, is important when considering primary prevention. Sports-related SCD numbers may be useful when creating an emergency action plan for an event or venue.

Sudden cardiac arrest (SCA) is also an important endpoint to consider. SCA is SCD prevented; most often because the athlete had a witnessed SCA with bystander access to a defibrillator. There is no mandatory reporting for SCA in the United States, and many cases of SCA are not reported in the media, making incidence numbers extremely difficult to ascertain. Reporting and tracking systems for SCA need to be improved to truly understand how often SCA occurs in athletes.

Football-Specific Incidence

There are groups of athletes that are at higher risk for SCA/D including male athletes, black athletes, football athletes, and male basketball athletes [1]. In studies that have reported on the incidence of SCD, football athletes have been consistently demonstrated as higher risk including studies in college and high school [1, 5–8] (Table 15.1).

Like other sports, SCD is the most common medical cause of death in football athletes, accounting for 12% of all deaths, 45% of medical deaths, and 42% of the deaths that occurred during exertion [9]. In studies not reporting incidence numbers but reporting the proportion of deaths attributable to football, football consistently represents a large proportion of the SCD, usually just behind male basketball athlete SCD [8, 10].

Table 15.1 Incidence of sudden cardiac death in athletes with a focus on football athletes

Study	Year	SCA/D or SCD?	Population	Incidence of SCD (in athlete-years)
Harmon	2015	SCD	NCAA athlete	1 in 53,703
			NCAA male athletes	1 in 37,790
			NCAA black athlete	1 in 21,491
			NCAA football athlete	1 in 35,951
			Black football athlete	1 in 21,987
			White football athlete	1 in 47,031
			NCAA male basketball athlete	1 in 8,978
Harmon	2016	SCA/D	High school athlete	1 in 67,064
			High school male athlete	1 in 44,832
			High school football athlete	1 in 86,494
Maron	2014		NCAA football athlete	1 in 39,060

Etiology of Sudden Cardiac Death

The etiology of SCD is important to consider, particularly when developing screening strategies. Initial studies of the causes of SCD suggested hypertrophic cardiomyopathy (HCM) occurred most commonly, accounting for 37% of cases; however, this data was likely skewed due to ascertainment bias (cases were collected through a HCM center), and cases which would be considered as autopsy-negative sudden unexplained death (AN-SUD) were not included in the cohort [11]. Later studies in NCAA athletes and athletes in Europe suggested the most common cause of death in athletes was AN-SUD [1, 12]. AN-SUD is thought to be secondary to arrhythmias or electrical disease.

Although these studies showed a lower incidence of strictly pathologically defined HCM, there is an increasing recognition of athletes dying with left ventricular hypertrophy (LVH) with fibrosis or cardiomyopathy that does not meet pathologic criteria for HCM [1, 12]. It is unclear if this is on the HCM continuum or is acquired from intense physical activity. If cases of LVH and possible cardiomyopathy are included with HCM, the incidence increases to around 25% [1, 12]. In a recent study including athletes 11–29 years old in the United States, HCM was the leading cause of death representing 16% of the cases, but when combined with LVH/possible cardiomyopathy represented 30% of all SCDs [10].

The etiology of SCD in football, specifically, is less often described. For the most part, the causes of death in NCAA football athletes paralleled the larger cohort of all NCAA athletes [1]. AN-SUD was the most common cause of death; however, there was a higher incidence of myocarditis (19%) and coronary artery disease (CAD) (13%) in football players compared to other NCAA athletes [1]. The increased incidence of CAD in football players may be related to the large body (and fat) masses of some of the players. HCM was responsible for 13% of SCD in football athletes; however when combined with LVH/possible cardiomyopathy represented 25% of the group. Interestingly, in men's basketball and men's soccer, HCM/LVH/possible cardiomyopathy caused 50% and 57% of SCDs, respectively. The reason for this differential is unclear. In the only other study looking at SCD in football, HCM represented 25% of SCD cases, which was similar to the proportion of HCM in male basketball players [10].

Screening

Since the 1960's when the American Medical Association (AMA) first called for screening young athletes prior to participation, the pre-participation evaluation (PPE) has been customary. In 1996, the American Heart Association (AHA) published cardiovascular screening recommendations stating that "some form of pre-participation cardiovascular screening for high school and collegiate athletes is justifiable and compelling, based on ethical, legal, and medical grounds" [13]. One in 300–400 athletes will have a cardiovascular condition that predisposes to SCD [14]. Primary prevention consists of screening for those conditions with the intent to manage and mitigate risk, while secondary prevention is treating an SCA once it has occurred. Both are important. The AHA and American College of Cardiology (ACC) state the purpose of the PPE is "to prospectively identify or raise suspicion of previously unrecognized and largely genetic congenital cardiovascular diseases known to cause SCA and sudden death in young people" [15]. Other organizations creating guidelines agree that the primary objective of the PPE is to detect potentially life-threatening conditions in athletes [16]. The benefits and drawbacks of various screening strategies are outlined below.

History of Physical Examination

History and physical examination has long been the mainstay of pre-participation screening. The AHA and the ACC have endorsed a screen which includes a personal and family history along with blood pressure measurement, cardiac auscultation, femoral artery pulse check, and examination for physical stigmata of Marfan syndrome as the "best available and most practical" strategy since their initial statement in 1996, affirming this position in both 2007 and 2014 while acknowledging "the standard history and physical examination intrinsically lack the capability to reliably identify many potentially lethal cardiovascular abnormalities" [13, 15, 17].

The recently published *Preparticipation Physical Evaluation Monograph, fifth Edition*, also endorses this recommendation [16]. However, recent statements from the NCAA and the American Medical Society for Sports Medicine (AMSSM) acknowledge that while the history and physical examination is pragmatic and widely practiced, it has limited ability to identify athletes at risk for SCA/D [18, 19].

Drawbacks of the history and physical as a detection strategy for underlying cardiovascular disease include a low sensitivity and a high false-positive rate. In an early study looking at 115 cases of SCD in athletes, only four athletes (3%) were suspected of having a cardiovascular condition and only one athlete (<1%) was correctly identified [20]. In a recent meta-analysis including almost 50,000 athletes, the sensitivity of history for cardiovascular conditions predisposing to SCD was 20% and physical exam was 9% [21]. It is not surprising that relying on a symptom-based questionnaire results in low sensitivity, as SCD is the presenting manifestation of underlying cardiovascular conditions in up to 80% of athletes SCDs. Low sensitivity is not the only concern; the recommended screening questions include symptoms which are fairly common in those without disease, with up to 67% of high school athletes and 33% of NCAA athletes answering affirmatively to at least one question, resulting in a high false-positive rate [14, 22].

The AHA/ACC recommendations for pre-participation cardiovascular screening in athletes do provide a standardized framework for evaluation and are considered the standard of care. Despite these recommendations being in place for over 20 years, they have not been widely implemented, with one study showing less than 6% of primary care physicians compliant with recommendations [23]. The benefits of the history and physical include wide accessibility. While cost is often cited as a benefit of history and physical compared to other screening strategies, this is typically in comparison to a pre-participation screen done at a school with volunteer workforce. Exams done in an office setting represent a significant cost. These volunteer screens may be widely accessible; however, they lack the ability to meet many of the other objectives of a PPE which are better accomplished within the medical home [16]. In the end, one must balance the low sensitivity and the high false-positive rate of history and physical examination with its wide accessibility and relatively low prevalence of SCD in many populations. It should not, however, be viewed as an effective screen for cardiovascular disorders.

Electro Cardiogram (ECG)

In 2005, the European Society of Cardiology recommended the addition of an ECG to the PPE based largely on the experience of the Italians who demonstrated an 89% reduction in athlete SCD after the implementation of a screening program including ECG [24, 25]. This has caused heated debate between proponents of ECG screening and those who oppose it. Recent statements from the NCAA and AMSSM recognize the statistical superiority of a screening strategy, which includes ECG while acknowledging barriers that include lack of infrastructure to adequately interpret the ECGs and access to appropriate follow-up cardiovascular care.

There has been an evolution in the criteria used to interpret ECG in athletes. Many findings which would be concerning in other settings should be considered normal in athletes and the result of physiological response to exercise. The false-positive rate using the latest criteria for interpretation of ECG in athletes, the International Criteria, is around 2% [26]. ECG can reliably detect the majority of conditions associated with SCD including hypertrophic cardiomyopathy (HCM) and electrical diseases such as long QT syndrome (LQTS) and Wolff-Parkinson-White (WPW) syndrome. ECG does not reliably detect coronary artery anomalies, atherosclerotic coronary artery disease, or aortic pathology, which accounted for 20% of the deaths in the NCAA cohort [1]. It is estimated that ECG identifies about two-thirds to three-fourths of cardiovascular conditions associated with SCD in most studies. In a recent study of elite English soccer players, ECG identified 86% of the cardiovascular conditions discovered [27]. In a meta-analysis comparing the sensitivity of history and physical examination and ECG in almost 50,000 athletes, ECG was 94% sensitive for the cardiovascular conditions identified [21].

ECG is superior to history and physical alone for the detection of cardiovascular conditions associated with SCD; however, it is unknown if this affects outcomes. Arguments against ECG include the low prevalence of cardiovascular disease in this population. Football players are at higher risk than other populations with an SCD risk of 1 in 36,000 athlete-years. Sixty-two percent of "Power 5" autonomy conferences include ECG as part of their cardiovascular screen; however, this may be impractical in other settings with fewer resources [28]. In a more recent 2019 survey [29] of head athletic trainers and team physicians at Autonomy Five schools, 72% (34/47) reported including ECG as part of their cardiovascular screen with 97% (33/34) of those screening all athletes from all sports. Ultimately, the decision to include ECG or not should depend on the physician's assessment of the risk-benefit ratio based on the resources available to them.

Echocardiogram

Echocardiogram (echo) is used in some settings as an adjunct to history and physical examination and ECG in cardiovascular screening. The type of echo varies from a full echo done on a hospital-grade ultrasound machine by a licensed cardiac sonographer to cardiac screening protocols administered by a sports physician using point-of-care ultrasound. Echocardiogram has the advantage of being able to visualize structural pathology including cardiomyopathies, aortic pathology, and some congenital artery abnormalities. Although echocardiography may identify serious disease in the absence of an abnormal ECG, the diagnostic yield from asymptomatic athletes with a normal history and physical examination and ECG is low [30]. Echocardiograms can identify congenital or structural conditions not associated with SCD, which may benefit from routine surveillance. The 2019 survey of Autonomy Five schools reported only 29.8% (14/47) obtain routine screening echo with 64% (9/14) of those screening all athletes from all sports [29].

The added value of echocardiogram compared to ECG to diagnose cardiomyopathy specifically has been questioned as the morphological alterations of exercise training can paradoxically cause changes in the cardiac structure that are difficult to differentiate from pathological changes, especially for non-experts [30]. Some have suggested that screening point-of-care echocardiograms could decrease the rate of referrals for further evaluations after a positive history and physical examination or ECG; however, this hypothesis remains unproven [31].

Two recent studies of collegiate football players have suggested that differentiating normal from abnormal echocardiographic findings can be challenging and indexing the interventricular septal diameter (IVSD) and left ventricular end-diastolic diameter (LVEDD) to body surface area (BSA) may provide a more specific measurement and limit false-positive findings [32] but does not appear to be applicable to the aortic root diameter (ARD) in these athletes [33].

Prevention

Even the best screening program will not identify all athletes with underlying cardiovascular disorders. Every school or institution that sponsors athletic activities should have a written and structured EAP (Chap. 14). Access to early cardiopulmonary resuscitation (CPR) and early defibrillation is the key to survival of SCA [34]. The EAP should be developed in conjunction with local emergency medical services, school or venue safety officials, likely first responders, and administrators. The EAP should be specific to each venue or field where football players practice or play and provide plans for a communication system, targeted first responders, the location of on-site automatic external defibrillators (AEDs), and transportation routes for arriving EMS. The EAP should be practiced at least annually by potential responders to SCA.

An identified team of targeted first responders (i.e., coaches, school health officials) should receive training in the recognition of SCA, CPR, and AED use. First responders in many situations are coaches. Recognition of SCA is the first step to response. Anyone who collapses and is unresponsive should be presumed to have had an SCA. Over 50% of athletes with SCA will have tonic-clonic movement of the limbs, which is often mistaken for a seizure causing critical delay. Agonal breaths or gasps should not be confused with respiration. Once SCA is recognized, CPR should be started and emergency medical services (EMS) should be activated. If there is a defibrillator on-site, it should be retrieved and placed on the athlete. On-site AED programs are ideal and the best means of achieving early defibrillation. Automated external defibrillators will not deliver a shock unless indicated. The target time from collapse to first shock should be less than 3 minutes.

Implantable Cardioverter-Defibrillators

Those deemed at high risk of future life-threatening ventricular arrhythmias sometimes have an implantable cardioverter-defibrillator (ICD) surgically implanted. This is a device that senses the rhythm and rate of the heart and will fire if life-threatening rhythms such as ventricular tachycardia or ventricular fibrillation are noted. Some athletes have returned to play after being diagnosed with a cardiac condition and receiving an ICD but only after achieving a thorough understanding of the risks and benefits being reviewed in a shared decision-making process [35]. Recent guidelines have recognized an evolving standard regarding return to play with an ICD; however, most experts consider it inadvisable to play football, a collision sport, with an ICD [36]. Damage to the device or the leads could cause malfunction. There is also a risk of inappropriate shock or failure of the device to abort lethal arrhythmias.

Potential Specific Causes of Cardiac Issues in American Football

Covered in this section are some of the most commonly encountered cardiac conditions in American football. Be aware that there are other relatively rare conditions not included and if concerned for these, cardiac specialist consultation and reference to the most recent consensus guidelines is recommended.

Structural

Hypertrophic Cardiomyopathy

Hypertrophic cardiomyopathy (HCM) is an inherited heterogeneous heart disease characterized most commonly by left ventricular hypertrophy (LVH) and is an important cause of arrhythmogenic sudden death and heart failure [37–39]. Best estimates conclude that the combination of HCM/idiopathic LVH/possible cardiomyopathy accounts for 24–36% of sudden cardiac deaths (SCD) in athletes [1, 10, 17].

HCM is diagnosed by a hypertrophied but nondilated LV chamber in the absence of another cardiac or systemic disease, such as hypertension (HTN), capable of causing the magnitude of hypertrophy seen [40]. LV wall thicknesses can range from mildly enlarged (13–15 mm) to massive with a thickness of up to 60 mm [40]. LVH is typically asymmetric with the anterior septum usually predominant [40]. When outflow tract obstruction occurs, it is usually from systolic anterior motion of the mitral valve [40].

Myocardial fibrosis is common [38] in HCM and, together with disorganized cellular architecture and expanded interstitial collagen, serves as life-threatening arrhythmogenic substrates [40]. The estimated phenotypic prevalence is 1 in 500 [37–39] with a possible genotypic prevalence of 1 in 200 [39]. Pathogenic mutations are transmitted in an autosomal dominant pattern, and more than 1500 different mutations have been identified within more than 11 different sarcomere- and myofilament-related genes, with more than 70% of mutations in just two genes, ß-myosin heavy chain (*β-MYH7*) and myosin-binding protein C (*MYBPC3*) [37, 41, 42].

With genetic testing, an increasing amount of HCM family members are recognized with pathogenic mutations (genotype positive) but in the absence of a clinical phenotype (phenotype-negative) [42]. When spontaneous conversion to phenotype-positive occurs, it is usually between 12 and 20 years of age [42] at the time of substantial LV remodeling during accelerated body growth during adolescence [40]. The phenotypic expression during this time is part of the rationale supporting pre-participation screening of high school and college athletes with interval repeat exams and history every several years [40].

HCM may be first suspected on routine history and physical or screening examination. However, frequently, SCD is the first clinical presentation of an athlete with HCM [37]. If an athlete presented in-season with symptoms concerning for HCM, it would usually be from a syncopal episode associated with exertion. Physical exam is frequently normal, but if an outflow tract obstruction exists, a systolic murmur may be heard best at the left lateral sternal border in positions that decrease preload, (Valsalva maneuver or squat-to-stand) emphasizing the importance of dynamic cardiac auscultation at physical exam.

Abnormalities on 12-lead ECG may precede development of overt structural cardiac disease [43–45]. If ECG abnormalities exist but the heart is found to be structurally normal, athletes should be allowed to participate but should be followed annually for the development of structural disease [43], as 6–7% of athletes with abnormal ECGs and initially structural normal hearts went on to develop structural pathology or cardiomyopathy at follow-up [44, 45].

Consultation of a cardiologist with expertise in sports cardiology should be sought for any athlete with suspected or known HCM. Routine diagnostic testing for those being evaluated for HCM includes an ECG, echocardiogram, exercise ECG test, and a minimum 24-hour Holter monitor test. If echocardiography is non-diagnostic or apical or antero-lateral HCM is suspected, contrast-enhanced cardiac MRI should be a standard component of the assessment as echocardiogram may not provide a reliable assessment of those areas. MRI provides a superior assessment of myocardial hypertrophy, and if gadolinium enhancement is present, can also suggest myocardial fibrosis [43]. Two-dimensional (2D) myocardial strain imaging is a new tool that has shown promise in discriminating subclinical functional differences in variant forms of left ventricular hypertrophy (LVH), like athlete's heart, from HCM [46, 47]. Detraining for 6 weeks to 6 months has been utilized as a method for distinguishing physiological LVH or "athlete's heart" from pathologic LVH or HCM, as most cardiac parameters regress and then completely normalize by 6 months of detraining [48, 49]. However, detraining is undesirable by athletes and not practical to implement, limiting its usefulness. Genetic screening and family evaluation may also be considered.

Treatment options depend on an individualized risk assessment for sudden death but include medication management (i.e., beta blockers), implantable defibrillators, surgical septal myectomy, and percutaneous alcohol septal ablation for outflow tract obstruction [37].

Currently, the risk for sudden death in the genotype-positive–phenotype-negative population appears very low, likely no higher than in the general population, and participation in competitive athletics is reasonable for this population [42]. For phenotype-positive HCM athletes, the current expert opinion is that they should not participate in competitive sports with the exception of low-intensity class IA sports (Table 15.2), which include bowling, golf, and yoga, even if treated medically or surgically [42] including an implantable defibrillator (See ICD under Screening and Prevention), given that intense exertion is a known arrhythmogenic substrate in a

Table 15.2 Classification of sports based on static/dynamic component [50]

	A. (Low dynamic < 50%)	B. (Moderate dynamic 50–75%)	C. High dynamic (>75%)
III. High static (>30%)	Gymnastics; Field (throwing); Martial arts; Weightlifting	Wrestling; Downhill skiing; Snowboarding; Bodybuilding	Boxing; Cycling; Rowing; Triathlon
II. Moderate static (10–20%)	Diving; Equestrian sports	*Football;* Field (jumping); Track (sprint)	Swimming; Track (mid-distance); Basketball; Lacrosse
I. Low static (<10%)	Golf; Yoga; Bowling	Softball; Volleyball	Soccer; Track (distance)/ Cross Country

patient with the impaired myocardial tissue of HCM. American-style football (ASF) is a class IIB sport (moderate static and dynamic components) [50]. There are genetic mutations associated with a higher risk of sudden SCD, including several *ß-MYH7* mutations and those involving the cardiac troponin T (*cTnT*) gene [41], and in general, sport participation recommendations for individuals with these mutations are dependent upon their phenotype status, as previously mentioned.

Aortic Diseases

Aortic dissection or rupture accounted for 5% of SCD in one decade-long study of collegiate athletes, but none were football athletes [1] and 6% of SCD in another study, over a 2-year duration, of middle school-aged through professional competitive athletes [10]. Aortopathies, including Marfan syndrome and a bicuspid aortic valve (BAV), are possible predisposing factors for aortic dissection.

Marfan syndrome (MFS) is an autosomal dominant (AD) condition with an estimated prevalence of 2–3 per10,000 individuals caused by abnormal fibrillin-1 due to mutations in the fibrillin-1 (*FBN1*) gene, of which approximately 75% are inherited and 25% are de novo mutations [51]. Marfan syndrome is a multisystem disorder of connective tissue, with cardiovascular manifestations a major cause of morbidity and mortality. The main features of MFS consist of aortic root aneurysm, ectopia lentis, and disproportionate long bone overgrowth [52]. The most common cardiovascular manifestation of MFS is ascending aorta dilatation at the level of the aortic sinuses [51]. Diagnosis is made using the revised Ghent criteria, which evaluates based on the presence of a dilated aorta, ectopia lentis, FBN1 mutation, systemic features of MFS, and family history [52, 53].

MFS would usually be suspected during pre-participation screening, as opposed to in-season, due to typical stigmata seen on physical exam.

The largest correctly measured aortic root diameter obtained from at least three transthoracic images should be corrected for body size and age and interpreted as a *Z*-score [52].

Individuals diagnosed with MFS typically have a transthoracic echocardiogram along with an ECG-gated CT scan of the entire aorta at the time of diagnosis followed by yearly echocardiograms to monitor; more frequently if the aortic diameter is approaching a surgical threshold [54]. Adults with repeatedly normal aortic root measurements may escalate to echocardiograms every 2–3 years [52]. Medication management with beta blockers, unless contraindicated, is the standard of care of prevention of complications, although there are research trials looking at other medications [52].

Prophylactic surgery should be considered when the aortic root diameter at the sinuses of Valsalva approaches 5.0 cm to prevent acute dissection of the ascending aorta which is a medical emergency [52].

Bicuspid aortic valve (BAV) is another often encountered aortic disease. It is one of the most common congenital heart defects with a prevalence of 0.5–2% in the general population [55–57] and may be associated with other aortic abnormalities such as aortic root and ascending aorta dilation, aneurysm, and coarctation [56, 57]. Aortic dilation can be found with BAV even in the absence of aortic valve stenosis or regurgitation and is believed to be due to abnormalities in the aortic media rather than primarily from hemodynamic alterations [56]. BAV may be suspected if a murmur is heard on physical exam, typically auscultated as an ejection murmur heart best at the apex. If symptoms present in-season, they are typically secondary to complications or associated conditions (i.e., aortic stenosis, aortic regurgitation, dissection).

Management of BAV consists of surveillance with serial echocardiography biannually or annually for those with aortic root diameters greater than 40 mm or valve lesions; medical therapy typically with beta-blockers to control blood pressure and reduce the pressure gradient across the valve, slowing progression of the disease; and surgical management for those meeting specific criteria [57].

One study showed ascending aortic dimensions were significantly larger in former National Football League (NFL) athletes compared to controls after adjusting for other factors; however, it is currently unknown if this translates to any increased risk [58].

Athletic participation decisions for those with abnormalities affecting the aorta should be made on an individual basis. A cardiologist experienced with athletes and an experienced cardiovascular surgeon should be consulted. Guidelines to consider when making a decision include the American Heart Association/American College of Cardiology (AHA/ACC) guidelines [59]. These guidelines recommend it is reasonable for athletes with MFS to participate in class IA and IIA competitive sports (see Table 15.2) provided they do not have any specified criteria placing them at higher risk [59]. In general, athletes with MFS should avoid contact sports and isometric activities involving a Valsalva maneuver [52], which precludes ASF.

The AHA/ACC guidelines [59] recommend athletes with BAV without a dilated aortic root or ascending aorta can participate in all competitive athletics. The function (stenosis, regurgitation) of the BAV also needs to be assessed. Athletes with BAV and dilated aortic dimensions should undergo serial aortic imaging to look for progression. Athletes with BAV and a mild to moderately dilated aorta may consider participation in low and moderate static and dynamic competitive sports with a low likelihood of bodily impact [59]. Athletes with BAV and a more severely dilated aorta should avoid any competitive sports that involve the potential for bodily collision and may consider participation in class IA (see Table 15.2) sports [59].

Coronary Artery Anomalies/Coronary Artery Disease

Anomalous coronary arteries are an important cause of SCD in sport with more recent estimates at prevalence as the etiology of 11% of SCD in the National Collegiate Athletic Association (NCAA) while Coronary Artery Disease (CAD) was the etiology in 9% [1]. In a cohort including a wider age range of athletes from middle school to professional, coronary artery anomalies accounted for 15.7% of cases of SCD over a 2-year period while CAD accounted for 2.4% of SCD [10].

Anomalous coronary arteries are a heterogeneous group of congenital anomalies involving an aberrant anatomy as they arise from the aortic root and sinuses of Valsalva. In one study of 27 cases of SCD in young athletes with anomalous coronary arteries, 85% had the left main coronary artery aberrantly from the right aortic sinus [60]. All of the athletes died either during (93%) or immediately following intense exertion [60]. Only 37% of those athletes had experienced premonitory symptoms which included syncope and/or chest pain, and if experienced, symptoms occurred within 2 years of their death [60]. Only two of the symptomatic athletes underwent echocardiography and all of the cardiovascular testing done on the symptomatic athletes was normal [60].

If anomalous coronaries are suspected, an experienced cardiologist and cardiothoracic surgeon should be consulted.

Imaging is needed to diagnose anomalous coronary arteries. The best methods include computed tomography angiography (CTA), magnetic resonance angiography (MRA) or coronary angiography [61]. However, in one study of intercollegiate athletes, the origin and proximal course of the coronary arteries were reliably and readily observed on echocardiogram, suggesting that if echocardiogram is performed, the protocol should include assessment of the coronary arteries [62].

In general, athletes with an anomalous coronary artery should be restricted from sports, with the possible exception of class IA (see Table 15.2), pending surgical repair [61]. After surgical repair of an anomalous coronary artery from the wrong sinus, sports participation may be considered 3 months post-surgery if symptom free with a normal exercise stress test [61].

There is increased concern about football players having an increased incidence of cardiovascular disease (CVD) due to a high prevalence of obesity and early HTN [63]. These concerns are increased in lineman who engage in short repetitive bouts of intense static activity, with little aerobic conditioning. Studies have actually shown a lower rate of CVD risk factors and mortality in several overall cohorts of retired NFL players [64, 65] compared to controls; however, ASF athletes are a heterogenous group with different cardiovascular demands depending on their position. When a position subgroup of defensive linemen were examined, they had a 42% higher CVD mortality compared to controls [64]. Retired NFL linemen also have shown a significant increased rate of moderate-to-severe subclinical atherosclerosis [66].

Athletes with CVD leading to CAD may present with chest pain, dyspnea, or decreased exercise tolerance, or they may experience "silent ischemia" seen only on provocative testing, or coronary artery calcification seen on imaging. The assumption for recommendations on participation in the risk of an exertion-related event is greater in those who have had a previous acute coronary syndrome [67].

As with all conditions, individual management and consultation with a cardiologist are recommended. General recommendations for athletes with atherosclerotic CAD include maximal exercise stress testing, an assessment of left ventricular (LV) function, and aggressive risk factor reduction including statin therapy to reduce the chance of plaque disruption [67]. Asymptomatic athletes with appropriate LV function, no inducible ischemia or electrical instability should generally be allowed to continue to participate in full ASF activity [67]. Symptomatic athletes, or those with impaired LV function, inducible ischemia or electrical instability should usually be restricted from ASF football, in addition to those <3 months out from an acute myocardial infarction or coronary revascularization procedure [67].

Electrical

Wolff-Parkinson-White Syndrome

Wolff-Parkinson-White syndrome (WPW) refers to ventricular pre-excitation which occurs due to one or more accessory pathways occurring between the atria and ventricles bypassing the atrioventricular (AV) node [68]. Sudden death can be provoked when atrial flutter and atrial fibrillation (AF) are rapidly conducted to the ventricle by the accessory pathway, triggering ventricular fibrillation (VF) [68, 69]. In one study looking at cause of SCD in NCAA athletes over a decade, WPW was responsible for 3% of deaths [1]. In another study on cause of sudden cardiac arrest/deaths (SCA/D) of competitive athletes 11–29 years of age, WPW was the etiology of 6.8% of cases. WPW syndrome can present with presyncope, lightheadedness, and palpitations caused by an atrioventricular reciprocating tachycardia (AVRT) or atrial tachycardia. It can also be diagnosed incidentally on an asymptomatic person on ECG done for screening or other purposes. The pathognomonic ECG findings include: (1) delta wave/slurred upstroke in the QRS complex, (2) short PR interval (<120 ms in adults) during sinus rhythm, (3) QRS duration >120 ms in adults, and (4) secondary ST and T-wave changes [70].

Once WPW is diagnosed, risk stratification must be performed to determine if an athlete has a high-risk pathway for lethal arrhythmias and sudden death or a low-risk pathway. Risk assessment is best completed through a referral to cardiology. Noninvasive tests used to help determine risk include echocardiogram (to look for structural heart disease associated with WPW), Holter monitor test (low risk if intermittent loss of pre-excitation at physiologic heart rates or high risk for multiple accessory pathway morphologies), and exercise stress test (EST) (low risk only with abrupt and complete loss of pre-excitation on EST) [68]. If a low-risk pathway cannot be confirmed with noninvasive testing, electrophysiological evaluation should be undertaken with ablation of the bypass tract if it is deemed high risk for SCD [71].

Transcatheter ablation offers a potential cure for WPW and is recommended for high-risk pathways and symptomatic athletes. An athlete who has undergone an ablation and is asymptomatic with normal follow-up ECG can usually return to sport within 1 week [68]. Asymptomatic athletes with low-risk pathways should be monitored for development of new symptoms [68].

Atrial Fibrillation

Atrial fibrillation (AF) is the most commonly encountered clinically significant arrhythmia [72]. Risk factors for AF include increasing age, hypertension (HTN), hyperthyroidism, structural heart disease, male sex, tall stature, left atrial remodeling, increased vagal tone, alcohol intake, endurance sport, and total lifetime exercise dose of over 1500–2000 hours [72–75]. When AF is not associated with known medical disease, it is termed lone atrial fibrillation (LAF).

Endurance sporting activity is a known, well-established risk factor for the development of AF, but Mont and colleagues [76] showed that the cumulated hours of moderate- and heavy-intensity sport activity and moderate occupational physical activity were also significantly higher in lone AF patients than in controls. Symptoms of AF may include palpitations, lightheadedness, and weakness. Most athletes (70%) present with "vagal AF" that occurs during rest or sleep, post-exercise, and post-prandial [73, 76]. Exercise-provoked symptoms, seen with "adrenergic AF," are less common and can also include fatigue and reduced exercise capacity [73]. AF usually presents initially as paroxysmal, occurring infrequently, and is self-limited, progressing to more frequent and prolonged over the years and then to persistent AF [72].

Evaluation of all athletes with AF should include blood pressure, thyroid function tests, ECG, echocardiograms, drug use (including illicit and performance-enhancing), supplement use, and alcohol use. Some athletes may warrant further testing such as cardiac magnetic resonance imaging and stress testing.

Athletes with AF that is well tolerated and self-terminating may participate in all competitive sports without therapy [71]. The need for anticoagulation for stroke prophylaxis should be determined for athletes the same as the general population, using a risk score such as CHA_2DS_2-VASc score. Most athletes are at low risk. When antithrombotic therapy, other than aspirin, is indicated, it is reasonable to consider the bleeding risk of sport prior to making clearance decisions [71]. This would preclude a football athlete from being able to participate while on antithrombotic therapy due to high risk of bleeding.

Management of AF in athletes includes rate or rhythm control. Rate control is not ideal for athletes due to the need to elevate heart rate for athletic performance. Rhythm control can be achieved with medication or ablation procedures, and ablation should be considered due to some evidence of sustained benefit, particularly in paroxysmal AF, and the risk of side effects with antiarrhythmic drug therapy [71].

In some cases, a reduction of physical activity can stabilize sinus rhythm and allow athletes to resume training after several months [72].

Long QT Syndrome

Long QT syndrome (LQTS) is an inherited cardiac ion channelopathy with electrocardiographic manifestations of QT prolongation and increased susceptibility to life-threatening arrhythmias such as torsades de pointes and ventricular fibrillation [77, 78]. The estimated prevalence is 1 in 2000 individuals [79]. It was responsible for 1% of SCD in NCAA athletes over a 10-year period [1] and 6% of SCA/D in competitive athletes between 11 and 29 years old over a 2-year period [10].

There are 17 currently known gene mutations associated with LQTS, of these LQT1, LQT2, and LQT3 account for 75% of cases [78]. LQT1 patients have an increased susceptibility to events with physical exertion, especially swimming, and emotional stress [80]. LQT2 are most often triggered by emotional stressors, followed by sleep and auditory events (alarm clocks), while LQT3 are most susceptible to events during sleep [80].

Athletes with LQTS can present with palpitations, presyncope, syncope, and cardiac arrest, or may be detected asymptomatically with prolonged QTc (men >470 ms, women >480 ms) on ECG.

Per the HRS/EHRA/APHRS Expert Consensus Statement on the Diagnosis and Management of Patients with Inherited Primary Arrhythmia Syndromes [81], LQTS can be diagnosed:

1. A. In the presence of an LQTS risk score ≥3.5 and in the absence of a secondary cause for QT prolongation

   B. In the presence of an unequivocally pathogenic mutation in one of the LQTS genes

   C. In the presence of a QT interval corrected for heart rate using Bazett's formula (QTc), ≥500 ms in repeated 12-lead electrocardiogram (ECG), and in the absence of a secondary cause for QT prolongation
2. In the presence of a QTc between 480 ms and 499 ms in repeated 12-lead ECGs in a patient with unexplained syncope in the absence of a secondary cause for QT prolongation and in the absence of a pathogenic mutation

All football athletes should be referred to a clinical (heart rhythm or genetic cardiologist) expert for an evaluation of risk [81].

Treatment of LQTS includes avoidance of QT-prolonging drugs; beta-blocker therapy with propranolol or nadolol is typically first-line treatment [77, 81]. Left cardiac sympathetic denervation (LCSD) is recommended for high-risk patients who cannot have either an implantable cardioverter-defibrillator (ICD) inserted or undergo beta-blocker therapy [81]. ICD is recommended for patients with LQTS who survive cardiac arrest [81].

It is recommended that suspected or symptomatic athletes from a cardiac channelopathy be restricted from sports until evaluation is complete, the patient and their family are well-educated about the treatment, the treatment is implemented, and the athlete is asymptomatic on therapy for 3 months [82]. It is reasonable for an asymptomatic athlete with genotype-positive/phenotype-negative LQTS to participate in football and competitive sports with appropriate precautionary measures [82]. For an athlete with symptomatic LQTS or ECG-manifest LQTS, competitive football and sport may be considered after institution of treatment and appropriate precautionary measures if the athlete has been asymptomatic on treatment for at least 3 months [82].

Situational/Other

Hypertension

Hypertension (HTN) is a major risk factor for CVD [83]. ASF athletes have consistently demonstrated a higher level of HTN than the general population. Compared with healthy controls, active NFL players had significantly higher incidence of prehypertension and HTN [63]. In collegiate ASF athletes, one season of participation was associated with significant increases in systolic blood pressure (SBP) and diastolic blood pressure (DBP), with the lineman position being one of the strongest independent predictors of postseason BP [84]. In a separate study of collegiate ASF athletes, the linemen also demonstrated a significantly larger increase in SBP than non-linemen in addition to a decreased (impaired) global longitudinal strain (GLS), suggesting a maladaptive remodeling at the lineman position [85].

In 2017, the ACC/AHA updated their guidelines on HTN and lowered the values for diagnosis (Table 15.3). The diagnosis should be based on an average of ≥2 readings on ≥2 separate occasions, and those with SBP and DBP in separate categories should be placed in the higher category [83].

The renaming of BP categories was based on the interpretation of data of the benefit of lowering BP in CVD risk and the earlier identification and intervention, even if with non-pharmacological treatment [83].

To diagnose HTN, blood pressure should be measured after the patient has been made to sit in a chair for more than 5 minutes with feet on the floor, relaxed, with an appropriate-sized cuff that encircles 80% of the arm (too small cuff leads to falsely elevated reading), and an average of ≥2 readings obtained on ≥2 occasions should be used [83].

Secondary causes of HTN should be evaluated for the onset of HTN in an athlete <30 years old or in the setting of history and physical exam findings suggestive of a secondary cause. The most common secondary causes of HTN include renal disease

Table 15.3 Categories of blood pressure in adults [83]

Blood pressure category	SBP		DBP
Normal	<120 mmHg	AND	<80 mmHg
Elevated	120–129 mmHg	AND	<80 mmHg
Stage 1 HTN	130–139 mmHg	OR	80–89 mmHg
Stage 2 HTN	≥140 mmHg	OR	≥90 mmHg

(especially fibromuscular hyperplasia in women), primary aldosteronism, obstructive sleep apnea, and drug or alcohol induced [83].

Initial testing for primary HTN should include fasting glucose; complete blood count; lipid profile; renal function; serum sodium, potassium, and calcium; thyroid-stimulating hormone; urinalysis; and ECG, while optional testing can include an echocardiogram, urinary albumin-to-creatinine ratio, and uric acid test [83].

Non-pharmacologic therapies such as exercise and healthy diet are typically not effective in athletes as they are typically already engaging in these behaviors, and weight loss is typically undesirable in football athletes. However, football athletes should be educated about these as they may be able to incorporate healthier behaviors both during and after their football career.

Pharmacological therapy is recommended for primary prevention of CVD in adults with no history of CVD, <10% atherosclerotic CVD (ASCVD) 10-year risk with Stage 2 HTN, or with an ASCVD 10 year risk >=10% and Stage 1 HTN, or for secondary prevention of recurrent CVD events in patients wtih clinical CVD and Stage 1 HTN [83].

Angiotensin-converting enzyme (ACE) inhibitors or aldosterone receptor blockers (ARB) are typically a first-line medication of choice for treating HTN in athletes due to their lack of negative effect on exercise performance or hydration and electrolyte status seen in some of the other classes of medications such as beta blockers and diuretics [86]. ACE inhibitors block the enzyme which coverts angiotensin I to angiotensin II, producing a vasodilatory effect. ARBs block the receptor for type 1 angiotensin II, which leads to vasodilation, decreased aldosterone, and decreased renal reabsorption of sodium and water. The most common side effect of ACE inhibitors is a dry cough which can be occur in up to 10% of people. This does not occur with ARBs. Calcium channel blockers should be considered first line in black athletes as they were found to be more effective in this population [86]. They should also be considered first line in females of child-bearing age because of potential teratogenic effects of ACE inhibitors [87].

It is reasonable to consider restriction from high static activities such as those lineman participate in and weightlifting for those with an SBP >160 mmHg or a diastolic BP >100 mmHg until HTN is controlled [88].

Myocarditis

Myocarditis is an inflammatory heart muscle disease associated with cardiac dysfunction and histologically with inflammatory infiltrates associated with myocyte degeneration and necrosis [89]. It has both infectious and noninfectious etiologies [89]. The most common noninfectious etiology is the hypersensitivity type from acute drug-related injury while infectious causes can include viral (coxsackievirus, adenovirus, HIV, coronavirus), bacterial (streptococcus), rickettsial (typhus, rocky mountain spotted fever), fungal, and parasitic agents [89].

Myocarditis accounted for 9% of NCAA athlete's SCD over a 10 year period but 19% of football players [1] and 4.3% of SCA/D in competitive athletes between 11 and 29 years of age over a 2-year period [10].

Myocarditis may present in many different ways, from mild symptoms of chest pain and palpitations to life-threatening cardiogenic shock and ventricular arrhythmia [90].

Endomyocardial biopsy (EMB) is the gold standard to diagnose myocarditis; however, this is not always practical nor recommended by current guidelines [90].

The AHA/ACC Eligibility and Disqualification Recommendations for Competitive Athletes with Cardiovascular Abnormalities [42] recommends diagnosis of acute myocarditis based on the presence of two clinical criteria: (1) A clinical syndrome that includes acute heart failure, angina-type chest pain, or myopericarditis for a duration of <3 months and (2) an otherwise unexplained elevation in serum troponin; ECG features of cardiac ischemia; otherwise unexplained high-degree AV block or arrhythmias; wall motion abnormalities; pericardial effusion on echocardiography or CMR imaging. Additional CMR findings that suggest myocarditis in the acute clinical setting include characteristic alterations in tissue signal on T2 or T1 weighted images and the presence of late gadolinium enhancement (LGE).

Myocarditis has been linked to sudden death, and strenuous physical exertion appears to increase that risk [42]. Athletes with suspected or diagnosed myocarditis should not participate in competitive sports while active inflammation is present independent of age, gender, and LV function [42].

Per the AHA/ACC Eligibility and Disqualification Recommendations for Competitive Athletes with Cardiovascular Abnormalities [42] before returning to competitive sports, athletes suspected of having an acute myocarditis should wait a minimum of 3–6 months before undergoing a resting echocardiogram, 24-hour Holter monitor, and exercise ECG. It is reasonable to consider resuming training if all of the following criteria are met:

- Ventricular systolic function has returned to normal.
- Serum markers of heart failure, myocardial injury, and inflammation have normalized.
- Clinically relevant arrhythmias are absent of Holter monitor and graded exercise ECG.

Guidelines, Shared Decision Making, and Institutional Risk

Medical decisions related to participation in athletics with cardiac conditions can be complicated, with particularly high stakes, given that the outcome could potentially be death. There are some guidelines that exist to help guide the decision-making process.

There are two recent consensus guidelines advising those caring for athletes with cardiac conditions. The 2015 Eligibility and Disqualification Recommendations for Competitive Athletes with Cardiovascular Abnormalities and A Scientific Statement from the American Heart Association and American College of Cardiology [36, 42, 50, 59, 61, 67, 71, 82, 88, 91–96] which is an update to the 2005 36th Bethesda Conference guidelines [97]. The European Society of Cardiology (ESC) also published guidelines in 2017 regarding Pre-participation cardiovascular evaluation for athletic participants to prevent sudden death [98].

Guidelines are just one factor a physician should consider while exercising best medical judgment, but should not be used in place of individualized recommendations regarding sports participation based on an athlete's medical short- and long-term best interests.

There are several precedent-setting cases involving student-athletes with cardiac conditions and medical disqualification. These specific cases involve basketball players but the principles apply to football athletes as well.

Knapp v. Northwestern University (cite) is a case in which a basketball student-athlete sued Northwestern University over the decision to medically disqualify him to play basketball at Northwestern due to a cardiac condition which had caused a previous cardiac arrest, claiming a violation of the Rehabilitation Act. The court ultimately ruled that a university has a legal right to establish legitimate physical qualifications for its student-athletes and Northwestern did not violate the Rehabilitation Act by accepting its team physician's reasonable medical determination [96].

It is required that a disqualification must have an individualized medical evaluation and a reasonable medical basis. An educational institution does not violate law in accepting its team physician's reasonable medical judgment or violate federal disability discrimination laws, even if other physicians disagree [96]. It is up to an individual institution to analyze the risk and make a medically reasonable decision.

Mobley v. Madison Square Garden LP (cite) is a separate case in which a federal district court ruled that Mobley, a former National Basketball Association player, may have a valid disability discrimination claim against the New York Knicks for his medical disqualification for hypertrophic cardiomyopathy during the 2008–2009 season, after having been medically cleared to play in 1999–2008 subject to his signing a liability waiver. The ruling in *Mobley* suggests it is possible some courts might consider an "athlete informed consent model" for professional athletes as opposed to the "team physician medical judgment model" seen in *Knapp* applied in a collegiate setting [96].

Ultimately, a physician has a duty to protect an athlete's health and safety, should provide sports participation recommendations based on best medical practice after an individualized assessment, and should not be forced to assume a medically unreasonable risk. There may be situations where a physician determines a cardiac condition does not carry a significant risk and medically clear the athlete to play. In these situations, written informed consent with the athlete, reviewing the possible risks of participation, is recommended.

Conclusions

Seemingly healthy football athletes may have cardiac disease ranging from hypertension to cardiovascular conditions that predispose to SCD. The incidence of SCD in football is higher than in most other sports except men's basketball. Screening for cardiovascular conditions that predispose to sudden death is a primary objective of the PPE. History and physical examination is the recommended screening strategy, although its sensitivity is low. Given that football is higher risk, some programs, typically at the college or professional level, have elected to include ECG or other advanced cardiac testing, which improves the ability to identify cardiovascular issues. The risks, benefits, and resources available need to be considered when deciding upon a screening strategy. The best screening program will not identify all cardiac conditions; therefore, it is important that EAPs be in place where athletes practice and play. Knowledge regarding specific cardiac conditions affecting football players is important for those who provide care. The process of shared decision-making in those identified with cardiovascular conditions has evolved in an attempt to balance prudence with patient autonomy. Decisions involving returning to play after a cardiac diagnosis have led to legal precedent which is important to be aware of.

References

1. Harmon K, Asif IM, Maleszewski JJ, Owens DS, Prutkin JM, Salerno JC, et al. Incidence, cause, and comparative frequency of sudden cardiac death in National Collegiate Athletic Association Athletes: a decade in review. Circulation. 2015;132(1):10–9.
2. Holst AG, Winkel BG, Theilade J, Kristensen IB, Thomsen JL, Ottesen GL, et al. Incidence and etiology of sports-related sudden cardiac death in Denmark – implications for preparticipation screening. Heart Rhythm. 2010;7(10):1365–71.
3. Risgaard B, Winkel BG, Jabbari R, Glinge C, Ingemann-Hansen O, Thomsen JL, et al. Sports-related sudden cardiac death in a competitive and a noncompetitive athlete population aged 12 to 49 years: data from an unselected nationwide study in Denmark. Heart Rhythm. 2014;11(10):1673–81.
4. Drezner JA, Harmon KG, Marek JC. Incidence of sudden cardiac arrest in Minnesota high school student athletes: the limitations of catastrophic insurance claims. J Am Coll Cardiol. 2014;63(14):1455–6.
5. Harmon KG, Asif IM, Klossner D, Drezner JA. Incidence of sudden cardiac death in National Collegiate Athletic Association athletes. Circulation. 2011;123(15):1594–600.
6. Maron BJ, Haas TS, Murphy CJ, Ahluwalia A, Rutten-Ramos S. Incidence and causes of sudden death in u.s. College athletes. J Am Coll Cardiol. 2014;63(16):1636–43.
7. Harmon KG, Asif IM, Maleszewski JJ, Owens DS, Prutkin JM, Salerno JC, et al. Incidence and etiology of sudden cardiac arrest and death in high school athletes in the United States. Mayo Clin Proc. 2016;91(11):1493–502.
8. Drezner JA, Peterson DF, Siebert DM, Thomas LC, Lopez-Anderson M, Suchsland MZ, et al. Survival after exercise-related sudden cardiac arrest in young athletes: can we do better? Sports Health. 2019;11(1):91–8.
9. Harmon KG, Drezner JA, Klossner D, Asif IM. Sickle cell trait associated with a RR of death of 37 times in National Collegiate Athletic Association football athletes: a database with 2 million athlete-years as the denominator. Br J Sports Med. 2012;46(5):325–30.
10. Peterson DF, Siebert DM, Kucera KL, Thomas LC, Maleszewski JJ, Lopez-Anderson M, et al. Etiology of sudden cardiac arrest and death in US competitive athletes: a 2-year prospective surveillance study. Clin J Sport Med. 2020;30(4):305–14.
11. Maron BJ, Doerer JJ, Haas TS, Tierney DM, Mueller FO. Sudden deaths in young competitive athletes. Analysis of 1866 deaths in the United States, 1980-2006. Circulation. 2009;119:1085–92.

12. Finocchiaro G, Papadakis M, Robertus JL, Dhutia H, Steriotis AK, Tome M, et al. Etiology of sudden death in sports: insights from a United Kingdom regional registry. J Am Coll Cardiol. 2016;67(18):2108–15.
13. Maron BJ, Thompson PD, Puffer JC, McGrew CA, Strong WB, Douglas PS, et al. Cardiovascular preparticipation screening of competitive athletes. A statement for health professionals from the Sudden Death Committee (clinical cardiology) and Congenital Cardiac Defects Committee (cardiovascular disease in the young), American Heart Association. Circulation. 1996;94(4):850–6.
14. Drezner JA, Owens DS, Prutkin JM, Salerno JC, Harmon KG, Prosise S, et al. Electrocardiographic screening in National Collegiate Athletic Association Athletes. Am J Cardiol. 2016;118(5):754–9.
15. Maron BJ, Friedman RA, Kligfield P, Levine BD, Viskin S, Chaitman BR, et al. Assessment of the 12-lead electrocardiogram as a screening test for detection of cardiovascular disease in healthy general populations of young people (12-25 years of age): a scientific statement from the American Heart Association and the American College of Cardiology. J Am Coll Cardiol. 2014;64(14):1479–514.
16. American Academy of Family Physicians, American Academy of Pediatrics, American College of Sports Medicine, American Medical Society for Sports Medicine, American Orthopaedic Society for Sports Medicine, American Osteopathic Academy Of Sports Medicine. The preparticipation physical evaluation. 5th ed. Elk Grove: American Academy of Pediatrics; 2019.
17. Maron BJ, Thompson PD, Ackerman MJ, Balady G, Berger S, Cohen D, et al. Recommendations and considerations related to preparticipation screening for cardiovascular abnormalities in competitive athletes: 2007 update: a scientific statement from the American Heart Association Council on Nutrition, Physical Activity, and Metabolism: endorsed by the American College of Cardiology Foundation. Circulation. 2007;115(12):1643–455.
18. Drezner JA, O'Connor FG, Harmon KG, Fields KB, Asplund CA, Asif IM, et al. AMSSM Position Statement on Cardiovascular Preparticipation Screening in Athletes: current evidence, knowledge gaps, recommendations and future directions. Br J Sports Med. 2017;51(3):153–67.
19. Hainline B, Drezner J, Baggish A, Harmon KG, Emery MS, Myerburg RJ, et al. Interassociation consensus statement on cardiovascular care of college student-athletes. Br J Sports Med. 2017;51(2):74–85.
20. Maron BJ, Shirani J, Poliac LC, Mathenge R, Roberts WC, Mueller FO. Sudden death in young competitive athletes. Clinical, demographic, and pathological profiles. JAMA. 1996;276(3):199–204.
21. Harmon KG, Zigman M, Drezner JA. The effectiveness of screening history, physical exam, and ECG to detect potentially lethal cardiac disorders in athletes: a systematic review/meta-analysis. J Electrocardiol. 2015;48(3):329–38.
22. Fudge J, Harmon KG, Owens DS, Prutkin JM, Salerno JC, Asif IM, et al. Cardiovascular screening in adolescents and young adults: a prospective study comparing the Pre-participation Physical Evaluation Monograph 4th Edition and ECG. Br J Sports Med. 2014;48(15):1172–8.
23. Madsen NL, Drezner JA, Salerno JC. Sudden cardiac death screening in adolescent athletes: an evaluation of compliance with national guidelines. Br J Sports Med. 2013;47(3):172–7.
24. Corrado D, Basso C, Pavei A, Michieli P, Schiavon M, Thiene G. Trends in sudden cardiovascular death in young competitive athletes after implementation of a preparticipation screening program. JAMA. 2006;296(13):1593–601.
25. Corrado D, Pelliccia A, Bjornstad HH, Vanhees L, Biffi A, Borjesson M, et al. Cardiovascular pre-participation screening of young competitive athletes for prevention of sudden death: proposal for a common European protocol. Consensus Statement of the Study Group of Sport Cardiology of the Working Group of Cardiac Rehabilitation and Exercise Physiology and the Working Group of Myocardial and Pericardial Diseases of the European Society of Cardiology. Eur Heart J. 2005;26(5):516–24.
26. Sharma S, Drezner JA, Baggish A, Papadakis M, Wilson MG, Prutkin JM, et al. International recommendations for electrocardiographic interpretation in athletes. J Am Coll Cardiol. 2017;69(8):1057–75.

27. Malhotra A, Dhutia H, Finocchiaro G, Gati S, Beasley I, Clift P, et al. Outcomes of cardiac screening in adolescent soccer players. N Engl J Med. 2018;379(6):524–34.
28. Miars CW, Stamatis A, Morgan GB, Drezner JA. Cardiovascular screening practices and attitudes from the NCAA autonomous "power" 5 conferences. Sports Health. 2018;10(6):547–51.
29. Allen G, Edenfield K, Fitch R, Hainline B, Altman J, Pitts N, Clugston J. Trends in pre-participation cardiac screening among NCAA division 1 autonomy five institutions. Clin J Sport Med. 2020;30(2):130.
30. Sharma S, Merghani A, Gati S. Cardiac screening of young athletes prior to participation in sports: difficulties in detecting the fatally flawed among the fabulously fit. JAMA Intern Med. 2015;175(1):125–7.
31. Yim ES, Basilico F, Corrado G. Early screening for cardiovascular abnormalities with preparticipation echocardiography: utility of focused physician-operated echocardiography in preparticipation screening of athletes. J Ultrasound Med. 2014;33(2):307–13.
32. Edenfield K, Reifsteck F, Carek S, Harmon K, Asken B, Dillon M, et al. Echocardiographic measurements of left ventricular end-diastolic diameter and interventricular septal diameter in collegiate football athletes at preparticipation evaluation referenced to body surface area. BMJ Open Sport Exerc Med. 2019;5:e000488.
33. Reifsteck F, Clugston J, Carek S, Harmon K, Asken B, Dillon M, et al. Echocardiographic measurements of aortic root diameter (ARD) in collegiate football Athletes at pre-participation evaluation. BMJ Open Sport Exerc Med. 2019;5:e000546.
34. Larsen MP, Eisenberg MS, Cummins RO, Hallstrom AP. Predicting survival from out-of-hospital cardiac arrest: a graphic model. Ann Emerg Med. 1993;22(11):1652–8.
35. Lampert R, Olshansky B, Heidbuchel H, Lawless C, Saarel E, Ackerman M, et al. Safety of sports for athletes with implantable cardioverter-defibrillators: long-term results of a prospective multinational registry. Circulation. 2017;135(23):2310–2.
36. Maron BJ, Harris KM, Thompson PD, Eichner ER, Steinberg MH. Eligibility and disqualification recommendations for competitive athletes with cardiovascular abnormalities: task force 14: sickle cell trait: a scientific statement from the American Heart Association and American College of Cardiology. J Am Coll Cardiol. 2015;66(21):2444–6.
37. Maron BJ, Maron MS. Hypertrophic cardiomyopathy. Lancet. 2013;381(9862):242–55.
38. Cooper RM, Raphael CE, Liebregts M, Anavekar NS, Veselka J. New developments in hypertrophic cardiomyopathy. Can J Cardiol. 2017;33(10):1254–65.
39. Semsarian C, Ingles J, Maron MS, Maron BJ. New perspectives on the prevalence of hypertrophic cardiomyopathy. J Am Coll Cardiol. 2015;65(12):1249–54.
40. Maron BJ. Hypertrophic cardiomyopathy: a systematic review. JAMA. 2002;287(10):1308–20.
41. Alcalai R, Seidman JG, Seidman CE. Genetic basis of hypertrophic cardiomyopathy: from bench to the clinics. J Cardiovasc Electrophysiol. 2008;19(1):104–10.
42. Maron BJ, Udelson JE, Bonow RO, Nishimura RA, Ackerman MJ, Estes NAM, et al. Eligibility and disqualification recommendations for competitive athletes with cardiovascular abnormalities: task force 3: hypertrophic cardiomyopathy, arrhythmogenic right ventricular cardiomyopathy and other cardiomyopathies, and myocarditis: a scientific statement from the American Heart Association and American College of Cardiology. J Am Coll Cardiol. 2015;66(21):2362–71.
43. Drezner JA, Sharma S, Baggish A, Papadakis M, Wilson MG, Prutkin JM, et al. International criteria for electrocardiographic interpretation in athletes. Br J Sports Med. 2017;51(9):704–31.
44. Schnell F, Riding N, O'Hanlon R, Axel Lentz P, Donal E, Kervio G, et al. Recognition and significance of pathological T-wave inversions in athletes. Circulation. 2015;131(2):165–73.
45. Pelliccia A, Di Paolo FM, Quattrini FM, Basso C, Culasso F, Popoli G, et al. Outcomes in athletes with marked ECG repolarization abnormalities. N Engl J Med. 2008;358(2):152–61.
46. Afonso L, Kondur A, Simegn M, Niraj A, Hari P, Kaur R, et al. Two-dimensional strain profiles in patients with physiological and pathological hypertrophy and preserved left ventricular systolic function: a comparative analyses. BMJ Open. 2012;2(4):e001390.
47. Wasfy MM, Weiner RB. Differentiating the athlete's heart from hypertrophic cardiomyopathy. Curr Opin Cardiol. 2015;30(5):500–5.

48. Basavarajaiah S, Wilson M, Junagde S, Jackson G, Whyte G, Sharma S, et al. Physiological left ventricular hypertrophy or hypertrophic cardiomyopathy in an elite adolescent athlete: role of detraining in resolving the clinical dilemma. Br J Sports Med. 2006;40(8):727–9; discussion 9.
49. Weiner RB, Wang F, Berkstresser B, Kim J, Wang TJ, Lewis GD, et al. Regression of "gray zone" exercise-induced concentric left ventricular hypertrophy during prescribed detraining. J Am Coll Cardiol. 2012;59(22):1992–4.
50. Levine BD, Baggish AL, Kovacs RJ, Link MS, Maron MS, Mitchell JH. Eligibility and disqualification recommendations for competitive athletes with cardiovascular abnormalities: task force 1: classification of sports: dynamic, static, and impact: a scientific statement from the American Heart Association and American College of Cardiology. J Am Coll Cardiol. 2015;66(21):2350–5.
51. Ammash NM, Sundt TM, Connolly HM. Marfan syndrome-diagnosis and management. Curr Probl Cardiol. 2008;33(1):7–39.
52. Loeys BL, Dietz HC, Braverman AC, Callewaert BL, De Backer J, Devereux RB, et al. The revised Ghent nosology for the Marfan syndrome. J Med Genet. 2010;47(7):476–85.
53. Braverman AC, Harris KM, Kovacs RJ, Maron BJ, American Heart Association Electrocardiography and Arrhythmias Committee of Council on Clinical Cardiology CoCDiY, Council on Cardiovascular and Stroke Nursing, Council on Functional Genomics and Translational Biology, and American College of Cardiology. Eligibility and disqualification recommendations for competitive athletes with cardiovascular abnormalities: task force 7: aortic diseases, including Marfan syndrome: a scientific statement from the American Heart Association and American College of Cardiology. Circulation. 2015;132(22):e303–9.
54. Radke RM, Baumgartner H. Diagnosis and treatment of Marfan syndrome: an update. Heart. 2014;100(17):1382–91.
55. Basso C, Boschello M, Perrone C, Mecenero A, Cera A, Bicego D, et al. An echocardiographic survey of primary school children for bicuspid aortic valve. Am J Cardiol. 2004;93(5):661–3.
56. Braverman AC. Aortic involvement in patients with a bicuspid aortic valve. Heart. 2011;97(6):506–13.
57. Yim ES. Aortic root disease in athletes: aortic root dilation, anomalous coronary artery, bicuspid aortic valve, and Marfan's syndrome. Sports Med. 2013;43(8):721–32.
58. Gentry JL, Carruthers D, Joshi PH, Maroules CD, Ayers CR, de Lemos JA, et al. Ascending aortic dimensions in Former National Football League Athletes. Circ Cardiovasc Imaging. 2017;10(11):e006852.
59. Braverman AC, Harris KM, Kovacs RJ, Maron BJ. Eligibility and disqualification recommendations for competitive athletes with cardiovascular abnormalities: task force 7: aortic diseases, including Marfan syndrome: a scientific statement from the American Heart Association and American College of Cardiology. J Am Coll Cardiol. 2015;66(21):2398–405.
60. Basso C, Maron BJ, Corrado D, Thiene G. Clinical profile of congenital coronary artery anomalies with origin from the wrong aortic sinus leading to sudden death in young competitive athletes. J Am Coll Cardiol. 2000;35(6):1493–501.
61. Van Hare GF, Ackerman MJ, Evangelista JK, Kovacs RJ, Myerburg RJ, Shafer KM, et al. Eligibility and disqualification recommendations for competitive athletes with cardiovascular abnormalities: task force 4: congenital heart disease: a scientific statement from the American Heart Association and American College of Cardiology. J Am Coll Cardiol. 2015;66(21):2372–84.
62. Hoyt WJ, Dean PN, Schneider DS, Conaway MR, Kramer CM, Battle RW. Coronary artery evaluation by screening echocardiogram in intercollegiate athletes. Med Sci Sports Exerc. 2017;49(5):863–9.
63. Tucker AM, Vogel RA, Lincoln AE, Dunn RE, Ahrensfield DC, Allen TW, et al. Prevalence of cardiovascular disease risk factors among National Football League players. JAMA. 2009;301(20):2111–9.

64. Baron SL, Hein MJ, Lehman E, Gersic CM. Body mass index, playing position, race, and the cardiovascular mortality of retired professional football players. Am J Cardiol. 2012;109(6):889–96.
65. Chang AY, FitzGerald SJ, Cannaday J, Zhang S, Patel A, Palmer MD, et al. Cardiovascular risk factors and coronary atherosclerosis in retired National Football League players. Am J Cardiol. 2009;104(6):805–11.
66. Basra SS, Pokharel Y, Hira RS, Bandeali SJ, Nambi V, Deswal A, et al. Relation between playing position and coronary artery calcium scores in retired National Football League players. Am J Cardiol. 2014;114(12):1836–40.
67. Thompson PD, Myerburg RJ, Levine BD, Udelson JE, Kovacs RJ. Eligibility and disqualification recommendations for competitive athletes with cardiovascular abnormalities: task force 8: coronary artery disease: a scientific statement from the American Heart Association and American College of Cardiology. J Am Coll Cardiol. 2015;66(21):2406–11.
68. Rao AL, Salerno JC, Asif IM, Drezner JA. Evaluation and management of Wolff-Parkinson-White in athletes. Sports Health. 2014;6(4):326–32.
69. Cohen MI, Triedman JK, Cannon BC, Davis AM, Drago F, Janousek J, et al. PACES/HRS expert consensus statement on the management of the asymptomatic young patient with a Wolff-Parkinson-White (WPW, ventricular preexcitation) electrocardiographic pattern: developed in partnership between the Pediatric and Congenital Electrophysiology Society (PACES) and the Heart Rhythm Society (HRS). Endorsed by the governing bodies of PACES, HRS, the American College of Cardiology Foundation (ACCF), the American Heart Association (AHA), the American Academy of Pediatrics (AAP), and the Canadian Heart Rhythm Society (CHRS). Heart Rhythm. 2012;9(6):1006–24.
70. Surawicz B, Childers R, Deal BJ, Gettes LS, Bailey JJ, Gorgels A, et al. AHA/ACCF/HRS recommendations for the standardization and interpretation of the electrocardiogram: part III: intraventricular conduction disturbances: a scientific statement from the American Heart Association Electrocardiography and Arrhythmias Committee, Council on Clinical Cardiology; the American College of Cardiology Foundation; and the Heart Rhythm Society. Endorsed by the International Society for Computerized Electrocardiology. J Am Coll Cardiol. 2009;53(11):976–81.
71. Zipes DP, Link MS, Ackerman MJ, Kovacs RJ, Myerburg RJ, Estes NAM. Eligibility and disqualification recommendations for competitive athletes with cardiovascular abnormalities: task force 9: arrhythmias and conduction defects: a scientific statement from the American Heart Association and American College of Cardiology. J Am Coll Cardiol. 2015;66(21):2412–23.
72. Calvo N, Brugada J, Sitges M, Mont L. Atrial fibrillation and atrial flutter in athletes. Br J Sports Med. 2012;46(Suppl 1):i37–43.
73. Raju H, Kalman JM. Management of Atrial Fibrillation in the athlete. Heart Lung Circ. 2018;27(9):1086–92.
74. Flannery MD, Kalman JM, Sanders P, La Gerche A. State of the art review: atrial fibrillation in athletes. Heart Lung Circ. 2017;26(9):983–9.
75. Chung MK, Eckhardt LL, Chen LY, Ahmed HM, Gopinathannair R, Joglar JA, et al. Lifestyle and risk factor modification for reduction of atrial fibrillation: a scientific statement From the American Heart Association. Circulation. 2020. https://doi.org/10.1161/CIR.0000000000000748.
76. Mont L, Tamborero D, Elosua R, Molina I, Coll-Vinent B, Sitges M, et al. Physical activity, height, and left atrial size are independent risk factors for lone atrial fibrillation in middle-aged healthy individuals. Europace. 2008;10(1):15–20.
77. Gomez AT, Prutkin JM, Rao AL. Evaluation and management of athletes with Long QT syndrome. Sports Health. 2016;8(6):527–35.
78. Schnell F, Behar N, Carré F. Long-QT syndrome and competitive sports. Arrhythm Electrophysiol Rev. 2018;7(3):187–92.
79. Schwartz PJ, Stramba-Badiale M, Crotti L, Pedrazzini M, Besana A, Bosi G, et al. Prevalence of the congenital long-QT syndrome. Circulation. 2009;120(18):1761–7.

80. Schwartz PJ, Priori SG, Spazzolini C, Moss AJ, Vincent GM, Napolitano C, et al. Genotype-phenotype correlation in the long-QT syndrome: gene-specific triggers for life-threatening arrhythmias. Circulation. 2001;103(1):89–95.
81. Priori SG, Wilde AA, Horie M, Cho Y, Behr ER, Berul C, et al. HRS/EHRA/APHRS expert consensus statement on the diagnosis and management of patients with inherited primary arrhythmia syndromes: document endorsed by HRS, EHRA, and APHRS in May 2013 and by ACCF, AHA, PACES, and AEPC in June 2013. Heart Rhythm. 2013;10(12):1932–63.
82. Ackerman MJ, Zipes DP, Kovacs RJ, Maron BJ. Eligibility and disqualification recommendations for competitive athletes with cardiovascular abnormalities: task force 10: the cardiac channelopathies: a scientific statement from the American Heart Association and American College of Cardiology. J Am Coll Cardiol. 2015;66(21):2424–8.
83. Whelton PK, Carey RM, Aronow WS, Casey DE, Collins KJ, Dennison Himmelfarb C, et al. 2017 ACC/AHA/AAPA/ABC/ACPM/AGS/APhA/ASH/ASPC/NMA/PCNA guideline for the prevention, detection, evaluation, and management of high blood pressure in adults: a report of the American College of Cardiology/American Heart Association task force on clinical practice guidelines. J Am Coll Cardiol. 2018;71(19):e127–248.
84. Weiner RB, DeLuca JR, Wang F, Lin J, Wasfy MM, Berkstresser B, et al. Exercise-induced left ventricular remodeling among competitive athletes: a phasic phenomenon. Circ Cardiovasc Imaging. 2015;8(12):e003651.
85. Lin J, Wang F, Weiner RB, DeLuca J, Wasfy MM, Berkstresser B, et al. Blood pressure and left ventricular remodeling among American Style Football Players. JACC Cardiovasc Imaging. 2016;9(12):1367–76.
86. Pelto H. Hypertensive medications in competitive athletes. Curr Sports Med Rep. 2017;16(1):45–9.
87. Niebauer J, Börjesson M, Carre F, Caselli S, Palatini P, Quattrini F, et al. Recommendations for participation in competitive sports of athletes with arterial hypertension: a position statement from the sports cardiology section of the European Association of Preventive Cardiology (EAPC). Eur Heart J. 2018;39(40):3664–71.
88. Black HR, Sica D, Ferdinand K, White WB. Eligibility and disqualification recommendations for competitive athletes with cardiovascular abnormalities: task force 6: hypertension: a scientific statement from the American Heart Association and the American College of Cardiology. J Am Coll Cardiol. 2015;66(21):2393–7.
89. Basso C, Carturan E, Corrado D, Thiene G. Myocarditis and dilated cardiomyopathy in athletes: diagnosis, management, and recommendations for sport activity. Cardiol Clin. 2007;25(3):423–9, vi.
90. Caforio AL, Pankuweit S, Arbustini E, Basso C, Gimeno-Blanes J, Felix SB, et al. Current state of knowledge on aetiology, diagnosis, management, and therapy of myocarditis: a position statement of the European Society of Cardiology Working Group on Myocardial and Pericardial Diseases. Eur Heart J. 2013;34(33):2636–48, 48a–48d.
91. Bonow RO, Nishimura RA, Thompson PD, Udelson JE. Eligibility and disqualification recommendations for competitive athletes with cardiovascular abnormalities: task force 5: valvular heart disease: a scientific statement from the American Heart Association and American College of Cardiology. J Am Coll Cardiol. 2015;66(21):2385–92.
92. Estes NAM, Kovacs RJ, Baggish AL, Myerburg RJ. Eligibility and disqualification recommendations for competitive athletes with cardiovascular abnormalities: task force 11: drugs and performance-enhancing substances: a scientific statement from the American Heart Association and American College of Cardiology. J Am Coll Cardiol. 2015;66(21):2429–33.
93. Link MS, Myerburg RJ, Estes NAM. Eligibility and disqualification recommendations for competitive athletes with cardiovascular abnormalities: task force 12: emergency action plans, resuscitation, cardiopulmonary resuscitation, and automated external defibrillators: a scientific statement from the American Heart Association and American College of Cardiology. J Am Coll Cardiol. 2015;66(21):2434–8.
94. Link MS, Estes NAM, Maron BJ. Eligibility and disqualification recommendations for competitive athletes with cardiovascular abnormalities: task force 13: commotio cordis: a scientific

statement from the American Heart Association and American College of Cardiology. J Am Coll Cardiol. 2015;66(21):2439–43.
95. Maron BJ, Levine BD, Washington RL, Baggish AL, Kovacs RJ, Maron MS. Eligibility and disqualification recommendations for competitive athletes with cardiovascular abnormalities: task force 2: preparticipation screening for cardiovascular disease in competitive athletes: a scientific statement from the American Heart Association and American College of Cardiology. J Am Coll Cardiol. 2015;66(21):2356–61.
96. Mitten MJ, Zipes DP, Maron BJ, Bryant WJ. Eligibility and disqualification recommendations for competitive athletes with cardiovascular abnormalities: task force 15: legal aspects of medical eligibility and disqualification recommendations: a scientific statement from the American Heart Association and American College of Cardiology. J Am Coll Cardiol. 2015;66(21):2447–50.
97. Maron BJ, Zipes DP. Introduction: eligibility recommendations for competitive athletes with cardiovascular abnormalities-general considerations. J Am Coll Cardiol. 2005;45(8):1318–21.
98. Mont L, Pelliccia A, Sharma S, Biffi A, Borjesson M, Brugada Terradellas J, et al. Preparticipation cardiovascular evaluation for athletic participants to prevent sudden death: position paper from the EHRA and the EACPR, branches of the ESC. Endorsed by APHRS, HRS, and SOLAECE. Eur J Prev Cardiol. 2017;24(1):41–69.

Exertional Sickling in Football Players with Sickle Cell Trait

16

Scott Anderson and E. Randy Eichner

Regarded as lazy and not living up to his full potential, John Anders' case report typifies exertion-related, nontraumatic fatality syndromes, wherein the basis of perception for failure is a lack of individual toughness, and the death Exertional Collapse Associate with Sickle Cell Trait (ES) is categorized as unrelated to sport participation. The team's day-1, 90-minute session was described as the "lightest day of opening football practice…ever…" with "a lot of running but no contact." In the early throes of death following collapse, he spoke of putting out 100%. Indeed, John was credited with having gone all out. Immediately recognized and treated as heat exhaustion, Anders died September 1, 1963, hours after his collapse. The called cause of death for the 225-pound wingback was not heat illness, but complications from sickle cell trait [1]. In death, Anders was dubbed one of the most promising athletes to ever don the institution's cherry and silver uniform.

Complication of exertional sickling (ES) as a fatality in football in an athlete with sickle cell trait (SCT) has been reported and recorded for decades. The most prominent early publication is Polie Portier in 1974 [2]. Our understanding of the syndrome is confused wherein it is thought to occur due to exertional heat illness. Prevention is confounded as ES, like other sport-related nontraumatic cause of death, is considered "indirect." Football fatality has long been classified direct or indirect with indirect defined as, "…football cannot be directly responsible for fatal injuries (heat stroke, heart failure, and so forth)." [3] Anders' case mirrors this errant causation classification, "…the activities on the athletic field very likely did not significantly contribute to his death…what precipitated that crisis I don't think

S. Anderson
Head Athletic Trainer, The University of Oklahoma, Norman, OK, USA
e-mail: sanderson@ou.edu

E. R. Eichner (✉)
Professor Emeritus of Medicine, University of Oklahoma Health Sciences Center, Oklahoma City, OK, USA
e-mail: reichner1@comcast.net

K. W. Farmer (ed.), *Football Injuries*,
https://doi.org/10.1007/978-3-030-54875-9_16

anyone can accurately say." [4] Greater than half a century after Anders' death, athlete SCT status is too often unknown and the ES syndrome remains controversial. Factors of causation are denied, signs and symptoms missed, and precautions go unheeded as preventable morbidity and mortality recurs.

There is a general lack of knowledge in the medical community regarding SCT. Unlike sickle cell disease, SCT causes no anemia. SCT has three associated clinical problems of which athletic healthcare providers should be aware. Gross hematuria, from sickling deep in the renal medulla, occurs in less than 5% of subjects with SCT. Over the years, this sickling may cause hyposthenuria (a loss in ability to concentrate urine). Hematuria, 80% of the time from the left kidney, can last for weeks. Those with SCT may also be at risk for deep vein thrombosis [5].

The primary clinical concern for athletes' health care providers and for football players with SCT is complications of intense exertion, which can be fatal. This threat has killed 24 youth, high school, and collegiate football players in the past 2 decades. In Athletic Medicine at the University of Oklahoma, the teachings of our colleague, E Randy Eichner MD, respecting SCT and the athlete, have been crafted into *The Eichner Quintus*, embodying the five manifestations of SCT in athletes: (1) asymptomatic, (2) ischemia, (3) ischemia with infarct, (4) rhabdomyolysis, and (5) metabolic death.

Asymptomatic

A condition of inheritance, SCT, is not a disease and is generally considered a benign trait. SCT inherits one gene for normal hemoglobin (A) and one gene for sickle hemoglobin (S). Each red blood cell in SCT typically has about 40% hemoglobin S and nearly 60% hemoglobin A, with trace amounts of minor hemoglobins such as hemoglobin F or A2. More than three million Americans have SCT and most live a normal, healthy life span and are rarely symptomatic. Because SCT protects against early death from malaria, SCT is "malarial," not racial, that is, it can be found in anyone whose heritage traces to malarial regions of our planet. So, skin phenotype does not predict hemoglobin genotype. SCT occurs in about 8% of African Americans, 0.5% of Hispanics, and 0.2% of Caucasians [6]. One can draw a general assumption of the percentage of football players with SCT based on an equivalent prevalence in the population. 6.7% of African American professional football players were SCT positive in one study [7]. One ES fatality in the dataset is a Caucasian football player. Co-inheriting the alpha thalassemia trait, present in up to one-third of African Americans, lowers the amount of hemoglobin S to <35% in each red blood cell and mitigates the risk of fatal ES in SCT [8].

SCT does not preclude participation in sports. Football players with SCT are rarely symptomatic in practices or games. Training activities purported to prepare players for football present a predictable risk for players with SCT.

Ischemia

Exertional sickling is the clinical concern in the athlete with SCT creating, for some, a grave risk. Individual cases of ES raise a question; "why the one?" But, when reviewed collectively, a common pattern emerges.

Football is a game of brief, intense, exertion followed by a comparative period of extended rest and recovery. Extended rest and recovery are protective for a player with SCT. Conversely, the tradition in football training is sustained, intense sprinting and/or drills demanding successive bouts of maximal exertion, all with little or no rest intervals [9]. Evidence suggests, in individuals with SCT subjected to such excess training, red blood cell sickling can begin within a few minutes of sustained, intense exertion. Strenuous exercise evokes four forces that in concert foster sickling in SCT: [1] severe hypoxemia, [2] metabolic (lactic) acidosis, [3] hyperthermia in working muscles, and [4] red blood cell dehydration, as red cells lose water traversing the hyperosmotic milieu of the working muscle [10]. Exercise physiology research shows that, in SCT, during intense exertion and hypoxemia, red blood cells containing hemoglobin S may elongate or "sickle," becoming "stiff" and "sticky" and so tend to "logjam" the microcirculation of the muscles. This exercise-induced sickling impedes capillary blood flow, causing ischemia. This phenomenon explains the ensuing complications of exertion in the athlete with SCT.

Ischemia in an exerting athlete manifests in muscle pain and, often, complaint of a "cramp." Allowed to set their own pace, the athlete invariably withdraws due to the self-limiting nature of the symptoms. Commonly presenting as shortness of breath, low back pain and/or leg pain and weakness, withdrawal from activity permits early opportunity for rest and recovery, accommodating cessation of the sickling process. As the sickled cells regain oxygen in the lungs, they tend to "unsickle," so symptoms can subside, and the athlete may resume activity. In this setting, ES typically is reversable [11].

"Why the one?" becomes the player with SCT pressed to continue the workout as signs and symptoms are unrecognized or ignored. Ischemia, unmanaged, progresses to infarct.

Ischemia with Infarct

Infarct in an athlete with SCT may be visceral or muscular.

Splenic infarct in travel with a jump in altitude warrants awareness in the SCT population. In such a setting, onset of abdominal pain, cramping, nausea, and vomiting mandates a differential diagnosis in an athlete with SCT, especially when coupled with the classic Kerr's sign of left upper quadrant pain radiating to the shoulder. Case reports, in the literature and media, document dismissal of signs and symptoms as gastroenteritis or splenic contusion [12]. Athletes with SCT exerting at high altitudes are predisposed to acute vaso-occlusive crisis. One high-profile case report is a National Football League (NFL) player with SCT playing a road game in the mile-high environs of Denver, Colorado. Sharp pain under his ribs in his first game in Denver as a visiting team player was diagnosed as a splenic contusion. With rest, missing the following game, the symptoms subsided, and he returned to play. The second event warranted removal from the team plane as he, again, experienced pain under his ribs. Detained in Denver, he was returned to the hotel for observation and treatment with pain medication. Multiple tests over multiple weeks followed upon his return home. Eventually, splenic infarct was diagnosed, and splenectomy ensued [13]. Newness to altitude, a jump in elevation of as little as 2000 feet, creates risk and becomes a point of awareness for the medical care team and a point of precaution for the athlete with SCT [14].

Muscular infarct due to ischemia in football players with SCT is the prevalent presentation. The pathophysiology is ischemic occlusion of the working muscle. Infarct has been identified in upper extremity muscle groups due to lifting, push-ups, etc. Lower extremity muscle groups at risk are thigh and anterior compartment. Muscular infarct can be a source of low back pain.

Compartments present risk as they are tightly confined due to bone and fascia. Though compartment syndromes occur apart from SCT, symptoms in an athlete with SCT, particularly atraumatic after exertion, warrant heightened cognizance. The normal pathophysiology of exercise serves to evoke sickling in an athlete with SCT and, potentially, the forces are exacerbated in compartments.

Reports of anterior lower extremity compartment syndrome in individuals with SCT exist but athlete-specific reports are rare. A pair of collegiate football case reports were presented within one symposium [15, 16]. Both were African American, National Collegiate Athletic Association (NCAA) Division I (DI) football players in winter conditioning. One player had completed day 2 of winter workouts. The other was in the last day of the team's winter out-of-season workouts. Fasciotomy for decompression was performed emergently in one case with a postoperative outcome of eventual full return to sport participation. Bilateral drop foot manifested in the second case. No fasciotomy was performed. Sport participation was compromised and there was a financial settlement with this athlete.

Acute lumbar paraspinal myonecrosis should be included in the differential diagnosis of a SCT football player reporting with acute low back pain. Like anterior compartment of the lower leg, the paraspinal compartments are tight. Their blood supply is from small branches of segmental arteries and the musculature in football players is large and well developed. Sickling, in weight training and conditioning, can cause acute lumbar paraspinal myonecrosis. Often greater one side versus the other, multifidus and rotatores have been identified as involved muscle groups. MRI is the "gold standard" for diagnosis, along with telltale clinical signs and symptoms and elevated serum creatine kinase (CK). Fasciotomy may be indicated in severe cases. In the authors' collection of case reports, no fasciotomy has been required. Return to participation progressions followed resolution of symptoms after 1–2 weeks [17].

Rhabdomyolysis

Rhabdomyolysis is the breakdown of skeletal muscle with release of intracellular contents into the bloodstream. Rhabdomyolysis was not in our sports medicine lexicon until year-round training for sport became the norm, circa 2000. Rhabdomyolysis was, however, in our sports medicine literature. The few mentions of rhabdomyolysis did not reference excesses in exertion producing outbreaks of individual athlete and team rhabdomyolysis that have brought the term to the forefront. Rather, the literature described rhabdomyolysis as a complication in athletes with SCT [5, 18].

Exercise physiology helps explain why exercise in sickle trait can cause rhabdomyolysis. In SCT, in which about 40% of hemoglobin in each red cell is hemoglobin S, strenuous exercise evokes the aforementioned four forces that foster “sickling,” or change of red-cell shape (when the red cell releases its oxygen) from round to quarter-moon or “sickle.” The metabolic acidosis and hyperthermia shift the oxygen dissociation curve to the right, displacing more oxygen from hemoglobin S. Dehydration of red cells traversing the hyperosmotic milieu of working muscles increases the concentration of hemoglobin S. And severe hypoxemia because of extreme muscle oxygen uptake completes the sickling foursome [19].

Military researchers showed that sickle cells accumulate in venous blood draining exercising muscles and in blood from the arm in recruits cycling with the legs. When SCT recruits cycled at high altitude, sickle cells in venous blood from the forearm rose to a mean of 9% and a maximum (in one man) of 28%. This suggests that as exercise stress and hypoxemia increase, SCT athletes can accumulate sickle cells in the arterial circulation—sickle cells that can go to the heart, brain, and muscles [11]. If too many sickle cells accumulate, they can “logjam” blood vessels and rob vital organs of blood [20].

Accumulation of sickle cells in muscle capillaries with ischemia, infarct, and myonecrosis can result in severe rhabdomyolysis in the athlete with SCT, a severity surpassing that of individual players in reported team outbreaks of exertional rhabdomyolysis. In a published review of collegiate football rhabdomyolysis occurring in an out-of-season weight lifting workout, the highest CK was 331,044 U/L in an athlete reported negative for SCT [21]. In contrast, a collegiate lineman with SCT, sprinting timed 300-m intervals, collapsed as he finished the prescribed 1500-m workout. Hospitalized for 17 days, his CK peaked at 880,000 U/L. Suffering acute renal failure, daily dialysis commenced on day 3 and was continued for nearly 2 months, until eventual discharge from a noncritical care facility. He lost half his renal function and 55 pounds of muscle [22]. Eventually, he returned to sport in brief, semi-professional play.

Metabolic Death

Although exertional rhabdomyolysis occurs in athletes without SCT, athletes suffering exertional heat stroke (EHS) (Chap. 15) die with rhabdomyolysis; athletes with SCT experiencing fulminant rhabdomyolysis die *from* rhabdomyolysis and its ensuing metabolic cascade. In other words, athletes with EHS die not from rhabdomyolysis, but from heat damage to the brain and liver. So, they die *with* some rhabdomyolysis, but not from rhabdomyolysis. In contrast, athletes with ES die directly from rhabdomyolysis. Death due to ES involves the following three components, with a caveat.

1. *Exertion is intense* and sustained for at least a few minutes. Hypoxemia occurs and red blood cells sickle. Sickled RBCs elongate and become stiff and sticky. Sickled cells adhere to each other and the vessel walls, "log jamming" downstream blood flow. Ischemia ensues, and the athlete starts to experience muscle pain and weakness, sometimes erroneously diagnosed as a "cramp."
2. *Exertion continues* despite these signs and symptoms of ischemia, resulting in muscular infarct and rhabdomyolysis. As exertion continues, "explosive" myonecrosis occurs, dumping myoglobin and potassium into the blood stream.
3. Enough myoglobin is released to damage ("plug") the kidneys, eventually inducing acute renal failure. Potassium excretion by the kidneys is severely reduced, and significant hyperkalemia results. Fatal cardiac ventricular fibrillation occurs because of the hyperkalemia.

CAVEAT: If the lactic acidosis and release of potassium are profound in condition 2, they can stop the normal heart even before myoglobin plugs the kidneys. In this setting, death can occur in 20, 40, or 60 min. The athlete loses their blood pressure; their heart rate becomes slower and slower, moving toward an agonal rhythm. Their rate of breathing becomes ever slower, and they lose all consciousness. The final arrhythmia in this situation is usually pulseless electrical activity, as a result of *metabolic storm.* [23] The automated external defibrillator (AED) says, "no shock advised."

Screening for SCT

Exertional sickling fatality in football players has been reported in youth as young as 12, occurs in high school football players, and has prevalence in collegiate NCAA DI football. ES fatality was the leading cause of death, whether traumatic or non-traumatic, in NCAA football, 2000–2018. Ten NCAA DI football players died due to ES, from 2000 to 2010. Effective August 1, 2010, the NCAA mandated SCT screening, documentation of prior screening, or declination of testing with a signed written release, during the pre-participation examination (PPE) for DI football [24]. From an average of one ES death per year to one ES death in NCAA DI football since its enactment, Bylaw 17.1.5.1 has resulted in a statistically significant reduction in fatalities [25]. A recent epidemiological study of fatality in high school and NCAA football evidenced Bylaw17.1.5.1, with targeted education and tailored precautions, has successfully reduced the risk (0.12) and incidence (3.34–0.4 per 100,000) of ES deaths in NCAA DI football athletes. Since implementation in 2010, through 2018, the Bylaw has spared the life of an estimated five NCAA DI football players [26]. At the HS level, though, there are no legislated ES guidelines. The "National Athletic Trainers' Association Consensus Statement: Sickle Cell Trait and the Athlete" is not football or level specific and offers guidance [27].

Though often misunderstood and underappreciated, complications of exertion in SCT athletes, including fatality, are preventable. The linchpin of prevention is knowledge of SCT status. SCT status can be known.

As of 2006, all 50 states and the District of Columbia screen for sickle hemoglobinopathies at birth. However, few in the young athlete demographic know their SCT status [28]. Positive newborn screens for SCT should be communicated to parents and recorded in the individual's medical record for communication to pediatricians and other primary care providers. If the natal screen is unavailable, screening should be repeated in the PPE at onset of sport participation with opportunity for counseling to the athlete and parents [29].

Despite its apparent success in preventing deaths among NCAA athletes, screening is not welcomed by all organizations, as the mandatory nature of screening in the PPE draws a perceived potential for stigmatization and discrimination against the athlete with SCT. The NFL and National Basketball Association screen absent criticism or fear careers are being compromised. The United States Navy, Air Force, and Marines screen in basic training. The US Army has foregone screening for recruits in basic training, believing ES is a condition of heat illness and universal precautions targeting heat illness are applicable to those with SCT. The United States military as a whole is, however, reassessing SCT screening and precautions based on a continuing pattern of ES death in warfighters, with attention being given to NCAA success in screening and lack of precautions preventing all ES fatalities.

Potential Modifiers

The insult creating the ES is sustained, intense activity. The are several conditions or modifiers worth noting which may make activities more intense, theoretically elevating risk of ES for the athlete with SCT. These modifiers are: incomplete acclimatization to ambient heat stress, exertion in sustained ambient heat, high body mass index (BMI), poor fitness, and football uniform heat retention. While modifiers are often presumed, in a retrospective review of ten NCAA DI football players dead due to ES described below, modifiers were rarely present. Sustained, intense activity was the constant:

- *Incomplete Acclimatization:* The acclimatization for two is indeterminate, but they were exerting in mid-80s temperature; one in August and one in September. Three died in winter workouts, indoors. Acclimatization is a 10-to-14-day process. Two were 6 weeks into their off-season regimen and one was week 5. So, only one of ten meets the incomplete acclimatization criteria.
- *Sustained Hot Weather:* Sustained exertion in hot weather induces elevated core temperature and the collapsed athlete suffers exertional heat illness, or so goes the premise. Only one of the ten exerted in a temperature in the 90s, the one

deemed lacking acclimation; his reported core temperature on collapse was 102 °F, lacking a clinical criterion for EHS but consistent with ES. Again, three were indoors. The remainder were in moderate climes, generally early in the workout, lacking climate and duration consistent with developing the sustained core temperature characteristic of EHS.

- *High BMI:* There is no reliable calculation of BMI in an athlete, given the inability of accepted formulas to account for athlete lean body mass. Our majority population of NCAA DI football ES dead are smaller skill players versus linemen.
- *Poor Fitness:* Fitness level is indeterminate in four of the ten. Even if one grants the benefit of doubt and says all four were deconditioned, "common" as a clinical theme, is still lacking as 60% were "fit." Four were weeks and months into their training. Fitness confers a margin of safety for the athlete with SCT. But, presuming only the unfit are at risk constitutes a dangerous dismissal of the syndrome. Fit athletes are placed at risk as they are pushed based on an assumption they have achieved a protective level of fitness.
- *Football Uniform:* Nine of the ten NCAA football players who died were working out in shorts and T-shirt; dress for the tenth is indeterminate. The high school football players who died due to ES had worn a mix of shorts and T-shirt, shorts and helmet, and one assumed to be in full football uniform. There is no knowledge that any of the athletes who died due to ES in youth football, high school basketball, college basketball, boxing, or collegiate track—save maybe one high school football player—were wearing anything other than shorts and T-shirt. The errant assumption football players are dying a nontraumatic death in and due to the football uniform simply does not withstand scrutiny.

Differentiating from Other Conditions

Not all exertional collapse is the same. Knowledge of SCT status becomes key. Athletic healthcare professionals in football must be able to differentially diagnose nontraumatic exertion-related syndromes. Differing characteristics of collapse in the varying syndromes is telling (Table 16.1).

Cardiac collapse (Chap. 16) is typified by an unprotected fall with no warning. There is an immediate loss of consciousness and unresponsiveness (over maybe 2–3 s). The victim is either limp or seizing. Death occurs quickly, within minutes, absent intervention with CPR, AED and emergent care. In contrast to sudden cardiac death, ES is a slow, conscious collapse (evolves over maybe 2–3 min).

Asthmatics have a history of diagnosis and a management plan. Often there is poor control with repetitive prior episodes of exertion-related struggles. The athlete in asthmatic collapse is breathless, gasping, panicky, on hand and knees, and likely holding their rescue inhaler. Upon auscultation, the athlete is moving little air.

Exertional heat stroke (EHS) (Chap. 15) is the common misdiagnosis of ES—in the field, in the emergency room, and in the morgue. Defining characteristics of EHS are sustained: elevated core temperature, 105 °F or greater, with central

Table 16.1 Differential of sudden, non-traumatic collapse in a football player

Non-traumatic collapse				
	ES	Cardiac	EHS	Asthma
Onset	Can occur early in workout	No warning	Usually occurs late in workout	Usually known asthma
	Slumps to ground	Unprotected fall	Can be in coma	Prior episodes, poor control
	Slow evolution to a conscious a collapse	Unconscious and unresponsive		Usually occurs after sprinting
Signs and symptoms	Responsive initially	Unresponsive	Fuzzy thinking	Breathless, may or may not wheeze
	Weakness > pain; low back and/or legs	Gasping, gurgling, snorting, or moaning	Bizarre behavior	Gasping, panicky, on hands/knees
	No palpable muscle cramp	Limp or seizing	Incoherent	Auscultate: moving little air
	Core Temperature < 103 °F	Core temperature irrelevant	Core temperature > 106 °F	Core temperature irrelevant
Management	High-flow O_2, 15 lpm non-rebreather mask	CPR, AED	Cold-water immersion	EpiPen, O_2
	If obtunded, EAP	EAP	Indicated medical referral—Cool first, transport second	EAP

nervous system dysfunction, that is, fuzzy thinking and bizarre behavior. EHS occurs almost wholly in linemen and rarely in skill players.

Symptom report in an athlete with SCT should trigger consideration of ES and removal from activity for assessment. Early withdrawal from exertion with rest and recovery may allow resolution of symptoms and return to activity, often within 15 or 20 min. Providing sideline supplemental oxygen may also be of benefit.

The ES syndrome is unique; characteristically, the player slumps to the ground as the legs give out. The player may have been a front runner, or off to a strong start, leading the sprint or drill. At some point before the collapse, the athlete will be noted as slowing down, falling behind, and struggling, complaining of shortness of breath and inability to recover. This is not the time to press the player to, "Finish!" They begin to lose smooth coordination; they evolve into an awkward running posture and gait, with legs that may look wooden or wobbly. They may complain of weakness, pain, and cramp in the low back and legs. The cramping in ES is distinct from the cramping of exercise-associated muscle cramping (EAMC); symptomatic muscles in ES are soft to palpation and do not "lock up," lacking the tetanic contracture common to EAMC. Weakness—legs like "jello"—is greater than pain. The pain of EAMC is generally excruciating; the hallmark of ES is weakness greater than pain. Core temperature in ES may be elevated,:103° F, consistent with exertion but inconsistent with EHS. Football players with SCT can suffer EHS; a differential diagnosis with indicated care is critical. (See Table 16.1 for differential of sudden, nontraumatic collapse in a football player.) Cold-water immersion is necessary for EHS but offers no salvation in ES, potentially, delaying care while hastening death.

Management

Exertional sickling is a medical emergency. A practiced emergency action plan (EAP) (Chap. 14) is a standard of care, certainly for NCAA sports. The EAP provides for personnel indicated equipment and emergency communication at a minimum. Upon an athlete with SCT presenting with symptoms suggestive of ES, high-flow oxygen, 15 liters per minute (lpm)_ via a non-rebreather mask, should be administered as vitals are monitored. As vitals decline or the athlete is obtunded, the EAP should be implemented; prepare for cardiopulmonary resuscitation. Alert the emergency Department physicians of SCT status and threat of explosive rhabdomyolysis. Absent awareness, early treatment may not be aggressive enough as the athlete's initial presentation may deceive as to the breadth and depth of their condition; often they are sicker than they appear. When ES is likely, emergency medical responders should consider giving calcium chloride (or gluconate) and sodium bicarbonate intravenously to mitigate the grave effects of soaring hyperkalemia and profound lactic acidosis on the heart. However, in many settings, regulations do not permit emergency medical responders to deliver these medications. Management in the emergency room includes aggressive fluid and electrolyte management and blood gas monitoring for metabolic acidosis. The early threat to life is pulseless electrical activity from the toxic metabolic storm; the cardiologist must be alerted to counter this threat. Later, a nephrologist may be needed for renal dialysis and an orthopedic surgeon may be needed to evaluate and treat muscle compartment syndromes [30, 31].

Prevention

Precautions and education greatly benefit players with SCT and may prevent or lessen the severity of ES events. Fifteen useful precautions are provided here:

Precautions for Athletes with Sickle Cell Trait

1. Ideally, athletes with SCT should set their own pace.
2. Engage in a slow and gradual preseason conditioning and lifting regimen.
3. Build up intensity slowly while training, for example, paced progressions.
4. Use adequate rest and recovery between repetitions, especially during serial sprints and intense station or mat drills.
5. No participation in "conditioning tests."

6. Be excused from performance tests such as timed serial sprints or miles, especially if these are not normal sports activities.
7. Not be urged to perform all-out exertion of any kind beyond 2–3 min without being offered a breather.
8. Stop activity immediately upon struggling, that is, at the earliest onset of any undue symptom, such as cramping, pain, weakness, breathlessness, or fatigue.
9. Report any symptoms to an athletic trainer or coach. Seek prompt medical care for any unusual distress.
10. Stay well hydrated, especially in hot and/or humid conditions.
11. Curb activity in very hot or humid conditions.
12. Curb activity when new at altitude, even a “jump” of only 2000 ft. Cut training effort, monitor closely, have ready access to supplemental oxygen.
13. Control asthma to cut risk of exertional sickling.
14. Decrease activity sharply during any illness, especially with fever, vomiting, or diarrhea.
15. Decrease activity after nights of poor sleep.

In the absence of SCT status knowledge, parents, physicians, athletic trainers, coaches, strength coaches, and athletes should be educated on the potentially lethal nature of this condition. If status is unknown, suspect SCT and screen players with a history of or evidencing struggle or collapse with intense, sustained exertion. [32] If identified, implement targeted education and tailored precautions. There is no evidence that any football player has ever died from ES when SCT status is known, athlete and staff are educated, and precautions are heeded. Knowledge beats ignorance.

References

1. Bearman L. Promising UNM Athlete is Dead. Albuquerque Journal C1. 1963, September 3.
2. (1974) Death of an Athlete with Sickle Cell Trait. Medical World News 15:44.
3. National Collegiate Athletic Association. NCAA sports medicine handbook. Indianapolis, IN: NCAA; 1981:17.
4. (1963, September 15). Illness Killed Anders. Albuquerque Journal C1.
5. Eichner ER. Sickle cell trait, heroic exercise, and fatal collapse. Phys Sportsmed. 1993;21(7):51–64.
6. Bonham VL, Dover GJ, Brody LC. Screening student athletes for sickle cell trait – a social and clinical experiment. N Engl Med. 2010;363:997–9.
7. Murphy JR. Sickle cell hemoglobin (Hb AS) in black football players. JAMA. 1973;225:981.
8. Kark JA, Ward FT. Exercise and hemoglobin S. Semin Hematol. 1994;31:181–225.
9. McGrew CA. NCAA football and conditioning drills. Curr Sports Med Rep. 2010;9:185–6.
10. Loosemore M, Walsh SB, Morris E, Stewart G, Porter JB, Montgomery H. Sudden exertional death in sickle cell trait. Br J Sports Med. 2012;46(5):312–4.
11. Martin TW, Weisman IM, Zeballos RJ, Stephenson SR. Exercise and hypoxia increase sickling in venous blood from an exercising limb in individuals with sickle cell trait. Am J Med. 1989;87(1):48–56.
12. Ortega JO. Nausea, vomiting, and abdominal pain in a collegiate basketball player. Clin J Sport Med. 2006;16:443a.

13. Kogod S Ryan Clark gets a pedicure and talks about the time he almost died. 2014. https://www.sbnation.com/nfl/2014/12/10/7361549/ryan-clark-pedicure-washington-football. Accessed 2019 May 03.
14. National Collegiate Athletic Association. NCAA sports medicine handbook. Indianapolis, IN: NCAA; 2014–15; 2014. p. 91–3.
15. Kessler D. 21 year old football conditioning problem with SCT. Park City: Presented at DJO Athletic Training/Sports Medicine Symposium; 2010.
16. Courson R. Acute lower leg compartment syndrome in a collegiate FB player. Park City: Presented at DJO Athletic Training/Sports Medicine Symposium; 2010.
17. Eichner ER, Schnebel B, Anderson S, Clugston JR, Hale MH, Michaudet C, Small JM. Acute lumbar paraspinal myonecrosis in football players with sickle cell trait: a case series. Med Sci Sports Exerc. 2017;49(4):627–32.
18. Browne RJ, Gillespie CA. Sickle cell trait: a risk factor for life threatening rhabdomyolysis? Phys Sportsmed. 1993;21(6):80–8.
19. Eichner ER. Sickle cell trait. J Sport Rehabil. 2007;16(3):197–203.
20. Smoot MK, Amendola A, Cramer E, Doyle C, Kregel KC, Chiang HY, Cavanaugh JE, Herwaldt LA. A cluster of exertional rhabdomyolysis affecting a division I football team. Clin J Sport Med. 2013;23(5):365–72.
21. Shelmadine BD, Baltensperger A, Wilson RL, Bowden RG. Rhabdomyolysis and acute renal failure in a sickle cell trait athlete: a case study. Clin J Sport Med. 2013;23(3):235–7.
22. Anzalone ML, Green VS, Buja M, Sanchez LA, Harrykissoon RI, Eichner ER. Sickle cell trait and fatal rhabdomyolysis in football training: a case study. Med Sci Sports Exerc. 2010;42:3–7.
23. National Collegiate Athletic Association. 2018-19 NCAA division I manual. Bylaw 17.1.5.1. Sickle cell solubility test. Indianapolis, IN: NCAA; 2018:242.
24. Eichner ER. "A stitch in time" and "If 6 was 9": preventing exertional sickling deaths and probing team Rhabdomyolysis outbreaks. Curr Sports Med Rep. 2016;15(3):122–3.
25. Boden BP, Fine KM, Breit, I, Lentz W, Anderson SA. Non-traumatic exertional fatalities in football: epidemiology and effectiveness of NCAA Bylaws, part I. (2020 submitted for publication).
26. National Athletic Trainers' Association. Consensus statement: sickle cell trait and the athlete. 2007. https://www.nata.org/sites/default/files/sicklecelltraitandtheathlete.pdf. Accessed 2019 May 03.
27. Taylor C, Kavanagh P, Zuckerman B. Sickle cell trait – neglected opportunities in the era of genomic medicine. JAMA. 2014;311(15):1495–6.
28. Treadwell MJ, McClough L, Vichinsky E. Using qualitative and quantitative strategies to evaluate knowledge and perceptions about sickle cell disease and sickle cell trait. J Natl Med Assoc. 2006;98(5):704–10.
29. Newman C, Fields KB. Atypical presentations of exertional collapse. Pediatr Emerg Care. 2019. [Ahead to print].
30. Eichner ER. Sickle cell trait in sports. Curr Sports Med Rep. 2010;9(6):347–51.
31. Koppes GM, Daly JJ, Coltman CA Jr, Butkus DE. Exertion-induced Rhabdomyolysis with acute renal failure and disseminated intravascular coagulation in sickle cell trait. Am J Med. 1977;63(2):313–7.

Brain Injuries in Football

17

Breton M. Asken, Brian D. Sindelar, James R. Clugston, and Julian E. Bailes

Introduction

American-style football (hereafter referred to as "football") carries a risk of traumatic brain injury (TBI), especially mild TBI (mTBI) or concussion. Unlike orthopedic injuries which have consistently been recognized as detrimental to football performance, career length, and general athlete health and accorded significant effort for their prevention, recognition, and rehabilitation, concussion has only garnered comparable attention in the past three decades. Medical research and public interest in concussion are now progressing quickly and contributions from diverse specialties like sports medicine, neurology, neuropsychology, neurosurgery, physical therapy, and occupational therapy are culminating in improved standards of care.

Traumatic brain injury broadly characterizes a complicated spectrum of head traumas with often confusing terminology. Concussion and mTBI are typically used interchangeably in medical literature. Generally, "concussion" is the preferred term in sports medicine settings, while more traditional medical settings use "mTBI" [1]. The term "sport-related concussion" (SRC) is now commonly used when describing concussion sustained during athletic activity and will be used throughout this chapter. The majority of the chapter will focus on SRC as it is the most common TBI

B. M. Asken (✉)
Department of Clinical and Health Psychology, University of Florida, Gainesville, FL, USA
e-mail: basken8@phhp.ufl.edu

B. D. Sindelar
Department of Neurosurgery, University of Florida, Gainesville, FL, USA

J. R. Clugston
Departments of Community Health & Family Medicine and Neurology, Team Physician, University of Florida, Gainesville, FL, USA

J. E. Bailes
Department of Neurosurgery, NorthShore University HealthSystem, Evanston, IL, USA

K. W. Farmer (ed.), *Football Injuries*,
https://doi.org/10.1007/978-3-030-54875-9_17

encountered in football but we will also consider several less common, but more severe conditions, which football clinicians must recognize. Finally, we will discuss potential long-term effects of football-related brain injury.

SRC: Characteristics, Biomechanics, and Pathophysiology

Characteristics

SRC definitions typically describe a transient disturbance in brain function induced by traumatic forces transmitted to the brain. The disturbance may manifest with common, nonspecific symptoms such as headache, dizziness, fatigue, fogginess, difficulty concentrating, blurry vision, nausea, etc. By definition, symptom presentation cannot be explained by other injuries, comorbid conditions, or medication/drug/substance use. SRC does not typically produce changes on standard brain imaging (computed tomography [CT] or magnetic resonance imaging [MRI] and thus traditionally has been termed a "functional" as opposed to "structural" injury. Complex, pathophysiologic changes presumably underlie the observed transient alteration of brain function and the typical acute onset of a variety of concussion-related symptoms, with or without loss of consciousness [LOC] [2, 3]. These definitions capture both the pathophysiologic and clinical (i.e., symptomatic) components of SRC; however, it is important to note that currently only the latter factors are applied in current diagnostic formulations (see section "Acute SRC Diagnosis").

Biomechanics and Pathophysiology

Football-related head impacts cause both linear and rotational forces that can mechanically deform, or strain, structures in the brain such as axons. Magnitude, acceleration, duration, location, and density (timing of recent impacts) are thought to influence risk. Giza and Hovda described the pathophysiology associated with concussion commonly referred to as the "neurometabolic cascade" [4]. Mechanical axon deformation opens membrane channels resulting in indiscriminate glutamate release, potassium efflux, and calcium and sodium influx. This creates a subsequently imbalanced electrical gradient that opens ion-gated channels and creates a "spreading depression-like" state. Restoring neuronal homeostasis requires increased energy use, but inefficiently functioning mitochondria and transiently reduced cerebral blood flow following concussion create a supply and demand mismatch. Ultimately, these neurometabolic alterations cause cytoskeletal damage to axons, dendrites, and astrocytes irrespective of the damage caused directly by the biomechanical forces of injury, termed "secondary injury."

Imaging

As alluded above, macroscopic pathophysiologic changes are rarely seen on current clinical imaging modalities such as standard MRI or CT. One study found acute, SRC-related findings on structural MRI in 1 out of 138 prospectively evaluated SRC cases (not football-specific), suggesting extremely low prevalence of standard MRI-detectable structural changes [5]. Therefore, CT and MRI are not considered necessary or standard of practice for SRC diagnosis and management, but they may be used at the clinician's discretion for ruling out more serious injuries (e.g., hemorrhage, skull fracture). More advanced neuroimaging, such as diffusion-weighted imaging, functional MRI, magnetic resonance spectroscopy, etc., may provide some characterization of the pathophysiologic effects of SRC but are not readily available and remain research tools not currently used as standard of care.

SRC Versus Civilian mTBI

Concussions sustained on the playing field may not be the same as those sustained off of it, and conventional neuroimaging outcomes highlight this dichotomy between athlete SRC and civilian mTBI samples. Standard CT/MRI imaging abnormalities, while still not diagnostic, are potentially far more common in nonathlete mTBI studies [6]. One might argue that athletes are therefore done a disservice by not receiving routine imaging after SRC. Presumably, if SRC and civilian mTBI are categorically equivalent injuries, athletes should show similar rates of abnormal CT/MRI. However, the prospective MRI study from Klein et al. refutes this [5]. Further, if abnormal CT/MRI findings were indeed present and pathologic in SRC cases, but not detected and managed, one would expect a high rate of SRC-related morbidity and mortality in athletes based on SRC frequency and the high rate of return to sport (often with further head impacts) in a relatively short time frame. Paradoxically, the opposite is true – athletes generally have better outcomes with more rapid recovery than that suggested by data from civilian mTBI studies.

Epidemiology and Risk of SRC in Football

Injury surveillance systems that track SRC prevalence and incidence have helped quantify SRC risk over the past decade. SRC risk is often expressed as a function of athlete exposures (AEs), which refer to one athlete participating in one athletic event such as a game or practice. Football is often, but not always, associated with the greatest SRC risk across participation levels relative to other sports. Overall, football-related SRC rates hover around 1/1000 AEs [7, 8]. SRC frequency in the National Football League (NFL) is approximately 0.4–0.7 per NFL game [9–11]. Professional-level practice rates are not available, but competition-related SRC rates are consistently higher than overall practice rates when compared directly at other participation levels. For example, Kerr and colleagues recently reported football SRC data from large high school and collegiate injury surveillance systems that showed competition SRC rates around 3/1000 AEs, which was almost 10× higher than practice rates [8, 12].

Importantly, the diverse structure of football practices and games underlies a current appreciation for SRC risk being nonuniform across football-related activities. Football practices vary drastically by intensity and contact level. More nuanced approaches evaluating different practice types in college football revealed an SRC risk in competition (4.5/1000 AEs) similar to the risk in preseason training camp practices (3.8/1000 AEs), which are often higher intensity and "game-like" [13]. Other work has similarly identified higher SRC rates throughout the season when focusing on practice types associated with more equipment and greater contact [7]. Within football games, special teams plays (e.g., kickoffs) have the greatest SRC risk [13, 14]. This sparked prevention efforts targeting reduction of high-risk plays, which initial reports show have been successful at decreasing SRC rates [15].

SRC risk variability among diverse football-related activities complicates interpretation of more general epidemiological estimates, but also introduces opportunities for more targeted risk-reduction strategies like the kickoff rule changes. Recent examples include mandates and recommendations for penalizing high-risk behaviors during games, reducing high-risk plays, restricting high-contact practices, and limiting exposure to specific high-risk drills [16–18].

One major caveat of SRC epidemiological data is that it relies significantly on athlete self-report, but SRC is often unrecognized by athletes and may not be apparent to supervising medical staff. In addition to poor recognition, intentional nondisclosure of SRC symptoms by athletes remains problematic and both suggest that prevalence/incidence rates underestimate true risk with upwards of half of all SRCs going unrecognized or unreported [19–21]. Conversely, any trends suggesting increased SRC rates over time may reflect improved awareness and diagnostic techniques, or cultural shifts toward increased willingness to report SRC symptoms [22].

Acute SRC Diagnosis

Acute SRC diagnosis is challenging for clinicians and often requires a high index of suspicion. Any athlete suspected of sustaining an SRC should be immediately removed from athletic activity and formally evaluated. Simultaneous consideration of other serious injuries such as cervical spine trauma and more severe head trauma is imperative and, if these are suspected, appropriate emergency action plans should be initiated (Chap. 14). In cases where overt signs such as LOC; tonic posturing; or gross abnormalities in memory, speech, gait, or behavior are present in combination with blunt trauma, SRC may be easy to detect but typically signs and symptoms are less obvious. Prior familiarity of the athlete is helpful in recognizing subtle changes in personality and speech. Initial questioning centers on what happened and what the athlete is feeling, followed by questions which assess the athlete's current memory, orientation, and concentration ability. Abbreviated assessments of balance, gait, vision, and vestibular-oculomotor function can also occur on the sideline in a timely manner, especially if they have been considered and rehearsed in advance by the sports health staff. If SRC is suspected after these initial evaluations, a more thorough examination, including a detailed neurological examination and performance of a battery of multimodal concussion testing (see section "Diagnostic Tools"), is usually performed. Sideline settings can be chaotic and removing the athlete to a less distracting environment such as a locker room or an athletic training facility for this secondary examination is prudent when possible. See Fig. 17.1 for a schematic representation of typical acute evaluation and Fig. 17.2 for the National Football League's (NFL) published "Concussion Game Day Checklist" [23]. The checklist is from the NFL's concussion diagnosis and management protocol, which is a peer-reviewed document describing football-specific concussion care at the professional level [23]. It, along with other position statements and organizational recommendations for SRC in general, provides detailed and applicable guidance on SRC management for football athletes.

It is important to note that the diagnosis of SRC can be made at any stage in this process based on the recognition of abnormal findings, and at that point, the process can be stopped if completion is not practical, such as when the clinician is needed for continued event coverage. The entire evaluation process should not be rushed or hurried and it is helpful to alert the athlete and coaches at the onset that a comprehensive examination will occur. Often removing a football athlete's helmet from the immediate surroundings helps reinforce this idea. If an athlete is diagnosed with SRC, there should be no same day return to athletic activity at any level of sport [2] (see section "Recovery and Rehabilitation").

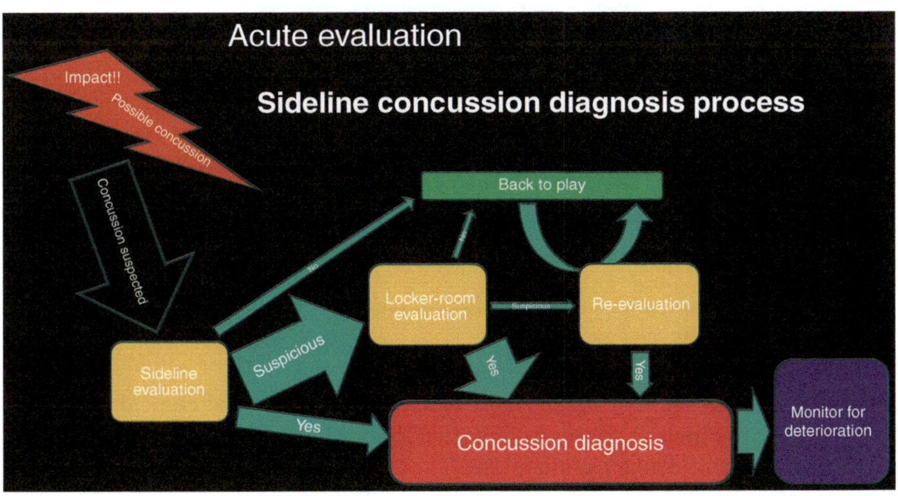

Fig. 17.1 Schematic representation of acute concussion evaluation

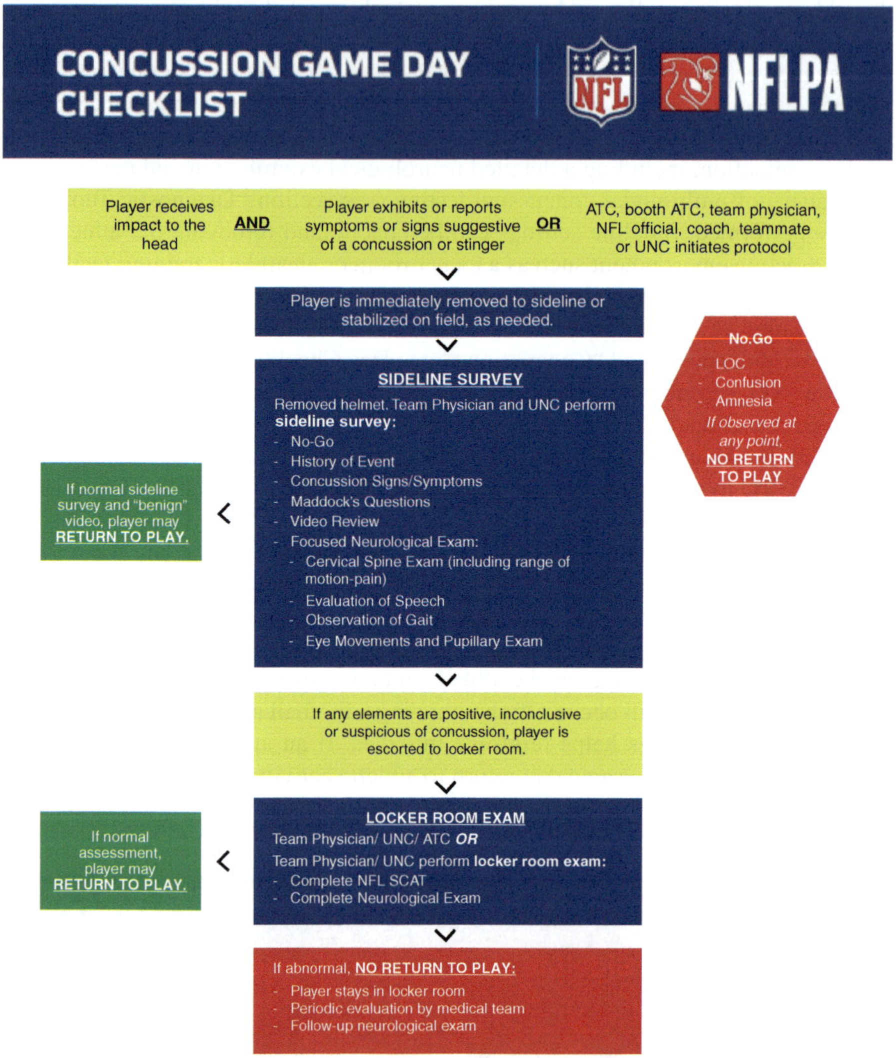

Fig. 17.2 NFL's concussion game day checklist [23]

Diagnostic Tools

As mentioned above, SRC diagnosis is based on a multifaceted clinical evaluation [3] that typically includes observed signs or reported symptoms and cognitive, balance, and vestibulo-ocular examinations. The clinical heterogeneity of SRC requires this multifaceted evaluation, and there are multiple tools, both open source and proprietary, that may help the clinician perform multimodal evaluations to arrive at the diagnosis of SRC.

Symptom reports are the most common information used to render SRC diagnosis [24]. Several reliable and validated concussion symptom questionnaires exist. The Concussion in Sport Group endorses the Sport Concussion Assessment Tool (SCAT-5) symptom evaluation for use in athletic settings [2, 25]. The SCAT-5 symptom evaluation includes 22 symptoms rated by the athlete on a 0–6 severity scale (0 – "symptom not present," 1–2 – "mild," 3–4 – "moderate," 5–6 – "severe"). SRC symptoms generally cluster into physical/somatic, cognitive, insomnia/sleep-related, emotional, and vestibulo-ocular domains [26–29]. Symptom inventories have strong sensitivity and specificity to SRC, presumably because the symptoms queried define SRC. However, they are limited by their reliance on subjective athlete report. Additional assessment tools supplement symptom inventories by providing a relatively more objective assessment of brain functions.

The Standardized Assessment of Concussion (SAC) is a brief cognitive screening tool assessing aspects of orientation, immediate memory, concentration, and delayed recall [30]. The most common postural stability test is the Balance Error Scoring System (BESS), which assesses the patient's balance in three stances while their eyes are closed and has demonstrated abnormalities in 24–37% of concussed athletes 24 hours post injury [31, 32]. The SAC, BESS, and SCAT-5 symptom evaluation are all components of the SCAT-5 (Echemendia et al., 2017), which is open source and now also includes an optional but more rigorous memory subtest of the SAC (10-word list instead of 5-word list). Early findings suggest that using the longer word list reduces ceiling effects and, presumably, improves detection of memory changes [33]. Other SRC assessments targeting vestibulo-ocular function, which is not incorporated into the SCAT-5, include the vestibulo-oculomotor screen (VOMS) [34] (open source), the King-Devick test [35] (proprietary), and eye trackers such as the newly FDA-approved EyeBOX [36] (proprietary) and EYE-SYNC (proprietary) devices. Additional technologies such as app-based balance measures, reaction timers, speech pattern analyzers, portable electroencephalograms, etc. are emerging but their acceptance is currently less widespread.

Computerized neurocognitive tests (CNTs) are also popularly used in non-acute sport settings such as during follow-up visits. Clinicians vary in how they implement their use, with some preferring CNTs as a confirmatory office-based diagnostic tool, while others may restrict administration to a "final clearance" before reinitiating physical activity; still others administer assessments serially throughout recovery as an objective measure. When used diagnostically, CNTs differentiate well SRC from non-SRC athletes acutely but show rapidly diminishing signal to SRC within the first few days to weeks after injury [37, 38]. Therefore, CNTs likely have greatest utility shortly after injury but provide minimal benefit as a measure of longer-term outcomes or cases of complicated recovery. For this reason, diagnosis and determination of a player's capacity to return to play typically requires a multimodal approach of various clinical tools to assess recovery.

Sports medicine clinicians often wonder about the importance or necessity of baseline SRC testing or preseason evaluations that purportedly capture each athlete's "healthy" performance to serve in post-suspected SRC comparison. Baseline testing can be costly, time-consuming, have poor reproducibility, demonstrate practice effects, and both intentionally and unintentionally be influenced by the athlete. The Concussion in Sport Group has consistently stated that broad implementation of baseline testing is not necessary for appropriate SRC management [2]. Baseline examinations are likely most useful for athletes suspected to fall outside of typical normative reference ranges for a given SRC test, or who belong to demographic groups that differ from the samples used to derive the normative ranges. This might include athletes with complicated developmental histories (e.g., attention-deficit hyperactivity disorder or learning disability), racial/ethnic minority groups, or those suspected to have well above or below average cognitive abilities. Asken et al. provide improved normative reference data for college-aged athletes that take many of these factors into account [39], but further work is needed across the athlete lifespan. Additional considerations for implementing baseline testing include access to resources for optimum testing environments (e.g., individual or small group testing in quiet, supervised environments) and trained professionals for test interpretation (e.g., neuropsychologists) as well as access to baseline information at the time of suspected SRC and location of the acute evaluation.

To summarize the diagnostic process and use of concussion testing as diagnostic tools, an athlete suspected of suffering an SRC may be confidently diagnosed based on affirmative acute symptom reporting linked to an injury mechanism. In this case, additional testing is not required but may provide supplemental information important for tracking recovery through serial administration over time after the injury. Athletes may also be diagnosed based on poor test performance despite being subjectively asymptomatic, particularly if the clinician feels the athlete may be motivated to withhold symptom reporting. For ambiguous cases where clinicians cannot definitively rule in or rule out SRC immediately upon suspected injury, err on the side of caution and monitor as time allows. Athletes diagnosed with SRC should be restricted from sport activities until resolution of symptoms and successful completion of rehabilitation protocols.

Recovery and Rehabilitation

Recovery time from SRC involves a symptomatic phase, which starts acutely after injury, symptom resolution and initiation of rehabilitation protocols, and asymptomatic progression through increasingly rigorous activities prior to full clearance for return to sport. Considering this general framework is important when interpreting existing data on "normal recovery" after SRC. Most (>85%) collegiate football athletes exhibit *symptom resolution* within 7–10 days, and only in a small minority persist >1 month [40]. Previously, due to lack of standard implementation of formalized return to sport protocols, symptom resolution time closely aligned with an athlete's timeline for clearance for return to sport [41]. As recently as the last decade, football athletes suffering an in-game SRC commonly returned to sport activity within a few days with expectations to be cleared for full activity for the following weekend's game. Therefore, implementation of a more formalized return to sport protocol with specific step-wise phases has contributed to longer rehabilitation phases, with a typical recovery time approaching 1–2 weeks. Throughout the path toward recovery, clinicians should serially administer the previously described tests throughout the rehabilitation protocols to objectively track recovery across multiple domains and further guide proper return to activity decision-making.

Return to activity protocols have existed for almost two decades. However, SRC rehabilitation has undergone arguably the greatest improvements and updates in the past few years. Past protocols focused only on returning to sport, while modern management plans include both a sport and academic component that incorporate similar rationale for progression. Return to sport (RTS; previously known as "return to play" or RTP) protocols for football are a six-step process: (1) symptom-limited activity, (2) light, aerobic exercise (e.g., walking or moderate stationary cycling), (3) sport-specific exercise, (4) non-contact, sport-specific training drills, (5) full contact practice, and (6) full return to sport (2). (See Table 17.1) Step 1 represents a marked shift in thinking away from prior protocols recommending strict rest until becoming asymptomatic and toward approaches emphasizing *symptom-limited activity*. Consensus guidelines recommend 24–48 hours of *relative physical and cognitive rest* prior to initiating the RTS and symptom-limited activities [42]. In other words, absolute rest and isolation (i.e., "cocoon therapy") has no place in the current protocol. After a brief period of relative rest, athletes are encouraged to engage in basic daily activities that are tolerable and do not exacerbate lingering symptoms. It is expected that athletes will be virtually asymptomatic or at least have stable (not worsening) symptoms prior to beginning Step 2, and that a minimum of 24 hours accompany each step in the progression thereafter. Each successive step incorporates more intense physical activities aimed at increasing heart rate, reintegrating with sport-specific activities, and, finally, exposure to activities with risk for head impacts. Any reemergence and/or exacerbation of SRC symptoms is accompanied by regression to the last successfully completed step, which will also extend recovery time. Expected timelines in younger football athletes may be longer, particularly during the symptomatic phase.

The first academic/cognitive corollary to the physical activity-based RTS protocol, the return to learn (RTL) protocol, was formalized in 2017 [2]. The basic components mimic the rationale of the RTS protocol, namely symptom-limited activity

Table 17.1 Basic components of a graduated return to sport protocol

Nonspecific example of graduated "return to sport" protocol		
Stage	*Aim*	*Activity*
0	Relative rest	24–48 h of relative physical and cognitive rest
1	Symptom-limited activity	Daily activities that do not provoke symptoms
2	Light aerobic exercise	Walking, stationary bike (slow-moderate pace); no resistance training
3	Sport-specific exercise	Running, swimming, skating; no head impacts
4	Non-contact training	Higher intensity training; progressive resistance training
5	Full contact training	Normal training activities
6	Return to sport	Normal game play without restrictions

Adapted from McCrory P, et al. BJSM 2017

and progression through gradual reintroduction to school-related activities (McCrory et al., 2017). Consideration of academic and cognitive activity is essential in SRC since most non-professional athletes are also students. Both the RTS and RTL protocols are freely available to clinicians in all medical settings [2]. It is generally accepted that no athlete be allowed to fully return to sport participation until they have first successfully completed the RTL progression.

Recently, in addition to returning to sport and academics, clinicians have begun to address the necessity of driving restrictions after SRC. Caution is recommended when counseling athletes on returning to drive in light of preliminary research demonstrating reduced reaction time or visuo-motor speed [43, 44] even when athletes report being asymptomatic. This situation may apply not only to athletes old enough to drive but also to those riding scooters or bicycles.

Rehabilitation planning for the acutely concussed athlete should begin at the time of SRC diagnosis. Educating the athlete on the importance of sleep for recovery and discussing sleep hygiene are important as well as counseling on the expectation of recovery [3]. As alluded to in the previous paragraphs, there is growing evidence supporting the safety and efficacy of aerobic exercise acutely after SRC [45]. The exercise can begin after a brief period of rest and its intensity should be below the level which produces symptoms termed "sub-symptom threshold." The idea of exercise as SRC treatment continues to gain momentum and will likely continue revolutionizing clinical management and rehabilitation of SRC in the coming years [46, 47]. As we discuss later, aerobic exercise protocols are also frequently beneficial for athletes with persistent SRC symptoms. Additionally, it is helpful to monitor for exacerbation of preexisting conditions such as headache disorder, mental health conditions, motion sickness etc., and treat them accordingly when they occur [3]. Clinicians may also find it helpful to consider individualized treatment recommendations based on clinical subtypes or "profiles" which have begun to be reported in the literature [3, 48] (See Fig. 17.3) and may provide more targeted treatments and inform prognosis [49].

Classifying and Treating Persistent Postconcussive Symptoms

A minority of athletes will experience SRC symptoms for longer than expected, otherwise known as persistent postconcussive symptoms. Some refer to these cases as having "postconcussion syndrome," but this term is decreasingly used, given the lack of agreement regarding the time frame and symptoms required for diagnosis. Arbitrary cutoffs created confusion because an athlete may be classified as having a "normal recovery" in one study, but "postconcussion syndrome" in another. Other athletes would fall outside the expected recovery window, but not experience symptoms long enough to be called "postconcussion syndrome," creating yet another classification gray area. For simplification, persistent postconcussive symptoms refer to any athlete experiencing SRC symptoms longer than expected. The Concussion in Sport Group defines protracted symptoms as those lasting longer than 10–14 days for adults and longer than 28 days for youth and adolescent athletes

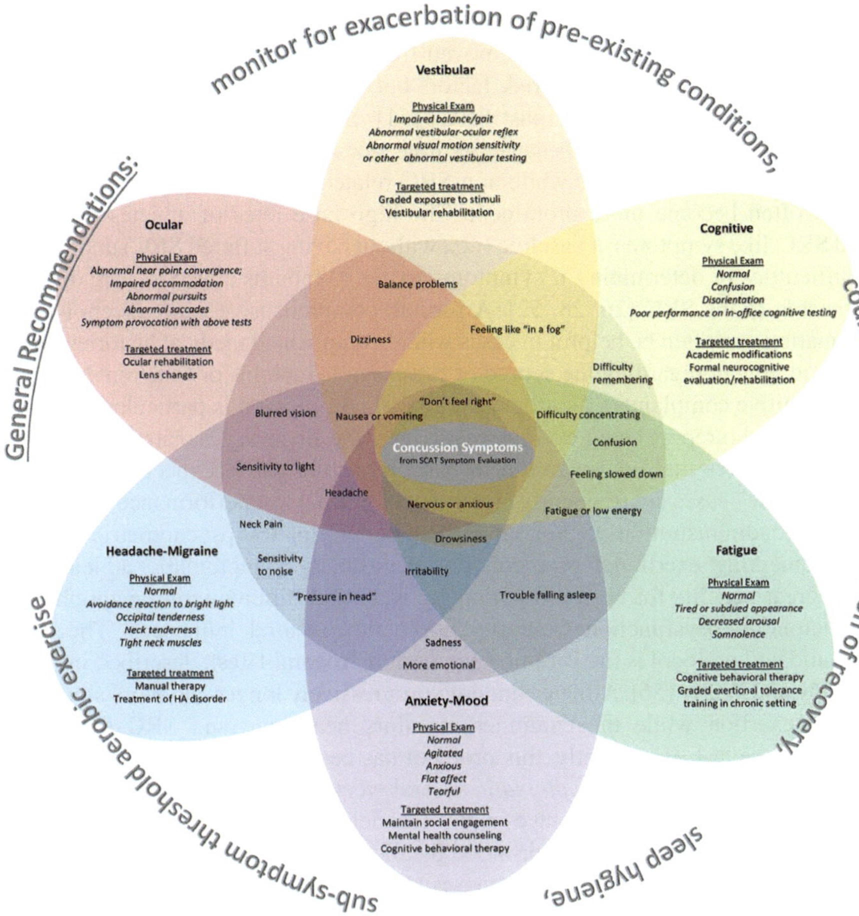

Fig. 17.3 From the 2019 AMSSM Position Statement on Concussion in Sport [3]. Overlapping clinical profiles: an emerging concept to facilitate individualized management after sport-related concussion. Most patients have features of multiple profiles. HA headache, SCAT Sports Concussion Assessment Tool.

[2]. Quantifying the frequency of athletes experiencing persistent SRC symptoms has proven challenging because of the lack of consistent application of these or other cutoffs. Identifying risk factors for prolonged recovery is likely a more helpful clinical approach to better identify those at higher risk and initiate aggressive early rehabilitation. We note, however, that data on these risk factors are inconsistent and complicated by study design variability.

Athletes may be considered "symptomatic" if they fail to return to baseline on select SRC assessments, continue reporting SRC-related symptoms, or both. Preexisting psychiatric conditions or psychiatric symptom reporting are among the most consistent and robust predictors of persistent SRC symptoms [50–52]. Accumulating data suggest that athletes who continue participating in athletic activity acutely after SRC, and are only later diagnosed with SRC, take longer to recover than athletes immediately removed from activity at the point of SRC [53–55]. Factors often thought of as risk factors but with more mixed findings include history of ADHD and multiple past SRCs [51]. Serial tracking of symptoms and functional status is essential because as time goes on after injury, confidence in symptom attribution dwindles while non-SRC-related influences (e.g., psychosocial factors) often become more prominent. The high base rates of athletes reporting broad SRC-like symptoms at baseline (i.e., without having suffered SRC) underscore the difficulties of determining if symptoms weeks to months after SRC are directly attributable to the SRC [26, 28, 52]. A formal, comprehensive neuropsychological examination can often be helpful in cases where complicated medical histories cloud clinical judgment regarding the source of persistent symptoms or functional deficits (e.g., cognitive complaints). Neuropsychological consultation is particularly helpful for athletes who report being asymptomatic but have lingering, isolated, and inconsistent test scores that do not return to baseline or normative expectations. These "symptomatic" cases are frequently an artifact of normal test performance variability over repeat administrations and/or suboptimal underlying test psychometrics.

Implementing exertional protocols for persistently symptomatic athletes has shown great benefits for both promoting recovery and differentiating pathophysiologic/autonomic dysfunction from psychosocial/behavioral influences. The most well-validated protocol is the Buffalo Concussion Treadmill Test, described in detail by Leddy and Willer [56]. Athletes undergo progressively longer and more strenuous physical exertion while the examiner monitors heart rate and SRC symptoms throughout the test. Importantly, this protocol has been demonstrated to be safe for patients who are *currently symptomatic* several weeks after SRC. Allowing athletes with persistent symptoms to engage in physical activity despite lingering symptoms often has profound impacts on their mood by alleviating frustrations associated with relative activity restrictions. The practice is also supported by research demonstrating the biological benefits of aerobic exercise after the acute window of SRC recovery [57, 58]. Conversely, prolonged inactivity has deleterious effects on the SRC recovery process and may further promote persistent SRC symptoms [42, 59].

Other common interventions for athletes with prolonged recovery are more symptom-specific. For example, vestibular therapy has proven extremely beneficial for athletes suffering from persistent dizziness or cervicogenic dysfunction [60, 61]. Traditional psychotherapy incorporating cognitive behavioral therapy (CBT) may help athletes struggling emotionally with their SRC recovery, or those that seemingly become hyperaware of presumed SRC symptoms, thus overly attributing all symptom experiences subsequent to the SRC as being directly and solely related to the SRC [62]. An analogous treatment, such as cognitive behavioral therapy for insomnia (CBTi), could specifically benefit athletes with lingering sleep difficulties. Sleep is commonly affected by SRC, and chronically, poor sleep can produce symptoms that mimic or exacerbate many SRC-like symptoms. CBTi or simply basic sleep hygiene recommendations can mitigate sleep-related complications in the recovery process, especially if psychiatric symptoms concurrently linger [63, 64]. Cognitive difficulties may be addressed initially with academic accommodations and in more recalcitrant cases, formal neurocognitive evaluation may be beneficial.

Pharmacological interventions for symptom management may be appropriate on a case-by-case basis, particularly for debilitating headaches or migraines; however, athletes must demonstrate symptom-free progression through rehabilitation stages *without* medication prior to being fully cleared for sport.

SRC Research with Fluid Biomarkers: A Work in Progress

Although much interest exists in finding objective markers of physiologic injury, a growing body of evidence demonstrates incomplete overlap of clinical and physiologic aspects of SRC [65] and suggests several potential avenues for advancing characterization of the latter using physiologic biomarkers [66]. Currently, however, SRC management is guided purely by its clinical manifestations.

The potential use of fluid (blood, cerebrospinal fluid [CSF], saliva) biomarkers in SRC has stirred hope for an objective measure for diagnosis as well as prognosis and recovery. Other biomarkers, like multimodal neuroimaging, are also advancing, but, at present, do not have the potential for rapid clinical application like fluid biomarkers due to cost, portability, ease of use, etc. Research has progressed exponentially in identifying various proteins, enzymes, and receptors to be used as biomarkers but has not yet validated the specific set of fluid biomarkers for clinical use in SRC management. The primary findings of this research thus far relate to the characterization of the pathophysiological response of the central nervous system following SRC as opposed to direct correlation to symptom burden. This is important, given recent conceptualizations that clearly demonstrate that clinical recovery from SRC (i.e., symptoms) does not completely overlap with physiologic recovery (i.e., underlying biologic alterations), with physiologic changes outlasting observable symptoms [65].

Fluid biomarkers in SRC research most commonly come from blood (either plasma or serum), while only a handful are obtained from CSF due to the invasiveness of sampling. Multiple brain injury-related proteins have been studied due to the presumed broad and heterogeneous impact of SRC on different aspects of the central nervous system (axons, glia, vasculature, etc.). Results have thus far been mixed and often vary based on study design, but generally, findings suggest borderline acceptable sensitivity and specificity to SRC [67–72]. Investigations of fluid biomarkers predicting recovery time have been similarly inconsistent [68, 73, 74]. More novel fluid biomarker sources in athletes include saliva for proteomic study and blood for both upregulation of micro-RNA and inflammatory markers post injury, all of which remain in their infancy [75–80].

Recent data demonstrated that factors rarely considered in biomarker studies to date, such as sex and race/ethnicity, significantly impact blood biomarker expression, [81] but these associations may be assay-dependent [71]. Further, there are concerns that levels of some biomarkers may elevate after both SRC and prolonged exertion or musculoskeletal injury [82–84], and that assessment of temporal fluctuations in biomarker levels acutely after SRC requires a panel-based, repeated sampling approach [85]. Readers are directed to McCrea et al. [66] and Papa et al. [85] for detailed reviews of biomarkers in SRC research.

Catastrophic Head Injuries

A significant part of this chapter focuses on SRC, the most common type of TBI occurring within football. However, participants in American football are also at risk for moderate-to-severe TBIs and, therefore, a brief discussion of them is warranted. Unlike the symptoms associated with SRC, moderate-to-severe TBIs are associated with significant neurological deficits like hemiplegia, comatose state, signs of cerebral herniation, (oculomotor nerve palsy, posturing, etc.) and even potentially death.

The Glasgow Coma Scale, or GCS, is a clinical scoring system that evaluates a traumatically injured patient and provides a crude but simple and rapid way to communicate the significance of injury based on their alertness, mentation, and functional abilities. This numerical score then assigns the patient as succumbing to either a "mild" (GCS 13–15), "moderate" (GCS 9–12), or "severe" (GCS 3–8) TBI. The lower the GCS score is, the more likely the athlete is to have greater extent and severity of both focal and/or diffuse cerebral pathologies. Clinicians rarely administer a GCS in SRC settings, but it is a valuable tool when more serious brain injuries are suspected.

The incidence of fatalities from cranial pathology in football has declined dramatically over the last 40 years. Recently, the National Center for Catastrophic Sport Injury Research reported a total of 26 such deaths between 2005 and 2014, or just under 3 per year, of which 46% were due to subdural hematoma [86]. In years past, the highest annual incidence reported was 17.2 deaths/year, which occurred between 1965 and 1969 [87]. Likely explanations for this precipitous drop include implementation of the modern football helmet along with energy-absorbing padding, chin strap, face mask, etc., in the early 1970s; increased awareness and preparation for on-field emergency response; and safety-related rule changes (e.g., penalizing dangerous hits like spearing).

Potentially catastrophic head injuries can arise from focal pathologies, which include subdural hematomas (SDHs), epidural hematomas (EDH), and traumatic intracerebral hemorrhage (TICH). An SDH occurs due to a rapid translation of the brain within the skull resulting in tearing of bridging veins and resultant blood accumulating in the space between the dura and the brain. CT imaging is significant for a hyperdense, concave/crescent-shaped lesion layering over the brain parenchyma (Fig. 17.4). Alternatively, an EDH is typically due to a fracture within the squamous portion of the temporal bone resulting in injury to either the middle meningeal artery or a dural sinus. The pathognomonic clinical presentation of an EDH involves a lucid interval followed by a dramatic neurological decline, but this is highly dependent on the size and location of the fracture, the patient's intracranial anatomy, and the rate of expansion of the hematoma. CT imaging for an EDH is significant for a hyperdense, convex/lentiform-shaped lesion that does not extend past suture lines because it is occurring between the dura and the periosteum (Fig. 17.5). With prompt surgical intervention, mortality for a EDH is estimated at 12%; however, due to the underlying parenchymal injury that occurs with SDH, SDHs typically predict a worse outcome than EDH [88]. Lastly, a TICH is due to a rapid

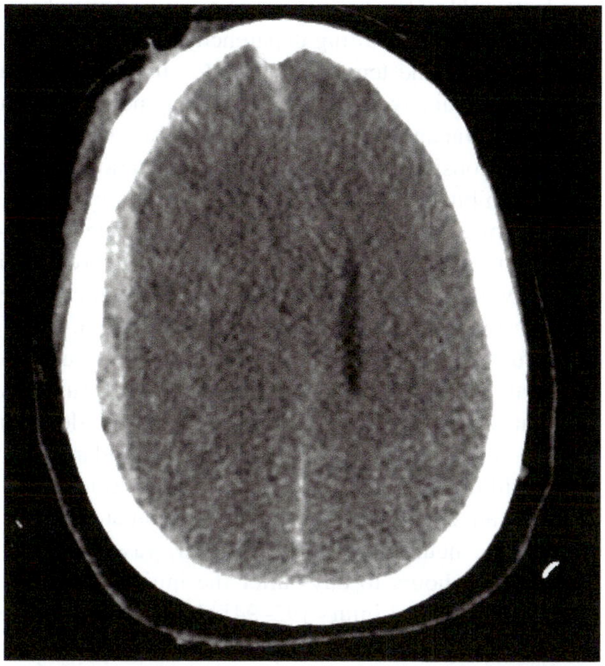

Fig. 17.4 Axial CT head demonstrating a right-sided acute pan-hemispheric subdural hematoma

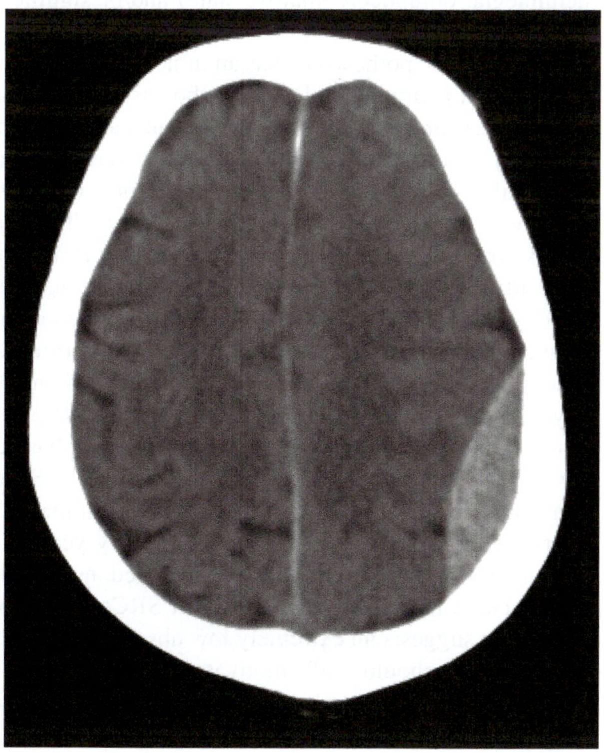

Fig. 17.5 Left-sided fronto-parietal epidural hematoma seen on an axial CT head

acceleration/deceleration event of the cranium where the brain strikes the bony edges of the skull resulting in parenchymal injury and hemorrhage, typically involving the frontal and temporal lobes. CT imaging demonstrates a hyperdense lesion within the brain parenchyma involving the cortical surface in coup-contra-coup locations. Management of focal mass lesions requires consultation to a neurosurgeon for consideration of surgical evacuation. Patients who are neurologically intact, exhibit minimal symptoms, and demonstrate a small lesion with minimal midline shift on CT imaging may be appropriate for nonoperative management with serial neurological examinations. Surgical intervention is indicated for athletes presenting with a neurological deficit and/or clinical deterioration, expansion of the mass, or with a substantially sized mass [89–91].

Diffuse brain injury is another potentially catastrophic event associated with head trauma in football. The most significant diffuse cerebral pathologies associated with catastrophic head injuries in football include diffuse axonal injury (DAI) and second impact syndrome. DAI occurs secondary to rotational strain on the long axons within the brain resulting in tearing (axotomy) or stretch injury to the nerves. If significant enough, this can result in a comatose state. Brain injury of all severities instigates a neurometabolic, chemical, vascular, and inflammatory cascade that evolves over hours to days after the initial insult and heightens susceptibility to secondary neuronal injury [92–94]. At the milder end of the spectrum (e.g., SRC), this can present clinically as headaches, confusion, neurocognitive deficits, etc., as described earlier. In more severe TBI, there can be significant neurological deficits (hemiplegia, obtunded/comatose state) and/or significant life-threatening cerebral edema, herniation, and death.

Some have hypothesized that an athlete returning to play prior to resolution of the disturbed neurometabolic state who sustains a repeat injury (even if mild) is at risk for a resulting hyperemic state with substantial cerebral vasodilation and edema, ultimately resulting in cerebral herniation and potential death [95–97]. Reported cases of this so-called second impact syndrome (SIS) typically involve young adult males who returned to contact sports (football, boxing, rugby, karate), within 4 weeks from initial brain injury [96, 98–100]. Brain imaging is significant for dramatic diffuse cerebral edema (cisternal obliteration, sulcal effacement, cerebral herniation) and occasionally smaller subdural hematomas or areas of traumatic subarachnoid hemorrhage. Only 20% of the reported deaths secondary to cranial injury in football had an SRC reported within 1 month of their death [86, 87]. This may suggest injury mechanisms unrelated to SIS per se. However, the proposed hypotheses underlying SIS-related mortality emphasize the importance of prompt SRC reporting and formal implementation of RTS guidelines. Data continually demonstrate high rates of SRC underreporting among athletes. Millions of collision sport athletes likely do not report SRCs every year and, presumably, then resume exposing their compromised brain to repeated insults. The number of confirmed SIS cases relative to the rate of unreported SRCs (i.e., those at greatest risk for SIS) fortunately suggests an extremely low absolute risk for SIS, but the potentially dire consequences should still motivate suspected SRC disclosure from athletes. Additionally, severe cerebral edema associated with isolated sport-related brain injury, even without an initial "priming event," has been described ("first impact syndrome") [101].

Management of a player that has sustained a significant cranial injury involves first a rapid on-field assessment followed by a more thorough assessment that includes evaluation of their "ABCs" with possible initiation of cardiopulmonary resuscitation, notification to local emergency response personnel, implementation of cervical spine precautions, and completion of a thorough neurological assessment. In-hospital management would include early, prompt cranial imaging consisting of a non-contrast head CT to evaluate for acute hemorrhage, cerebral edema, and the need for possible neurosurgical intervention. Though beyond the scope of this chapter, management of severe head trauma is focused around prevention of further secondary neuronal injury, specifically by avoiding hypoxia, hypotension, hypoglycemia, hypocarbia (unless life-threatening cerebral herniation is evident necessitating hyperventilation en route to the operating room), and periods of elevated intracranial pressure [102, 103]. Pharmacological agents to be considered acutely after suspected severe TBI include anti-epileptics like phenytoin (Dilantin) or levetiracetam (Keppra) for prevention of early posttraumatic seizures [102–104]. Conversely, steroids are contraindicated due to their associated increased risk of morbidity. A multidisciplinary approach with neurosurgery and neurocritical care is needed to medically and, potentially, surgically address elevations in intracranial pressure. The process typically requires stepwise intracranial pressure monitoring and may require aggressive sedation, analgesia, hypertonic therapy and/or mannitol, paralytics, ventricular drainage, and possible decompressive hemicraniectomy [102, 103, 105–107]. Due to the likely significant neurological deficits in an athlete with a severe TBI and need for long-term rehabilitation, return to contact sports is highly unlikely.

Long-Term Effects of Football-Related Head Trauma

American football somewhat uniquely exposes participants to repetitive head trauma, frequently referred to as "subconcussive" or "subclinical impacts", where an athlete sustains a blow to the head but does not exhibit signs or symptoms of SRC [108]. These impacts may occur hundreds to thousands of times over the course of a football season, with the linemen typically experiencing the highest frequency [109, 110]. Over the last 15 years, there have been renewed concerns about the potential negative influence on neurologic health posed by extensive exposure to subclinical impacts and, often, multiple SRCs. These concerns mostly center on chronic traumatic encephalopathy (CTE), a neurodegenerative disease characterized primarily by irregular tau protein deposition; however, CTE typically presents as a mixed proteinopathy [111–113]. Preliminary neuropathologic diagnostic criteria now exist and may be applied at autopsy [114] but will likely be refined in the coming years through prospective validation and systematic characterization of varying disease severities. The clinical syndrome associated with CTE remains ill-defined, and symptoms observed antemortem have not been adequately correlated in athletes harboring CTE pathology at autopsy. Given the relative infancy of both neuropathologic and syndromic diagnostic approaches, epidemiological data on CTE prevalence, incidence, and risk factors are unsurprisingly elusive. However, clinicians involved in football athlete health and safety can still take important steps toward reducing presumed risks for later-life neurological impairment.

Prevailing theories identify repetitive subclinical impacts as the primary culprit for CTE risk rather than number of SRCs per se. These theories require a great deal more research before drawing confident conclusions, but a conservative risk management approach would ideally target activities that have a high risk of exposure to *both* repetitive impacts and SRC. Most repetitive impacts occur in practice settings, and recent data highlight the uneven spread of impacts (based on both frequency and magnitude) across different drills. Minor modifications to the highest risk drills may result in significant exposure reductions. One study estimated that non-linemen and linemen could avoid 300 and 1000 practice-related head impacts, respectively, over the course of a college football career by reducing participation in high-risk drills by 1–3 min per practice [18]. Research in younger football players further describes successful modifications to practice structures that limited head impact exposure [17]. Practice settings offer a unique opportunity to control the amount and type of exposure but will almost certainly require collaboration with coaches who initially may be resistant to changes perceived as negatively impacting player development. Regulations of number of total and contact practice sessions as well as in-game rule changes such as decreasing number of kickoff returns and increasing targeting penalties may also lessen this risk.

A second scenario where sports medicine clinicians can intervene occurs when football athletes develop concerns about their neurological health while actively playing or after their retirement. The current climate surrounding CTE concerns understandably heightens player awareness if or when they perceive changes in their cognition, mood, or behavior. All athletes expressing worries about such symptoms or about having CTE should be strongly encouraged to seek appropriate medical care, such as consultation with neurology and neuropsychology [3]. Many symptoms associated with CTE are nonspecific but often have other treatable etiologies. Additionally, active and former elite football athletes disproportionately possess several risk factors other than repetitive brain trauma for expressing such symptoms, such as chronic pain, dysregulated sleep, mental health issues, and substance use, among others [115–117]. Recent and ongoing CTE-related research now incorporates prospective, longitudinal designs that involve comprehensive clinical evaluations and advanced biomarkers [118, 119]. Such work will help unravel the many lingering questions about CTE and the long-term effects of football-related head trauma [120–122].

Summary of Brain Injury in Football

Football is associated with a high risk for SRC, and although rare, the potential for moderate to severe TBI.

Therefore, sports medicine clinicians covering football must be prepared to recognize and manage SRC as well as have emergency action plans in place to reduce risks for catastrophic outcomes linked to hematomas and other severe cranial injuries. Appropriately trained medical providers diagnose SRC using a multifaceted clinical examination, and any athlete with suspected SRC should be immediately removed from athletic participation. Rehabilitation protocols exist for gradual reintegration of the athlete back into academics in concert with a systematic, stepwise progression of physical exertion following an SRC in efforts to return to sport. Evidence supports limiting strict rest after SRC while encouraging symptom-limited activities and aerobic exercise as tolerated. Exercise interventions and specialist referral (neuropsychology, neurology, vestibular therapy, etc.) may be especially helpful for athletes suffering from persistent SRC symptoms. Currently, clinical symptoms drive SRC management, but through our improved understanding of pathophysiologic correlates, the future of SRC diagnosis and management (rehabilitation and return to play) could potentially be supplemented by more objective markers of injury.

The long-term risks associated with football participation remain poorly characterized and further understanding is needed through prospective studies. In the interim, head impact exposure and unsafe playing styles should be eliminated wherever possible in order to reduce risk. Also, reassurance and appropriate referral for comprehensive evaluation and treatment options should occur in current or former athletes concerned about perceived changes in cognition, mood, or behavior.

References

1. Tator CH. Let's standardize the definition of concussion and get reliable incidence data. Can J Neurol Sci. 2009;36(4):405.
2. McCrory P, Meeuwisse W, Dvorak J, Aubry M, Bailes J, Broglio S, et al. Consensus statement on concussion in sport—the 5th international conference on concussion in sport held in Berlin, October 2016. Br J Sports Med. 2017:bjsports-2017-097699.
3. Harmon K, Clugston J, Dec K, Hainline B, Herring S, Kane S, et al. American Medical Society for Sports Medicine position statement on concussion in sport. Br J Sports Med. 2019;53(4):213–25.
4. Giza CC, Hovda DA. The new neurometabolic cascade of concussion. Neurosurgery. 2014;75(suppl_4):S24-S33.
5. Klein AP, Tetzlaff JE, Bonis JM, Nelson LD, Mayer A, Huber DL, et al. Prevalence of potentially clinically significant MRI findings in athletes with and without sport-related concussion. J Neurotrauma. 2019(ja).
6. Yuh EL, Mukherjee P, Lingsma HF, Yue JK, Ferguson AR, Gordon WA, et al. Magnetic resonance imaging improves 3-month outcome prediction in mild traumatic brain injury. Ann Neurol. 2013;73(2):224–35.
7. Wasserman EB, Coberley M, Anderson S, Grant M, Hardin JA. Concussion rates differ by practice type and equipment worn in an autonomy five collegiate football conference. Clin J Sport Med. 2018;30:366.
8. Kerr ZY, Wilkerson GB, Caswell SV, Currie DW, Pierpoint LA, Wasserman EB, et al. The first decade of web-based sports injury surveillance: descriptive epidemiology of injuries in United States high school football (2005–2006 through 2013–2014) and National Collegiate Athletic Association Football (2004–2005 through 2013–2014). J Athl Train. 2018;53(8):738–51.
9. Clark MD, Asken BM, Marshall SW, Guskiewicz KM. Descriptive characteristics of concussions in National Football League games, 2010–2011 to 2013–2014. Am J Sports Med. 2017;45(4):929–36.

10. Pellman EJ, Powell JW, Viano DC, Casson IR, Tucker AM, Feuer H, et al. Concussion in professional football: epidemiological features of game injuries and review of the literature–part 3. Neurosurgery. 2004;54(1):81–94; discussion –6.
11. Yengo-Kahn AM, Johnson DJ, Zuckerman SL, Solomon GS. Concussions in the National Football League: a current concepts review. Am J Sports Med. 2016;44:801.
12. Kerr ZY, Comstock RD, Dompier TP, Marshall SW. The first decade of web-based sports injury surveillance (2004–2005 through 2013–2014): methods of the National Collegiate Athletic Association Injury Surveillance Program and High School Reporting Information Online. J Athl Train. 2018;53(8):729–37.
13. Houck Z, Asken B, Bauer R, Pothast J, Michaudet C, Clugston J. Epidemiology of sport-related concussion in an NCAA division I football bowl subdivision sample. Am J Sports Med. 2016;44(9):2269–75.
14. Ocwieja KE, Mihalik JP, Marshall SW, Schmidt JD, Trulock SC, Guskiewicz KM. The effect of play type and collision closing distance on head impact biomechanics. Ann Biomed Eng. 2012;40(1):90–6.
15. Wiebe DJ, D'alonzo BA, Harris R, Putukian M, Campbell-McGovern C. Association between the experimental kickoff rule and concussion rates in Ivy League football. JAMA. 2018;320(19):2035–6.
16. Hosick M. DI council votes to eliminate football two-a-days www.ncaa.org2017. Available from: http://www.ncaa.org/about/resources/media-center/news/di-council-votes-eliminate-football-two-days.
17. Broglio SP, Williams RM, O'Connor KL, Goldstick J. Football players' head-impact exposure after limiting of full-contact practices. J Athl Train. 2016;51(7):511–8.
18. Asken BM, Brooke ZS, Stevens TC, Silvestri PG, Graham MJ, Jaffee MS, et al. Drill-specific head impacts in collegiate football practice: implications for reducing "friendly fire" exposure. Ann Biomed Eng. 2018;47:2094.
19. Kroshus E, Garnett B, Hawrilenko M, Baugh CM, Calzo JP. Concussion under-reporting and pressure from coaches, teammates, fans, and parents. Soc Sci Med. 2015;134:66–75.
20. Kerr ZY, Register-Mihalik JK, Kay MC, DeFreese J, Marshall SW, Guskiewicz KM. Concussion nondisclosure during professional career among a cohort of former National Football League athletes. Am J Sports Med. 2018;46(1):22–9.
21. McCrea M, Hammeke T, Olsen G, Leo P, Guskiewicz K. Unreported concussion in high school football players: implications for prevention. Clin J Sport Med. 2004;14(1):13–7.
22. Kerr ZY, Register-Mihalik JK, Marshall SW, Evenson KR, Mihalik JP, Guskiewicz KM. Disclosure and non-disclosure of concussion and concussion symptoms in athletes: review and application of the socio-ecological framework. Brain Inj. 2014;28(8):1009–21.
23. Ellenbogen RG, Batjer H, Cardenas J, Berger M, Bailes J, Pieroth E, et al. National Football League Head, neck and spine Committee's concussion diagnosis and management protocol: 2017-18 season. Br J Sports Med. 2018;52(14):894–902.
24. Garcia GP, Broglio SP, Lavieri MS, McCrea M, McAllister T, Investigators CC. Quantifying the value of multidimensional assessment models for acute concussion: an analysis of data from the NCAA-DoD care consortium. Sports Med. 2018;48(7):1739–49.
25. Echemendia RJ, Meeuwisse W, McCrory P, Davis GA, Putukian M, Leddy J, et al. The sport concussion assessment tool 5th edition (SCAT5). Br J Sports Med. 2017:bjsports-2017-097506.
26. Asken BM, Snyder AR, Smith MS, Zaremski JL, Bauer RM. Concussion-like symptom reporting in non-concussed adolescent athletes. Clin Neuropsychol. 2017;31(1):138–53.
27. Fazio VC, Lovell MR, Pardini JE, Collins MW. The relation between post concussion symptoms and neurocognitive performance in concussed athletes. NeuroRehabilitation. 2007;22(3):207–16.
28. Iverson GL, Silverberg ND, Mannix R, Maxwell BA, Atkins JE, Zafonte R, et al. Factors associated with concussion-like symptom reporting in high school athletes. JAMA Pediatr. 2015;169(12):1132–40.

29. Kontos AP, Elbin R, Schatz P, Covassin T, Henry L, Pardini J, et al. A revised factor structure for the post-concussion symptom scale: baseline and postconcussion factors. Am J Sports Med. 2012;40(10):2375–84.
30. McCrea M, Kelly JP, Randolph C, Kluge J, Bartolic E, Finn G, et al. Standardized assessment of concussion (SAC): on-site mental status evaluation of the athlete. J Head Trauma Rehabil. 1998;13(2):27–35.
31. Riemann BL, Guskiewicz KM. Effects of mild head injury on postural stability as measured through clinical balance testing. J Athl Train. 2000;35(1):19–25.
32. Carney N, Ghajar J, Jagoda A, Bedrick S, Davis-O'Reilly C, du Coudray H, et al. Concussion guidelines step 1: systematic review of prevalent indicators. Neurosurgery. 2014;75(Suppl 1):S3–15.
33. Norheim N, Kissinger-Knox A, Cheatham M, Webbe F. Performance of college athletes on the 10-item word list of SCAT5. BMJ Open Sport Exerc Med. 2018;4(1):e000412.
34. Mucha A, Collins MW, Elbin R, Furman JM, Troutman-Enseki C, DeWolf RM, et al. A brief vestibular/ocular motor screening (VOMS) assessment to evaluate concussions: preliminary findings. Am J Sports Med. 2014;42(10):2479–86.
35. Oride M, Marutani JK, Rouse MW, Deland PN. Reliability study of the Pierce and King-Devick saccade tests. Am J Optom Physiol Optic. 1986;63(6):419–24.
36. Samadani U, Ritlop R, Reyes M, Nehrbass E, Li M, Lamm E, et al. Eye tracking detects disconjugate eye movements associated with structural traumatic brain injury and concussion. J Neurotrauma. 2015;32(8):548–56.
37. Nelson LD, LaRoche AA, Pfaller AY, Lerner EB, Hammeke TA, Randolph C, et al. Prospective, head-to-head study of three computerized neurocognitive assessment tools (CNTs): reliability and validity for the assessment of sport-related concussion. J Int Neuropsychol Soc. 2016;22(1):24–37.
38. Karr JE, Areshenkoff CN, Garcia-Barrera MA. The neuropsychological outcomes of concussion: a systematic review of meta-analyses on the cognitive sequelae of mild traumatic brain injury. Neuropsychology. 2014;28(3):321.
39. Asken BM, Houck ZM, Schmidt JD, Bauer RM, Broglio SP, McCrea MA, et al. A normative reference vs. baseline testing compromise for ImPACT: the CARE consortium multiple variable prediction (CARE-MVP) norms. Sports Med. 2020;50:1533.
40. Meehan WP 3rd, d'Hemecourt P, Comstock RD. High school concussions in the 2008-2009 academic year: mechanism, symptoms, and management. Am J Sports Med. 2010;38(12):2405–9.
41. McCrea M, Guskiewicz KM, Marshall SW, Barr W, Randolph C, Cantu RC, et al. Acute effects and recovery time following concussion in collegiate football players: the NCAA concussion study. JAMA. 2003;290(19):2556–63.
42. Schneider KJ, Leddy JJ, Guskiewicz KM, Seifert T, McCrea M, Silverberg ND, et al. Rest and treatment/rehabilitation following sport-related concussion: a systematic review. Br J Sports Med. 2017;51(12):930–4.
43. Schmidt JD, Hoffman NL, Ranchet M, Miller LS, Tomporowski PD, Akinwuntan AE, et al. Driving after concussion: is it safe to drive after symptoms resolve? J Neurotrauma. 2017;34(8):1571–8.
44. Schmidt JD, Lynall RC, Lempke LB, Weber ML, Devos H. Post-concussion driving behaviors and opinions: a survey of collegiate student-athletes. J Neurotrauma. 2018;35:2418.
45. Leddy JJ, Haider MN, Ellis MJ, Mannix R, Darling SR, Freitas MS, et al. Early subthreshold aerobic exercise for sport-related concussion: a randomized clinical trial. JAMA Pediatr. 2019;173:319.
46. Leddy JJ, Haider MN, Ellis M, Willer BS. Exercise is medicine for concussion. Curr Sports Med Rep. 2018;17(8):262–70.
47. Leddy JJ, Haider MN, Ellis MJ, Mannix R, Darling SR, Freitas MS, et al. Early subthreshold aerobic exercise for sport-related concussion: a randomized clinical trial. JAMA Pediatr. 2019;173:319.

48. Kontos AP, Sufrinko A, Sandel N, Emami K, Collins MW. Sport-related concussion clinical profiles: clinical characteristics, targeted treatments, and preliminary evidence. Curr Sports Med Rep. 2019;18(3):82–92.
49. Collins MW, Kontos AP, Okonkwo DO, Almquist J, Bailes J, Barisa M, et al. Statements of agreement from the targeted evaluation and active management (TEAM) approaches to treating concussion meeting held in Pittsburgh, October 15-16, 2015. Neurosurgery. 2016;79(6):912–29.
50. Nelson LD, Tarima S, LaRoche AA, Hammeke TA, Barr WB, Guskiewicz K, et al. Preinjury somatization symptoms contribute to clinical recovery after sport-related concussion. Neurology. 2016;86(20):1856–63.
51. Iverson GL, Gardner AJ, Terry DP, Ponsford JL, Sills AK, Broshek DK, et al. Predictors of clinical recovery from concussion: a systematic review. Br J Sports Med. 2017;51(12):941–8.
52. Asken BM, Snyder AR, Clugston JR, Gaynor LS, Sullan MJ, Bauer RM. Concussion-like symptom reporting in non-concussed collegiate athletes. Arch Clin Neuropsychol. 2017;32(8):963–71.
53. Asken BM, Bauer RM, Guskiewicz KM, McCrea MA, Schmidt JD, Giza CC, et al. Immediate removal from activity after sport-related concussion is associated with shorter clinical recovery and less severe symptoms in collegiate student-athletes. Am J Sports Med. 2018;46(6):1465–74.
54. Asken BM, McCrea MA, Clugston JR, Snyder AR, Houck ZM, Bauer RM. "Playing through it": delayed reporting and removal from athletic activity after concussion predicts prolonged recovery. J Athl Train. 2016;51(4):329–35.
55. Elbin R, Sufrinko A, Schatz P, French J, Henry L, Burkhart S, et al. Removal from play after concussion and recovery time. Pediatrics. 2016:e20160910.
56. Leddy JJ, Willer B. Use of graded exercise testing in concussion and return-to-activity management. Curr Sports Med Rep. 2013;12(6):370–6.
57. Griesbach GS, Tio DL, Nair S, Hovda DA. Recovery of stress response coincides with responsiveness to voluntary exercise after traumatic brain injury. J Neurotrauma. 2014;31(7):674–82.
58. Leddy J, Hinds A, Sirica D, Willer B. The role of controlled exercise in concussion management. PM&R. 2016;8(3):S91–S100.
59. Thomas DG, Apps JN, Hoffmann RG, McCrea M, Hammeke T. Benefits of strict rest after acute concussion: a randomized controlled trial. Pediatrics. 2015:peds. 2014–0966.
60. Schneider KJ, Meeuwisse WH, Nettel-Aguirre A, Barlow K, Boyd L, Kang J, et al. Cervicovestibular rehabilitation in sport-related concussion: a randomised controlled trial. Br J Sports Med. 2014;48(17):1294–8.
61. Ellis MJ, Leddy JJ, Willer B. Physiological, vestibulo-ocular and cervicogenic post-concussion disorders: an evidence-based classification system with directions for treatment. Brain Inj. 2015;29(2):238–48.
62. Al Sayegh A, Sandford D, Carson AJ. Psychological approaches to treatment of postconcussion syndrome: a systematic review. J Neurol Neurosurg Psychiatry. 2010;81(10):1128–34.
63. Stepanski EJ, Wyatt JK. Use of sleep hygiene in the treatment of insomnia. Sleep Med Rev. 2003;7(3):215–25.
64. Taylor DJ, Pruiksma KE. Cognitive and behavioural therapy for insomnia (CBT-I) in psychiatric populations: a systematic review. Int Rev Psychiatry. 2014;26(2):205–13.
65. Kamins J, Bigler E, Covassin T, Henry L, Kemp S, Leddy JJ, et al. What is the physiological time to recovery after concussion? A systematic review. Br J Sports Med. 2017;51(12):935–40.
66. McCrea M, Meier T, Huber D, Ptito A, Bigler E, Debert CT, et al. Role of advanced neuroimaging, fluid biomarkers and genetic testing in the assessment of sport-related concussion: a systematic review. Br J Sports Med. 2017;51(12):919–29.
67. Meier TB, Nelson LD, Huber DL, Bazarian JJ, Hayes RL, McCrea MA. Prospective assessment of acute blood markers of brain injury in sport-related concussion. J Neurotrauma. 2017;34(22):3134–42.

68. Asken BM, Bauer RM, DeKosky ST, Svingos AM, Hromas G, Boone JK, et al. Concussion BASICS III: serum biomarker changes following sport-related concussion. Neurology. 2018:https://doi.org/10.1212/WNL. 0000000000006617.
69. Shahim P, Tegner Y, Wilson DH, Randall J, Skillbäck T, Pazooki D, et al. Blood biomarkers for brain injury in concussed professional ice hockey players. JAMA Neurol. 2014;71(6):684–92.
70. Meier TB, Bergamino M, Bellgowan PS, Teague T, Ling JM, Jeromin A, et al. Longitudinal assessment of white matter abnormalities following sports-related concussion. Hum Brain Mapp. 2016;37(2):833–45.
71. Asken B, Yang Z, Xu H, Weber A, Hayes RL, Bauer RM, et al. Acute effects of sport-related concussion on serum GFAP, UCH-L1, total tau, and neurofilament light measured by a multiplex assay. J Neurotrauma. 2020;37:1537.
72. McCrea M, Broglio SP, McAllister TW, Gill J, Giza CC, Huber DL, et al. Association of blood biomarkers with acute sport-related concussion in collegiate athletes: findings from the NCAA and Department of Defense CARE Consortium. JAMA Network Open. 2020;3(1):e1919771-e.
73. Gill J, Merchant-Borna K, Jeromin A, Livingston W, Bazarian J. Acute plasma tau relates to prolonged return to play after concussion. Neurology. 2017:https://doi.org/10.1212/WNL. 0000000000003587.
74. Shahim P, Linemann T, Inekci D, Karsdal MA, Blennow K, Tegner Y, et al. Serum tau fragments predict return to play in concussed professional ice hockey players. J Neurotrauma. 2016;33(22):1995–9.
75. Johnson JJ, Loeffert AC, Stokes J, Olympia RP, Bramley H, Hicks SD. Association of salivary microRNA changes with prolonged concussion symptoms. JAMA Pediatr. 2018;172(1):65–73.
76. LaRocca D, Barns S, Hicks SD, Brindle A, Williams J, Uhlig R, et al. Comparison of serum and saliva miRNAs for identification and characterization of mTBI in adult mixed martial arts fighters. PLoS One. 2019;14(1):e0207785.
77. Di Pietro V, Porto E, Ragusa M, Barbagallo C, Davies D, Forcione M, et al. Salivary MicroRNAs: diagnostic markers of mild traumatic brain injury in contact-sport. Front Mol Neurosci. 2018;11:290.
78. Di Battista AP, Churchill N, Rhind SG, Richards D, Hutchison MG. Evidence of a distinct peripheral inflammatory profile in sport-related concussion. J Neuroinflammation. 2019;16(1):17.
79. Gill J, Merchant-Borna K, Lee H, Livingston WS, Olivera A, Cashion A, et al. Sports-related concussion results in differential expression of nuclear factor-κB pathway genes in peripheral blood during the acute and subacute periods. J Head Trauma Rehabil. 2016;31(4):269–76.
80. Svingos AM, Asken BM, Bauer RM, DeKosky ST, Hromas GA, Jaffee MS, et al. Exploratory study of sport-related concussion effects on peripheral micro-RNA expression. Brain Inj. 2019;33:1–7.
81. Asken BM, Bauer RM, DeKosky ST, Houck ZM, Moreno CC, Jaffee MS, et al. Concussion Biomarkers Assessed in Collegiate Student-Athletes (BASICS) I: normative study. Neurology. 2018:https://doi.org/10.1212/WNL. 0000000000006613.
82. Bouvier D, Duret T, Abbot M, Stiernon T, Pereira B, Coste A, et al. Utility of S100B serum level for the determination of concussion in male rugby players. Sports Med. 2017;47(4):781–9.
83. Kiechle K, Bazarian JJ, Merchant-Borna K, Stoecklein V, Rozen E, Blyth B, et al. Subject-specific increases in serum S-100B distinguish sports-related concussion from sports-related exertion. PLoS One. 2014;9(1):e84977.
84. Schulte S, Podlog LW, Hamson-Utley JJ, Strathmann FG, Strüder HK. A systematic review of the biomarker S100B: implications for sport-related concussion management. J Athl Train. 2014;49(6):830–50.
85. Papa L, Ramia MM, Edwards D, Johnson BD, Slobounov SM. Systematic review of clinical studies examining biomarkers of brain injury in athletes after sports-related concussion. J Neurotrauma. 2015;32(10):661–73.

86. Kucera KL, Yau RK, Register-Mihalik J, Marshall SW, Thomas LC, Wolf S, et al. Traumatic brain and spinal cord fatalities among high school and college football players – United States, 2005–2014. MMWR Morb Mortal Wkly Rep. 2017;65(52):1465–9.
87. Boden BP, Breit I, Beachler JA, Williams A, Mueller FO. Fatalities in high school and college football players. Am J Sports Med. 2013;41(5):1108–16.
88. Rivas JJ, Lobato RD, Sarabia R, Cordobes F, Cabrera A, Gomez P. Extradural hematoma: analysis of factors influencing the courses of 161 patients. Neurosurgery. 1988;23(1):44–51.
89. Bullock MR, Chesnut R, Ghajar J, Gordon D, Hartl R, Newell DW, et al. Surgical management of traumatic parenchymal lesions. Neurosurgery. 2006;58(3 Suppl):S25–46; discussion Si-iv.
90. Bullock MR, Chesnut R, Ghajar J, Gordon D, Hartl R, Newell DW, et al. Surgical management of acute epidural hematomas. Neurosurgery. 2006;58(3 Suppl):S7–15; discussion Si-iv.
91. Bullock MR, Chesnut R, Ghajar J, Gordon D, Hartl R, Newell DW, et al. Surgical management of acute subdural hematomas. Neurosurgery. 2006;58(3 Suppl):S16–24; discussion Si-iv.
92. Hovda DA. The neurophysiology of concussion. Prog Neurol Surg. 2014;28:28–37.
93. Giza CC, Hovda DA. The neurometabolic cascade of concussion. J Athl Train. 2001;36(3):228–35.
94. Giza CC, Hovda DA. The new neurometabolic cascade of concussion. Neurosurgery. 2014;75(Suppl 4):S24–33.
95. Cantu RC. Second-impact syndrome. Clin Sports Med. 1998;17(1):37–44.
96. Cantu RC, Gean AD. Second-impact syndrome and a small subdural hematoma: an uncommon catastrophic result of repetitive head injury with a characteristic imaging appearance. J Neurotrauma. 2010;27(9):1557–64.
97. McCrory PR, Berkovic SF. Second impact syndrome. Neurology. 1998;50(3):677–83.
98. Hebert O, Schlueter K, Hornsby M, Van Gorder S, Snodgrass S, Cook C. The diagnostic credibility of second impact syndrome: a systematic literature review. J Sci Med Sport. 2016;19:789.
99. Mori T, Katayama Y, Kawamata T. Acute hemispheric swelling associated with thin subdural hematomas: pathophysiology of repetitive head injury in sports. Acta Neurochir Suppl. 2006;96:40–3.
100. McLendon LA, Kralik SF, Grayson PA, Golomb MR. The controversial second impact syndrome: a review of the literature. Pediatr Neurol. 2016;62:9–17.
101. Bailes J, Patel V, Farhat H, Sindelar B, Stone J. Football fatalities: the first impact syndrome. J Neurosurg Pediatr. 2016;19:116.
102. Surgeons ACo. Best practices in the management of traumatic brain injury. TQIP. 2015;30
103. Carney N, Totten AM, O'Reilly C, Ullman JS, Hawryluk GW, Bell MJ, et al. Guidelines for the management of severe traumatic brain injury, fourth edition. Neurosurgery. 2016;80:6.
104. Roberts I, Yates D, Sandercock P, Farrell B, Wasserberg J, Lomas G, et al. Effect of intravenous corticosteroids on death within 14 days in 10008 adults with clinically significant head injury (MRC CRASH trial): randomised placebo-controlled trial. Lancet (London, England). 2004;364(9442):1321–8.
105. Guidelines for the management of severe traumatic brain injury. J Neurotrauma. 2007;24 Suppl 1:S1–106.
106. Cooper DJ, Rosenfeld JV, Murray L, Arabi YM, Davies AR, D'Urso P, et al. Decompressive craniectomy in diffuse traumatic brain injury. N Engl J Med. 2011;364(16):1493–502.
107. Hutchinson PJ, Kolias AG, Timofeev IS, Corteen EA, Czosnyka M, Timothy J, et al. Trial of decompressive craniectomy for traumatic intracranial hypertension. N Engl J Med. 2016;375(12):1119–30.
108. Bailes JE, Petraglia AL, Omalu BI, Nauman E, Talavage T. Role of subconcussion in repetitive mild traumatic brain injury: a review. J Neurosurg. 2013;119(5):1235–45.
109. Crisco JJ, Wilcox BJ, Beckwith JG, Chu JJ, Duhaime A-C, Rowson S, et al. Head impact exposure in collegiate football players. J Biomech. 2011;44(15):2673–8.

110. Mihalik JP, Bell DR, Marshall SW, Guskiewicz KM. Measurement of head impacts in collegiate football players: an investigation of positional and event-type differences. Neurosurgery. 2007;61(6):1229–35.
111. Mez J, Daneshvar DH, Kiernan PT, Abdolmohammadi B, Alvarez VE, Huber BR, et al. Clinicopathological evaluation of chronic traumatic encephalopathy in players of American football. JAMA. 2017;318(4):360–70.
112. Turner RC, Lucke-Wold BP, Robson MJ, Lee JM, Bailes JE. Alzheimer's disease and chronic traumatic encephalopathy: distinct but possibly overlapping disease entities. Brain Inj. 2016;30(11):1279–92.
113. Armstrong RA, McKee AC, Stein TD, Alvarez VE, Cairns NJ. Cortical degeneration in chronic traumatic encephalopathy and Alzheimer's disease neuropathologic change. Neurol Sci. 2018;40:529–33.
114. McKee AC, Cairns NJ, Dickson DW, Folkerth RD, Keene CD, Litvan I, et al. The first NINDS/NIBIB consensus meeting to define neuropathological criteria for the diagnosis of chronic traumatic encephalopathy. Acta Neuropathol. 2016;131(1):75–86.
115. Asken BM, Sullan MJ, Snyder AR, Houck ZM, Bryant VE, Hizel LP, et al. Factors influencing clinical correlates of chronic traumatic encephalopathy (CTE): a review. Neuropsychol Rev. 2016;26(4):340–63.
116. Mannes ZL, Waxenberg LB, Cottler LB, Perlstein WM, Burrell LE, Ferguson EG, et al. Prevalence and correlates of psychological distress among retired elite athletes: a systematic review. Int Rev Sport Exerc Psychol. 2018;12:265–94.
117. Schwenk TL, Gorenflo DW, Dopp RR, Hipple E. Depression and pain in retired professional football players. Med Sci Sports Exerc. 2007;39(4):599–605.
118. Omalu B, Small G, Bailes J, Ercoli L, Merrill D, Wong K, et al. Postmortem autopsy-confirmation of antemortem [F-18] FDDNP-PET scans in a football player with chronic traumatic encephalopathy. Neurosurgery. 2018;82:237–46.
119. Mez J, Solomon TM, Daneshvar DH, Murphy L, Kiernan PT, Montenigro PH, et al. Assessing clinicopathological correlation in chronic traumatic encephalopathy: rationale and methods for the UNITE study. Alzheimers Res Ther. 2015;7(1):62.
120. Smith DH, Johnson VE, Trojanowski JQ, Stewart W. Chronic traumatic encephalopathy—confusion and controversies. Nat Rev Neurol. 2019;15:179.
121. Asken BM, Sullan MJ, DeKosky ST, Jaffee MS, Bauer RM. Research gaps and controversies in chronic traumatic encephalopathy: a review. JAMA Neurol. 2017;74(10):1255–62.
122. Manley G, Gardner AJ, Schneider KJ, Guskiewicz KM, Bailes J, Cantu RC, et al. A systematic review of potential long-term effects of sport-related concussion. Br J Sports Med. 2017;51(12):969–77.

Mental Health Considerations in Football

18

Timothy Neal

Introduction

The full range of mental health concerns found in the general student population are also found in football players at all levels of competition. Football players, like all students, are adapting to a new environment, are responsible for managing their time, and attempting to meet the demands of coursework to stay eligible. The football player is starting to explore their new-found freedom at the collegiate level, and are making choices regarding their personal behavior regarding sexuality, alcohol, and drug use [1–3]. Many football players define themselves by their identity as a football player [1–4]. Threats to that identity may come in the form of a struggling performance level, or a chronic, career-ending, or time-loss injury. Other concerns are conflicts with coaches and teammates, or simply losing the passion for playing their sport [1–4]. These challenges and other associated factors may put the football player in a position to experience a mental health issue, or exacerbate an existing mental health concern [1–4].

Prevalence of Mental Health Disorders

Studies are starting to reveal the growing prevalence in the types, severity, and percentage of mental illnesses in adolescents and young adults age 14–25. This age range includes secondary school and college football players [5]. Given the number of overall National Collegiate Athletic Association (NCAA) student-athlete participation rates of over 450,000 in the 2011–2012 year, of which are well over a 100,000 football players, [6] the probability of encountering a football player, or players, with a mental health challenge is a certainty at the intercollegiate level. Given the

T. Neal (✉)
Concordia University, Ann Arbor, MI, USA

K. W. Farmer (ed.), *Football Injuries*,
https://doi.org/10.1007/978-3-030-54875-9_18

higher number of secondary school football players, it is also a concern at the secondary school level.

The American Psychiatric Association's Diagnostic and Statistical Manual of Mental Disorders (DSM) states that "a mental disorder is conceptualized as a clinically significant behavioral or psychological syndrome or pattern that occurs in an individual and that is associated with present distress or disability or with a significantly increased risk of suffering death, pain, disability, or loss of freedom" [7]. The definition also states that a mental disorder, syndrome, or pattern, "must not be merely an expectable and culturally sanctioned response to a particular event (e.g., the death of a loved one). Whatever its original causes, it must currently be considered a manifestation of a behavioral, psychological, or biological dysfunction of the individual".

Data indicate that approximately one in every four to five youth and adults in America meets criteria for a mental health disorder, with severe impairment across a lifetime [8]. Nearly one in three adolescents (31.9%) met criterion for anxiety disorder, 19.1% were affected by behavioral disorders, 14.3% experienced mood disorders, and 11.4% in the study had substance use disorders [8]. Data also document the early onset of major classes of mental disorders [8]. Of affected adolescents, half experienced their disorders by age 6 for anxiety disorders, by age 11 for behavioral disorders, by age 13 for mood disorders, and age 15 for substance use disorders [8]. Comorbidity rates of affected individuals have been reported at 40%, while 22.2% in the study reported having a mental disorder with severe impairment and/or distress that interfered with daily life [8].

Studies have also shown that the average age of onset of major depression and dysthymia is between 11 and 14 years of age [9]. Another study discovered the rate of outpatient treatment for depression in the United States increased between 1987 and 1997, and that 75.3% of those individuals being treated for depression were using antidepressant medication in 2007 [10]. Studies are showing an early onset of mental disorders, and that most seriously impairing and persistent mental disorders found in adults are associated with child and adolescent onsets with high comorbidity [11]. A study on adversity in childhood and its relationship to developing a mental illness reported that adolescents aged 13–17 years, that had experienced a childhood adversity of either parental loss, parental maltreatment, parental maladjustment, or economic adversity highly occurring in that age group, was strongly associated with the onset of psychiatric disorders [12]. The range of disorders went from 15.7% having fear disorders, to 40.7% having behavioral disorders. Of all onsets of psychiatric disorders, 28.2% were associated with one or more childhood adversity [12]. This suggests that a football player coming from a socioeconomic disadvantage or challenging parental home as a youth is at risk for a mental health disorder in adolescence or young adulthood. Football players coming onto the team with this background should be monitored for developing a mental health disorder.

Epidemiological surveys estimate that as many as 30% of the adult population in the United States meet criteria for a yearlong DSM-mental disorder [13, 14]. Fewer than 50% of individuals diagnosed with a mental disorder receive treatment [15, 16]. The range of mental disorders are widespread, with serious cases concentrated in a relatively small proportion of cases with high comorbidity [17]. Anxiety disorders are reported often in mental disorder surveys [17] and appear to exact significant and independent tolls on health-related quality of life [18]. These statistics outline the need for early recognition and referral of the football player, exhibiting signs or symptoms of a mental health disorder.

Football players participating at the intercollegiate level are students as well as athletes. In a study of college students, there is general report of high levels of stress. In 2012, the American College Health Association reported a survey on the health of the general college student population [19]. The Reference Group Executive Summary reported on a wide range of health topics, including mental health. The undergraduate students surveyed reported the following experiences within the last 12 months:

- 31.6% felt so depressed that it was difficult to function.
- 86.8% felt overwhelmed by all they had to do.
- 58.4% felt very lonely.
- 81.9% felt exhausted (not from physical activity; participation in football may exacerbate).
- 46.5% felt things were hopeless.
- 61.9% felt very sad.
- 38.1% felt overwhelming anger.
- 51.3% felt overwhelming anxiety.
- 7.5% seriously considered suicide.

Psychiatric disorders, particularly alcohol use disorders, are common in the college-aged population. Though treatment rates varied across disorders, overall, fewer than 25% of individuals with a mental disorder sought treatment during the past year for consumption of alcohol in a survey taken by Columbia University [20]. The secondary school football player is also at risk for developing a mental health disorder, according to studies of adolescent mental health. Approximately 22.2% (one in five teens) in the United States suffer from a mental disorder that is severe enough to impact their daily activities, either currently or at some point in their lives. The prevalence of many emotional and behavioral disorders in children and adolescents is higher than many of the well-known physical ailments, like asthma and diabetes, in the same age group. Anxiety disorders, such as panic disorders and social phobia, are the most common conditions, with 31.9% of teens with the diagnosis. The next most common is behavior disorders, 19.1% of teens, which includes ADHD. Mood disorders, including major depressive disorder, were third with 14.3% and substance use disorders fourth with 11.4% [8].

Comorbidity (experiencing two or more mental health disorders at the same time) is a significant issue in the adolescent age group, as nearly 40% of subjects with one class of disorder also met the criteria for a second class of disorders at some point in their life. In a review of several community survey studies from across the world, it appears that approximately one-fourth of all youth experienced a mental disorder during the past year, and about one-third did so across their lifetime [21].

Incidence of depression increases with age, as the depression rate at age 13 of 1–2% climbs to 3–7% at age 15, and continues to increase throughout early adulthood. Thus, if a football player who reports as a freshman with a history of depression, their rate of depression may well trend upward in the ensuing years. Results are mixed when it comes to the effect of social class, race, and ethnicity. Although rare in children, bipolar disorder, mania, and hypomania range from 0% to 0.9% in those age 14–18 years with lifetime prevalence rates from 0% to 2.1%. As far as comorbidity, both major depressive disorder and bipolar are associated with multiple other disorders, including ADHD, anxiety disorders, oppositional defiant disorder and conduct disorder [22, 23]. Suicide is the third leading cause of death among adolescents, and half of all adult mental disorders have their onset during adolescence [24]. If a football player is suffering from a mental health disorder(s), and is experiencing heightened signs and symptoms of their disorder, the athletic trainer and team physician need to be vigilant for suicide ideation in that player.

Children with a physical illness are more likely to develop depression, and those with emotional disorders have an increased risk of developing physical disorders [25, 26]. If a secondary school football player sustains an injury, the athletic trainer, team physician, parent, and coach should be aware of any depressive signs and symptoms in that player. Also, if a football player has a mental health disorder, they are susceptible for injury.

Stressors

Participation in intercollegiate and secondary school football imposes additional demands and stressors on the student-athlete. These demands range from the physical (e.g., physical conditioning, participating with injuries, environmental conditions), to the mental (e.g., game strategy, meeting coaching expectations, attention from media and fellow students, time spent in sport, community service requirements, and diminishing personal and family time). These and other demands of being a football player, coupled with the requirements of being a student (e.g., classes, study time, projects, papers, midterm and final examinations, attaining and maintaining a grade point average to remain academically eligible, and maintaining or pursuing a scholarship), present a continuum of expectations on a student-athlete [27–35]. Intercollegiate football players are typically separated from the rest of the campus community, in that they live together, eat together, and work out together. Often, athletic facilities are separate from the general student population [4].

Pressure on the football player is widely seen in the "no off-season" approach to training. The football player is exposed to a predictable pattern and lack of sleep and under-recovery, putting the player at risk for anxiety and depression [36–48]. Football player overtraining is often the main feature of a "well-developed" training plan; in three separate samples found 21–45% of all student-athletes reported staleness (physical, mental, and emotional disturbances and a precursor to burnout) [49]. Recovery factors are closely related to factors of well-being and performance, and that many student-athletes are in consistent syndromes of chronic fatigue [50]. For football players, the complex relationship of long-term training and uncontrollable life variables often leads to overtraining and puts them at risk for physical, mental, and emotional health problems.

Some football players couple the stress of being an athlete with risky activities, thus raising their stress level with their behavior, as evidenced by a report that student-athletes participated in risk-taking behaviors, with male contact sports student-athletes such as football taking more risks. Student-athletes that had one risk-taking behavior were more likely to have multiple risk-taking behaviors, such as not wearing seatbelts, alcohol consumption, use of smokeless tobacco, unsafe sexual practices, and involvement in physical fights [51]. Football players engaging in risky behaviors should have an earnest discussion on their stressors and mental health and wellness.

Keep in mind that the stressors of being a football player can "trigger" a mental health disorder, or exacerbate or initiate a recurrence of a past mental disorder.

Bullying and Hazing

Bullying unfortunately is present in some athletic settings, especially at the secondary school level. Bullying is a type of youth violence and can cause physical, social, emotional, and academic issues. The harm done by bullying not only affects the victim but can also affect families and friends, and the overall health and safety of schools and neighborhoods. The Centers for Disease Control and Prevention defines *bullying* as any unwanted aggressive behavior(s) by another youth or group of youths who are not siblings or current dating partners that involves an observed or perceived power imbalance and is repeated multiple times or is highly likely to be repeated. Bullying may inflict harm or distress on the targeted youth, including physical, psychological, social, or educational harm [52].

A young person can be a bully, a victim, or both. Bullying can take place via physical, verbal, or social methods. Each form of aggression can occur in person or through technology (cyberbullying). In football players, signs of being bullied include the loss of focus, playing or performing tentatively, feeling anxious, dropping out of tournaments or competitions, or quitting sports altogether. In addition, adolescent athletes are frequently reluctant to tell their parents or coaches they have been bullied due to embarrassment, shame, and wanting to remain 'part of the team [53, 54]. It is imperative that all football players, especially secondary school level, have their behavior monitored to discourage, prevent, and discipline any form of bullying.

Mental Health Care Team

It is useful to have a team in place to address the psychological concerns of football players and all athletes. This team includes the team physician(s), athletic trainers, campus counseling at the intercollegiate level, guidance counseling and mental health professionals at the secondary school, and community-based mental health care professionals (clinical psychologists and psychiatrists). It is helpful to also have point persons overseeing various issues such as substance abuse and eating disorders programs. For mental health incidents where a football player violates a code of conduct within an athletic department or school, point persons for code of conduct violations may be part of a general plan. Code of conduct violations usually occur with a threat of, or acts of, harm toward oneself, others, or property. Check with state and school guidelines to establish a code of conduct violation definition [4].

Team physicians are called upon to meet with and evaluate a football player for a reported mental health concern. Some team physicians prescribe medications to football players for mental disorders, and encourage the referral for counseling by a mental health care professional. In many cases, the team physician is seeing a student-athlete for a mental health disorder on the recommendation of the athletic trainer, coach, or parent of the player. The team physician should rely on their experience and limitation in expertise in evaluating and managing a football player for a mental health disorder, and working with mental health care professionals in developing the appropriate plan of care relative to medication or counseling for the student-athlete [4].

Physicians practicing sports medicine frequently encounter mental health disorders in football players. Physicians also discuss mental health issues with injured football players fairly frequently, although their comfort and perceived competence vary widely [55].

At the secondary school level, school counselors can be an excellent source of information for the athletic trainer and team physician. If a student has permitted the school counselor to discuss personal information with the athletic trainer or team physician, as dictated by the local and district policies, the athletic trainer and team physician can use that information to best serve the student playing football. The athletic trainer should meet with the school counseling staff early in the year to obtain information that could be critical in working with student-athletes. In the case of emergent referrals for mental health problems, the athletic trainer can obtain the contact information for the local crisis intervention specialists. The athletic trainer should meet with the school counselors and school nurse to educate them regarding the symptoms of concussions and post-concussion sequelae. If the school counselors are aware that a football player has sustained a concussion, they can notify the student-athlete's teachers to consider making academic adjustments [4, 56].

The athletic trainer should establish a network within the secondary school and school district [56]:

- Make connections and become oriented with the school nurse and school counselor.
- Learn the district's policies and procedures for referrals. Discuss a plan of action should a referral be warranted.
- Include the nurse and counselor in the referral plan (introducing them if necessary). Ask for their input and feedback on various scenarios. This is no different than the process of creating a required Emergency Action Plan.

The athletic trainer should determine what resources are available at the secondary school, and how and when to access the resource. Many school districts provide school nurses and counselors only on certain days of the week and at certain times of the day. An early meeting between the athletic trainer and the school-based health team facilitates efficient communication protocols. Knowing when, where, and how to access the school nurse and counselor is essential for the athletic trainer and team physician to execute a plan of action. In addition, the school nurse and counselor can advise the athletic trainer and team physician regarding legal limitations, confidentiality considerations, and the school's current plan of action. They will also be able to identify youth mental health resources within the community. The athletic trainer and school health team can then expand the plan of action to incorporate the athletic trainer's scope of care per their respective state practice act, protocols for after-school hours, procedures for contacting parents, and district policy regarding contracted employees, as needed. The school health team can also advise the athletic trainer, regarding circumstances in which a parent may be the source of the problem or a barrier to the child's access to mental health care. Given that until children reach age 18, legal guardians have the authority to make decisions on virtually all aspects of their health care, so relying on the school administration for this type of intervention will be critical [56]. The indications for referral can differ, depending on the mental health issue being addressed, and it is useful to err on the side of safety when considering the speed in which an evaluation should be scheduled [4, 56].

If possible, for a nonemergency referral, assist the football player in making the initial appointment for a mental health care evaluation. This is where having a relationship with campus, secondary school, or community mental health care professionals prior to utilizing their services are important. Having a prior relationship may help access their services more expeditiously than having the football player try and make the initial appointment for an evaluation. In some cases, speaking with the counselor while making the appointment for the football player is advantageous if you know the mental health care professional. Oftentimes, the mental health care professional may want to know some context for the referral and trusts the judgment of the person making the referral. This helps the mental health care professional have a better understanding of the dynamics facing the football player going for the initial appointment. Ask the football player to report back to you that they have made their initial appointment, and ask if there is anything you, as the athletic trainer, can do to help expedite their appointments. Emphasize to the football player that whatever is discussed between the student-athlete and the mental health care professional is confidential. If the football player shares what is discussed at their appointments, unless it is of a nature that indicates harm to themselves or others, reassure the football player that the information shared will be kept confidential [4, 56].

The Pre-participation Physical Examination and the Student-Athlete's Mental Health History

The pre-participation physical examination is an optimal time to ask about a history of mental health problems and to screen for common mental health conditions such as depression, anxiety, learning disabilities, and eating disorders. Questions related to nutrition, weight, performance, learning disabilities, eating disorders, and other mental disorders should be included in the health history. The pre-participation physical examination offers an opportunity to ask open-ended questions, demonstrate openness, and destigmatize mental health concerns by including mental health as an important aspect of overall health. Suggestions for "yes," "no" mental health screening questions during the pre-participation physical examination are [4]:

- I often have trouble sleeping.
- I wish I had more energy most days of the week.
- I think about things over and over.
- I feel anxious and nervous much of the time.
- I often feel sad or depressed.
- I struggle with being confident'.
- I don't feel hopeful about the future,
- I have a hard time managing my emotions (frustration, anger, impatience).
- I have feelings of hurting myself or others.

Any affirmative answers to these questions should be brought to the attention of the physician for a discussion with the football player to ascertain whether follow-up evaluation, care, or medication is required. The vast majority of secondary school football players are minors; therefore, parental notification of discussions and referrals is recommended [56].

Behaviors to Monitor

The athletic trainer, team physicians, and others in the athletic department (athletic administrators, coaches, strength and conditioning staff, academic support staff, equipment staff) are in positions to observe and interact with football players daily. In most cases, athletic department personnel have the trust of the football player, and are someone the player turns to for advice or assistance during personal issues or crisis. Other football players may seek out teammates or non-athletic students on campus, a professor, a friend, or family member for help during a personal or psychological concern. Some football players, however, will not be aware of how a stressor is affecting them, or if they are aware of their potential mental health disorder, will not inform anyone, but may well act out in a non-verbal way to alert others that something is bothering them [1–4, 56]. Oftentimes, when a football player, athletic trainer, team physician, coach, teammate, or parent considers a student-athlete's "health," they think primarily of a physical health without considering "mental health." [57] However, both physical and mental health are equally important for the football player, and some medical problems often have psychological consequences that affect the personal life of the player as well as their playing status.

Recognition and Referral for Mental Health Evaluation and Care

Changes in mood and mental states of a sub-clinical nature impact football players and require further attention by sports medicine personnel. Traditional markers of personal distress, incapacitation, maladaptive behavior, and odd or erratic behaviors can begin with sub-clinical symptoms. When taking into account sub-clinical states of health and the aforementioned markers, it is often best to understand movements away from health in volume and intensity. Movements away from the football player's baseline of well-being shift from soft and subtle to consistent and loud. These changes in mental status when identified early (in their soft and subtle tones) create opportunities for remediation and thus enhance the return to premorbid functioning. Similarly, changes to the football player's wellness can also be due to environmental changes, such as changes to team members, coaches, support staff, or with their family of origin. The sensitivity to identify and refer, when situational changes/stress occur, strengthens the possibility to move football player's toward resilience and significant wellness [4, 56].

Inversely, the nature of mental health issues all along the continuum of personal welfare to performance can impact others, especially when team cohesion is a goal and an expectation. Thus, the stress created by negative mental health states, clinical or subclinical, are important to anticipate and address so it does not spread. This is no different than using situational play and practice to inoculate, protect, and assist in helping football players more resilient in the face of predictable stress of competition. Football player welfare requires prevention at each point along the welfare–performance continuum, not just when symptoms are consistent and intense. Vigilance with the identification, education, and treatment process enhances the opportunity to move toward overall health, reducing chances of injury, underperformance, and the reduction of the student-athletes quality of life.

The vulnerabilities/challenges identified within this population lead us to propose that student-athletes encounter a different set of risks than non-athletes, and, more importantly, we believe that the extreme nature of the work student-athletes do under extreme conditions is often under-acknowledged. Whether we are looking at changes which are diagnosable or not, prevention is key at all points along the welfare–performance continuum.

Approaching a football player with a concern over their mental well-being can be an uncomfortable experience for the athletic trainer or team physician. However, the health and wellness of the football player is the primary duty of the health care professional. It is important to have facts correct, with context, relative to the behavior of concern, before arranging a private meeting with the player. The conversation should focus on the football player as a person, not as an athlete. Empathetic listening and encouraging the student- athlete to talk about what is happening is essential [4, 56]. Encouraging a football player to consider a mental health evaluation can be challenging, given the stubborn stigma that is attached to receiving mental health care [58]. Though football players experience as much or more psychological distress as non-athletes, research indicates student-athletes, in general, use professional mental health services less than non-athletes [59].

A helpful component in football players receiving a mental health evaluation and care is convincing them to start the process. Pointing out that mental health is as important as physical health is one line of reasoning that may help the reticent player to seek help for their mental health issue. Assisting the player in accessing the mental health care system at the institution, secondary school, or community through the pre-arrangement of services eases the transition from deciding to go for help to meeting a mental health care professional and is the second component of getting a player for help for their mental health concern. It is important to note that in most cases, unless there is an imminent risk of harm to them and/or others, a football player cannot be compelled to report for a mental health evaluation. In the event a football player is reluctant to go for a mental health evaluation, the following suggestions may be made to the student-athlete [4]:

- Express confidence in the mental health profession.
- Clarify what counseling is and how it could help the student-athlete's overall health.
- Offer to accompany the student-athlete to the appointment if desired.
- Emphasize the confidentiality of mental health care and referral.
- Be persistent, but not pushy, in recommending a mental health evaluation.

If a football player at the intercollegiate level reports that they have independently sought out mental health care without prior knowledge by the athletic trainer or team physician, encourage the player to continue with their care, and assure the player that confidentiality of this arrangement will be maintained as long as there are no threats of harm to oneself or others [4].

Confidentiality

The issue of informing the football player's coach or parents invariably comes up. Some football players may believe that their coach, teammates, or parent may perceive receiving care for a mental health challenge is a sign of weakness, and are reluctant to inform anyone they are receiving mental health care.

In a routine referral, inform the player that while their referral is confidential, it may be helpful if they informed their coach and parents of their mental health care. They are not compelled to do so, but emphasize that coaches and parents are concerned about the welfare of the player, and keeping them informed of their mental health care is no different from any other forms of physical care [4, 58]. Encourage the football player to inform their coach or parents, but do not insist. Due to the minor age of most secondary school football players, secondary school districts must develop referral protocols for psychological concerns to ensure compliance with state law regarding the care of minor children [56]. This includes emergent mental health care evaluations in the event of a threat or actual incident of self-harm, harm to others, or destruction of property. Defer to risk management or general counsel on confidentiality matters regarding an under-aged student-athlete's mental health care [56]. In most cases, once a threat of harm to oneself or others is made, the confidentiality of that discussion is null and void, requiring the athletic trainer and team physician to enact the emergency mental health plan and informing officials, parents, and other stakeholders in the safety and wellness of the football player of this threat.

When referring to community-based mental health care professionals where the football player's private medical insurance may be utilized, it is important to inform the player that their parents or guardians will receive notification of their mental health care treatment from their insurance company in the form of an explanation of benefits (EOB) notification. Encourage the football player to inform their parents or guardians of their impending care so it is not a surprise to the parents or guardians when they are notified by their insurance carrier of the player's mental health care costs [4, 56].

Emergent Mental Health Referral

In the event that a football player demonstrates or voices an imminent threat to themselves, others, or property (which in many cases rises to a code of conduct violation); reports feeling out of control; unable to make sound decisions; and is incoherent, confused, or expresses delusional thoughts, an emergent mental health referral is highly recommended. The aforementioned list isn't all inclusive; other troubling symptoms, severity, or number of symptoms affecting the player should also be given weight when considering a routine or emergent mental health referral is in order. Consider the following steps when developing an emergent mental health referral protocol:

- Obtain and have available in your plan the institutional protocol for emergent mental health evaluations for students. Follow the protocol. Contact the university Public Safety Department or the Office of Student Affairs to obtain a copy.
- If the player appears or acts violently, call for campus and/or local law enforcement and seek immediate assistance and steps to protect bystanders from harm.
- If the football player's behavior is not violent, do not leave them alone. Call for assistance per the institutional protocol. Wait for instructions on how and where the player will be taken for an assessment. Offer to accompany the player to the place of evaluation—this may help reassure and calm the player during the assistance process.
- Contact your supervisor of sports medicine, school administration, athletics administration, Office of Student Affairs, team physician, and the student-athlete's coach to alert them to an emergent incident.

- Get all phone numbers of those caring for the player for any follow-up circumstances or questions by the parents/guardians and team physician.
- Seek advice or assistance with athletic administration, Office of Student Affairs, or general counsel on contacting the player's family and informing them of this incident.

Suicide in Student-Athletes

Suicide has been identified as the third leading cause of death among NCAA student- athletes [60]. While most people with a mental issue or challenge do not harm themselves or others, over 60% of all people who die by suicide suffer from major depression. With over 30% of all undergraduate students reporting feeling so depressed that it was difficult to function [19], and that few youth or young adults receive adequate mental health care [8], the specter of suicide in young adults, and in student-athletes, is present. Approximately 4700 young people between the ages of 14 and 24 die by suicide annually in the United States [61]. In addition, 1 in 6 high school students seriously consider attempting suicide, and 1 in 13 high school students attempt suicide one or more times [61].

A combination of individual, relational, community, and societal factors may contribute to the risk of suicide. Risk factors are those characteristics associated with suicide; they may or may not be direct causes [4, 56].

Risk factors:
- Family history of suicide.
- Family history of child maltreatment.
- Previous suicide attempt(s).
- History of mental disorders, particularly clinical depression.
- History of alcohol and substance abuse.
- Feelings of hopelessness.
- Impulsive or aggressive tendencies.
- Cultural and religious beliefs (e.g., belief that suicide is the noble resolution of a personal dilemma).
- Local epidemics of suicide.
- Isolation, a feeling of being cut off from other people.
- Barriers to accessing mental health treatment.
- Loss (relational, social, work, or financial).
- Physical illness.
- Easy access to lethal methods.
- Unwillingness to seek help due to the stigma attached to mental health and substance abuse disorders or to suicidal thoughts.

Protective factors buffer the individual from suicidal thoughts and behavior. To date, protective factors have not been studied as rigorously as risk factors. Identifying and understanding protective factors are, however, as important as researching risk factors.

Protective factors:

- Effective clinical care for mental, physical, and substance abuse disorders.
- Easy access to a variety of clinical interventions and support for help-seeking.
- Family and community support (connectedness).
- Support from ongoing medical and mental health care relationships.
- Skills in problem-solving, conflict resolution, and nonviolent ways of handling disputes.
- Cultural and religious beliefs that discourage suicide and support instincts for self-preservation.

Psychology of Injury

The psychological response to an injury is something the athletic trainer, physician, and coach should consider when a football player is injured. An injury, no matter how minor, is a cause of stress. Each player is different from another, so one sign or symptom described by a player may not be what another player experiences [4, 56].

Given the stressors placed on a football player, adding an injury, particularly one that is time-limiting, season ending, career ending, or life threatening, may be a huge source of stress. A football player may respond many ways to injury stress. Some may handle it well, with little impact, while others struggle, physically or emotionally. Some players may experience a personal injury for the first time while participating at the secondary or collegiate level, so there is a learning curve on handling the physical and emotional response to pain and disability that the athletic trainer must take into account and help the football player through. It is during this time of psychological and physical stress of injury that the football player should be observed for behaviors to monitor. Detecting any symptoms of psychological concern is part of the comprehensive care for the football player [62]. For example, the athletic trainer may be on the alert for a player who presents with a problematic emotional reaction to an injury or injuries: injuries that do not resolve no matter the correct diagnosis and care, symptoms that worsen over time without explanation, or the player's reaction to the severity or symptoms of an injury that seems excessive.

Football players often fear reinjury upon their return to participation [63]. The athletic trainer should be aware of this situation, reassure the player of their readiness to return to participation. The psychological response to an injury is something the athletic trainer, physician, and coach should consider when a football player is injured.

Concussions

The evolving awareness of the aftereffects of concussions includes the cognitive and psychological impact on student-athletes sustaining concussions [64–69] (see Chap. 18, Brain Injuries). Football players sustaining a concussion should be monitored for any changes in behavior or self-reported psychological difficulties while symptomatic, and after their return to activity following a concussion. It is also recommended that football players, once asymptomatic and cleared to resume physical activity by a physician, follow the return-to-play protocol in its Concussion Management Plan for student-athletes, as mandated by NCAA legislation 3.2.4.17 [70]. To return fully from a concussion is important; repeated concussions, especially during the same competitive season, puts the football player at risk for a mental health disorder as well as persistent post-concussion symptoms.

Psychosocial Skills

The athletic trainer can assist the football player by utilizing psychosocial skills. Psychosocial skills integrate psychology and sociology within the injury and healing processes [71]. The interplay between psychology and sociology best captures situational and individual factors [71]. These skills can be used for an injured player or for a player dealing with mental health issues. Pain is both physical and psychological. Often, the cognitive and emotional efforts in recovering from an injury are underappreciated. The athletic trainer should familiarize themselves with the basic principles of psychosocial skills to provide holistic care for the injured football player or to properly assess and refer the player suffering from a mental health disorder. Following are some psychosocial skills that the athletic trainer may employ to assist the football player [71]:

Sociocultural Aspects of Injury and the Injury Response

There are physical, environmental, psychological, and sociocultural risk factors in participating in football. The sport of football has a "sport ethic" [72, 73] that includes making personal sacrifices for the game, accept the risk of playing with pain, striving for distinction for being the best football player, and overcoming obstacles in the pursuit of excellence as a football player.

Psychosocial Antecedents to Injury

Understanding how stress and the player's response to stressors psychologically is important for the athletic trainer and team physician to know. Knowing that a football player's response to a stressor is either physiological or cognitive is vital in providing holistic care. The response to injury stress may take the form of adherence or nonadherence to the rehabilitation plan, which should be taken into account, especially during the competitive football season when the player is trying to return from a time-limiting injury.

Emotional Responses to Injury

Common emotional responses associated with injury include confusion, fear and anxiety, depression, isolation, and loss of identity as a football player. One common practice that needs examination is the isolation of injured football players from practice or team meetings. Each head football coach has his own way of approaching the injured football player. Knowing the devastating effects of feeling isolated from their support unit (teammates and position coaches), some consideration should be given to have the time-loss or season-ending injured football players attend meetings or parts of practice, in order to maintain their sense of belonging and reduce feelings of isolation, which could exacerbate other negative emotional responses to their injury.

Communication and Education

It is vital that the athletic trainer develop and enhance their communication skills to better care for and educate injured football players. Realizing that communication occurs nonverbally as well as with words is important. Demonstrating empathy and providing feedback through paraphrasing help the athletic trainer's communication with the injured football player, coach, and parents.

Identification of Psychosocial Distress and Referral

The athletic trainer and team physician are in unique positions to observe and interact with football players. Developing rapport with the player is helpful in determining when a behavior is demonstrating that the player is suffering from a potential mental health disorder or challenge. Being aware of red flags to a player's behavior is something the athletic trainer and team physician should know. Being able to approach the player with a concern over the player's mental health is critical. Having a referral plan in place to address routine and emergency mental health evaluations and care is part of holistic care for the football player.

Pain Management

Football is a high-velocity impact sport where injuries occur routinely. With injury comes pain. However, pain is both a physical and emotional experience. Pain is very subjective but very real to the injured football player. Realize that emotional stress can exacerbate physical pain symptoms. Acute and chronic pain bring their own set of physical symptoms, and the athletic trainer and team physician can better educate the football player through these processes to reduce the psychological as well as physiological impact of injury.

Psychosocial Aspects of Rehabilitation

There are many elements to consider in the psychological aspect of rehabilitation. Personal factors, cognitive factors, and emotional and behavioral factors, all must be contemplated and evaluated along with the range-of-motion and strengthening exercises. Whenever a football player is not adhering to the rehabilitation attendance or protocol, psychosocial factors should be considered.

Social Support

Helping the football player cope with their injury effectively is a primary duty of the athletic trainer. Promoting a sense of support to the football player during their recovery is part of holistic care. The athletic trainer wants to set up a trusting environment, where the football player feels comfortable in seeking help not only with the physical element of their care but also in the mental aspect of recovery.

Psychosocial Aspects of Return to Participation

Some football players may feel their identity as a football player is at risk when injured. Even as they recover, there may be anxieties as the player reaches a return to participation. Three key areas to instill in the recovering football player are competence, relatedness, and autonomy. Educate and demonstrate through testing to the player that, physically, the player is ready to return to participation, that they are competent to resume the rigors of football. Help the player in their relatedness with teammates by integrating the player gradually back to full activity. This keeps the player around their teammates and feeling a part of the team. Finally, as appropriate, have the football player have input and some control over their return to activity. This ensures the autonomy that is so important in the holistic approach to care.

Developing a Mental Health Plan

Considerations in building a recognition and referral plan for any student-athlete as well as a football player regarding a mental health concern are [4, 56]:

1. Establish the need for a plan on recognizing and referring student-athletes with psychological concerns. Start the process with a memorandum to administration outlining the prevalence of mental disorders in college-age students, the stressors found in student-athletes, and the availability of mental health care at the institution and community. Once the decision has been made to create a plan, initiate a draft of a document. Consider using the information contained in this NATA Inter-Association Consensus Statements on Developing Plans to Address Psychological Concerns in Athletes as a starting point [4, 56]..

2. Once the draft of the document is finished, share it with athletics administration, the counseling center, health services, risk management, Office of Student Affairs, (secondary school administration if the setting is the secondary school level), and general counsel for review and approval. Have all stakeholders review, amend, and approve the plan for legal and procedural purposes. Be sure to include the college or secondary school emergency mental health plan in the event of suicide ideation. No one plan can contain guidance on every situation. Each institution will have a variation of the plan based on their particular dynamics.
3. Once the plan is approved, send it to all sports medicine staff, physicians, coaches, and administrators, and secondary school officials (if developed for a secondary school) along with all approving departments for use. Encourage each person to carry the document with them at all times; no one can tell when a football player may report a mental health problem or crisis; having a plan in front of you to help navigate the process is helpful. Ensure that all relevant staff receives instructions regarding the plan. Review and update your plan annually or as necessary.

Utilizing the information contained in the NATA Inter-Association Consensus Statements on Developing a Plan to Address Psychological Concerns [4, 56] will assist the athletic trainer and team physician at an institution or secondary school in developing a plan and assisting football players with their mental health issues. Variables such as institutional human resource guidelines, state or federal laws, statutes, rules, and regulations (especially in working with minor children at the secondary school level) may affect the development and implementation of these recommendations.

References

1. NCAA Guideline 2o, Mental health: interventions for intercollegiate athletics, 2012–2013 NCAA sports medicine handbook; NCAA.org/health-safety.
2. Neal TL. Recognizing the signs. Train Condition. 2012;23(3):36–43.
3. Neal TL. Game changers: mental-health issues can impair a student-athlete's performance, so support is critical. Adv Phys Ther Rehabil Med. 2010;21:32–3.
4. Neal TL, Diamond AB, Goldman S, et al. Inter-association recommendations for developing a plan to recognize and refer student-athletes with psychological concerns at the collegiate level: an executive summary of a consensus statement. J Athl Train. 2013;48(5):716–20.
5. Substance Abuse & Mental Health Services Administration, Results from the 2010 National Survey on drug use and health: mental health findings, NSDUH series H-42, HHS publication no. (SMA) 11–4667. Rockville: Substance Abuse and Mental Health Services Administration; 2012.
6. NCAA Champion Magazine, Fall 2012, page 15.
7. American Psychiatric Association. Diagnostic and statistical manual of mental disorders. 5th ed. Arlington: American Psychiatric Association; 2013.
8. Merikangas KR, Jian-ping H, Burstein M, et al. Lifetime prevalence of mental disorders in U.S. adolescents: results from the national comorbidity survey replication-adolescent supplement (ncs-a). J Am Acad Child Adolesc Psychiatry. 2010;49(10):980–9.

9. Lewinsohn PM, Rohde P, Seeley JR. Major depressive disorder in older adolescents: prevalence, risk factors, and clinical implications. Clin Psychol Rev. 1998;18:765–94.
10. Marcus SC, Olfson M. National trends in the treatment for depression from 1998 to 2007. Arch Gen Psychiatry. 2010 Dec;67(12):1265–73.
11. Kessler RC, Wang PS. The descriptive epidemiology of commonly occurring mental disorders in the United States. Annu Rev Public Health. 2008;29:115–29.
12. McLaughlin KA, Greif GJ, Gruber MJ, et al. Childhood adversities and first onset of psychiatric disorders in a national sample of US adolescents. Arch Gen Psychiatry. 2012;69(11):1151–60.
13. Kessler RC, McGonagle KA, Zhao S, et al. Lifetime and 12-month prevalence of DSM-III-R psychiatric disorders in the United States: results from the National Comorbidity Survey. Arch Gen Psychiatry. 1994;51(1):518–9.
14. Reiger DA, Kaelber CT, Rae DS, et al. Limitations of diagnostic criteria and assessment instruments for mental disorders: implications for research and policy. Arch Gen Psychiatry. 1998;55(2):109–15.
15. Kessler RC, Berglund PA, Bruce ML, et al. The prevalence and correlates of untreated serious mental illness. Health Serv Res. 2001;3(6):987–1007.
16. Kessler RC, Zhao SK, Katz SJ, et al. Past-year use of outpatient services for psychiatric problems in the National Comorbidity Survey. Am J Psychiatry. 1999;15(6):115–23.
17. Kessler RC, Chiu WT, Demler O, Walters EE. Prevalence, severity, and comorbidity of 12-month DSM-IV disorders in the National Comorbidity Survey Replication. Arch Gen Psychiatry. 2005;62(6):617–27.
18. Comer JS, Blanco C, Hasin DS, et al. Health-related quality of life across the anxiety disorders: results from the national epidemiological survey on alcohol and related conditions (NESARC). J Clin Psychiatry. 2011;72(1):43–50.
19. American College Health Association. American college health association-National College Health Assessment II: undergraduate reference group executive summary spring 2012. Hanover: American College Health Association; 2012.
20. Blanco C, Okuda M, Wright C, Hasin DS, Grant BF, Lui SM, Olfson M. Mental health of college students and their non-college-attending peers: results from the National Epidemiologic Study on alcohol and related conditions. Arch Gen Psychiatry. 2008;65(12):1429–37.
21. Merikangas KR, Nakamura EF, Kessler RC. Epidemiology of mental disorders in children and adolescents. Dialogues Clin Neurosci. 2009;11(1):7–20.
22. Lewinsohn PM, Moerk KC, Klein DN. Epidemiology of adolescent depression. Econom Neurosci. 2000;2:52–68.
23. Lewinsohn PM, Duncan EM, Stanton AK, et al. Age at first onset for nonbipolar depression. J Abnorm Psychol. 1986;95(4):378–83.
24. Belfer ML. Global burden of child mental disorders. J Child Psychol Psychiatry. 2008;49(3):226–36.
25. Cohen P, Pine DS, Must A, et al. Prospective associations between somatic illness and mental illness from childhood to adulthood. Am J Epidemiol. 1998;147(3):232–9.
26. Parry-Langdon N, Clements A, Fletcher D, et al. Three years on survey of the development and emotional well-being of children and young people. Office for National Statistics: Newport; 2008.
27. Etzel EF, Ferrante AP, Pinkney JW. Counseling college student-athletes: issues and interventions. 2nd ed. Morgantown: Fitness Information Technology; 1996.
28. Etzel EF. Understanding and promoting college student-athlete health: essential issues for student-affairs professionals. J Stud Affairs Res Pract. 2006;43(3):894–922.
29. Humphrey JH, Yow DA, Bowden WW. Stress in college athletics: causes, consequences, coping. New York: Haworth Half-Court Press; 2000.
30. Kohlstedt SES. 2012. Psychosocial development in college students: a cross-sectional comparison between athletes and non-athletes. PhD diss., American University.
31. Raglin JS, Wilson GS. Overtraining in athletes (pp. 191–207). In: Hanin Y, editor. Emotions in sport. Champaign: Human Kinetics; 2000.

32. Weiss SM. A comparison of maladaptive behaviors of athletes and nonathletes. J Psychol. 1999;133(3):315–22.
33. Wilson G, Pritchard M. Comparing sources of stress in college student athletes and non- athletes. Athletic insight: the online journal of sport psychology. 2005. Retrieved July 6 2008: http://www.athleticinsight.com/Vol7Iss1/StressAthletesNonathletes.htm.
34. Zaichkowsky L, Kane MA, Blann W, Hawkins K. Career transition needs of athletes: a neglected area of research in sport psychology. Proceedings: 8th World Congress of Sport Psychology (pp. 785–7), Lisbon, 1993.
35. Etzel EF, Watson JC, Visek AL, Maniar SD. Understanding and promoting college student-athlete health: essential issues for student affairs professionals. NASPA J. 2006;43(3):518–46.
36. Derman W, Schwellnus MP, Lambert MI, Emms M, Sinclair-Smith C, Kirby P, Noakes TD. The 'worn-out athlete': a clinical approach to chronic fatigue in athletes. J Sports Sci. 1997;15(3):341–51.
37. Gould D. Personal motivation gone awry: burnout in competitive athletes. Quest. 1996;48(3):275–89.
38. Gould D, Dieffenbach K. Overtraining, under-recovery, and burnout in sport (pp. 25–35). In: Kellmann M, editor. Enhancing recovery: preventing underperformance in athletes. Champaign: HumanKinetics; 2002.
39. Hanin Y. Individually optimal recovery in sports: an application of the IZOF model (pp. 199–217). In: Kellmann M, editor. Enhancing recovery: preventing underperformance in athletes. Champaign: Human Kinetics; 2002.
40. Kellmann M, Kallus KW. Mood, recovery-stress state, and regeneration (pp. 101–17). In: Lehmann M, Foster C, Gastmann U, Keizer H, Steinacker JM, editors. Overload, fatigue, performance incompetence, and regeneration in sport fatigue, performance incompetence, and regeneration in sport. New York: Plenum; 1999. pp. 101–17
41. Kellmann M. Psychological assessment of under-recovery (pp. 37–55). In: Kellmann M, editor. Enhancing recovery: preventing underperformance in athletes. Champaign: Human Kinetics; 2002.
42. Puffer JC, McShane JM. Depression and chronic fatigue in athletes. Clin Sport Med. 1992;11(2):327–38.
43. Raedeke TD. Is athlete burnout more than just stress? A sport commitment perspective. J Sport Exerc Psychol. 1997;19(4):396–417.
44. Shuer ML, Dietrich MS. Psychological effects of chronic injury in elite athletes. WJM. 1997;166(2):104–9.
45. Silva JM. An analysis of the training stress syndrome in competitive athletics. J Appl Sport Psychol. 1990;2(1):5–20.
46. Tsuno N, Besset A, Ritchie K. Sleep and depression. J Clin Psychiatry. 2005;66(10):1254–69.
47. Voelker R. Stress, sleep loss, and substance abuse create potent recipe for college depression. JAMA. 2004;291(18):2177–9.
48. Yang J, Peek-Asa C, Corlette JD, Cheng G, Foster DT, Albright J. Prevalence of and risk factors associated with symptoms of depression in competitive collegiate student athletes. Clin J Sport Med. 2007;17(6):481–7.
49. Silva JM. An analysis of the training stress syndrome in competitive athletes. J Appl Sport Psychol. 1990;2(1):5–20.
50. Gould D. Personal motivation gone awry: burnout in competitive athletes. J Sports Sci. 1997;15(3):341–51.
51. Nattiv A, Puffer JC, Green GA. Lifestyles and health risks of collegiate athletes: a multi-center study. Clin J Sport Med. 1997;7(4):262–72.
52. Eating disorders. National Institute of Mental Health Website. http://www.nimh.nih.gov/health/topics/eating-disorders/index.shtml#3. Accessed May 10 2019.
53. Youth risk behavior surveillance: United States, 2011. Centers for Disease Control and Prevention Web site. http://www.cdc.gov/MMWR/PDF/SS/SS6104.PDF. Accessed May 10 2019.

54. Gladden RM, Vivolo-Kantor AM, Hamburger ME, Lumpkin CD. Bullying surveillance among youths: uniform definitions for public health and recommended data elements, version 1.0. Centers for Disease Control and Prevention Web site. http://www.cdc.gov/violenceprevention/pdf/bullying-definitions-final-a.pdf. Published 2014. Accessed May 10 2019.
55. Mann BJ, Grana WA, Indelicato PA, O'Neill DF, George SZ. A survey of sports medicine physicians regarding psychological issues in patient-athletes. Am J Sports Med. 2007;35(12):2140–7.
56. Neal TL, Diamond AB, Goldman S, et al. Inter-association recommendations for developing a plan to recognize and refer student-athletes with psychological concerns at the secondary school level: a consensus statement. J Athl Train. 2015;50(3):231–49.
57. NCAA Managing student-athletes' mental health issues. Available online at http://www.NCAA.org/health-safety.
58. Schwenk TL. The stigmatization and denial of mental health illness in athletes. Br J Sports Med. 2000;34(1):4–5.
59. Pinkerton RS, Hinz LD, Barrow JC. The college student-athlete: psychological considerations and interventions. J ACH. 1989;37(5):218–26.
60. Harmon KG, Asif IM, Klossner D, Drezner JA. Incidence of sudden cardiac death in National Collegiate Athletic Association Athletes. Circulation. 2011;123:1594–600.
61. Kann L, Kinchen S, Shanklin SL, et al. Youth risk behavior surveillance: US, 2013. MMWR Morbid Mortal Wkly Rep. 2013;63(SS04):1–168.
62. Ray R, Wiese-Bjornstal DM. Counseling in sports medicine. Champaign: Human Kinetic Books; 1999.
63. Ardern CL, Taylor NF, Feller JA, Webster KE. A systematic review of the psychological factors associated with returning to sport following injury. Br J Sports Med. 2001;45(7):596–606.
64. Giza CC, Hoyda DA. The neurometabolic cascade of concussion. J Athl Train. 2001;36(3):228–35.
65. Schoenhuber R, Gentilini M. Anxiety and depression after mild head injury: a case control study. J Neurol Neurosurg Psychiatry. 1988;51:722–4.
66. Guskiewicz KM, Marshall SW, Bailes J, McCrea M, Cantu RC, Randolph C, Jordan BD. Association between recurrent concussion and late-life cognitive impairment in retired professional football players. Neurosurgery. 2005;57(4):719–26.
67. Karzmark P, Hall K, Englander J. Late-onset post-concussion symptoms after mild brain injury: the role of premorbid, injury-related, environmental, and personality factors. Brain Inj. 1995;9(1):21–6.
68. Kerr ZY, Marshall SW, Harding HP, Guskiewicz KM. Nine-year risk of depression diagnosis increases with increasing self-reported concussions in retired professional football players. Am J Sports Med. 2012;40(10):2206–12.
69. Chen JK, Johnston KM, Petrides M, Ptito A. Neural substrates of symptoms of depression following concussion in male athletes with persisting post-concussion symptoms. Arch Gen Psychiatry. 2008;65(1):81–9.
70. NCAA Guideline 2i: Concussion or Mild Traumatic Brain Injury (TBI) in the Athlete. 2014-2015 NCAA sports medicine handbook. NCAA.org/health-safety.
71. Granquist M, Hamson-Utley J, Kenow LJ, Stiller-Ostrowski J. Psychosocial strategies for athletic training. Philadelphia: FA Davis Company; 2015.
72. Coakley J. Sports in society: issues and controversies. 10th ed. New York: McGraw Hill; 2009.
73. Hughes R, Coakley J. Positive deviance among athletes: the implications of over conformity to sport ethic. Sociol Sport J. 1991;8:307–25.

Infectious Disease Concerns in Football

19

Robert G. Hosey, M. Kyle Smoot, and Cameron D. Straughn

Introduction

Infectious diseases commonly occur among the general population as well as football athletes, and, consequently, make up a large portion of training room visits, cause time away from sport, and effect on-field performance. Unique stresses may be placed on football athletes, especially at upper levels, including significant travel requirements, meetings, group meals, residential housing, and consistent exposure to highly populated areas such as practice and competition sites. These factors increase disease exposure and often do not allow for isolation conditions for sick individuals.

Epidemiologic studies of infectious disease, in relation to amount of training, have focused mainly on the endurance of the athlete population. These results can be extrapolated to American football, as training times and exertional expenditures are similar. Nieman et al. showed that 98% of athletes experience at least one illness over the 2-month period in winter. There is a J-shaped epidemiologic curve (Fig. 19.1) for frequency of illness, specifically upper respiratory infection (URI)-type infections in relation to exercise levels [1]. This has been hypothesized to be due to suppression of the immune system for several hours post vigorous exercise.

The febrile athlete should have special consideration, as this is an altered physiologic state. Fever is a physiologic response of the immune system aimed at shortening the course of an infection by release of cytokines and inflammatory markers. Unfortunately, this immune response has many ill effects on the body. These include increasing insensible fluid losses, dehydration, metabolic demands, and dysregulation of body temperature. Increased production of adrenaline occurs, which

R. G. Hosey (✉) · M. K. Smoot
Department of Orthopedic Surgery and Sports medicine, University of Kentucky College of Medicine, Lexington, KY, USA
e-mail: rhosey@uky.edu; kyle.smoot@uky.edu

C. D. Straughn
Department of Sports Medicine, James Madison University, Harrisonburg, VA, USA
e-mail: straugcd@jmu.edu

K. W. Farmer (ed.), *Football Injuries*,
https://doi.org/10.1007/978-3-030-54875-9_19

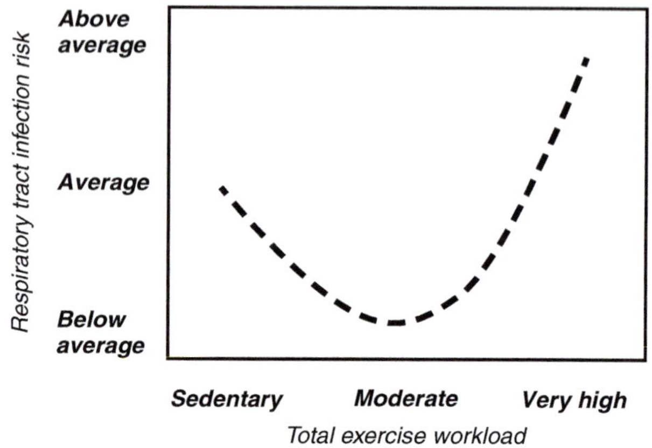

Fig. 19.1 The J-shaped curve, found by Niemen et al., showing the epidemiologic relationship between level of exercise and risk of URTI. The model suggests that extremely high levels of exercise may increase risk, while moderate exercise is protective, with permission from Niemen et al. [1]

increases metabolic rate, heart rate, and muscle tone. There is approximately a 10% increase in metabolic rate for every degree Celsius increase in body temperature. Fever also produces a stimulus for glycolysis and peripheral vasoconstriction, which, in turn, plays a part in decreasing the amount of free glucose available in circulation. Glycolysis then shifts metabolism toward lipolysis and proteolysis, leading to muscle catabolism [2, 3].

The athlete's hydration status is key when dealing with fever. The body will decrease production of antidiuretic hormone (ADH), which potentiates dehydration. If exercise is continued, the increased heat can promote further fluid loss and potentiate dehydration or hyperthermia.

Fever has also been correlated with reduced exercise tolerance, decreased endurance, and muscle strength. This decrease can be explained by muscle catabolism through the febrile period. Often, complete recovery can take several weeks. The magnitude of these losses and recovery time is correlated to the time in the acute phase response. Of note, motor skills, precision, and coordination are also affected and should be taken into account in terms of injury prevention and return to sport (RTS) [4].

Upper Respiratory Infections: Above the Neck

Upper respiratory infections (URIs) are the most common acute illnesses in the general population. In particular, athletes have been seen to be at an increased risk for contracting URIs due to the high levels of activity, group settings, extended travel, and general increase in exposure to pathogens. These have a wide range of severity and return-to-play considerations.

Common Cold

Viral URIs are generally benign and self-limiting conditions, manifesting as rhinorrhea, cough, and fever lasting 5–14 days. There are multiple viral families that can cause this, but they are most commonly rhinovirus, coronaviruses, and respiratory syncytial virus (RSV) in that respective order. These are spread via person-to-person particle contact, and time of exposure is the main risk factor for transmission. It has been shown that 40–90% of persons with a cold will have viral particles on their hands; therefore, personal hygiene and appropriate separation of the athlete are important [5].

URIs are diagnosed clinically and have nonspecific physical exam findings. Generally, these are treated symptomatically, and antibiotics do not have a role in treatment unless complicated by secondary infection. The athlete can typically continue to participate unless febrile or having general malaise. These can be signs that the body is undergoing a systemic response and therefore can be subject to the previously discussed physiologic responses limiting exercise. Medical follow-up should be every 2–3 days until symptoms resolve to ensure resolution or to treat accordingly if worsening [15, 17].

Viral myocarditis, though rare, is a well-known complication of viral URIs and most commonly associated with Coxsackie virus. Despite limited human data suggesting exercise increases the likelihood of myocarditis, the potential outcome is significant. The basis of this idea stems from murine models infected by Coxsackie virus, in which exercise increases the rate of viral replication and morbidity associated with myocarditis [4]. Viral myocarditis is associated with sudden cardiac death and accounts for 3–5% of known cases in young athletes [8]. Though low in occurrence, this is a significant outcome and has received a large amount of publicity. Due to the associated morbidity, myocarditis should receive due thought; however, fear of this uncommon outcome should not be the predominant factor that affects return to sport and participation in activity during viral URIs.

Sinusitis

Acute sinusitis, which is generally defined as inflammation of the paranasal sinuses, is most commonly associated with viral infections, lasting from 7 to 10 days. Generally, acute bacterial sinusitis also has a self-limiting course, but without treatment, it can last upwards of a month. Bacterial sinusitis has the opportunity to lead to more severe complications such as intracranial or orbital infections [6, 14].

Though the symptoms of sinusitis are nonspecific, there is a correlation between persistent purulent rhinorrhea and facial pain with a bacterial etiology. Lab and imaging studies are not usually necessary for diagnosis. With this said, if needed for differentiation of worrisome intra-nasal pathologies, CT scan is the test of choice [6].

Treatment is based around symptomatic management. If the athlete has a history of allergic rhinitis, then antihistamines or intra-nasal steroids can significantly reduce duration and severity of symptoms, though these agents do not play a role in patients without allergic rhinitis [9]. Antibiotics are useful if the athlete has severe symptoms (fever/myalgia), has no improvement within 10 days, or a worsening of symptoms from the 5th- to 7th-day mark. It should be noted that side effects increase considerably with antibiotic use. If the athlete is afrebrile, sport/physical activity can still be considered. If severe symptoms (myalgias, extreme headache, fever) occur, exercise should be avoided until improved.

Acute Pharyngitis

Acute pharyngitis is another very common occurrence among the general population and athletic population, with a general constellation of symptoms, including pharyngeal swelling, erythema, and pharyngeal exudate. The etiologic causes are diverse with the virus causing roughly 50% of cases, and Group A *Streptococcus* (GAS) accounting for 10–15% and 30% of cases in the adult and pediatric population, respectively [10]. In the young athletic population, other pathogens must be considered, including *Neisseria gonorrhea*, herpes simplex, and Epstein Barr, as these can produce similar clinical syndromes. The other important etiologies to differentiate from acute pharyngitis are peritonsillar and retropharyngeal abscesses [18, 19].

Classically, the Centor criteria have been used for the clinical diagnosis of GAS. Unfortunately, even at its best, the positive predictive value (PPV) is only around 50% if four of the variables are present [11]. The six variables used in the criteria listed from highest predictive value to lowest were tonsillar exudates, swollen tender anterior cervical nodes, temperature greater than 101 orally, pharyngeal exudates, lack of cough, and swollen posterior cervical nodes [12].

The largest incentive for antibiotic prescriptions for GAS is generally expedient reduction of symptoms and prevention of acute rheumatic fever with its many possible complications. With this said, the incidence of rheumatic fever has significantly decreased since the original epidemiologic studies in the 1960s; therefore, empirical antibiotic treatment without testing is no longer recommended. Rapid streptococcal antigen testing has improved and currently has sensitivity between 80% and 90% and specificity from 90% to 100%. Despite these statistics, throat culture remains the gold standard for diagnosis [6]. If GAS is identified, then appropriate antibiotic therapy is recommended. For non-GAS pharyngitis, symptomatic treatment is still the mainstay of therapy. Anti-inflammatories are helpful for symptomatic reduction, but they should be used under close supervision and individualized for the severity of illness. Nonsteroidal anti-inflammatory drugs (NSAIDs) have the potential for gastrointestinal (GI) upset and adverse renal effects. Corticosteroids have been seen to provide initial relief, but they, generally, will not shorten the total illness course [13]. It is also important to note that in GAS, the athlete is contagious for the first 24 h on antibiotics. There is some thought that the athlete should be held from participation during this time; however, if symptomatic improvement is occurring in the first 24-hr period and no fever is present, then participation is feasible under close supervision [6].

Influenza

The clinical disease of flu is caused by the influenza virus and has a multitude of strands. It should be considered specifically during the winter months with abrupt onset of fever, headache, myalgia, malaise, nausea, and vomiting. Often, cough and sore throat accompany the classic symptomatology. The morbidity and mortality of influenza are often associated with disease complications, such as pneumonia, meningitis, myocarditis, myositis, rhabdomyolysis, and Guillain-Barre syndrome. There are no specific physical exam findings that help differentiate influenza from other URTI's. The lab diagnosis is usually made from nasal or throat swabs, but clinical suspicion is still extremely important. Depending on the brand of test, sensitivity is only between 50% and 70% [62].

For continued symptomatic treatment, there are two types of antivirals used, neuraminidase inhibitors (zanamivir and oseltamivir) and M2 inhibitors (amantadine and rimantadine). Neuraminidase inhibitors are the most commonly used, as they are active against both influenza A and B [21, 22]. These medications should be started within the first 48 h of illness and generally will decrease symptom duration by roughly 48 h if taken at the recommended treatment doses [22]. Due to the close living quarters and regular interactions with teammates, if an outbreak of influenza begins, the entire team and training staff can be given prophylactic dosing to limit the spread. Even with prophylaxis, the affected athlete should be quarantined away from the team for 5 days, given a minimum of 48 h of treatment with a neuraminidase inhibitor, and should be afebrile prior to returning to the team. Once these conditions are met, the athlete can then return to the team, and as long as they are symptomatically improving, athletic participation can begin. Due to its superior evidence-based side-effect profile, oseltamivir has been the most common drug used. It is fairly well tolerated with the most common side effect being GI upset with or without vomiting [23].

With the severity of the clinical course and the virility of influenza, justification for vaccination is fairly simple. Unfortunately, efficacy of the influenza vaccine is variable from year to year. There are multiple different formulations and ways to administer the vaccine. The antigens are produced in eggs, which though rare can lead to side effects to egg-allergic athletes. It has been hypothesized that due to increased geographic exposure of athletes, the quadrivalent vaccine is the best ratio of benefit with limiting side effects [24]. Timing and anatomic location of administration should be taken into consideration, based on sport and position. For most football players, arm or leg administration would not matter; however, for quarterbacks, gluteal injections may be better, and as for kickers, upper arm injections may be preferable. Local irritation is common after administration, as is muscular pain after intramuscular (IM) injection. There should be some care taken to ensure the injection is IM and not into a bursal area such as the subdeltoid bursa, which can lead to weeks and possibly months of pain. Possibility of further side effects, such as fever, headache, and fatigue, should be taken into consideration when planning the timing of vaccination during the course of the season or practice week. Vaccines should be given either post game or at a time when recovery is already taking place.

Mononucleosis

Infectious mononucleosis (IM) is classically the primary infection of the Epstein–Barr Virus (EBV). It is now most common in the second decade of life with 30–75% of college freshman being seronegative for EBV [30]. Generally, there is a prodrome of malaise, fever, and chills followed by sore throat, fever, sweating, headache, stiff neck, anorexia, abdominal discomfort, pharyngitis, exudative tonsillitis, palatal petechiae, and general lymphadenopathy [29, 30]. Other features may include periorbital edema (33%), hepatomegaly (25%), jaundice (10%), and rash (<25%). Of these, the most common presenting signs are pharyngitis, fever, malaise, and classically posterior cervical chain lymphadenopathy [32]. This being said, there are multiple organisms or viruses that can produce a similar clinical picture, especially GAS. Therefore, testing for both is essential as one is an indication for antibiotics, which can cause complications with the other [30].

Testing was originally done with heterophile antibodies, but the monospot test has since taken its place being slightly more sensitive and specific. Other abnormalities to be aware of are marked lymphocytosis with atypical lymphocytes, mildly elevated liver enzymes, and, finally, often most talked about in athletics, is splenomegaly. Splenomegaly has been proposed to be a common occurrence with mono (8–100%) [30, 34], and the possibility of splenic rupture though rare (0.1–0.2%) in contact sports has significant morbidity and mortality. Hosey et al. demonstrated an increase in spleen size in all athletes with IM via US measurement. Previous estimates of the increase in splenic size made by physical exam were anywhere from 8% to 25%. The majority of case reports of splenic ruptures have been within the first 3 weeks of illness. In concordance with this, the rate of splenic size increase was demonstrated to peak within the first 12 days [34]. Also, the absolute splenic size peaked within the first 3.5 weeks from illness onset and decrease in size was consistently seen after this initial peak. Clinically following splenic size is a complicated, difficult task that is often futile. A single US examination for determining splenomegaly is of limited value as there is a large variation in normal splenic size [33]. Unfortunately, based on this, without a baseline splenic size, it is difficult to interpret a single measurement to inform decisions on return-to-play protocols (Fig. 19.2).

Treatment for athletes with IM is symptomatic in nature. There is no cure for EBV, and antiviral treatment has not been supported [30]. There have been several studies looking at corticosteroid treatment, showing a difference in length and severity of initial symptoms. Though clinical improvement was seen, significant

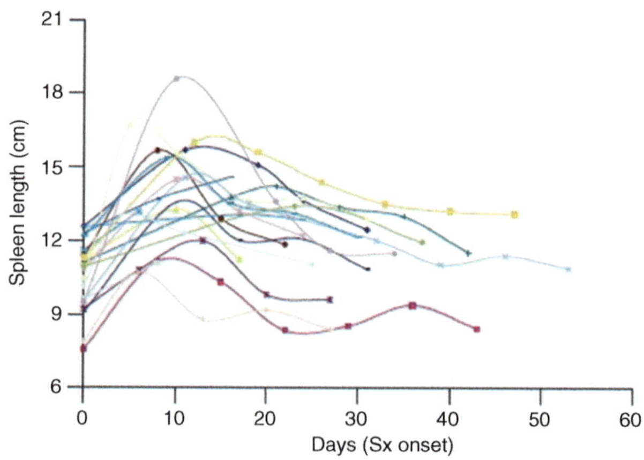

Fig. 19.2 Illustration of splenic length versus time from onset of symptom in 20 patients with Mononucleosis (Day 0 reflects baseline measurement, with permission from Hosey et al. [33]

disease course modification was not observed. Iatrogenic complications should be avoided and the athlete counselled on appropriate use of medications. Specific examples of iatrogenic complications include worsening of bleeding-related complications with aspirin and rashes associated with penicillin derivatives given for presumed GAS [30, 31].

In regard to return to play after IM, there are multiple elements to take into consideration. The initial symptomatic illness is generally between 5 days and 7 days. Then the fatigue, that can be severe, often lasts up to a month after initial illness. Due to the associated mortality and morbidity, the risk of splenic rupture must be considered. The RTS decision should be individualized, based on the athlete's recovery, though based on the abovementioned findings and case reports, it is presumed to be safe to return to contact sport at the 3-week mark if the athlete is otherwise able to participate [25–28].

Lower Respiratory Infections: Below the Neck

Acute Bronchitis

Acute bronchitis is defined by inflammation of the large airways and almost always characterized by cough. Viruses are the dominant etiologic cause of bronchitis, most notably being influenza, RSV, and parainfluenza. Known bacterial causes include *Bordetella pertussis*, *Chlamydia pneumoniae*, and *Mycoplasma pneumoniae* [35, 36]. Cough is the predominant symptom; therefore, if fever is present, differential should be more oriented toward an influenza-type illness. Also as vaccination rates dwindle, pertussis should be considered in athletes with 2–3 weeks of cough. If this diagnosis is being considered, pertussis can be confirmed with a nasopharyngeal swab followed by polymerase chain reaction (PCR). The differential for bronchitis also includes gastroesophageal reflux disease (GERD), asthma, and allergic rhinitis. Generally, beyond testing for aggressive causes such as influenza or pertussis, there is not currently anynecessary testing for bronchitis. Treatment is based on symptoms, generally starting with antitussives. Therapy tailored around the other differentials can be tried based on the athlete's risk factors, H_2 blockers for GERD, corticosteroids for allergic rhinitis, etc. Return-to-play guidelines are based off of the possibility for worsening pulmonary infection, febrile guidelines, and hydration status. Athletes should be counselled on the possibly of worsening infection (roughly 30%), progressing to further pulmonary infection. The athlete should know that even if time away is needed for recovery, 4–5 days of inactivity is needed before physical deconditioning begins [16, 37].

Community-Acquired Pneumonia

Pneumonia is an acute infection of the pulmonary parenchyma and termed community-acquired pneumonia (CAP) when the patient-athlete has not been hospitalized or in a long-term care facility for 14 days prior to symptom onset. CAP's most common etiology is *Streptococcus pneumoniae*; however, the etiology of CAP is becoming increasingly broad. Viral pneumonias, specifically due to influenza, are increasing with secondary bacterial infections such as *Staphylococcus aureus* commonly seen post influenza. Atypical infections, including *Haemophilus influenza*, *Moraxella catarrhalis*, and *Pseudomonas aeruginosa*, occur in patients with underlying lung disease or chronically taking glucocorticoids [39].

In the young athletic population, the constellation of fever, cough, sputum production, and shortness of breath (SOB) with a new infiltrate noted on chest X-ray is diagnostic for CAP. Traditionally, blood and sputum cultures are used for identification of the organism. Due to these tests' limitations, large medical centers often use PCR for identification of difficult-to-culture organisms, such as viral etiologies and atypical infections [41, 42].

Whenever talking about CAP, severity scoring is important and is generally used to determine in- or outpatient management. For the athletes, the Pneumonia Severity Index is the most commonly used, but it is beyond the scope of this chapter [40]. For treatment in the outpatient setting, if the patient does not have any comorbid conditions and the community pneumococcal macrolide resistance is less than 25%, the recommendation is to start with either a macrolide or doxycycline. Though if the athlete has a coexisting illness, recently used a macrolide, or community pneumococcal resistance is >25%, then a beta-lactam plus a macrolide can be used or levofloxacin as monotherapy cautiously considered. It should be noted that the fluoroquinolone antibiotics should rarely, if ever, be used in the athletic population due to the increased risk of tendon rupture (Fig. 19.3) [38, 39].

Most of the outcome data about CAP are mortality data, and there are limited RTS data. Based on general populace data, 67% of patients had resolution of

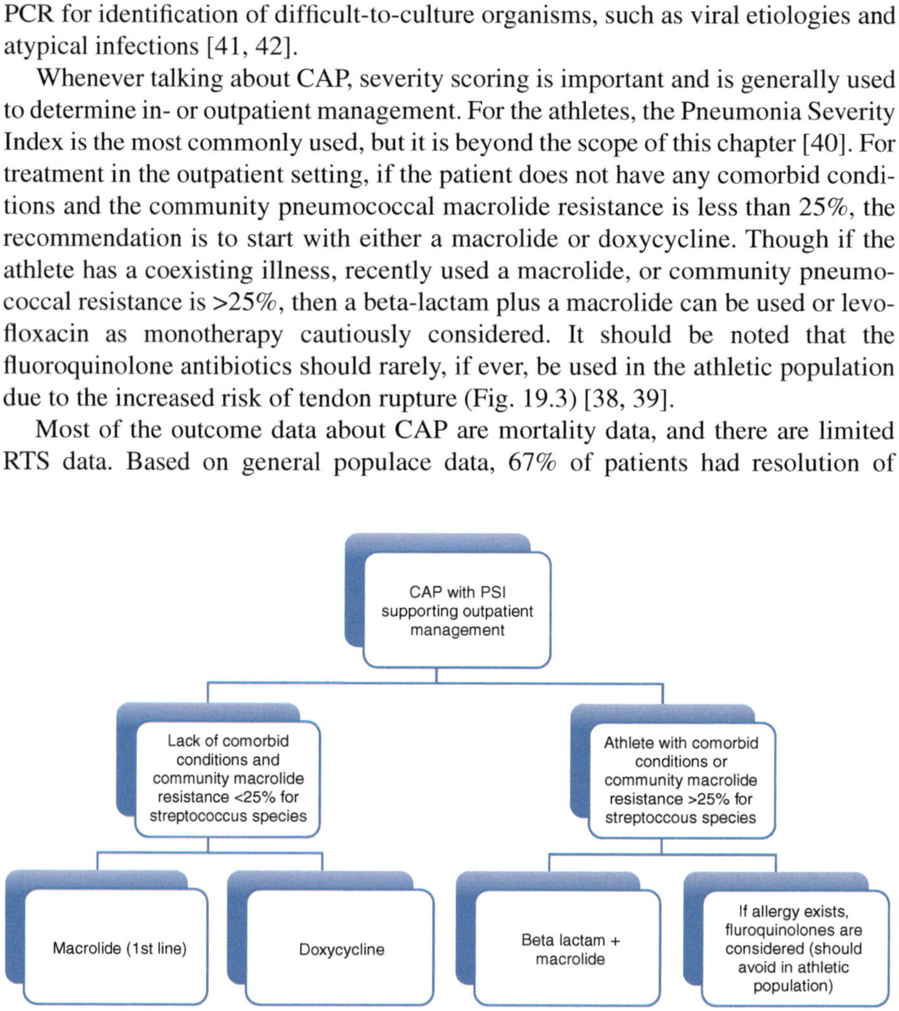

Fig. 19.3 Pneumonia outpatient treatment algorithm, adapted from the treatment algorithm outlined by Musher et al. [39] and MK Smoot and RG Hosey [37]

symptoms by day 14, and the median return to work was 6 days. Also of note, 35% still had at least once symptom at day 28 [43]. If these findings are extrapolated to the football setting, it can be expected that RTS should be similar to the return-to-work data, but the athlete could continue to have residual symptoms for a month after initial onset, and level of play could be affected. During the recovery process, both bronchitis and CAP can cause airway hypersensitivity, which can be somewhat ameliorated by broncho-dilating agents. The athlete should be informed of the estimated time frame to return to activity, and mild exertional training can theoretically be attempted as soon as 2–3 days, depending on symptom resolution [7, 16, 21].

Gastroenteritis

In the general and athletic population, GI infections are extremely common, but thankfully through the progression of the twentieth century, the morbidity and mortality associated with them have greatly decreased. This has occurred due to clean water sources becoming the rule and not the exception. For athletic teams, GI infections can still become problematic and often debilitating. With the close proximity of the team, especially while traveling, these infections can spread quickly through athletes and staff. While foodborne illnesses are often the first thing thought of, these only make up a small percentage of the incidence of GI infections, while transmission by way of water or person-to-person contact is much more common. Thankfully, based on the epidemiologic data by Peterson et al. [46], the athletic-age population has the lowest mortality associated with these infections. With this being said, there have been several widespread outbreaks over university campuses and collegiate football teams, which have affected gameplay and, in extreme circumstances, the ability of a team to field enough players to participate [44, 45].

The most likely viral etiology for GI infections in the athlete is the Norovirus (Norwalk-like) or Norwalk viral illness, accounting for 96% of acute nonbacterial outbreaks in the United States [47]. More specific to Football, in 1998, a North Carolina football team had an outbreak of norovirus while traveling to Florida, which was transferred via improper food handling. Though over 40 players on the North Carolina team were sick, the game was played with the team from Florida winning easily. After the game, multiple players from Florida contracted a similar illness [45]. There have been several other episodes where a Norovirus or Noro-like virus sidelined teams for multiple practices or games were cancelled. These viruses, part of the Caliciviridae family, cause nausea, vomiting, abdominal pain/cramping, diarrhea, and can cause fever and fatigue. The illness can last anywhere from 12 to 60 h and is contagious at any point during the symptomatic illness. Transmission is generally fecal contamination of water or a food source, though person-to-person contact through the same particles can spread the infection in a game setting. Treatment is focused around rehydration strategies and symptom relief. Due to the possibility of spread and significant risk for worsening of a dehydration state, symptomatic players are held from team activities. Hydration should be the main focus and should be followed clinically and objectively with regular weigh-ins. Return to play can be considered once the patient is asymptomatic and afebrile. Generally, the course is self-limited, and further testing or hospitalization is rare. Reasons to pursue further workup include grossly bloody stools, profuse diarrhea with dehydration, passage of more than six unformed stools in 48 h, fever, severe abdominal pain, or diarrhea in an immunocompromised individual [44, 45].

The other leading causes of GI infections are bacterial and parasitic. As most cases of GI-related illness resolve spontaneously, only key facts will be discussed later in this chapter. Several red flag symptoms and characteristics will be examined as key aspects of the athlete's history or physical exam that may point toward another etiology. Generally, these will warrant further workup, which should be pursued prior to the athlete worsening [44, 46, 49].

Salmonella is one of the leading causes of food poisoning in the United States and is associated with poultry, beef, milk, or egg contamination. In the majority of cases, salmonella has a self-limited course of nausea, vomiting and non-bloody diarrhea. In contrast, the typhoid type can lead to a prolonged febrile illness, splenomegaly, delirium, and severe abdominal pain. Antibiotic use is limited to patients with signs of focal infection (abscess), the immune-deficient or septic patients [44, 48].

Shigella is also related to food-borne illness, but it is not as common as salmonella. It is highly infective and can easily spread in close quarters in a fecal-oral manner. The clinical illness initially begins as watery diarrhea, then, as the bacteria migrate to the colon, mucosal sloughing occurs causing small-volume bloody and sometimes mucoid stools. The illness is generally self-limited, but it should be noted that the patient could become toxic with high fever and severe diarrhea [44, 48]. If this occurs, a higher level of care is needed.

Campylobacter jejuni is the most common cause of bacterial GI infection in the world. Symptoms occur with acute diarrhea, often bloody; abdominal pain; fever; and malaise. Symptoms are usually caused by toxins and sometimes, but less commonly, mucosal invasion of the bacteria. These cases can often mimic inflammatory bowel disease with the presence of bloody stools and abdominal pain. *Campylobacter* is transmitted by the fecal-oral route and is associated with contaminated water or food (classically chicken) by an infected food handler [44, 48].

Escherichia coli (*E. coli*) produces several different types of illnesses. Enterohemorrhagic *E. coli* (EHEC) is the leading cause of infectious bloody diarrhea in the world. The most well-known subtype O157:H7 causes hemorrhagic colitis and can lead to hemolytic uremic syndrome (HUS). Though this is only 5–10% epidemiologically of *E. coli*, the outcomes are severe. If the abdomen is distended, especially with focal right lower quadrant tenderness (this may be generalized) and bloody stools, this must be on the differential diagnosis. If EHEC is suspected, further testing is warranted and a higher level of care is likely necessary [44, 48].

There are five other forms of *E. coli* that produce enteric infection. Enterotoxic *E. coli* (ETEC) is the other relevant kind, as it is commonly known as traveler's diarrhea or Montezuma's revenge. This is associated with contaminated drinking water and is endemic to tropical environments. Generally, though self-limited, this can last for several days, and the athlete must be watched closely for clinical signs of worsening [44, 48].

Previously, *Clostridium difficile* (*C. difficile*) was almost explicitly a nosocomial infection. More recently, *C. difficile* has an increased incidence in the community setting and should be considered in the setting of recent antibiotic use. If *C. difficile* is on the differential, testing should be obtained using a stool antigen. Signs of systemic infection should be evaluated for, but if the athlete is not showing toxic signs, generally, the patient can be managed in an outpatient setting with metronidazole. For any acute diarrheal episode, hydration status is extremely important and should be monitored closely. With *C. difficile*, the use of anti-diarrheal medications, such as loperamide, are not recommended. These medications have the potential to slow the clearance of the bacterial toxin, which can lead to megacolon and potential perforation [44, 46, 48]. Return-to-play considerations should be made on a clinical basis. Adequate hydration status is a necessity as is control of the patient's nausea and diarrhea. The athlete should be improving and have recovered enough to be able to put forth the necessary effort to participate in an athletic competition.

Methicillin-Resistant *Staphylococcus aureus* (MRSA)

The athletic population has a very high incidence of methicillin-resistant *Staphylococcus aureus* (MRSA) infections. The collegiate population has almost twice the incidence for MRSA colonization as the general population [51]. Per Braun et al., the MRSA infection rate of the contact athletic population (football, wrestling) is roughly tenfold higher than the general population. If an athlete is colonized with MRSA, they have a seven times higher risk of developing MRSA-linked infections than non-colonized colleagues. Cellulitis and abscesses are generally the pathologic manifestations of MRSA infections. It should be noted that *Streptococcus* and methicillin-sensitive *Staphylococcus aureus* (MSSA) are also common causative agents. Cellulitis usually forms an erythematous patch that causes the skin to be firm. There is no fluctuance associated with cellulitis; in contrast, an abscess possesses discernable fluctuance. The treatment of choice for abscess is incision and drainage (I&D) if the lesion is large enough; if I&D is undertaken, wound culture should be obtained. Small lesions can be considered for treatment with warm compresses multiple times a day and close follow-up [50–52]. When considering treatment for cellulitis, the causative bacteria should be considered. This determination can be difficult, as often there is no clinical indicator to determine the correct bacteria [56]. If concomitant abscess is present, wound culture is helpful; however, skin culture is unreliable for cellulitis alone. For difficult infections to obtain a culture, intra-nasal swab can be helpful, as 82% of patients who developed bacteremia have identical strains that can be isolated from within the nares [57]. Empiric antibiotic treatment should be undertaken, and the risk factors for MRSA infection should be considered. Topical therapies can be helpful, but, unfortunately, there is increasing mupirocin resistance with recent epidemiologic data, putting resistance as high as 28%. Though mupirocin can be helpful in preventing spread from MRSA carriers within an athletic department, there are several oral antibiotics that are currently used for treatment of MRSA. The most commonly used outpatient antibiotics are trimethoprim-sulfamethoxazole (TMP–SMX) and clindamycin. It should be noted that there is increasing antibiotic resistance to these medications, and the local antibiotic resistance statistics should be known prior to prescription [53–56].

The only hard-and-fast rules for participation with cellulitis or abscess are in wrestling, though multiple medical colleges have proposed following those guidelines for other contact sports. If the lesions can be adequately covered, bandages changes regularly, and adequate hygiene undertaken, superficial infections without systemic signs generally do not cause athletes to miss time. In reference to abscesses after I&D, the wound should be packed and covered with the packing and bandage changed prior to and directly after participation in athletic events whether practice or game. If the athlete starts to develop systemic signs (fever, malaise, chest pain, shortness of breath, or altered mental status), then urgent referral should be made for a higher level of care [56–60].

There has been much debate in the literature about decolonization strategies for the prevention of spread, as the athletic population is particularly susceptible to the spread of MRSA and subsequent outbreaks of infections. While successful decolonization is highly effective in the short term, unfortunately the effect is transient and the risk of infection remains high. Mupirocin is often used for elimination of MRSA intra-nasally. However, the recolonization rate is greater than 50% at the 1-year mark, based on data by Reagan et al. and Doebblin et al. [60, 61]. It is still thought that the best prevention is through education strategies, adequate hygiene, and avoidance of actively draining wounds. There have been several studies showing that adequate handwashing can dramatically decrease MRSA transmission [58, 59]. Hygiene is a difficult subject, as new habits and responsible practices are challenging to implement. Limited resources within an athletic department often compound this already difficult situation. Multiple epidemiologic studies have shown that athletes will often share towels, razors, and other non-hygienic items. It is of utmost importance to educate all levels of participants on personal hygiene and ways to limit MRSA spread. It is imperative to identify and treat MRSA infections in a timely manner to limit risk to other participants (Fig. 19.4).

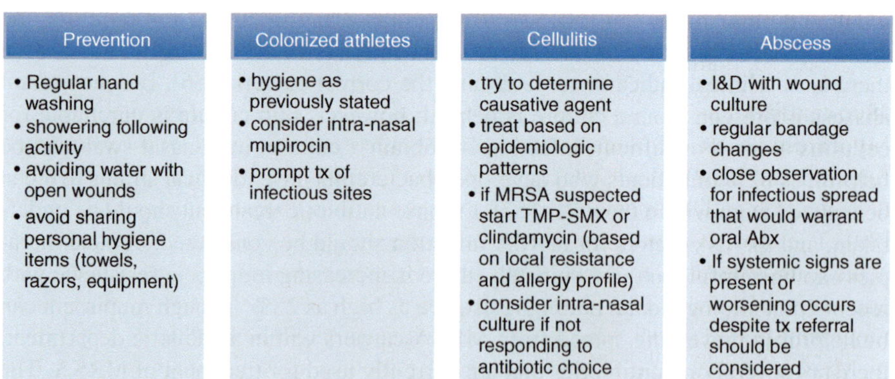

Fig. 19.4 Football specific MRSA treatment algorithm based on stages of infection

Conclusion

There are multiple ways that infectious diseases present challenges to the in-season team physician. Keeping an athlete on the field and participating at a high level is as much an art as it is a science. Therefore, each case should be treated uniquely. However, treatment guidelines when available should be followed for streamlined and effective medical treatment of each condition. Often, athletes can continue to train or participate with common infections of upper respiratory system, following the above-the-neck and no fever rule. Infections of the lower respiratory system and GI systems should be monitored closely and treated according to the clinical signs of the patient. It is important to identify early red flag symptoms, as this will likely change management prior to athletes worsening during travel situations or prior to game participation. Not only is it important for the health of the affected athlete to quickly identify infectious processes, it is important to the health of the entire team and opposing team. Prevention and limitation of spread should be the team physician's goal when dealing with athletes and the athletic training staff, who are often the primary contact for the affected athlete.

References

1. Nieman D. Risk of upper respiratory tract infection in athletes: an epidemiologic and immunologic perspective. J Athl Train. 1997;32:4; Social Science Premium Collection.
2. Malm C. Suspectibility to infections in elite atheletes: the S-curve. Scand J Med Sci Sports. 2006;16:4–6.
3. Dick N, Diehl J. Febrile illness in the athlete. Sports Health. 2014;6:3.
4. Ilback NG, Fohlman J, Friman G. Exercise in coxsackie B3 myocarditis: effects on heart lymphocyte subpopulations and the inflammatory reaction. Am Heart J. 1989;117:1298Y302.
5. Kendall EJ, Bynoe ML, Tyrell DA. Virus isolations from common colds occurring in a residential school. Br Med J. 1962;2(5297):82.
6. Page C, Diehl J. Upper respiratory infections in athletes. Clin Sports Med. 2007;26:345–59.
7. Scharhag J, Meyer T. Return to play after acute infectious disease in football players. J Sports Sci. 2014;32(13):1237–42.
8. Maron BJ, Epstein SE, Roberts WC. Causes of sudden death in the competitive athlete. J Am Coll Cardiol. 1986;7:204–14.
9. Piccirillo JF. Clinical practice. Acute bacterial sinusitis. NEJM. 2004;351:902–10.
10. Cooper RJ, Hoffman JR, Bartlett JG, et al. Principles of appropriate antibiotic use for acute pharyngitis in adults: background. Ann Intern Med. 2001;134:509.
11. Centor RM, Witherspoon JM, Dalton HP, et al. The diagnosis of strep throat in adults in the emergency room. Med Decis Making. 1981;1(3):239–46.
12. Lindbaek M, Hoiby EA, Lermark G, et al. Clinical symptoms and signs in sore throat patients with large colony variant [beta]-haemolytic streptococci groups C or G versus group A. Br J Gen Pract. 2005;55:615–9.
13. Thomas M, Del Mar C, Glaziou P. How effective are treatments other than antibiotics for acute sore throat? Br J Gen Pract. 2000;50:817–20. Search date 1999; primary sources Medline and Cochrane Controlled Trials Registry.
14. Gwaltney JM Jr, Scheld WM, Sande MA, Sydnor A. The microbial etiology and antimicrobial therapy of adults with acute community-acquired sinusitis: a fifteen-year experience at the University of Virginia and review of other selected studies. J Allergy Clin Immunol. 1992;90(3 pt 2):457–61.

15. Spence L, Brown W, Pyne D, et al. Incidence, etiology, and symptomatology of upper respiratory illness in elite athletes. Med Sci Sports Exerc. 2007;39(4):577–68.
16. Smoot MK, Hosey R. Pulmonary infections in the athlete. Curr Sports Med Rep. 2009;8(2):71.
17. Lanza DC, Kennedy DW. Adult rhinosinusitis defined. Otolaryngol Head Neck Surg. 1997;117(3 pt 2):S1–7.
18. Wilckens JH, Glorioso JE. Risk assessment and management of nonorthopaedic conditions; viral disease. In: DeLee JC, Drez D, Miller MD, editors. Orthopaedic sports medicine principles and practice. 2nd ed. Philadelphia: WB Saunders; 2002. p. 251–63.
19. Bisno AL. Acute pharyngitis. NEJM. 2001;344(3):205–11.
20. Kruse RJ, Cantor CL. Pulmonary and cardiac infections in athletes. CSM. 2007;26:361–82.
21. Kamali A, Holodniy M. Influenza treatment and prophylaxis with neuramidase inhibitors: a review. Infect Drug Resist. 2013;6:187.
22. Abramowicz M. Antiviral drugs for prophylaxis and treatment of influenza. Med Lett Drugs Ther. 2005;47:93–5.
23. Nicholson KG, Aoki FY, Osterhaus ADME, et al. Efficacy and safety of oseltamivir in treatment of acute influenza: a randomized controlled trial. Lancet. 2000;355:1845–50.
24. Gartner B, Meyer T. Vaccination in elite athletes. Sports Med. 2014;44:1361–76.
25. Crawford DH. Epstein-Barr virus. Principles and practices of clinical virology. 5th ed. 1994:109–24.
26. Papesch M, Watkins R. Epstein-Barr virus infectious mononucleosis. Clin Otolaryngol. 2001;26(1):3–8.
27. Maki DG, Reich RM. Infectious mononucleosis in the athlete. Diagnosis, complications, and management. Am J Sports Med. 1982;10(3):162–73.
28. MacKnight JM. Infectious mononucleosis: ensuring a safe return to sport. Phys Sportsmed. 2002;30(1):27–8.
29. Hoagland RJ. Infectious mononucleosis. Prim Care. 1975;2:295–307.
30. Luzuriaga K, Sullivan J. Infectious mononucleosis. NEJM. 2010;362:1993–2000.
31. Farley DR, Zietlow SP, Bannon MP, Farnell MB. Spontaneous rupture of the spleen due to infectious mononucleosis. Mayo Clin Proc. 1992;67:846–53.
32. Tamayo SG, Rickman LS, Mathews WC, Fullerton SC, Bartok AE, Warner JT, et al. Examiner dependence on physical diagnostic tests for the detection of splenomegaly: a prospective study with multiple observers. J Gen Intern Med. 1993;8(2):69–75.
33. Hosey RG, Quarles JD, Kriss VM, Mattacola CG. Spleen size in athletes - a comparison of BMI, gender, race, and past history of mononucleosis. Med Sci Sports Exerc. 2004;36(5):S-312.
34. Hosey RG, et al. US assessment of spleen size in collegiate athletes. BJSM. 2006;40:251–4.
35. Macfarlane J, Holmes W, Gard P, et al. Prospective study of the incidence, aetiology and outcome of adult lower respiratory tract illness in the community. Thorax. 2001;56(2):109–14.
36. Louie JK, Hacker JK, Gonzales R, et al. Characterization of viral agents causing acute respiratory infection in a San Francisco University Medical Center Clinic during the influenza season. Clin Infect Dis. 2005;41(6):822–8.
37. Smoot MK, Hosey RG. Pulmonary infections in the athlete. Curr Sports Med Rep. 2009;8(2):71–5.
38. Lorenc TM, Kernan MT. Lower respiratory infections and potential complications in athletes. Curr Sports Med Rep. 2006;5(2):80Y6.
39. Musher DM, Thorner AR. Community-acquried pneumonia. NEJM. 2014;371(17):1619–28.
40. Fine MJ, Auble TE, Yealy DM. A prediction rule to identifty low risk patients with community-acquired pneumonia. N Engl J Med. 1997;336:243–50.
41. Portiz MA, Blaschke AJ, Byington CL. FilmArray, an automated nested multiplex PCR system for multi-pathogen detection: development and application to respiratory tract infection. PLoS One. 2011;6:e26047.
42. Chartrand C, Leeflang MM, Minion J, Brewer T, Pai M. Accuracy of rapid influenza diagnostic tests: a meta analysis. Ann Intern Med. 2012;156:500–11.
43. Metlay JP, Fine MJ, Schulz R, et al. Measuring symptomatic and functional recovery in patients with community-acquired pneumonia. J Gen Intern Med. 1997;12(7):423Y30.

44. Karageanes SJ. Gastrointestinal infections in the athlete. Clin Sports Med. 2007;26:433–48.
45. Becker DM, Moe CL, Southwick KL, MacCormack JN. Transmisison of Norwalk virus during a football game. NEJM. 2000;343(17):1223–7.
46. Peterson CA, Calderon RL. Trends in enteric disease as a cause of death in the United States, 1989–1996. Am J Epidemiol. 2003;157:58–65.
47. Fankhauser RL, Noel JS, Monroe SS, Ando T, Glass RI. Molecular epidemiology of "Norwalk-like viruses" in outbreaks of gastroenteritis in the United States. J Infect Dis. 1998;178:1571–8.
48. Musher DM, Musher BL. Contagious acute gastrointestinal infections. N Engl J Med. 2004;351(23):24172427.
49. Adachi AA, Backer HD, DuPont HL. Infectious diarrhea from wilderness and foreign travel. In: Auerbach PS, editor. Wilderness medicine. 4th ed. St. Louis: Mosby; 2001. p. 1237–70.
50. Karanika S, et al. Colonization with MRSA and risk for infection among asymptomatic athe-letes: review and Metaanalysis. Clin Infect Dis. 2016;63:195–204.
51. Braun T, et al. Community associated MRSA infection rates and management among Student-Athletes. Med Sci Sports Exerc. 2018;50:1802–9.
52. Stevens DL, Bisno AL, Chambers HF, et al. Practice guidelines for the diagnosis and management of skin and soft tissue infections: 2–14 update by the Infectious Diseases Society of America. CID. 2014;59(15):e10–52.
53. Zinder SM, Basler RS, Foley J, Scarlata C, Vasily DB. National Athletic Trainers' Association position statement: skin diseases. J Athl Train. 2010;45(4):411–28.
54. Talan DA, Mower WR, Krishnadasan A, et al. Trimethoprim-sulfamethoxazole versus placebo for uncomplicated skin abscess. N Engl J Med. 2016;374(9):823–32.
55. Pate AJ, Terribilini RG, Ghobadi F, et al. Antibiotics for methicillin-resistant *Staphylococcus aureus* skin and soft tissue infections: the challenge of outpatient therapy. Am J Emerg Med. 2014;32(2):135–8.
56. Benjamin HJ, Nikore V, Takgishi J. Practical management: community-associated methicillin-resistant Staphyloccus aureus (CA-MRSA): the latest sports epidemic. Clin J Sport Med. 2007;17:393–7.
57. Von Eiff C, Becker K, Machka K, et al. Nasal carriage as a source of Staphylococcus aureus bacteremia. N Engl J Med. 2001;344:11–6.
58. Archibald LK, Shapiro J, Pass A, Rand K, Southwick F. Methicillinresistant Staphylococcus aureus infection in a college football team: risk factors outside the locker room and playing field. Infect Control Hosp Epidemiol. 2008;29(5):450–3.
59. Romano R, Lu D, Holtom P. Outbreak of community-acquired methicillin-resistant Staphylococcus aureus skin infections among a collegiate football team. J Athl Train. 2006;41(2):141–5.
60. Reagan DR, Doebbeling BN, Pfaller MA, et al. Elimination of coincident Staphylococcus aureus nasal and hand carriage with intranasal application of mupirocin calcium ointment. Ann Intern Med. 1991;114:101–6.
61. Doebbeling BN, Reagan DR, Pfaller MA, et al. Long-term efficacy of intranasal mupirocin ointment. A prospective cohort study of Staphylococcus aureus carriage. Arch Intern Med. 1994;154:1505–8.
62. Call SA, Vollenweider MA, Hornung CA. Does this patient have influenza? JAMA. 2005;293:987–97.

Chest and Abdominal Injuries in Football

20

R. Warne Fitch and Dwayne D'Souza

Chest Injuries

An important part of a team physician's responsibilities is the ability to understand, diagnose, and treat chest injuries. In addition, physicians must have a clear understanding of return-to-play guidelines after these injuries occur. Recognition of the mechanism of injury is key, as well as the ability to perform a quick assessment of airway, breathing, and circulation (ABCs), following Advanced Trauma Life Support (ATLS) guidelines. In the acute setting, it is critical to establish a patent airway and follow spine precautions if necessary. Next, the athlete's breathing and circulation should be assessed, and any life-threatening injuries should be both identified and immediately treated during the primary survey. Once ABCs have been stabilized, a secondary survey can be performed after exposing the athlete and doing a quick neurological exam and focused exam on the area of interest.

Most injuries that occur on the field consist of muscle strains and soft tissue contusions that require supportive care [1]. However, there are life-threatening conditions that occasionally occur such as tension pneumothorax, commotio cordis, fractures, and pulmonary contusions that require further evaluation and treatment in an emergent fashion. A thorough exam of the chest, at a minimum, requires exposure of the chest wall by removing shoulder pads, palpation of the injured area to look for deformity or crepitus, and auscultation of the heart and lungs, checking for diminished breath sounds or new murmurs. On the field, resources such as advanced imaging and diagnostic workups are limited. Therefore, players should be transferred to a higher level of care if these injuries are suspected, based on mechanism

R. W. Fitch (✉)
Department of Emergency Medicine and Department of Orthopaedic Surgery and Rehabilitation, Vanderbilt University, Nashville, TN, USA
e-mail: robert.fitch@vumc.org

D. D'Souza
Department of Emergency Medicine, Vanderbilt University, Nashville, TN, USA

K. W. Farmer (ed.), *Football Injuries*,
https://doi.org/10.1007/978-3-030-54875-9_20

of injury, physical exam, and vital signs. Although chest injuries in football are rare, these injuries do carry significant delays in return to play, with less than 50% of athletes returning to play in 1 week [2]. High-risk injuries that require further acute evaluation are highlighted next.

Rib Fracture/Sternum Fracture

Most rib and sternum fractures are due to a direct blow to the thorax from a helmet, shoulder pads, or the ground when a player has arms flexed above shoulder level. Rib fractures occur more frequently on the lateral aspects of the chest wall due to positioning and exposure during tackling. The injured athlete will usually complain of chest pain during respiration or will have point tenderness on direct palpation over the injured area. Skin crepitus may be palpated as well. One exam maneuver that can indicate an underlying rib fracture is compressing the sternum and the posterior spine with the palms of the examiner's hands. If positive, the athlete will usually complain of lateral rib pain. In order to fully evaluate for rib and sternum fractures, multiple imaging modalities can be used. Chest X-rays can be diagnostic (Fig. 20.1). Furthermore, ultrasound can be utilized to evaluate for cortical defects, pneumothorax, or pulmonary contusion. If both X-ray and ultrasound are negative but a high clinical suspicion remains, a CT scan should be utilized due to its higher sensitivity for detecting sternum and rib fractures [3, 4]. Additional injuries such as pneumothorax, pulmonary contusion, and spleen or liver lacerations should be considered and ruled out.

Treatment consists of supportive care with acetaminophen, nonsteroidal anti-inflammatory drugs (NSAIDs), nerve blocks, splint tape, or protective pads over the

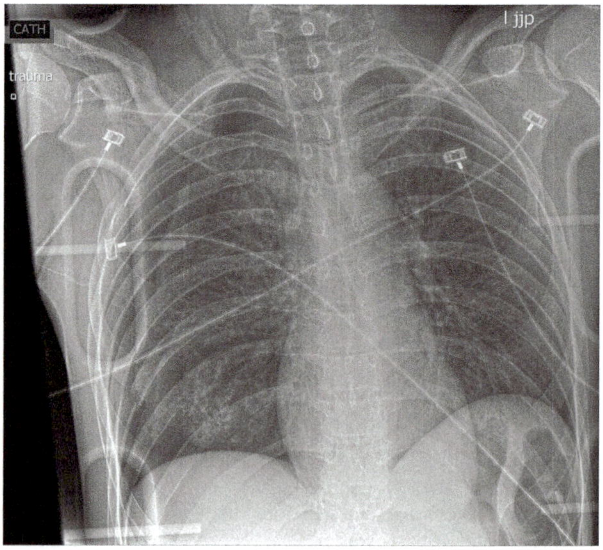

Fig. 20.1 Chest radiograph demonstrating right-sided rib fractures with pneumothorax

injured ribs. Most fractures heal on their own; however, in cases where patients have prolonged pain, underlying injuries, or compromised cardiac or pulmonary function, operative stabilization of the fracture may be indicated. Depending on extent of injury, contact activity should be limited during the initial recovery phase for about 2 to 3 weeks. Some athletes will benefit from a rib protector for 6 to 8 weeks after injury [5].

Sternoclavicular Joint Dislocation

Sternoclavicular (SC) joint dislocations are rare and usually the result of a direct blow to the anterior chest wall or from a fall on the lateral aspect of the shoulder. A recent study showed that SC joint dislocations occur in about 5% of shoulder injuries [6]. The two main types of dislocations are anterior and posterior, with anterior dislocations being more common. However, a posterior SC dislocation leads to more complications due to compression of the mediastinum. Posterior dislocations can potentially cause lung, cardiac, tracheal, aortic, or esophageal injuries, depending on degree of displacement. On exam, patients tend to have deformity, swelling, bruising, and pain on direct palpation of the SC joint. They can also have referred pain to the SC joint when the glenohumeral joint is manipulated. Advanced imaging is necessary to make the diagnosis and a special X-ray view called the serendipity view AP X-ray can be utilized (Fig. 20.2). Ultimately, computed tomography (CT) scan is the gold standard for diagnosis.

Anterior dislocations can usually be reduced (uncommon) or left in-situ and then treated conservatively without a need for surgery. The rare posterior dislocation should not be reduced in a low-resource setting. Instead, the athlete should be taken to the operating room for open versus closed reduction by an orthopedic surgeon, and a thoracic surgeon should be available for backup in the unlikely event that removing pressure from the mediastinum causes acute decompensation. Athletes may return to play without restrictions in 4 to 6 weeks after reduction, but this varies greatly based on symptoms. Prior to return to full participation, the athlete should be asymptomatic and have no instability [5]. If either occurs, further workup is necessary, and stabilization of the SC joint may be indicated.

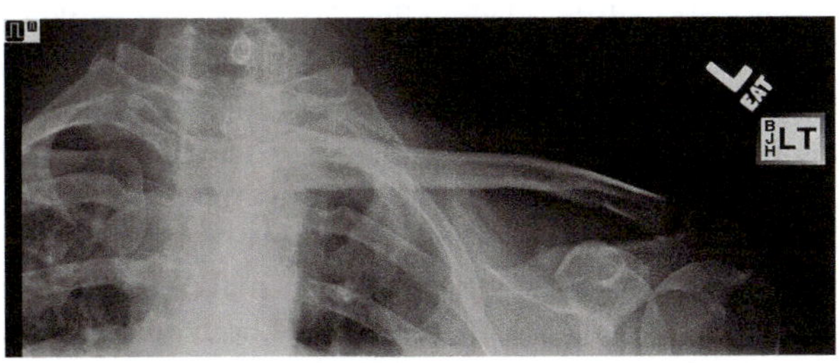

Fig. 20.2 Serendipity view demonstrating a left sternoclavicular dislocation

Pulmonary Contusion

Pulmonary contusions may occur as a result of blunt trauma to the chest. These injuries are rare, given the protective equipment worn by football players; however, like rib fractures, pulmonary contusions can occur. Younger athletes are more susceptible to this injury pattern since their ribs are more pliable and tend to fracture less. Therefore, the force from a direct hit to the chest is transferred to the lungs underneath the rib cage [7, 8]. Clinical presentation and exam can be variable, and the diagnosis requires a high degree of suspicion on the provider's part. Some presentations are delayed as edema increases in the damaged lung. Athletes may complain of shortness of breath, hemoptysis, tachypnea, or pleurisy. Athletes can even be hypoxic or splint when taking deep breaths secondary to pain. Exam may have crackles or slight wheezing on auscultation, but more commonly, the exam is completely normal [1]. Chest X-ray, ultrasound, and CT imaging can be used to confirm the diagnosis. X-ray and ultrasound findings may take 4 to 48 hours to show infiltrate or edema as the damaged lung is starting to heal. CT scan is currently the gold standard for pulmonary contusions, as it shows the pulmonary contusion early and in more detail [9]. (Figs. 20.3a, b).

Treatment for this injury is supportive, with pain control being the primary objective. It is important to make sure the athlete does not have an underlying pneumothorax during an evaluation for a pulmonary contusion. In acute cases, supplemental oxygen can be used as needed. For most individuals, the symptoms resolve within 1 to 2 weeks, and repeat chest X-ray can be used to track resolution of the pulmonary contusion [5, 8, 10].

Pneumothorax/Tension Pneumothorax

A pneumothorax is the result of air becoming trapped in between the chest wall and the pleura of the lung. There are multiple causes, but athletes are more likely to develop them spontaneously or due to direct blunt injury to the chest wall. A tall, thin male is more susceptible to a spontaneous apical pneumothorax from running, weight lifting, or forceful coughing [11]. A traumatic pneumothorax can be associated with rib fractures, as the fractured fragments cause separation between the chest wall and the pleura (Fig. 20.1). A pneumothorax that develops via tension physiology is called a tension pneumothorax, and this type of pneumothorax is immediately life threatening. In this condition, a one-way air-leak develops in the thoracic cavity, and air becomes trapped compressing the mediastinum. If the pressure increases greater than the venous return to the heart, athletes can suffer acute cardiopulmonary arrest if the injury is not dealt with immediately [12]. A high degree of suspicion is necessary to make the diagnosis as athletes present with shortness of breath and occasional chest pain. On exam, the provider may find decreased breath sounds on the side of the pneumothorax. Physical exam alone can miss a pneumothorax. Individuals with a tension pneumothorax will present in severe respiratory and cardiac distress. These individuals tend to be uncomfortable

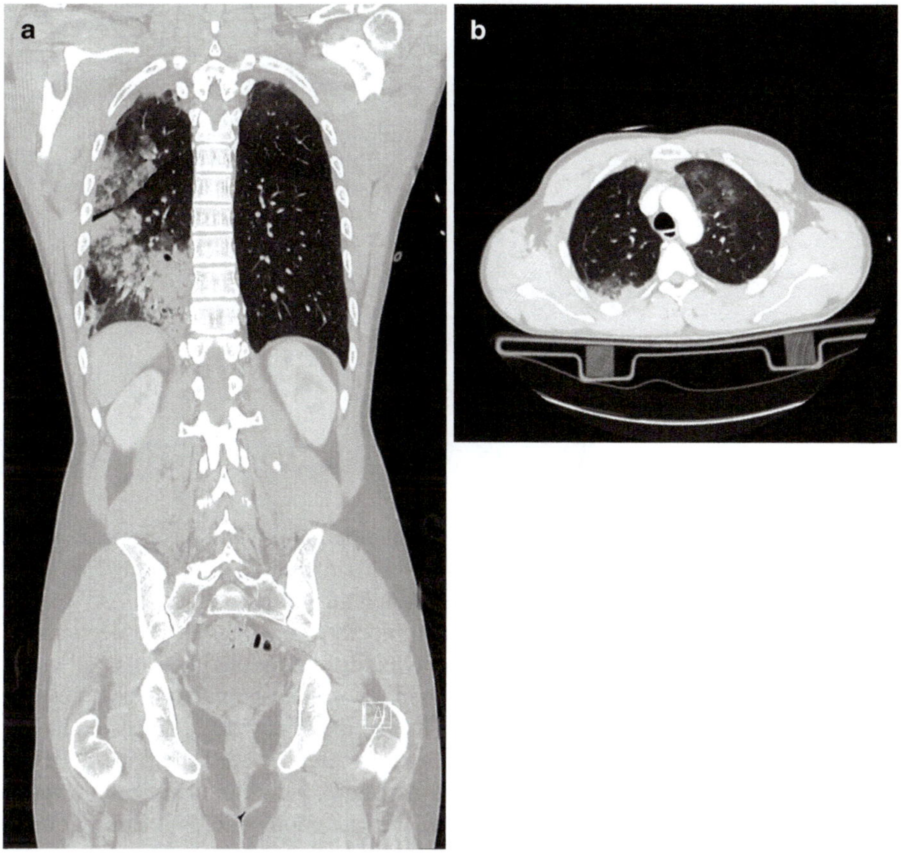

Fig. 20.3 (**a**) Coronal CT scan demonstrating a right-sided pulmonary contusion, (**b**) Axial CT scan demonstrating right- and left-sided pulmonary contusions

with unstable vital signs. In addition, they may have absent lung sounds, hypoxia, hypotension, tachypnea, tachycardia, distended neck veins, and, possibly, tracheal deviation away from the injured lung. If suspicion is high for a tension pneumothorax, emergent treatment should be performed and not delayed for imaging. Point-of-care ultrasound used on the field or in the training room is becoming more common, as it has higher sensitivities and specificities compared to chest X-ray and can be done immediately [13, 14]. Chest X-ray can be used and should be checked for deviation of the mediastinum in tension physiology or for lung markings that do not extend all the way to the chest wall (Fig. 20.4). Ultimately, CT scan is the gold standard to diagnose a pneumothorax if other modalities do not show evidence and the diagnosis is uncertain.

Treatment depends on the size of the pneumothorax and the stability of the patient. If the pneumothorax involves <20% of the lung, athletes can be given supplemental oxygen and observed. Repeat chest X-ray should be performed to make

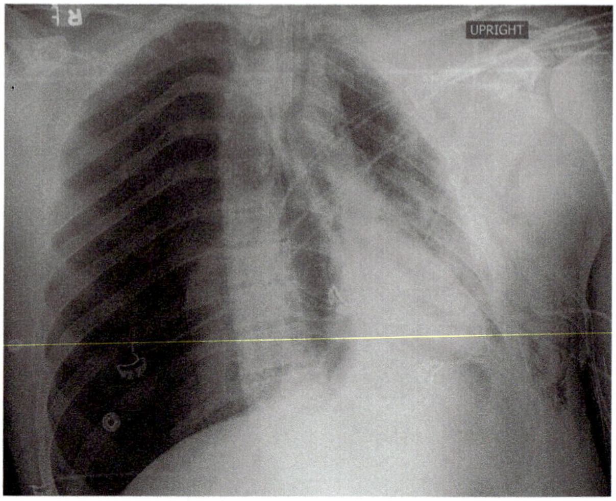

Fig. 20.4 Chest radiograph demonstrating a right-sided tension pneumothorax

sure the pneumothorax is not expanding. Supplemental oxygen has been shown to increase the rate of absorption of the pneumothorax to around 4% per day compared to 1.25% per day in patients not receiving supplemental oxygen [15]. Any patient suspected of having a tension pneumothorax needs immediate needle decompression of the second intercostal space, midclavicular line on the injured side, and/or immediate chest tube placement at the fifth intercostal space midaxillary line [12]. These patients require immediate transfer to an emergency department for further evaluation. All athletes should refrain from return to play until the pneumothorax has completely resolved on chest X-ray. Furthermore, they should not be allowed to fly for 2 weeks after complete resolution of the pneumothorax, as it can redevelop due to acute changes in pressure [16].

Commotio Cordis

Commotio Cordis is Latin for "agitation of the heart" and is defined as sudden cardiac death secondary to chest wall impact. The exact incidence is difficult to ascertain, but some studies believe it to be the second leading cause of death in young athletes after hypertrophic cardiomyopathy [17]. Even though these injuries appear to be due to traumatic injury, many experts believe commotio cordis is mainly due to an electrical event with ventricular fibrillation, occurring immediately on chest wall impact. Therefore, multiple variables, including velocity of impact, location of impact (over the cardiac silhouette), and timing of impact during the cardiac electrical cycle are believed to play a role [18, 19]. Athlete presentation is immediately after impact, and most athletes will be unresponsive in cardiopulmonary arrest with no pulse. Diagnosis is presumptive, based on the above factors, and treatment should begin immediately following ATLS guidelines and focusing on airway, breathing, and circulation. In the past, outcomes were much poorer; however, with more awareness, bystander cardiopulmonary resuscitation (CPR), and use of the automatic external defibrillators with early defibrillation, there have been more successful resuscitations recently [12, 18]. Patients should be transferred to the nearest emergency department, and survivors should undergo electrocardiogram (EKG), cardiac ultrasound, cardiac magnetic resonance imaging (MRI), and exercise stress testing [20]. Per the American Heart Association and the American College of Cardiology, athletes who have survived commotio cordis can resume training and competition if they have a completely negative workup after being evaluated by a cardiologist.

Abdominal Injuries

While the overall incidence of abdominal injuries due to sports participation is rare, it does account for 10% of all abdominal injuries presenting to emergency departments, second only to car accidents [21]. A study using the National Pediatric Trauma Registry reviewed injuries related to contact sports over a 10-year period of time and found that the spleen (50%) was the most common organ injured followed by kidney (22%), liver (6.8%), pancreas (5.8), and testis (0.5). American football was the most common sport associated with abdominal injury, with 49.7% of all sports-related abdominal injuries occurring in football athletes [22]. In a review of the emergency department presentation of American football injuries, Smart et al. found internal injuries only accounted for 0.25% of all football injuries, but accounted for the longest hospital stay (3.4 days) [23]. The lower ribs provide limited protection, and mandatory protective equipment in football leaves the abdomen largely unprotected from injury. Injuries can occur from direct trauma from falls and collisions, as well as from contact at high velocity. These injuries are infrequent; however, life-threatening emergencies can occur, so rapid assessment and treatment are critical to ensure a positive outcome. Sideline assessment and management should be focused on the potential diagnosis and rapid stabilization. Prompt transportation to the emergency department for advanced imaging and definitive treatment should be a priority. These injuries can rapidly deteriorate and be life threatening. While most team physicians will not provide definitive care to the athletes with these injuries, team physicians must be familiar with the recognition, workup, treatment, and return-to-play criteria for common abdominal and genitourinary injuries that may be encountered on the football field.

Solar Plexus Injuries

A solar plexus injury, also known as "getting the wind knocked out," is the most common abdominal injury in contact and collision sports. This can occur from a direct blow to the midepigastrium or back that irritates the celiac plexus, resulting in diaphragmatic spasm. Athletes may complain of mild abdominal pain with difficulty catching their breath, though minimal abdominal pain will be detected upon palpation of the abdomen. These symptoms are transient, lasting seconds to a couple of minutes and may improve with knee and hip flexion. Athletes can return to play once symptoms and exam normalize. Persistent abdominal pain and symptoms require prompt workup for additional internal injury, and athletes should be withheld from play until completely asymptomatic.

Rectus Sheath Hematoma

A rectus sheath hematoma is caused by a direct blow to the anterior abdominal wall, which results in bleeding from injury to the epigastric vein or artery into the rectus abdominis sheath. Patients will present with persistent and often worsening abdominal wall tenderness with bruising noted over the rectus abdominis musculature. Examination of the abdomen will reveal ecchymosis localized within the rectus musculature, and pain should be limited to this area as well. The athlete will have pain with flexion of the abdominal muscles, but he/she should not have pain on palpation elsewhere in the abdomen (Carnett's Sign) and should not have peritoneal signs [24]. Ultrasound can be useful on the sideline or in the training room to assess the hematoma; however, CT scan imaging remains the gold standard imaging modality of choice and can show additional injuries [25] (Fig. 20.5). Most rectus sheath hematomas will self-tamponade with ice, rest, and gentle compression. Surgical evacuation and ligation of the involved vessels is rarely required. Athletes with rectus sheath hematomas should be withheld from play until pain and symptoms have resolved. Protective padding should be used to minimize repeat injury to the area.

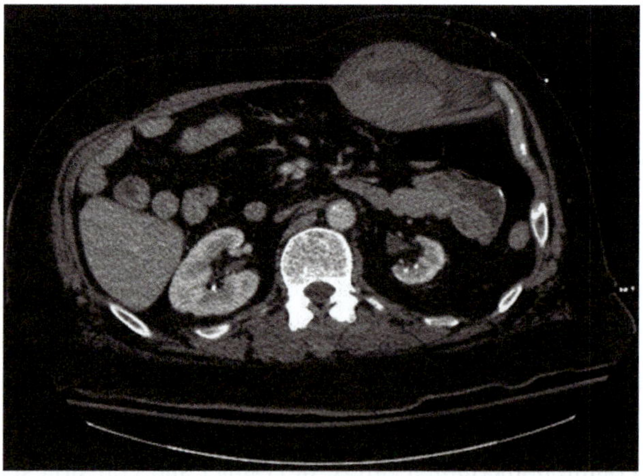

Fig. 20.5 Axial CT demonstrating a left rectus-sheath hematoma

Spleen Injuries

The spleen is the most commonly injured abdominal organ during sports due to blunt trauma [22]. The spleen has some protection from the ninth through 11th ribs in adults, while in children the spleen is only partially covered. Athletes with splenomegaly due to mononucleosis may be at an increased risk for injury, as both spontaneous and traumatic ruptures have been reported in this population [26] (see Chap. 20). Patients will typically present with abdominal pain localized to the left upper quadrant with abdominal tenderness with rebound and guarding on exam. Some patients may have referred left shoulder pain from diaphragmatic irritation (Kehr's sign). Serial abdominal exams should be routinely performed if the clinician suspects a spleen injury since early symptoms may be mild. Hypotension and tachycardia may be present, but they typically occur later. The use of ultrasound on the sideline and in the training room can be helpful if available. The focused assessment with sonography in trauma (FAST) exam can be used to detect hemoperitoneum related to a splenic laceration. Normal initial studies do not exclude a spleen injury, so repeat exams should be performed since sensitivity increases with serial exams. A negative FAST exam does not exclude a spleen injury; therefore, rapid transportation to the emergency department is still indicated in patients with persistent abdominal pain. An abdominal CT scan remains the imaging study of choice and is used to grade the severity of the injury on a scale of 1–5 (Fig. 20.6). All patients with splenic injuries should be admitted to the hospital for observation and management. Length of stay varies on symptoms but is typically 1 day longer than the grade of injury [27]. Surgical intervention is based on hemodynamic instability and should be considered in higher-grade injuries. While non-operative management is preferred, risk of delayed rupture can occur in up to 6% of cases [28]. Healing rates vary, based on the grade of injury, with higher-grade injuries taking longer. Serial ultrasound and CT scans are not typically recommended to follow healing progression. Most splenic injuries recover in 3–4 months, and decisions

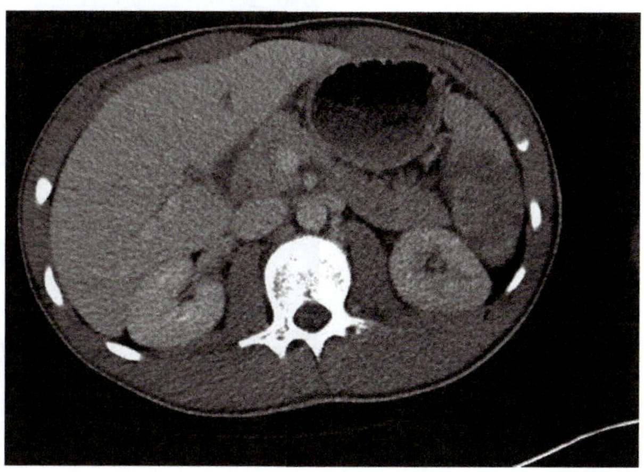

Fig. 20.6 Axial CT demonstrating a spleen laceration

regarding return to play and activity should be discussed jointly with the treating trauma surgeon [29–32]. Athletes who undergo splenectomy must receive vaccinations for encapsulated organisms, including *Haemophilus influenza*, *Neisseria*, and *Pneumococcus*.

Liver Injuries

Liver injuries can occur with a direct blow to the abdomen, causing a crush-type injury, as well as from rapid deceleration causing lacerations to the thin capsule and attached parenchyma. Patients will present with abdominal pain localized to the right upper quadrant, often with referred pain to the right shoulder (Kehr's sign). Serial abdominal exams should be performed, and the presence of persistent or worsening abdominal pain or any rebound, guarding, or peritoneal signs warrants a transfer to the emergency department for CT scan imaging. Vital signs have been reported to be normal initially in 50% of patients with liver injuries, while tachycardia and hypotension are late, ominous findings [33]. The FAST exam can be used to assess for hemoperitoneum with 85% sensitivity, though CT scan imaging remains the gold standard in assessing liver injuries [34] (Fig. 20.7).

Liver injuries are graded 1 through 5, based on severity. While this system can be helpful in classifying injuries, it is not used to guide therapy. Many liver injuries can be treated non-operatively, and surgical management should be based on hemodynamic instability and case-by-case clinical situations. Non-operative management is common and successful in 94% of hemodynamically stable patients [35, 36]. Healing rates of liver injuries vary, depending on grade and severity with most taking 3 to 6 months to fully recover. Serial CT and ultrasound scans have been used to

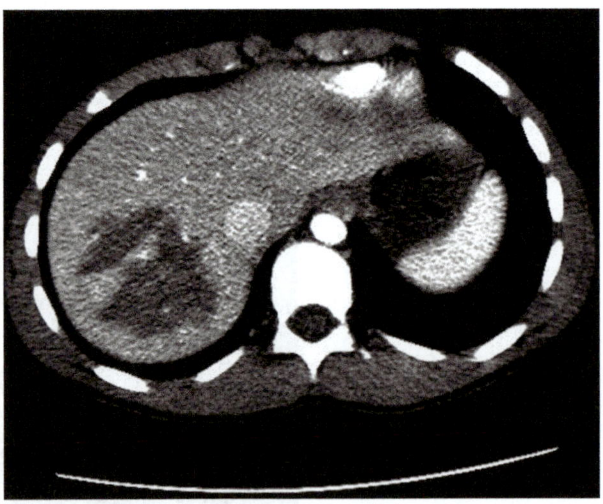

Fig. 20.7 Axial CT demonstrating a liver laceration

follow injury healing; however, these studies are not routinely recommended unless clinically indicated [33, 37–39]. Most athletes can return to light aerobic activity by 3 months and return to contact at 5 to 6 months. Athletes should have normalization of their liver function studies, and return to sport should be made in conjunction with the treating trauma surgeon.

Kidney Injuries

Kidney is the second most commonly injured abdominal organ in sports. Most kidney injuries occur from direct trauma to the back or flank and may be associated with rib or spinous process fractures. Athletes with kidney injuries may complain of back or flank pain with or without associated bruising and tenderness on palpation. Hematuria is present in 98% of kidney injuries, and team physicians suspicious for an injury should obtain a urinalysis [40, 41]. On-field and training room assessment should include vital signs and assessment of other injuries. A FAST scan can be helpful in assessing blood around the kidney; however, as with other abdominal injuries, CT scan imaging is the study of choice (Fig. 20.8). Kidney injuries are graded 1–5 based on severity. Lower-grade injuries can be successfully treated non-operatively. Most injuries typically heal within 6 to 8 weeks. Athletes should have resolution of hematuria prior to return to play, and it is encouraged that urology be involved with final clearance to return to contact sports [42]. Athletes with a solitary kidney or kidney dysfunction should be warned about the risks of returning to a contact or collision sport, and appropriate padding and flap jackets should be used [42, 43].

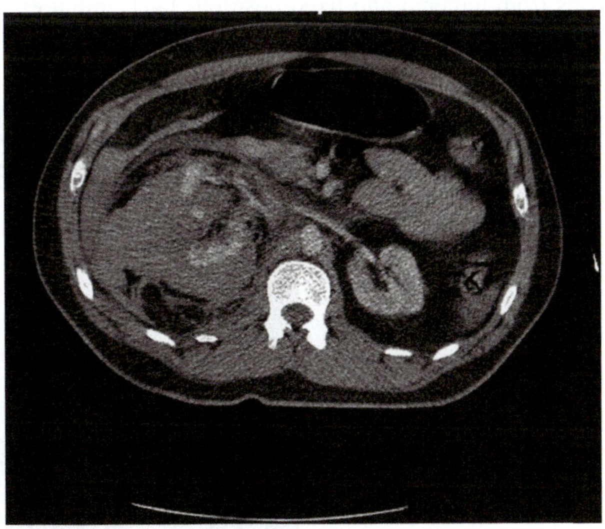

Fig. 20.8 Axial CT demonstrating a right kidney laceration

Pancreas Injuries

Pancreatic injuries are rare in sports, comprising <5% of solid organ abdominal injuries. While these injuries are rare, they are associated with high morbidity and mortality. Blunt abdominal trauma is the classic mechanism of injury with the pancreas body levered across the vertebral spinous body. Patients will present complaining of abdominal pain, although tenderness noted on abdominal exam and onset of symptoms may be minimal and delayed as the pancreas sits retroperitoneal. Rebound and guarding on exam may be noted <10% of the time [44]. FAST exam is not beneficial, and CT scan imaging of the abdomen and pelvis is the study of choice (Fig, 20.9). Unfortunately, initial CT scan imaging may miss pancreatic injuries, with one study showing a sensitivity of only 71% [44]. Serum amylase and lipase levels should be checked and are elevated in 89% of cases [45]. If clinically indicated and symptoms persist, repeat CT scan imaging should be encouraged [46]. Treatment options vary depending on the location and severity of the pancreatic injury. Return-to-play options and timing have not been well established in the literature and should be made in conjunction with the treating trauma physician.

Bowel Injuries

Hollow viscous injuries are rare in sports and account for only 1.1% of sports-related abdominal injuries, with small intestine injuries being more common than large intestine injuries [22]. Blunt abdominal trauma can result in a crush injury between the spine and a rigid object, closed loop of bowel bursts, and shearing injuries from tethered and fixed positions [47]. Initial exam findings may be minimal with mild abdominal pain on exam; however, serial exams will show eventual

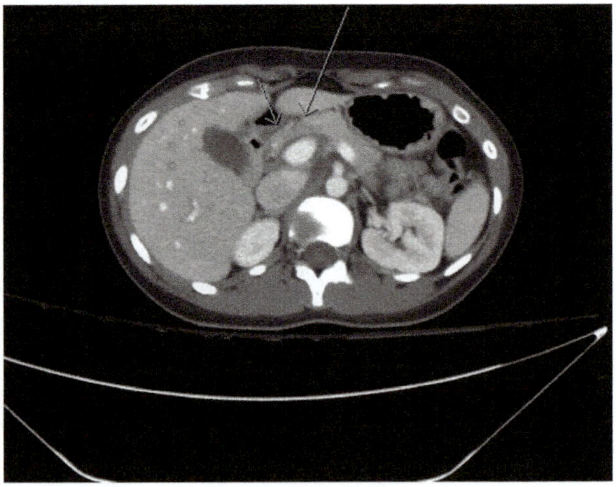

Fig. 20.9 Axial CT scan demonstrating a pancreatic neck laceration

peritoneal signs with associated nausea, tachycardia, rebound, or guarding, while hypotension with fever occurs late. Labs will show an elevated white blood cell count, while X-ray and CT scan imaging will show free air and free fluid (Fig. 20.10). Patients with bowel injuries require admission to the hospital with intravenous (IV) antibiotics and surgical management. Delays in diagnosis and management may be associated with higher morbidity and mortality. Return-to-play criteria are case based, but most athletes following bowel surgery are able to return to sport within 6 weeks.

Testicular Injuries

Scrotal and testicular injuries are rare in sports accounting for <1% of all sports-related injuries. Most occur as a result of blunt trauma to the groin. Athletes will present with scrotal and testicular pain, swelling, and possibly ecchymosis. Labs may show hematuria. Any athlete suffering from testicular trauma with swelling and ecchymosis should undergo an emergent testicular ultrasound with Doppler to assess for testicular rupture, blood flow abnormalities, and scrotal hematomas. Early surgical intervention can help preserve the testis. Prompt recognition with an emergent ultrasound and emergent surgical exploration and stabilization are important for a successful treatment [48–50]. Athletes may be cleared to play within 2 to 4 weeks after surgical intervention. Athletes with a solitary testicle may return to sport but should be cautioned regarding future fertility in the event of another injury, and should be encouraged to use protective athletic cups.

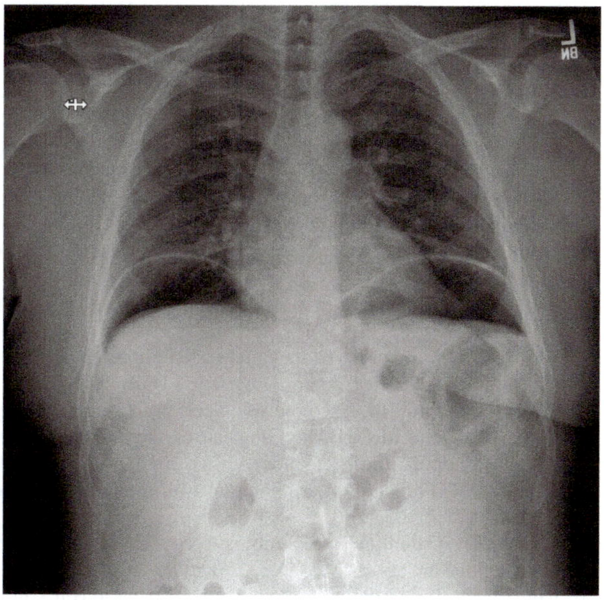

Fig. 20.10 Chest radiograph demonstrating free air under the diaphragm

References

1. Phillips NR, Kunz DE. Chest trauma in athletic medicine. Curr Sports Med Rep. 2018;17:90–6.
2. Johnson BK, Comsock RD. Epidemiology of chest, rib thoracic spine, and abdomen injuries among United States high school athletes, 2005/2006 to 2013/2014. Clin J Sport Med. 2017;27:388–93.
3. Chan SS. Emergency bedside ultrasound for the diagnosis of rib fractures. Am J Emerg Med. 2009;27:617–20.
4. Turk F, Kurt AB, Saglam S. Evaluation by ultrasound of traumatic rib fractures missed by radiography. Emerg Radiol. 2010;17:473–7.
5. Thomas RD, De Luigi AJ. Chest trauma in athletes. Curr Sports Med Rep. 2018;17:251–3.
6. Chaudhry S. Pediatric posterior sternoclavicular joint injuries. J Am Acad Orthop Surg. 2015;23:468–75.
7. Meese MA, Wayne JS. Pulmonary contusion secondary to blunt trauma in collegiate football player. Clin J Sport Med. 1997;7:309–10.
8. Lively MW, Stone D. Pulmonary contusion in football players. Clin J Sport Med. 2006;16:177–8.
9. Trupka A, Waydhas C, Hallfeldt KK, et al. Value of thoracic computed tomography in the first assessment of severely injured patients with blunt chest trauma: results of a prospective study. J Trauma. 1997;43:405–11.
10. Feden JP. Closed lung trauma. Clin Sports Med. 2013;32:255–65.
11. Partridge RA, Coley A, Boeie R, Woolard RH. Sports related pneumothorax. Ann Emerg Med. 1997;30:539–41.
12. Advanced Trauma Life Support, Ninth edition. 2013.
13. Sharma A, Jindal P. Principles of diagnosis and management of traumatic pneumothorax. J Emerg Trauma Shock. 2008;1:34–41.
14. Ianniello S, Di Giacoma V, Sessa B, Miele V. First line sonographic diagnosis of pneumothorax in major trauma: accuracy of e-FAST and comparison with multi-detector computed tomography. Radiol Med. 2014;119:674–80.
15. Chadha TS, Cohn MA. Non invasive treatment of pneumothorax with oxygen inhalation. Respiration. 1983;44:147.
16. Aerospace Medical Association Medical Guidelines Task Force. Medical guideline s for airline travel, 2nd edition. Aviat Space Environ Med. 2003;74(Suppl 5):A1–19.
17. Maron B. Sudden death in young athletes. N Engl J Med. 2003;349:1064–75.
18. Maron B, Mark Estes IIINA. Commotio Cordis. N Engl J Med. 2010;362:917–27.
19. Link MS. Commotio cordis: ventricular fibrillation triggered by chest impact-induced abnormalities in repolarization. Circ Arrhythm Electrophysiol. 2012;5(2):425–32.
20. Eligibility and Disqualification Recommendations for Competitive Athletes With Cardiovascular Abnormalities: Task Force 13: Commotio Cordis: A Scientific Statement From the American Heart Association and American College of Cardiology. Circulation 2015, 132(22):339–342.
21. Bergqvist D, Hedelin H, et al. Abdominal trauma during thirty years: analysis of a large case series. Injury. 1981;13:93–9.
22. Wan J, Corvino T, et al. Kidney and testicle injuries in team and individual sports: data from the National Pediatricc Trauma Registry. J Urol. 2003;170(4):1528–32.
23. Smart BJ, Haring RS, Asemota AO, Scott JW, Canner JS, Nejim BJ, George BP, Alsulaim H, Kirsch TD, Schneider EB. Tackling causes and costs of ED presentation for American football injuries: a population-level study. AJEM. 2016;34(7):1198–204.
24. Thomson H, Francis DM. Abdominal wall tenderness: a useful sign in the acute abdomen. Lancet. 1977;2:1053–4.
25. Johnson R. Abdominal wall injuries: rectus abdominis strains, oblique strains, rectus sheath hematoma. Curr Sports Med Rep. 2006;5:99–103.
26. Kindernecht JJ. Infectious mononucleosis and the spleen. Curr sports Med Rep. 2002;1:116–20.

27. Gaines BA. Intra-abdominal solid organ injury in children: diagnosis and treatment. J Trauma. 2009;67:135–8.
28. Cocanour CS, Moore FA, Ware DN, et al. Delayed complications of non-operative management of blunt adult splenic trauma. Arch Surg. 1998;133:619–24.
29. Pearl RH. Splenic injury: a 5 year update with improved results and changing criteria for conservative management. J Ped Surg. 1989;24:428–31.
30. Savage SA. The evolution of blunt splenic injury: resolution and progression. J Trauma. 2008;64:1085–92.
31. Pranikoff T, Hirschl RB. Resolution of splenic injury after nonoperative management. J Pediatric Surg. 1994;29:1366–9.
32. Lynch JM, Meza MP, Newman B, Gardner MJ, Albanese CT. Computed tomography grade of splenic injury is predictive of the time required for radiographic healing. J Ped Surg. 1997;32:1093–5.
33. Juyia RF, Kerr HA. Return to play after liver and spleen trauma. Sports Health. 2014;6(3):239–45.
34. McKenney MG, Martin L, et al. 1000 consecutive ultrasounds for blunt abdominal trauma. J Trauma. 1996;40(4):607–12.
35. Rifat SF, Gilfydis RP. Blunt abdominal trauma in sports. Curr Sprts Med Rep. 2003;2:93–7.
36. Pachter HL. The current status of nonoperative management of adult blunt hepatic injuries. Am J Surg. 1995;169:442–54.
37. Karp MP. The nonoperative management of pediatric hepatic trauma. J Pediatric Surg. 1983;18(4):512–8.
38. Tiberio GA. Evaluation of the healing time of non-operatively managed liver injuries. Hepato-Gastroenterology. 2008;55:1010–2.
39. Ray R, Lemire J. Liver laceration in an intercollegiate football player. J Athl Training. 1995;30:324–6.
40. Diamond DL. Sports related abdominal trauma. CJSM. 1989;8:91–9.
41. Miller KS, McAninch JW. Radiographic assessment of renal trauma: our 15 year experience. J Urol. 1995;154:352–5.
42. McAleer MJ. Renal and testis injuries in team sports. J Urol. 2002;168:1805–7.
43. Papagiannopoulos D, Gong E. Revisiting sports precautions in children with solitary kidneys and congenital anomalies of the kidney and urinary tract. Urology. 2016;101:9–14.
44. Bradley EL, Young PR, et al. Diagnosis and initial management of blunt pancreatic trauma. Guidelines from a multi-institutional review. Ann Surg. 227(6):861–9.
45. Echlin K. Pancreatic injury in the athlete. Curr Sports Med Rep. 2005;4:96–101.
46. Zaydfudim V, Cotton BA, Kim BD. Pancreatic transection after sports injury. J Trauma. 2010;69(4):33.
47. Hughes TM, Elton C. The pathophysiology and management of bowel and mesenteric injuries due to blunt trauma. Injury. 2002;33:295–302.
48. Wang Z, Yang JR, et al. Diagnosis and management of testicular rupture after blunt scrotal trauma: a literature review. Int Urol Nephrol. 2016;48:1967–76.
49. Freehill MT, Gorbachinsky I, Lavender JD, et al. Presumed testicular rupture during a college baseball game. Sport Health. 2015;7(2):177–80.
50. Chen AW, Archbold CS, Huthchinson M, Domb B. Sideline management of non musculoskeletal injuries by the orthopedic team physician. J AAOS. 2018;27(4):1–10.

Pain Management in Football

21

Robert G. Hosey, Kyle Smoot, and Srikanth Nithyanandam

Introduction

"No pain, no gain" is an exercise motto every coach and athlete has utilized to stay motivated through the challenges of athletic training and participation. In a contact sport like football, pain is inevitable. Studies have shown that there is pain hyposensitivity among athletes when compared to nonathletes, an inherited and developed trait from sports participation [1, 2]. Pain management in the sports training and competition environment can be a challenging issue to differentiate and potentially treat for clinicians, given the "no pain, no gain" culture of American football.

Pain is defined as an "unpleasant sensory and emotional experience associated with actual or potential tissue damage or described in terms of such damage" [3]. Pain is classified into various types that includes nociceptive pain, neuropathic pain, nociplastic/algopathic/nocipathic pain, and pain of unknown origin [3, 4].

Nociceptive Pain

Nociceptors are a specialized sense of receptors that communicate pain to our central nervous system (CNS). Tissue damage from a sport results in a cascade of events that results in sensitization of the nociceptors, causing the aversive discomfort for the athlete that can result in loss of participation, poor performance, or

R. G. Hosey · K. Smoot
Department of Orthopedic Surgery and Sports medicine, University of Kentucky College of Medicine, Lexington, KY, USA
e-mail: rhosey@uky.edu; kyle.smoot@uky.edu

S. Nithyanandam (✉)
Department of Family and Community Medicine, University of Kentucky College of Medicine, Lexington, KY, USA
e-mail: sri.nisi89@uky.edu

K. W. Farmer (ed.), *Football Injuries*,
https://doi.org/10.1007/978-3-030-54875-9_21

changes in movement patterns, increasing the risk for further injuries [3]. In a contact sport like football, nociceptive pain encompasses the major bulk of pain in athletes from acute versus overuse injuries.

Neuropathic Pain

Neuropathic pain is secondary to a lesion of the somatosensory system—pain following direct trauma to the nerve roots, peripheral nerve, or spinal cord. Examples include stingers or sciatica [3].

Nociplastic/Algopathic/Nocipathic Pain

Nociplastic pain does not appear to have an association with activation of nociceptors from damage or inflammation but rather hypersensitivity/disruptive nociceptive function. When pain persists long term beyond the tissue healing time, this type of pain should be considered. As a clinician, it is important to be aware of this type of pain, as these patients should be managed through a multidisciplinary team [3].

Pain experts have noted a dearth of medical literature in a proper way of managing pain in an athlete, and most of the treatments are based on expert opinions [4]. Clinicians should be equipped with medical knowledge to serve the interest of athlete safely and aggressively to expedite their return to play. In this chapter, we will focus on non-pharmacological and pharmacological management of pain and their current literature, highlighting the effectiveness of their management.

Assessment of Pain

Pain assessment should include the player position, the location of pain, mechanism of injury, aggravating and relieving factors, pain intensity, and limitation of activities. The game season should be noted as the injury treatment may differ between off-season and in-season. History of previous injuries should be noted as pain from past injury can lead to abnormal movement proximal to the kinetic chain, leading on to compensatory pain. Clinicians should be aware of the training load and periodization as athletes with poor periodization are more vulnerable to injury [3]. While well-localized pain is secondary to nociceptive pain, pain in a dermatomal distribution is likely neuropathic pain; poorly localized pain can be secondary to nociplastic pain. Psychological factors, sleep, nutrition, stress, and social factors could also contribute to the risk of injury as well as pain modulation and should be a part of the history taking while assessing pain [3].

Non-pharmacological Pain Management

Cupping

Cupping has become popular, especially with the use by American Sports. The theory behind dry cupping includes improved vasodilation, microcirculation by causing localized ischemia, and buildup of lactate. Bloodletting cupping involves skin incision and thought to be removing stagnant blood containing toxins [5]. Based on a recent systematic review, no explicit recommendation could be used for or against the use of cupping in athletes. Studies that were included in that review had a high risk of bias [5].

Acupressure

Acupressure uses a firm pressure on the acupoints on the body's meridians. Recent randomized control trial using acupressure as a symptom management modality for acute pain resulting from musculoskeletal injuries such as sprain, strain, and fractures resulted in improved metrics decreasing moderate pain to mild pain [6].

Acupuncture

Role of acupuncture in the treatment of acute musculoskeletal pain has inconclusive evidence. Recent meta-analysis highlights very-low-quality evidence in pain reduction [7, 8]. There is small, low-quality evidence that acupuncture is beneficial in the treatment of tendinopathy by increasing local blood flow with vasodilation and increasing collagen proliferation [9]. Traditional acupuncture was noted to be beneficial in carpal tunnel syndrome when compared to oral steroid treatment and also for Achilles tendinopathy when compared with exercise [10]. Adverse effects include organ or tissue injuries, infections, local adverse events, syncope, and dizziness [10]. As mortalities can be associated with adverse events, it is imperative to advise patients the risks of acupuncture treatment and to explore practitioner's knowledge and experience before referring athletes.

Laser Therapy, Iontophoresis, and Electrical Stimulation

Low-level laser therapy (LLLT) has been used in the treatment of acute pain reduction. A recent meta-analysis has shown LLLT to be an effective treatment modality in the treatment of acute musculoskeletal pain, and adherence to world therapy laser guidelines seems to enhance the effect [11].

There is good evidence to recommend ice, electrical stimulation, and iontophoresis, although little evidence for a faster return to play is noted [12, 13].

Casting and Splinting

Upper extremity injuries are common in a sport like football, threatening the loss of playing time [14]. Nathan et al. conducted a retrospective review in the National Football League (NFL) over a 10-year period and found that metacarpal fractures and proximal interphalangeal joint dislocation were the two most common injuries [15]. Return to play with a hand injury is possible with protective techniques, but athletes should be aware that playing with an unstable injury is risky and chances of delayed healing or nonunion in case of a fracture are inherent risks [14]. In case of a fracture, it is necessary to wait for 10 days until fracture becomes stable with callus formation before taking up the sport. Most athletic associations require athletes to wear a rigid cast or splint to have the entire area covered in no less than 0.5-inch-thick closed-cell slow-recovery foam padding to protect both the injured athlete and opponents [14, 16]. A temporary game cast molded for game functionality should be separate from the original cast available to the athletes [14]. Common examples of game casts include thumb Spica cast, ulnar gutter cast, prefabricated plastic splints for the distal interphalangeal joint injuries, etc. [16]. Frequent follow-ups than the general population are recommended to avoid missing progression of the pathology.

Return to play is position specific in a sport like football. Defensive lineman can return to sport easily with a cast, but it is not so for a wide receiver, offensive lineman, or quarterback [16].

Pharmacological Pain Management

Topical Medications

Topical Nonsteroidal Anti-inflammatory Drugs (NSAIDs)

Topical NSAIDs are absorbed intradermally, resulting in sub-therapeutic doses without associated systemic side effects [17]. Topical diclofenac and ketoprofen have been widely used in studies, and a recent Cochrane review found good evidence in its usefulness for acute sprains and strains [18]. There was around 50% pain reduction and number needed to treat for acute (maximum length of treatment—1 week) and chronic conditions (maximum length of treatment—2 weeks) were around 3.9 and 3.1, respectively [18, 19].

Transdermal NSAID Patches

Patches allow controlled delivery of medication for around 12–24 h [20]. Diclofenac and Ketoprofen patches are not inferior to topical medications, and they have almost similar effectiveness in terms of pain reduction [13, 21, 22].

Lidocaine Patches

Practitioners have used lidocaine patches anecdotally for pain relief, but there are no studies to date, demonstrating efficacy for lidocaine patches for athletic injuries [12].

Compounding Formulations

In contrast to using single pain medications, compounded medications use low-dose multiple concomitant and complimentary therapies. Warner et al. surveyed practicing prescribers who use compounding creams, and majority mentioned it to be effective and safe [23]. However, there are around 6% incidence of side effects from the compounding creams, of which majority are rashes that occur likely from the compounding base [24]. Topical compound creams are most commonly used for neuropathic pain and musculoskeletal pain [23]. Table 21.1 shows classes of medications that are often used in compounding creams. When using topical lidocaine, it is important to avoid use on widespread areas under occlusion. Since there is paucity of literature on this, we need future studies to collect data on professional compounding practices [25].

Oral Medications

Acetaminophen

Acetaminophen (ACT) has analgesic and antipyretic properties similar to NSAIDs, but contrary to previous belief, ACT has weak anti-inflammatory properties based on new evidence of their cyclooxygenase (COX)-inhibiting mechanisms [26]. This drug has been placed on all three steps of pain management intensity in the World Health Organization ladder of pain. A single dose should not exceed 1 g/day, and a daily dose of 4 g is safe. With new research, there is evidence that there is inhibition of prostaglandins like NSAIDs at a dose more than 2 g/day, which theoretically puts them at risk of gastrointestinal (GI) side effects [26]. However, there is a paucity of randomized controlled trials (RCTs), highlighting bleeding side effects from ACT. Therefore, caution is recommended when combining NSAIDs with ACT. Lower dosage ≤2 g/day is advised. Doses of Tylenol more than 4 g/day increases the risk of hepatotoxicity [27]. It is important to educate athletes to correctly identify ACT-containing products over the counter to avoid unintentional harm. Laboratory studies in a controlled environment have documented safety with appropriate dosage for clinicians to keep in mind during usage in sports, while other factors are involved such as concomitant NSAID use, caffeine, hot/humid conditions, hydration status, etc., which could potentially increase the risk of gut injury through their COX-inhibiting effects [27]. Even though ACT is a safe drug

Table 21.1 Common medications used in compounding creams

Class	Drug
NSAIDs	Diclofenac, ketoprofen, piroxicam, ibuprofen, and indomethacin
Anesthetics	Ketamine, lidocaine, bupivacaine, prilocaine, and tetracaine
Opioids	Morphine, methadone, levorphanol, fentanyl, hydrocodone, and buprenorphine
CNS agents	Amitriptyline, gabapentin, baclofen, doxepin, prochlorperazine, carbamazepine, and phenytoin
Miscellaneous	Capsaicin, aspirin, and caffeine

Modified from Shawaqfeh and Harrington [25]

compared to their counterparts, clinicians should always assess the risks and benefits of this drug before prescribing to the elite athlete.

Studies have shown ACT's role as an ergogenic aid to enhance exercise performance, as evidenced by an increase in power output and reduced time to exhaustion [28]. Given its easy accessibility, misuse may be common in athletes.

Nonsteroidal Anti-Inflammatory Drugs (NSAIDs)

NSAIDs are a class of medications that has anti-inflammatory properties through inhibition of COX-1 and COX-2 pathways [22, 29]. NSAIDs have been highly effective in the treatment of pain compared to placebo [22].

NSAIDs are associated with gastrointestinal bleeding, increased risk of cardiovascular disease (CVD), acute kidney injury (AKI) secondary to hemodynamic instability, or interstitial nephritis [29–31]. Gastrointestinal (GI) side effects are approximately three times when compared to nonusers, and the risk increases for patients with the previous history of gastrointestinal side effects [32].

COX −2 inhibitors have superior GI safety profile but offset by their increased risk for cardiovascular side effects [30]. However, new evidence shows that all NSAIDs increases the risk of cardiovascular side effects and therefore should be used cautiously, especially in a patient with heart disease or at risk for heart disease [31]. A meta-analysis shows a similar risk of AKI among all traditional NSAIDs, and the risk is increased in the setting of intravascular volume depletion and chronic kidney disease [29].

In spite of side effects mentioned earlier, a survey of American football players showed that one out of seven high school athletes took NSAIDs daily, and 29% of college athletes took them as a prophylactic medication on the game day [33]. Stache et al. surveyed Division II and Division III college athletes and found that Division I football athletes have higher rates of misuse of nonprescription medications [34].

Of note, based on retrospective cohort studies among college football athletes, the prevalence of hypertension is 19.2% compared to 7% among non-football athletes [35]. At a single Division III University of College Football, the lineman was associated with elevated cardiovascular disease risk [36]. Increased risk of CVD is well documented in patients with a previous history of heart disease; sports medicine clinicians should always explain the risks and benefits to the patient [31]. Athletes are also more prone to intravascular volume depletion that puts them at risk for NSAID-induced kidney injury. However, one study using survey data from 210 college football athletes did not report any evidence of acute kidney injury [22]. It is alarming to know from the same study that 50% of football athletes used NSAIDs daily or weekly once during in-season. Seven players reported side effects that was not related to GI bleeding or AKI [22]. Case reports highlight acute renal failure from using NSAIDs during endurance competition, but there are no meta-analysis studies to strengthen the evidence [37]. Recent randomized control trial did not show evidence of renal stress from endurance training in heat after intake of Ibuprofen 600 mg when compared to placebo [38].

Preliminary evidence highlights that NSAIDs enhance exercise performance likely through analgesics but hamper chronic training adaptation [39]. Evidence toward NSAIDs as an ergogenic aid is very weak [28]. Still, Warner et.al found in his study that athletes perceived NSAIDs as a potential performance improvement drug [40].

There is always a risk of post-traumatic hemorrhage in a contact sport like football while taking NSAIDs [20]. NSAIDs should be avoided in the first 72 hours after a concussion because of a theoretical risk of bleeding. Tylenol is considered safe in this setting [41].

There is a gap in knowledge whether short-term use of NSAIDs delay tissue healing [4, 42]. Impaired fracture healing secondary to NSAID exposure remains speculative. Animal studies have shown evidence of impaired fracture healing, but human studies have shown contradictory outcomes [43]. A recent systematic review evaluating the research quality of the NSAID use in fracture studies showed substantial variability and, therefore, their outcomes. However, the mean number of clinical studies that cited that NSAIDs were safe were higher [44]. Given the lack of consensus on the safe use of NSAIDs in fracture healing, it is recommended to avoid using them, or discuss the risks versus benefits with the patient before prescribing them, especially for completed fractures and high-risk stress fractures [43].

Based on studies, our conclusion is to use the lowest dose of NSAIDs and for the shortest time possible [29–31]. Due to their analgesic effects, premature return to play is possible.

Since NSAIDs and paracetamol are easily accessible and may be used as an ergogenic aid, coaches and athletic trainers should adequately counsel on the long-term side effects of these medications. Table 21.2 lists the commonly used non-opioid medications and their dosing.

Oral Steroids

Corticosteroids exert potent anti-inflammatory effects by inhibiting phospholipase A2 resulting in decreased leukotrienes, prostaglandins and thromboxanes, part of the inflammatory pathway [45]. In addition to inhibiting inflammation, they also inhibit granulation tissue formation, collagen precursor ground substance sulfation, fibroblast and blood vessel formation, and collagen tissue repair, which theoretically can predispose healthy tendons to tendinopathy [46, 47]. Also, some of the tendinopathy conditions are found to be degenerative rather than inflammatory and have questioned the role of steroids in these conditions [48]. Even sometimes, suppressing inflammation may have negative consequences detrimental to tissue healing, and analgesic effect of these medications could mask worsening injury [48]. World anti-doping agency (WADA) has prohibited the use of glucocorticoids when administered by oral, intramuscular, intravenous, or rectal routes because of the strong evidence of its potential as an ergogenic aid [Table 21.3] [28, 49].

Oral corticosteroids (OCS) administered as a steroid burst, in which an initial high dose is tapered rapidly over 5–14 days, is a common practice by clinicians, usually prescribed for inflammatory disorders such as dermatitis and chronic obstructive pulmonary disease/asthma exacerbation [46]. Until now, there are no

Table 21.2 Commonly used non-opioid medications

Generic	Brand	Dosing
Acetaminophen (oral)	Tylenol	Adults: 325–650 mg every 4–6 h. maximum dose: 4 g/day
Aspirin (oral)		Adults: 325–650 mg every 4–6 h. maximum dose: 4 g/day
Ibuprofen (oral)	Advil, Motrin	Adults: 400–800 mg every 6–8 h. maximum dose: 3200 mg/day Children: 30–40 mg/kg/day in 3–4 divided doses
Naproxen (oral)	Alleve	Adults: 250–500 mg every 12 hours. Maximum dose: 1500 mg/day Children and adolescents: 12 yrs. or older: 220 mg orally every 8–12 h. maximum dose: 440 mg (in any 8–12 h period); 660 mg (in any 24 h period)
Diclofenac (oral)	Voltaren XR	Adults: 75 mg every 12 h daily. Maximum dose: 150 mg/day Children and adolescents – Safety not established
Diclofenac (topical)	Voltaren 1% gel	4gm for each joint in lower extremities, every 6 h daily. Maximum dose: 16 g/day 2 g for each joint in upper extremities, every 6 h daily. Maximum dose: 8 g/day
Meloxicam (oral)	Mobic	Adults: 7.5 mg once daily. Maximum dose: 15 mg/day Children and adolescents: 0.125 mg/kg/dose. Maximum dose: 7.5 mg/day
Ketorolac (IV/IM)	Toradol	Adults weighing 50 kg or more: 30 mg (IV/IM) every 6 h. maximum dose: 120 mg/day Adults weighing less than 50 kg: 15 mg (IV/IM) every 6 h. maximum dose: 60 mg/day Limit systemic use for 5 days Children and adolescents: 0.5 mg/kg/dose (IV/IM). Maximum dose: 30 mg/dose. Limit use for 48–72 h
Ketorolac (oral)		Usually used as continuation therapy after IV/IM dose Adults weighing 50 kg or more: 20 mg as the initial dose and 10 mg every 4–6 h. maximum dose: 40 mg/day Adults weighing less than 50 kg: 10 mg every 4–6 h. maximum dose 40 mg/day
Ketorolac (intranasal)		Adults weighing 50 kg or more: 1 spray (15.75 mg/spray) in each nostril (total dose of 31.5 mg) every 6–8 h. maximum dose: 8 sprays/day Adults weighing less than 50 kg: 1 spray (15.75 mg/spray) in one nostril every 6–8 h. Maximum dose: 4 sprays/day

Drugs.com [Internet]. c2000–2020 [Updated: 4 May 2020, Cited: 11 May 2020]. Available from: https://www.drugs.com
Children and adolescents: 2–16 yrs., *XR* extended release, *IV/IM* intravenous/intramuscular

studies that have investigated the efficacy of systemic steroids in the treatment of athletic injuries [46, 50]. However, there is some good-quality evidence that oral steroids improve pain and function for low back pain with sciatica due to lumbar disk herniation [51].

The rationale behind the use of oral steroids in athletic injuries is to control inflammation; rehabilitation will be enhanced and return to play expedited [52]. Harmon et al. conducted a survey study, asking primary care physicians regarding their use of oral steroids in the management of athletic injuries and found 58.6%

Table 21.3 Substances banned by World Anti-Doping Agency

	Substances always prohibited
S0	Non-approved substances
S1	Anabolic agents
S2	Peptide hormones, growth factors, related substances, and mimetics
S3	Beta-2 agonists
S4	Hormone and metabolic modulators
S5	Diuretics and masking agents
	Methods
M1	Manipulation of blood and blood components
M2	Chemical and physical manipulation
M3	Gene and cell doping
	Substances prohibited in competition
S6	Stimulants
S7	Narcotics
S8	Cannabinoids
S9	Glucocorticoids
	Substances prohibited in particular sports
P1	Beta-blockers

Prohibited list by WADA for 2019 is available on https://www.wada-ama.org/en/content/what-is-prohibited

prescribed oral steroids for musculoskeletal injuries [52]. Prednisone 60 mg was a commonly prescribed medication [52]. Those who received additional fellowship training in sports medicine were more often to prescribe for non-discogenic pain. Some physicians indicated that the severity of the injury was the reason for their decision-making toward using steroids [52]. Physicians who did not use steroids cited a lack of evidence as the reason [52].

Methylprednisolone Dosepak is a commonly used medication in the NFL [53]. Langer et al. conducted a survey study regarding prescription of methylprednisolone Dosepak by members of Arthroscopic Association of North America (AANA) and the American Orthopedic Society for Sports Medicine (AOSSM) in 2005. 41% completed the survey, and among them 47% had prescribed Medrol Dosepak for sports injuries. Post-injury was the common indication for prescribing steroids, and glucose intolerance was the most common side effect noted [53]. Most common reasons cited for not prescribing oral steroids include fear of osteonecrosis, lack of proven efficacy, and fear of malpractice [53]. A large proportion of cases of osteonecrosis due to multiple possible etiologies, not reported in the study were seen by physicians who had responded that they prefer not to prescribe steroids, implicating that their clinical experience of severity and complex management of osteonecrosis could have cautioned them against prescribing steroids.

Madanagopal et al. conducted a survey study in 2006 to question the use of oral corticosteroid by orthopedic physicians in high school and college athletes. A total of 34% of physicians prescribed oral steroids in the last 24 months, of which 66% prescribed to both high school and college athletes [54]. Four to seven days' treatment were common, and around 11% reported prescribing steroids to skeletally immature athletes [54]. Half of the physicians who completed the survey felt that the patient benefited from treatment. Only 6% of physicians reported the occurrence of medical complications associated with the use of short-term oral corticosteroids in the competitive high school or college athletes [54]. No case of avascular necrosis was reported in a 2-year recall period [54]. Physicians who prescribed multiple cycles of OCS and usage of OCS in a skeletally immature athlete were more prone for complications. A total of 90% of respondents used a tapered dose [54]. Future studies are required to assess the recent practice among sports medicine physicians.

Controlled/Illegal Substances

Opioids

According to Centers for Disease Control and Prevention, on average, 130 Americans die every day from opioid overdose. Veliz et al. conducted a longitudinal study, showing that male adolescents who continually participate in organized sports have higher odds of medical use and misuse of opioid medications [55]. Schwenk et al. conducted a survey data on retired football players, finding that around 50% suffer from chronic pain and around 85% suffering from depression [56]. Cottler et al. conducted a study using survey data from retired NFL players registered in Retired Players Association in 2010. Overall, 52% used opioids during their NFL career with 71% reporting misuse [57]. Past-month opioid prescription misuse by retired NFL players was reported to be 7%, which is 4.5 times the aged-matched rate of opioid prescription misuse (1.6%) in the general population at the time of the study which is alarming [57]. Approximately one in four retired NFL athletes previously exposed to prescription pain medication during their playing career is currently using prescription opioids, with half of those reporting misuses or abuse of the prescription drugs [58]. Former NFL players currently misusing opioids are three times more likely to be involved in at-risk drinking [58]. Athletes using opioids during their NFL career for "relax/relieve stress" were 1.5 times more likely to abuse opioids currently [58]. Information presented here should alert the clinician before prescribing opioids for the management of pain in athletes.

Tramadol and Codeine use is allowed by WADA (Table 21.3). Tramadol has a dual mechanism of action, being both a mu-opioid receptor agonist and serotonin and norepinephrine reuptake inhibitor [28]. It is possible that tramadol could be used as ergogenic aid, given its action on serotonin and norepinephrine reuptake inhibitors, although there are no studies to date to back up theoretical claims. Codeine is like morphine. After ingestion, a small amount of codeine is converted into morphine. Mechanism of action of codeine is not known, but they also bind to opioid receptors in the brain, decreasing the pain sensation [28].

Cannabis

Cannabis use is illegal in many states and is prohibited in Sport according to WADA [59]. According to the National Survey on Drug Use and Health, the prevalence of marijuana use between ages 12–17 years and 18–25 years is around 15% and 52%, respectively. It is the second most common recreational drug behind alcohol and ahead of tobacco [60]. In recent years where marijuana is being legalized in many states, people's notion of their safety may have changed that has led to increased prevalence.

Cannabis has 9-tetrahydrocannabinol (THC), a partial agonist at the cannabinoid receptors, CB-1 and CB-2 receptors [59, 61, 62]. Through its effects, it causes impaired short-term memory, impaired motor coordination, altered judgment, and, in high doses, increased risk of psychosis [63]. Long-term users increase the risk of addiction, diminished life satisfaction, chronic bronchitis, and chronic psychosis [63]. Cannabis comes under two predominant forms illegally—botanical marijuana and synthetic cannabinoid [62]. A synthetic cannabinoid is a full agonist of the cannabinoid receptors when compared to botanical marijuana that is only a partial agonist, and therefore the acute effects are more exaggerated [61, 62].

Based on the study among college athletes, the prevalence rate was around 28% and was common around Division III school [64]. A recent study among college athletes reported around 2% of lifetime use of synthetic cannabis use [65]. Potential risk factors being male athletes, Caucasian, athletes who use sports performance-enhancing drug for recreation [60]. Some studies have pointed that less than 1% of athletes use marijuana as a performance-enhancing agent, although there is no scientific data to support its ergogenic effects, and athletes should be properly informed of this [59]. Marijuana has been widely implicated in the treatment of chronic pain and as an anti-inflammatory agent in the treatment of conditions such as rheumatoid arthritis. However, collegiate athletes have not pointed out these reasons for their use [63]. Anecdotally, cannabis was used for symptom management for chronic traumatic encephalopathy, and therefore use among athletes may increase as the prevalence of post-concussion syndrome increase [66]. With the myriad of potential questionable benefits, it would be of no surprise that the prevalence may continue to rise, and as a sports medicine clinician, we must educate our athletes properly.

Injectable Medications

Ketorolac (Toradol)

Toradol is a nonsteroidal anti-inflammatory drug that has potent analgesic and anti-inflammatory properties [67]. It can be administered orally, intramuscularly, intravenously, and nasally. Ketorolac reaches its peak plasma concentration within 20 minutes when taken orally and within 45 minutes when administered via an intramuscular (IM) route [68]. Oral bioavailability is 100%, and therefore the dose equivalent of oral and IM dose is the same except the time to its peak effects [68]. Relative bioavailability of intranasal route compared to IM route at a dose of 15 mg and 30 mg is around 75% and 67%, respectively [69].

Ketorolac increases the risk of internal bleeding by inhibition of platelets [67]. Niemi et al. conducted a study comparing the platelet function using ketoprofen, ketorolac, and diclofenac and found that they caused reversible platelet dysfunction. Diclofenac had the mildest effect, while platelet dysfunction was seen even after 24 h after the beginning of ketorolac [70]. Like other NSAIDs, ketorolac increases the risk of acute kidney injury. However, when studied in hospitalized patients, it did not increase the risk of acute renal failure if used for less than 5 days [71].

Ketorolac is indicated for short-term (< 5 days) management of moderately severe acute pain that requires analgesia at the opioid level [67]. This consensus comes after a meta-analysis study, assessing the pain outcome after ketorolac injection in post-operative pain, and found 60 mg of ketorolac had opioid-sparing benefits [72]. However, until now, there are no randomized controlled studies to point ketorolac superiority compared to other NSAIDs in the treatment of acute musculoskeletal pain [73, 74].

Toradol use is common in the NFL, as described in a 2002 study by Powell et al., where most medical staffs believed that Toradol provided 50–75% pain relief that lasted 1–2 days. Of the 28 teams that used Toradol, 6 teams reported minor complications such as gastrointestinal irritation, generalized soreness, and muscle injuries (including strains and worsening contusions). Significant bleeding and renal complications were not reported, but several teams saw "psychological addiction" to game-day Toradol injections [75]. Overall, 93% of NFL physicians in the USA reported administering injectable ketorolac as often as once per week during the 2000 season, with 21% of teams reporting an adverse experience [76].

John B et al. conducted a survey where 32 NFL head team physicians were contacted between 2008 and 2016, regarding their use of Toradol injections. It was noted that the proportion of team physicians using Toradol injections before football games continued to decrease, from 93% of physicians in 2008 to less than half in 2016, and its decrease is believed to be the result of NFL task force recommendations [77]. Gregory et al. conducted a survey in 2011 involving team physicians and found 49% used IM Toradol in the care of the athletes [78]. In that study, Toradol usage was highest among football and almost twice when compared to other sport such as basketball and soccer [78]. Around 75% of physicians frequently administered 6 h before the event. Most frequently cited reasons for not using Toradol was fear of renal and bleeding complications [78]. Bleeding and renal problems were 2.9% and 1.9%, respectively in this study. However, the severity was not addressed [78].

Given the nature of sport and the increased risk of bleeding due to contact and acute renal failure due to dehydration, NFL Task Force Recommendations were developed for Toradol that came into effect in 2012 [67]. Task force recommendations are as follows:

- Ketorolac should be administered only under the direct supervision and order of a team physician.
- Ketorolac should not be used prophylactically as a means of reducing anticipated pain either during or after participation in NFL games or practices.
- Ketorolac use should be limited to those players diagnosed with an injury or condition and listed on the team's latest injury report, or following a physician-diagnosed injury or condition that occurs after the last injury report has been submitted to the NFL before the competition.

- Ketorolac should be given in the lowest effective therapeutic dose and should not be used in any form for more than 5 days. There is no evidence that an increase in dosage is necessary for players with larger body mass.
- Ketorolac should be given in its oral preparation under typical circumstances, as it is recognized that the oral preparation has a faster onset of action than the IM preparation, has a duration of action that is equivalent to the intramuscular (IM) and intravenous (IV) forms, and has a plasma concentration-time curve that is nearly identical to the IM and IV preparations.
- IM and IV injection of ketorolac should not be used, except following an acute, game-related injury where significant visceral or central nervous system bleeding is not expected and where other oral or IM pain medications are inadequate or not tolerated. If IM or IV ketorolac is felt to be appropriate by the treating physician, the lowest possible dose should be used.
- Ketorolac should not be taken concurrently with other NSAIDs.
- Ketorolac should not be taken by those players with a history of allergic reaction to ketorolac, other NSAIDs, or aspirin.
- Player with a history of significant GI bleeding, renal compromise, or a history of complications related to NSAIDs should not take ketorolac.

Joint/Bursal/Peri-Tendinous Injections

Injectable Corticosteroids and Local Anesthetics

During the 1960s, corticosteroids started being widely used by the sports medicine clinicians [46]. They have reported being effective in short-term pain management for many conditions, including supraspinatus tendinitis, lateral epicondylitis, Iliotibial band syndrome, acromioclavicular joint sprain, foot tendinopathies, De Quervain's tenosynovitis, osteitis pubis, bucket handle tears of the medial plica, plantar fasciitis, and Achilles tendinitis [46].

Various formulations are available, and actions vary based on their water solubility. There is an inverse relationship between water solubility and length of action [45, 48], and more insoluble concentration remains at the site longer, possibly increasing the benefit [45, 48]. Less soluble, particulate steroids such as betamethasone acetate and triamcinolone are often used in peritendinous and intra-articular sites [48]. Local anesthetics are often combined with steroid injections to provide short-term relief and also to add diagnostic value to the injection [48]. Basic science investigations point to evidence of chondrotoxicity predominantly from local anesthetics used in the injection [45]. Some investigations have shown chondrotoxicity association only with epinephrine-containing local anesthetics [79, 80]. With these evidence, experts recommend less than four injections per year [45].

Andrew et al. performed a systematic review of almost 18 studies noting the complications associated with steroid injections and found tendon rupture and plantar fascial rupture were the predominant complications reported. Plantar fascia rupture was most common followed by patellar/Quadriceps, Achilles tendon rupture and biceps tendon rupture [46]. The incidence of these side effects is alarming as athletes are further predisposed given the amount of stress they place on tissues.

Mcelindon et al. conducted a randomized control trial studying the effects of steroids in patients with knee osteoarthritis and found a greater significant cartilage volume loss based on annual MRI but no significant difference in knee pain [81].

Although these studies may not be relevant to the athletic population, adverse findings of steroids remain to be considered, keeping in mind the longevity of the joint and careful consideration before intra-articular injection. Bursal injections, including those at the greater trochanter, subacromial space, pes anserine, and iliopsoas, have only low-quality evidence supporting its use, and the extent of its benefit is variable [48].

Coombes et al. performed a systematic review, showing that steroid improves pain only in the short-term but reversed at intermediate and long-term outcome [82]. Information is also needed regarding the effect of multiple corticosteroid injections on long-term tissue damage, other risks, and patient outcomes [4, 42].

Absolute contraindications to local steroid injection include local infection, bacteremia, fracture, joint prosthesis, tumor, Achilles or patellar tendinopathy, and history of allergy to corticosteroids [45]. Reported incidence of septic arthritis varies from 1:10,000–16,000 [45]. Corticosteroid flare reaction is more common. No exact etiology is properly determined but likely due to rapid intracellular ingestion of microcrystalline corticosteroid ester [45]. In vivo studies regarding the association of tendon ruptures have been highlighted predominantly in case reports [45]. The rupture rate of plantar fasciitis after corticosteroid injection ranged from 2.4% to 6.7% in two retrospective studies [83, 84]. Cochrane review found inconclusive evidence to support the use of steroid injections in the treatment of Achilles tendinopathy [85]. There are case reports of osteonecrosis from intra-articular as well as systemic corticosteroids and need to be further studied [45].

Given the adverse effects of steroids, it is important to follow certain rules to decrease the risk of complications.

- Corticosteroids should not directly be injected into tendon, ligament, or fascia, given the risk of rupture. Corticosteroids should not be injected into joints in the setting of intra-articular fracture [48].
- Corticosteroid should be avoided both immediately after an injury and immediately before sports participation, especially in weight-bearing joints [48, 49].
- World Anti-Doping Agency has proposed for 2017 that "intra-articular, intrabursal, periarticular, peritendinous, epidural" injections are prohibited less than 72 hours before the start of the competition, unless a therapeutic use exemption is obtained [49].

Injection should serve as only one aspect of a comprehensive rehab program and return to play.

One study that is worth mentioning here that is contradictory to usual practice is a study by Levine et al., where they successfully treated 58 players with hamstring injuries using 3 ml of 1% lidocaine hydrochloride and 1 ml of dexamethasone sodium phosphate (4 mg,) and they directly injected into the hamstring muscle. Only 6 of 58 players were immediately able to play after the injury, but there were no complications reported, and there were no strength deficits [86]. Using the NFL database, they did not find a recurrence of hamstring injuries in these athletes. It should be noted that this study did not have a control group or blinding and therefore cannot be generalized that this treatment was effective and safe [86].

Local anesthetics alone is commonly used in the management of professional athletes to provide immediate pain relief, so that an injured player may either continue participating in matches or allow them an earlier return.

Mark et al. conducted a retrospective review in NFL league over a three-season period and found 14% of the athletes required injection for musculoskeletal sprain and strain [87]. All corticosteroid injections were administered 1–2 days before the game, and local anesthetic injections were administered within 1 hour of the beginning of the game, using local and ultrasound guidance [87]. The ankle was the most common location of the 14 anatomical sites that were injected [87]. In these series, there were no infections, tendon ruptures, or progression of the injury in severity in those 3-year reviews. Corticosteroids were safely used to treat acromioclavicular joint sprains, ankle sprains, forefoot, midfoot and medial collateral ligament of the knee and elbow [87]. It was also safely used to treat strain, involving the hamstring, adductor longus, quadriceps, biceps brachii, rectus femoris, gastrocnemius, and peroneus longus [87]. In a descriptive case series involving three professional football teams, they used local anesthetic injections to hasten a return to play in 238 injuries. Some of the injections were performed on the match day [88]. Major complications were 2% that includes distal clavicle osteolysis, partial rupture of Achilles tendon, adductor muscle strain, prepatellar bursitis, scapholunate ligament tear [88]. However, it should be noted that distal clavicle excision was also present in athletes who did not receive injection, but there was a 3% decrease in their incidence compared to receiving injections [88]. Tendon injuries were likely secondary to pushing through the pain.

Based on literature, injecting local anesthetic for acromioclavicular joint sprain, phalangeal injuries and metacarpals 2–5, rib and sternum injuries, bruised iliac crests and chronic plantar fasciitis are considered as low-risk conditions (Tables 21.4, 21.5, and 21.6) [88, 89]. MRI is recommended to assess the health of the articular cartilage before considering local anesthetic injection into joints [88]. Caution should be exercised while injecting a tendon as it may predispose to rupture and also before injecting bursa as it may predispose to infection [88]. Scaphoid fractures should always be ruled out before considering first metacarpophalangeal (MCP) joint injection [88].

There have been no studies that have compared the short- and long-term safety of local anesthetic injections compared with other treatment options, and that provides the best relative safety in situations where pain relief is required to continue in elite sporting competition [4, 89]. There is no compulsory notification regulation in a sport like football, regarding the use of local anesthetics, and therefore its use remains a private matter and makes it difficult to assess the long-term outcome of these injections [89].

Table 21.4 Injuries for which local anesthetic could be used in professional football with routine caution (i.e., where the benefits will usually outweigh the risks)

Injury	Notes
Acromioclavicular joint sprain	Block is usually very successful. There may be an increased risk of requiring distal clavicle resection at end of season, which is not usually a significant threat to a player's career
Phalangeal injuries (toes 2–5 and fingers) and metacarpals 2–5	Block is easy to perform. Vasoconstrictors should not be used. Some injuries may lead to degenerative arthritis of interphalangeal joints, although in most cases this is acceptable to a professional football player. The major factors to assess are loss of range of motion and whether the player has any pursuit outside football that involves fine use of the hands, such as playing a musical instrument
Rib and sternum injuries	Block is usually successful when rib injuries are lateral or posterior. Sternum, sternoclavicular joint, and anterior injuries to high ribs are very hard to adequately block. Pneumothorax is a possible complication, but it usually occurs in conjunction with acute injury
Bruised iliac crest	Block usually provides major relief from this very painful but self-resolving injury. The only common complication is sensory nerve block (lateral femoral cutaneous nerve)
Plantar fasciitis	Injection is very painful. Rupture of the plantar fascia origin is likely, but this may, in fact, "cure" the chronic condition

With Permissions from Rights link/Springer nature Orchard [89]

Table 21.5 Examples of injuries for which local anesthetic should only be used in professional football, with extra caution, when the rewards are very high (as risks are also high)

Injury	Notes
Ankle sprains	Magnetic resonance imaging scan is indicated to assess the state of articular cartilage, and injection (even extra-articular) is best avoided if there is any significant articular damage
Tendon injuries	Tendon ruptures are likely when a local block is performed to relieve pain arising from the tendon. In certain circumstances (particularly tendons with many agonists), this risk may be acceptable.
Prepatellar and olecranon bursa	Infection is a likely complication of injection of these bursae. In the case of prepatellar bursa (or any other extra-articular knee injury), documentation should be made, perhaps with a witness, to specifically note that the injection was extra-articular, in case the player experiences a serious knee injury during the game Likely to worsen and require surgery, but surgery is usually curative
Iliotibial band syndrome First metacarpal and radiocarpal injuries (other than scaphoid injuries)	Thumb and wrist are more critical hand structures, and degenerative conditions should not be accepted lightly in these regions. Scaphoid fractures should always be excluded by imaging prior to block of this area

With Permissions from Rights link/Springer nature Orchard [89]

Table 21.6 Examples of injuries for which local anesthetic is generally unsafe, even in professional football, as the risks of major complications are very high

Injury	Notes
Intra-articular knee injuries	Risk of possibly causing or worsening knee osteoarthritis
Shoulder rotator cuff and glenohumeral injuries	Risk of rotator cuff rupture or intra-articular shoulder injury
Intra-articular ankle injuries	Risk of possibly causing or worsening ankle osteoarthritis
Achilles and patellar tendon injuries	Risk of Achilles or patellar tendon rupture, which although repairable, can be career-limiting
Adductor tendinopathy and osteitis pubis	Risk of adductor tendon rupture, irreversible pubic symphysis degeneration, and femoral or obturator nerve block
Hamstring, quadriceps, and calf muscle strains or hematomas	Block is unlikely to be successful, nerve block is likely, and compartment syndrome may result
Foot injuries (other than phalanges 2–5 and plantar fascia)	Risk of degenerative osteoarthritis of foot joints
Scaphoid fractures and scapholunate ligament injuries	Risk of irreversible scaphoid nonunion and/or scapholunate ligament collapse

With Permissions from Rights link/Springer nature Orchard [89]

With the above discussion on non-pharmacological and pharmacological pain management, analgesic ladder created by "World Health Organization" for cancer pain has been modified to be used as a general guideline for the management of pain in athletes (Fig. 21.1).

Ethical Issues and Pre-Game Decision-Making Principles

In a professional sport like American football, sports medicine clinicians are faced with unique challenges standing between the athlete's autonomy in making his own decisions and physician's role in promoting health. There is no acceptable code of ethics in the field of sports medicine [90]. International Federation of Sports Medicine reports the duties of a sports medicine clinician is always to make the health of the athlete a priority, never do harm, and allow the athlete to make his/her own decisions. It is always imperative that physicians explain all treatment alternatives, their risks and benefits of any treatment, and patient chooses without any external influence.

Sports medicine clinicians should be aware of the conflicts of interest in deciding for the athlete. Examples include paternalistic approach because of physician's involvement in winning the game, pressure from coaches, and also to make sure that the athlete is free of any influence in making his own decisions [90]. Although we want our patients to make their own decisions, in the field of sports medicine, the patient is influenced by many factors in making his decisions that may impose long-term problems. Examples include losing a spot in the team, scholarships, fame, or pressure from the coaches to opt one treatment over the other that may be inferior for athlete's long-term health outcome. Even an astute clinician may not always be aware of the external influence in the athlete's decision-making.

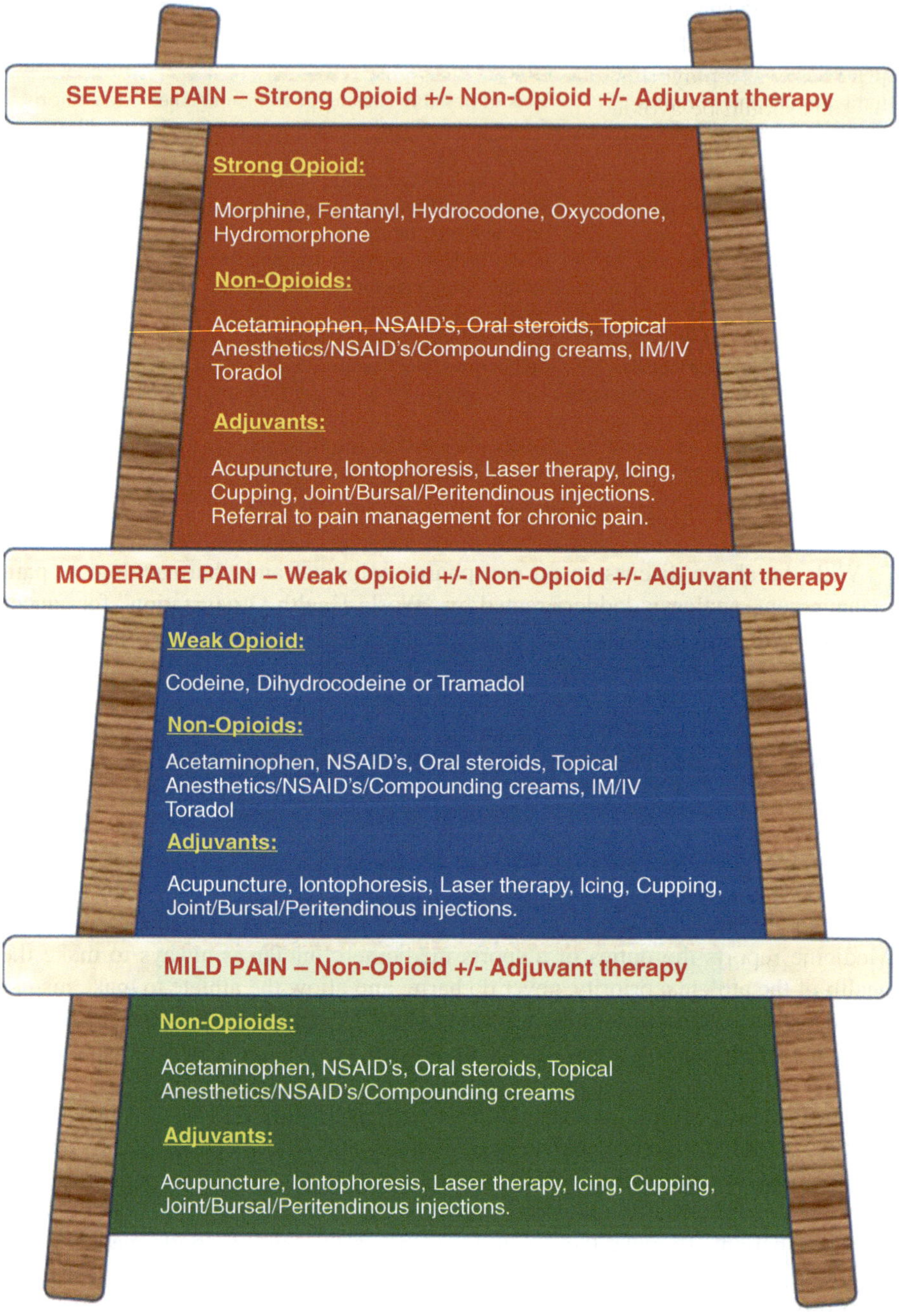

Fig. 21.1 Analgesic ladder for the management of pain in athletes

The timing of season influences a lot of treatment decisions before the game. For example, using local anesthetics for acromioclavicular joint sprain may be considered if this was a playoff game compared to an off-season game. Taking last-minute decisions should be avoided. Involving the entire health care for the athlete is recommended in caring for the athlete before pre-game. Informed consent is an essential process before undertaking any procedures for the athlete, ensuring that the consent is voluntary [90]. All NFL players are enrolled in college and therefore understanding the consent form is not an obstacle.

As highlighted throughout this chapter, most of the available interventions in the field of sports medicine consist predominantly of evidence on their short-term effectiveness but lack long-term data regarding their long-term outcomes. Sports Medicine Physicians should be equipped with current knowledge and provide care to athletes based on best professional judgment, considering their lack of evidence and should not influence their decisions based on short-term outcomes alone [90].

Chronic Pain in Athletes

Anecdotally, many athletes report pain that persists beyond tissue healing times, resulting in chronic pain. We need to have more data on the prevalence of chronic pain among football athletes and find if there is a correlation between intervention during sporting career and the resulting chronic pain etiology [3, 4]. There are increased gaps in our knowledge of how cognitive or psychosocial issues related to pain and performance limitations in elite athletes [4]. Cognitive behavioral therapy has become very popular and effective in the treatment of chronic pain. However, there is a lack of medical literature of its use in the athletic population [4].

References

1. Assa T, Geva N, Zarkh Y, Defrin R. The type of sport matters: Pain perception of endurance athletes versus strength athletes. Eur J Pain (London, England). 2018.
2. Thornton C, Sheffield D, Baird A. A longitudinal exploration of pain tolerance and participation in contact sports. Scand J Pain. 2017;16:36–44.
3. Hainline B, Turner JA, Caneiro JP, Stewart M, Lorimer MG. Pain in elite athletes-neurophysiological, biomechanical and psychosocial considerations: a narrative review. Br J Sports Med. 2017;51(17):1259–64.
4. Zideman DA, Derman W, Hainline B, Moseley GL, Orchard J, Pluim BM, et al. Management of pain in elite athletes: identified gaps in knowledge and future research directions. Clin J Sport Med. 2018;28(5):485–9.
5. Bridgett R, Klose P, Duffield R, Mydock S, Lauche R. Effects of cupping therapy in amateur and professional athletes: systematic review of randomized controlled trials. J Altern Complement Med (New York, NY). 2018;24(3):208–19.
6. Macznik AK, Schneiders AG, Athens J, Sullivan SJ. Does acupressure hit the mark? A three-arm randomized placebo-controlled trial of acupressure for pain and anxiety relief in athletes with acute musculoskeletal sports injuries. Clin J Sport Med. 2017;27(4):338–43.

7. Yuan QL, Wang P, Liu L, Sun F, Cai YS, Wu WT, et al. Acupuncture for musculoskeletal pain: a meta-analysis and meta-regression of sham-controlled randomized clinical trials. Sci Rep. 2016;6:30675.
8. Cox J, Varatharajan S, Cote P, Optima C. Effectiveness of acupuncture therapies to manage musculoskeletal disorders of the extremities: a systematic review. J Orthop Sports Phys Ther. 2016;46(6):409–29.
9. Neal BS, Longbottom J. Is there a role for acupuncture in the treatment of tendinopathy? Acupunct Med. 2012;30(4):346–9.
10. Chan MWC, Wu XY, Wu JCY, Wong SYS, Chung VCH. Safety of acupuncture: overview of systematic reviews. Sci Rep. 2017;7(1):3369.
11. Clijsen R, Brunner A, Barbero M, Clarys P, Taeymans J. Effects of low-level laser therapy on pain in patients with musculoskeletal disorders: a systematic review and meta-analysis. Eur J Phys Rehabil Med. 2017;53(4):603–10.
12. Smith BJ, Collina SJ. Pain medications in the locker room: to dispense or not. Curr Sports Med Rep. 2007;6(6):367–70.
13. Bolin DJ. Transdermal approaches to pain in sports injury management. Curr Sports Med Rep. 2003;2(6):303–9.
14. Carruthers KH, O'Reilly O, Skie M, Walters J, Siparsky P. Casting and splinting management for hand injuries in the in-season contact sport athlete. Sports Health. 2017;9(4):364–71.
15. Mall NA, Carlisle JC, Matava MJ, Powell JW, Goldfarb CA. Upper extremity injuries in the National Football League: part I: hand and digital injuries. Am J Sports Med. 2008;36(10):1938–44.
16. Almekinders LC, Tao MA, Zarzour R. Playing hurt: hand and wrist injuries and protected return to sport. Sports Med Arthrosc Rev. 2014;22(1):66–70.
17. Singh P, Roberts MS. Skin permeability and local tissue concentrations of nonsteroidal anti-inflammatory drugs after topical application. J Pharmacol Exp Ther. 1994;268(1):144–51.
18. Derry S, Wiffen PJ, Kalso EA, Bell RF, Aldington D, Phillips T, et al. Topical analgesics for acute and chronic pain in adults - an overview of Cochrane Reviews. Cochrane Database Syst Rev. 2017;5:Cd008609.
19. Moore RA, Tramer MR, Carroll D, Wiffen PJ, McQuay HJ. Quantitative systematic review of topically applied non-steroidal anti-inflammatory drugs. BMJ. 1998;316(7128):333–8.
20. Ziltener JL, Leal S, Fournier PE. Non-steroidal anti-inflammatory drugs for athletes: an update. Ann Phys Rehabil Med. 2010;53(4):278–82, 82-8
21. Esparza F, Cobian C, Jimenez JF, Garcia-Cota JJ, Sanchez C, Maestro A. Topical ketoprofen TDS patch versus diclofenac gel: efficacy and tolerability in benign sport related soft-tissue injuries. Br J Sports Med. 2007;41(3):134–9.
22. Holmes N, Cronholm PF, Duffy AJ 3rd, Webner D. Nonsteroidal anti-inflammatory drug use in collegiate football players. Clin J Sport Med. 2013;23(4):283–6.
23. Warner M, Tuder D. A brief survey on prescriber beliefs regarding compounded topical pain medications. Int J Pharm Compd. 2014;18(3):182–8.
24. Cline AE, Turrentine JE. Compounded topical analgesics for chronic pain. Dermatitis. 2016;27(5):263–71.
25. Shawaqfeh MS, Harrington C. Pain: systematic review of pharmacy compounding of pain medication. Int J Pharm Compd. 2018;22(1):19–24.
26. Jozwiak-Bebenista M, Nowak JZ. Paracetamol: mechanism of action, applications and safety concern. Acta Pol Pharm. 2014;71(1):11–23.
27. Esh CJ, Mauger AR, Palfreeman RA, Al-Janubi H, Taylor L. Acetaminophen (paracetamol): use beyond pain management and dose variability. Front Physiol. 2017;8:1092.
28. Holgado D, Hopker J, Sanabria D, Zabala M. Analgesics and sport performance: beyond the pain-modulating effects. PM R. 2018;10(1):72–82.
29. Ungprasert P, Cheungpasitporn W, Crowson CS, Matteson EL. Individual non-steroidal anti-inflammatory drugs and risk of acute kidney injury: a systematic review and meta-analysis of observational studies. Eur J Intern Med. 2015;26(4):285–91.

30. Hermann M, Ruschitzka F. Cardiovascular risk of cyclooxygenase-2 inhibitors and traditional non-steroidal anti-inflammatory drugs. Ann Med. 2007;39(1):18–27.
31. Pepine CJ, Gurbel PA. Cardiovascular safety of NSAIDs: additional insights after PRECISION and point of view. Clin Cardiol. 2017;40(12):1352–6.
32. Gabriel SE, Jaakkimainen L, Bombardier C. Risk for serious gastrointestinal complications related to use of nonsteroidal anti-inflammatory drugs. A meta-analysis. Ann Intern Med. 1991;115(10):787–96.
33. Tricker R. Painkilling drugs in collegiate athletics: knowledge, attitudes, and use of student athletes. J Drug Educ. 2000;30(3):313–24.
34. Stache S, Close JD, Mehallo C, Fayock K. Nonprescription pain medication use in collegiate athletes: a comparison of samples. Phys Sportsmed. 2014;42(2):19–26.
35. Karpinos AR, Roumie CL, Nian H, Diamond AB, Rothman RL. High prevalence of hypertension among collegiate football athletes. Circ Cardiovasc Qual Outcomes. 2013;6(6):716–23.
36. Wright CJ, Abbey EL, Brandon BA, Reisman EJ, Kirkpatrick CM. Cardiovascular disease risk profile of NCAA Division III intercollegiate football athletes: a pilot study. Phys Sportsmed. 2017;45(3):280–5.
37. Lange ML, Skansing TB. Acute renal failure after participation in high endurance sport. Ugeskr Laeger. 2016;178(3):V08150682.
38. McDermott BP, Smith CR, Butts CL, Caldwell AR, Lee EC, Vingren JL, et al. Renal stress and kidney injury biomarkers in response to endurance cycling in the heat with and without ibuprofen. J Sci Med Sport. 2018;21(12):1180–4.
39. Lundberg TR, Howatson G. Analgesic and anti-inflammatory drugs in sports: implications for exercise performance and training adaptations. Scand J Med Sci Sports. 2018;28(11):2252–62.
40. Warner DC, Schnepf G, Barrett MS, Dian D, Swigonski NL. Prevalence, attitudes, and behaviors related to the use of nonsteroidal anti-inflammatory drugs (NSAIDs) in student athletes. J Adolesc Health. 2002;30(3):150–3.
41. Scorza KA, Cole W. Current concepts in concussion: initial evaluation and management. Am Fam Physician. 2019;99(7):426–34.
42. Chan KM, Fu SC. Anti-inflammatory management for tendon injuries – friends or foes? Sports Med Arthrosc Rehabil Ther Technol. 2009;1(1):23.
43. Mehallo CJ, Drezner JA, Bytomski JR. Practical management: nonsteroidal antiinflammatory drug (NSAID) use in athletic injuries. Clin J Sport Med. 2006;16(2):170–4.
44. Marquez-Lara A, Hutchinson ID, Nunez F Jr, Smith TL, Miller AN. Nonsteroidal anti-inflammatory drugs and bone-healing: a systematic review of research quality. JBJS Rev. 2016;4(3):01874474.
45. Honcharuk E, Monica J. Complications associated with intra-articular and extra-articular corticosteroid injections. JBJS Rev. 2016;4(12):01874474.
46. Nichols AW. Complications associated with the use of corticosteroids in the treatment of athletic injuries. Clin J Sport Med. 2005;15(5):370–5.
47. Dean BJ, Lostis E, Oakley T, Rombach I, Morrey ME, Carr AJ. The risks and benefits of glucocorticoid treatment for tendinopathy: a systematic review of the effects of local glucocorticoid on tendon. Semin Arthritis Rheum. 2014;43(4):570–6.
48. Olafsen NP, Herring SA, Orchard JW. Injectable corticosteroids in sport. Clin J Sport Med. 2018;28(5):451–6.
49. Fitch K. Glucocorticoids at the Olympic Games: state-of-the-art review. Br J Sports Med. 2016;50(20):1267.
50. Dvorak J, Feddermann N, Grimm K. Glucocorticosteroids in football: use and misuse. Br J Sports Med. 2006;40(Suppl 1):i48–54.
51. Goldberg H, Firtch W, Tyburski M, Pressman A, Ackerson L, Hamilton L, et al. Oral steroids for acute radiculopathy due to a herniated lumbar disk: a randomized clinical trial. JAMA. 2015;313(19):1915–23.
52. Harmon KG, Hawley C. Physician prescribing patterns of oral corticosteroids for musculoskeletal injuries. J Am Board Fam Pract. 2003;16(3):209–12.

53. Langer P, Fadale P, Hulstyn M, Fleming B, Brady M. Survey of orthopaedic and sports medicine physicians regarding use of medrol dosepak for sports injuries. Arthroscopy. 2006;22(12):1263–9.e2.
54. Madanagopal SG, Kovaleski JE, Pearsall AW. Survey of short-term oral corticosteroid administration by orthopaedic physicians in college and high school athletes. J Sports Sci Med. 2009;8(1):37–44.
55. Veliz P, Epstein-Ngo QM, Meier E, Ross-Durow PL, McCabe SE, Boyd CJ. Painfully obvious: a longitudinal examination of medical use and misuse of opioid medication among adolescent sports participants. J Adolesc Health. 2014;54(3):333–40.
56. Schwenk TL, Gorenflo DW, Dopp RR, Hipple E. Depression and pain in retired professional football players. Med Sci Sports Exerc. 2007;39(4):599–605.
57. Cottler LB, Ben Abdallah A, Cummings SM, Barr J, Banks R, Forchheimer R. Injury, pain, and prescription opioid use among former National Football League (NFL) players. Drug Alcohol Depend. 2011;116(1–3):188–94.
58. Dunne EM, Striley CW, Mannes ZL, Asken BM, Ennis Formerly Whitehead N, Cottler LB. Reasons for prescription opioid use while playing in the national football league as risk factors for current use and misuse among former players. Clin J Sport Med: official journal of the canadian academy of sport medicine. 2018. https://doi.org/10.1097/jsm.0000000000000628.
59. Ware MA, Jensen D, Barrette A, Vernec A, Derman W. Cannabis and the health and performance of the elite athlete. Clin J Sport Med. 2018;28(5):480–4.
60. Brisola-Santos MB, Gallinaro JG, Gil F, Sampaio-Junior B, Marin MC, de Andrade AG, et al. Prevalence and correlates of cannabis use among athletes-a systematic review. Am J Addict. 2016;25(7):518–28.
61. Akram H, Mokrysz C, Curran HV. What are the psychological effects of using synthetic cannabinoids? A systematic review. J Psychopharmacol. 2019;33:271–83.
62. Chase PB, Hawkins J, Mosier J, Jimenez E, Boesen K, Logan BK, et al. Differential physiological and behavioral cues observed in individuals smoking botanical marijuana versus synthetic cannabinoid drugs. Clin Toxicol (Phila). 2016;54(1):14–9.
63. Volkow ND, Baler RD, Compton WM, Weiss SR. Adverse health effects of marijuana use. N Engl J Med. 2014;370(23):2219–27.
64. Green GA, Uryasz FD, Petr TA, Bray CD. NCAA study of substance use and abuse habits of college student-athletes. Clin J Sport Med. 2001;11(1):51–6.
65. Egan KL, Erausquin JT, Milroy JJ, Wyrick DL. Synthetic cannabinoid use and descriptive norms among collegiate student-athletes. J Psychoactive Drugs. 2016;48(3):166–72.
66. Russo EB. Cannabis therapeutics and the future of neurology. Front Integr Neurosci. 2018;12:51.
67. Matava M, Brater DC, Gritter N, Heyer R, Rollins D, Schlegel T, et al. Recommendations of the national football league physician society task force on the use of toradol((R)) ketorolac in the national football league. Sports Health. 2012;4(5):377–83.
68. Buckley MM, Brogden RN. Ketorolac. A review of its pharmacodynamic and pharmacokinetic properties, and therapeutic potential. Drugs. 1990;39(1):86–109.
69. McAleer SD, Majid O, Venables E, Polack T, Sheikh MS. Pharmacokinetics and safety of ketorolac following single intranasal and intramuscular administration in healthy volunteers. J Clin Pharmacol. 2007;47(1):13–8.
70. Niemi TT, Taxell C, Rosenberg PH. Comparison of the effect of intravenous ketoprofen, ketorolac and diclofenac on platelet function in volunteers. Acta Anaesthesiol Scand. 1997;41(10):1353–8.
71. Feldman HI, Kinman JL, Berlin JA, Hennessy S, Kimmel SE, Farrar J, et al. Parenteral ketorolac: the risk for acute renal failure. Ann Intern Med. 1997;126(3):193–9.
72. De Oliveira GS Jr, Agarwal D, Benzon HT. Perioperative single dose ketorolac to prevent postoperative pain: a meta-analysis of randomized trials. Anesth Analg. 2012;114(2):424–33.
73. Eichner ER. Intramuscular ketorolac injections: the pregame Toradol parade. Curr Sports Med Rep. 2012;11(4):169–70.

74. Turturro MA, Paris PM, Seaberg DC. Intramuscular ketorolac versus oral ibuprofen in acute musculoskeletal pain. Ann Emerg Med. 1995;26(2):117–20.
75. Powell ET, Tokish JM, Hawkins RJ. Toradol use in the athletic population. Curr Sports Med Rep. 2002;1(4):191.
76. Tokish JM, Powell ET, Schlegel TF, Hawkins RJ. Ketorolac use in the national football league: prevalence, efficacy, and adverse events. Phys Sportsmed. 2002;30(9):19–24.
77. Schrock JB, Carver TJ, Kraeutler MJ, McCarty EC. Evolving treatment patterns of NFL players by orthopaedic team physicians over the past decade, 2008-2016. Sports Health. 2018;10(5):453–61.
78. Sawyer GA, Anderson BC, Raukar NP, Fadale PD. Intramuscular ketorolac injections in the athlete. Sports Health. 2012;4(4):319–27.
79. Dragoo JL, Korotkova T, Kanwar R, Wood B. The effect of local anesthetics administered via pain pump on chondrocyte viability. Am J Sports Med. 2008;36(8):1484–8.
80. Dragoo JL, Korotkova T, Kim HJ, Jagadish A. Chondrotoxicity of low pH, epinephrine, and preservatives found in local anesthetics containing epinephrine. Am J Sports Med. 2010;38(6):1154–9.
81. McAlindon TE, LaValley MP, Harvey WF, Price LL, Driban JB, Zhang M, et al. Effect of intra-articular triamcinolone vs saline on knee cartilage volume and pain in patients with knee osteoarthritis: a randomized clinical trial. JAMA. 2017;317(19):1967–75.
82. Coombes BK, Bisset L, Vicenzino B. Efficacy and safety of corticosteroid injections and other injections for management of tendinopathy: a systematic review of randomised controlled trials. Lancet. 2010;376(9754):1751–67.
83. Acevedo JI, Beskin JL. Complications of plantar fascia rupture associated with corticosteroid injection. Foot Ankle Int. 1998;19(2):91–7.
84. Kim C, Cashdollar MR, Mendicino RW, Catanzariti AR, Fuge L. Incidence of plantar fascia ruptures following corticosteroid injection. Foot Ankle Spec. 2010;3(6):335–7.
85. Kearney RS, Parsons N, Metcalfe D, Costa ML. Injection therapies for Achilles tendinopathy. Cochrane Database Syst Rev. 2015 (5):Cd010960.
86. Levine WN, Bergfeld JA, Tessendorf W, Moorman CT 3rd. Intramuscular corticosteroid injection for hamstring injuries. A 13-year experience in the National Football League. Am J Sports Med. 2000;28(3):297–300.
87. Drakos M, Birmingham P, Delos D, Barnes R, Murphy C, Weiss L, et al. Corticosteroid and anesthetic injections for muscle strains and ligament sprains in the NFL. HSS J. 2014;10(2):136–42.
88. Orchard JW. Benefits and risks of using local anaesthetic for pain relief to allow early return to play in professional football. Br J Sports Med. 2002;36(3):209–13.
89. Orchard JW. Is it safe to use local anaesthetic painkilling injections in professional football? Sports Med. 2004;34(4):209–19.
90. Testoni D, Hornik CP, Smith PB, Benjamin DK Jr, McKinney RE Jr. Sports medicine and ethics. Am J Bioethics. 2013;13(10):4–12.

Index

K. W. Farmer (ed.), *Football Injuries*,
https://doi.org/10.1007/978-3-030-54875-9

F

GPSR Compliance

The European Union's (EU) General Product Safety Regulation (GPSR) is a set of rules that requires consumer products to be safe and our obligations to ensure this.

If you have any concerns about our products, you can contact us on ProductSafety@springernature.com

In case Publisher is established outside the EU, the EU authorized representative is:

Springer Nature Customer Service Center GmbH
Europaplatz 3
69115 Heidelberg, Germany

Batch number: 10732076

Printed by Printforce, the Netherlands